Reduced Port Laparoscopic Surgery

Toshiyuki Mori • Giovanni Dapri

Editors

Reduced Port
Laparoscopic Surgery

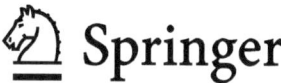 Springer

Editors
Toshiyuki Mori
Kyorin University
Tokyo, Japan

Giovanni Dapri
Saint-Pierre University Hospital
Brussels, Belgium

ISBN 978-4-431-54600-9   ISBN 978-4-431-54601-6 (eBook)
DOI 10.1007/978-4-431-54601-6
Springer Tokyo Heidelberg New York Dordrecht London

Library of Congress Control Number: 2014930159

Printed on acid-free paper

Springer is part of Springer Science+Business Media (www.springer.com)

Memorial Tribute to Professor Motoo Yamagata

This is not, by all means, an obituary. This is a eulogy and a memorial tribute to our dear friend, Prof. Motoo Yamagata. He was adored by many colleagues and friends both in Japan and across the world. He was a prominent figure and led the field of endoscopic surgery, always striving to move onwards and upwards.

Professor Yamagata has long been a dear friend, a colleague and a companion of mine. He dedicated his life for his patients as a surgeon, a teacher, and a researcher. He is the key person of this book not only for his pioneering work in minimally invasive surgery but for his role to get surgeons and researchers together, and most of all, for his effort for the international collaboration in this field.

Professor Motoo Yamagata was born on May 18, 1956 at Surugadai Nihon University Hospital (which would later, rather coincidentally, turn out to be his work place) as the eldest son to Kozo and Kiwako Yamagata. His father owns Nihonbashi Yamagataya, a renowned tailor, established in 1890.

As a surgeon, he showed his ability to the fullest and shared his knowledge and talent with many academics across different fields (including achalasia, breast cancer and single port laparoscopic surgery) at academic conferences such as the Japan Society for Endoscopic Surgery, while always projecting strong traits of leadership and a frontier spirit.

He was a co-founder of Japanese Society of Single-Port Surgery (TANKO) and chaired the third meeting of TANKO on February 19, 2011. At this meeting, he stressed as follows. "As life expectancy increases, patients may need surgery for a second or third time. Reduced port laparoscopic surgery (RPLS), which causes minimal abdominal wall damage and has a relatively low risk of postoperative adhesion, will become even more vital going forward. Don't think only in the present. We need to think about 5 years, even 10 years from now. It is not just for a cosmetic reason. We have to develop this technique right now."

These are the distinguished thoughts of Prof. Yamagata, who always put his patients first, above everything else.

Professor Giovanni Dapri, who was a close friend of Prof. Yamagata, visited Japan for the first time to give a hands-on course and lectures in that meeting. Impressed with TANKO development in Japan, Prof. Dapri promised to Prof. Yamagata to

introduce TANKO in Europe. Professor Yamagata was later selected as course director, along with Prof. Dapri, of the postgraduate course, "Single-Port Laparoscopic
Surgery—joined with TANKO (Japanese Society of Single-Port Surgery)" at the 20th
International Congress of EAES (European Association for Endoscopic Surgery),
which was held in Brussels, Belgium, in June 2012. In this way, Prof. Yamagata
helped to transmit Japanese RPLS to the rest of the world. It was also the time
when this international project to publish recent advancement in minimally invasive
surgery, namely RPLS, was first discussed.

However, Prof. Yamagata, in the most sudden and unexpected way, passed away
at Boston's Massachusetts General Hospital on January 31, 2013 at the age of 56,
without seeing publication of this book. This was something that no one had anticipated in any way. His family, who was hoping for his full recovery, as well as his
loving friends and colleagues, were stunned at this sudden loss.

The all-night vigil on February 13, 2013, followed by the funeral on February 14,
2013, was attended by 2,000 people, who shed tears of sorrow and mourned the loss
of this great man.

He was truly an irreplaceable figure, both within Japan and in the wider international community. This illustrates the extent to which he was loved, adored and
respected by all. The deep love and affection which Prof. Yamagata expressed was
felt by all and this love was also returned to him from those around him.

As many of you may know, his knowledge of food was seemingly infinite, he had
personal connections across a vast array of fields and sectors. It is clear that even
outside of his life as a surgeon, he had a very special life.

On August 3, 2013, the "Memory of Prof. Motoo Yamagata" memorial event was
held at the Reduced Port Surgery Forum in Morioka. In commemoration and recognition of his great achievements, his name will be eternalized through the Yamagata
Prize, which will be awarded to acknowledge the most outstanding figures in the
field at the Reduced Port Surgery Forum from 2013.

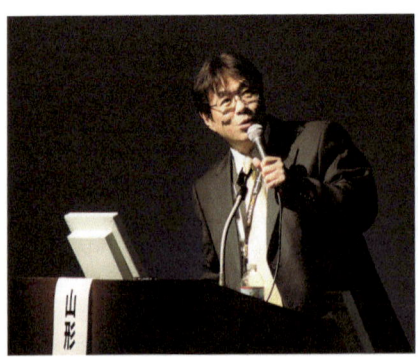
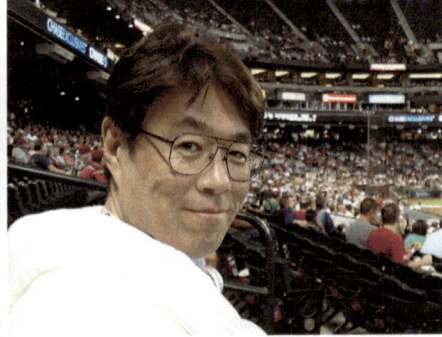

Finally, I would like to finish by writing briefly about "Moto-chan." This is a nickname that I lovingly gave Prof. Yamagata as a sign of my affection and respect for him.

Professor Yamagata would sometimes speak and act in a superhuman way; during these times, I believed that he was a messenger chosen by God.

It seems like Prof. Yamagata was working 24 h a day, 365 days a year, when considering all of the work he did at his hospital, his academic contributions, and his undertakings outside of work.

Although Prof. Yamagata lived a short life of only 56 years, he achieved more in that short time than any ordinary person could achieve in over 100 years.

We are extremely fortunate to have lived at the same time and to have come in contact with this great man. Professor Yamagata will be sorely missed. But greater than the sorrow from his passing is the joy that he spread in his life. Just as he guided every one of us, his wisdom and love will continue to guide each one of us throughout our lives. His humility, integrity, and hard work continue to inspire those who knew him.

On behalf of the editors and contributors, I would like to dedicate this book to Prof. Yamagata, or rather, "Moto-chan." You taught us to keep our sunny side up, so we will. Moto-chan, we all love you and miss you very much. I am certain that your spirits will stay alive with this book, forever.

Adachi Kyosai Hospital, Tokyo, Japan   Manabu Yamamoto

Foreword

Reduced port laparoscopic surgery (RPLS) is laparoscopic surgery performed with the minimum possible number of ports and/or small-sized ports. Considering that the basic principle of laparoscopic surgery is minimal invasiveness, RPLS is a natural objective for surgeons in this field to pursue. In fact, surgery performed via a reduced number of ports or via small ports (called needlescopic surgery) has been attempted since the early days of laparoscopic surgery, but such procedures have not gained widespread acceptance. For safe and easy performance of laparoscopic surgery, the following are important: (1) a laparoscope system that provides strong illumination and high resolution, (2) various energy sources, suturing devices, and forceps with high operability, and (3) appropriate triangulation. It has been generally believed that these conditions could not be fully met with ports reduced in number or size. Since its introduction, laparoscopic surgery has gradually expanded to more difficult procedures. However, with more difficult surgeries, there is generally a need to increase the number as well as the size of the ports.

Somewhat unexpectedly, RPLS has attracted recent attention. This attention followed the 2008 report of single-incision laparoscopic surgery (SLS), which is the ultimate form of minimal incision surgery, in the United States. SLS garnered a great deal of interest among patients due to the promise of an invisible scar. Because almost all abdominal surgeries can now be performed laparoscopically, minimizing the scarring and abdominal pain associated with the ports of entry has become a new objective in the field. The efforts to accomplish this objective are supported by the development of new laparoscopes and surgical instruments, which have made it possible to perform operations easily and safely via fewer and smaller ports. SLS and needlescopic surgery are referred to collectively as RPLS, and various techniques have been developed. RPLS has been applied to almost all procedures in a very short time.

Surgeons who wish to perform RPLS should not forget the following points. First of all, an improved cosmetic outcome is the only evidence-based advantage of this method. The reduced port method requires more advanced techniques than the standard laparoscopic method requires, and thus it involves a new learning curve. Therefore, surgeons who use this method should be careful to avoid telling patients that it is superior to conventional laparoscopic surgery by repeating unproven claims (e.g., claims that the method reduces wound pain and invasion). Also, RPLS should be performed only by surgeons who are experienced in conventional laparoscopic surgery. For patients undergoing surgery for a malignant tumor, this method should not be employed if there is any risk of lessening the radicality of treatment. If difficulties are encountered during RPLS or if there is any danger, additional ports should be placed or small ports should be switched to larger ports without hesitation.

In Japan, the TANKO Society (TANKO is an acronym that comes from the Japanese words for Single Port Surgery) was established by Dr. Masazumi Okajima, Dr. Toshiyuki Mori, and other practitioners in 2009, and the first study meeting was held on February 20, 2010. Subsequent TANKO study meetings have been held semi-annually. Since 2012, the study meeting has been called the Reduced Port Surgery Forum and has been held in conjunction with the Needlescopic Surgery Meeting. The 7th meeting was held August 2–3, 2013, and attendees numbered more than 700. This meeting covered all areas of laparoscopic surgery. Thanks to the efforts of many surgeons, it is believed that Japan currently leads the world in the field of RPLS.

This book contains 43 chapters, 27 of which were written by Japanese surgeons who are pioneers in the field of RPLS. Another 16 experienced surgeons from Europe, the United States, South America and Asia have contributed to this book. The book covers the history of RPLS, as well as its terminology, pros and cons, instruments and equipment, suture methods, robotic surgery, and details of the various operative procedures. When procedures are explained, numerous diagrams and photographs are provided to facilitate understanding. In short, this is the most up-to-date text written by leading laparoscopic surgeons, and it is a must-read book for all operators who wish to perform RPLS.

Fujinomiya City General Hospital, Shizuoka, Japan   Taizo Kimura

Preface

Few phenomena have changed the face of surgery like the widespread introduction of videoscopic technologies in the 1980s. For one thing, the technology allowed all members of the surgical team to view, on a video monitor, the same image of the surgical field inside the patient's body cavity. More importantly, the surgeons' hands were freed for more complex maneuvers. Thus, a dramatic increase in the adoption of laparoscopic surgery occurred in the late 1980s and early 1990s. The method represented a less invasive alternative to the conventional open wound method and gained acceptance as the standard of care for many diseases.

Laparoscopic surgery is performed via access channels (ports). Decreased disruption of the normal structure of the abdominal wall, attributed to the dramatic reduction in surgical invasiveness, resulted from performance of laparoscopic surgery. Patients who underwent laparoscopic procedures experienced less pain, required a shorter hospital stay, and returned to their normal activities much faster than those who underwent open procedures. It did not take long for pioneering surgeons to put effort into minimizing the number and size of the ports and the caliber of the devices with a belief that less destruction of the abdominal wall would result in further reduction of the surgical invasiveness. One of the main goals became SLS, in which access to the body cavity was to be achieved via a small wound (i.e. umbilical access). Natural orifice translumenal endoscopic surgery (NOTES) has been considered the ultimate goal in terms of minimal invasion. Theoretically NOTES precludes any injury to the intact abdominal wall. Currently, NOTES stands as a promising option for which the instrumentation and technicalities remain to be worked out.

Another approach to reducing abdominal wall injury is needlescopic surgery, for which a small caliber scope and small caliber instruments (<3 mm) are used.

Although the term remains ambiguous, "reduced port laparoscopic surgery (RPLS)" is generally accepted to refer to a scenario in which minimally invasive surgical methods are mixed. Many surgeons have noticed that the pros and cons of single-incision and needlescopic surgery are complementary and that mixed use of the two techniques markedly resolves the difficulty of performing single-incision surgery. Interestingly, introduction of RPLS gave birth to the hybrid use of other minimally invasive surgical methods such as robotic surgery and NOTES.

This book was designed to describe the latest applications of RPLS. We have been fortunate to assemble authors who are acknowledged authorities in the field. They are true experts in both clinical performance and surgical education. Many were involved in the development and dissemination of the procedures they describe. We are much indebted to them for their contribution to this volume.

We have aimed this text at all levels of students of surgery—from surgical interns to well-established surgical practitioners. Enough pearls and wisdom are contained herein to enhance the readers' technical ability to treat patients by means of RPLS.

We dedicate this book to Prof. Motoo Yamagata, who also served as director of the first EuroTANKO (Japanese Society of Single Port Surgery), held in Brussels, Belgium in June 2012. Collaboration between European and Japanese surgeons began there and resulted in this textbook.

We also express our deepest gratitude to our Copy Editor, Ms. Tina Tajima, for her invaluable and precise editing work. She was extraordinarily tolerant and supportive throughout the editing process. Her constructive comments and suggestions were invaluable. Without her consistency, accuracy and persistent help this textbook would not have been possible.

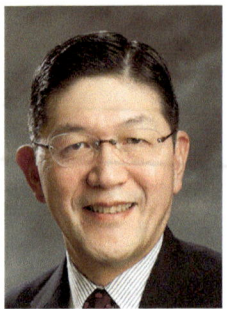

Tokyo, Japan   Toshiyuki Mori

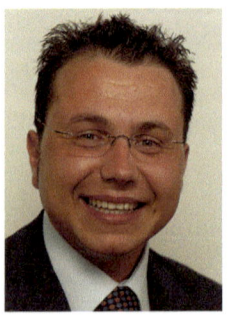

Brussels, Belgium   Giovanni Dapri

Contents

Contributors

Isaias Alarcón Hospital Universitario Virgen del Rocío, Sevilla, Spain

Francisco Almeida Red Cross University Hospital, Curitiba, Brazil

Riccardo Autorino Second University of Naples, Naples, Italy

Shigeaki Baba Iwate Medical College, Morioka, Japan

Carmen Balague University Autonomous of Barcelona, Barcelona, Spain

Marcus Vinícius Dantas De Campos Martins Estacio de Sa University, Rio de Janeiro, Brazil

Eugene P. Ceppa Duke University Medical Center, Durham, NC, USA

Giovanni Dapri Saint-Pierre University Hospital, Brussels, Belgium

Marco De Sio Second University of Naples, Naples, Italy

Yuichiro Doki Osaka University, Osaka, Japan

Guillermo Dominguez Fundación Hospitalaria Private Children's Hospital, Buenos Aires, Argentina

Hidenori Fujii Fukui Red Cross Hospital, Fukui, Japan

Masaki Fukunaga Juntendo University Urayasu Hospital, Urayasu, Japan

Toshiharu Furukawa Keio University, Tokyo, Japan

Ken Hagiwara Nihon University, Tokyo, Japan

Aiichiro Higure University of Occupational and Environmental Health, Kitakyusyu, Japan

Chih-Kun Huang Bariatric and Metabolic International Surgery Centre, E-Da Hospital, Kaohsiung, Taiwan

Atsushi Iida Fukui University, Fukui, Japan

Noriyuki Inaki Ishikawa Prefectural Central Hospital, Kanazawa, Japan

Aya Kamei Medical Topia Soka, Saitama, Japan

Noriaki Kameyama International Goodwill Hospital, Yokohama, Japan

Goro Kaneda National Hospital Organization, Sagamihara Hospital, Sagamihara, Japan

Eiji Kanehira Medical Topia Soka, Saitama, Japan

Kazunori Kasama Yotsuya Medical Cube, Tokyo, Japan

Goutaro Katsuno Juntendo University, Juntendo Urayasu Hospital, Urayasu, Japan

Yo Kawarada Tonan Hospital, Hokkaido, Japan

Iwaho Kikuchi Juntendo University, Tokyo, Japan

Guowei Kim National University, Singapore, Singapore

Yuko Kitagawa Keio University, Tokyo, Japan

Masaya Kitamura National Hospital Organization, Sagamihara Hospital, Sagamihara, Japan

Shuji Kitashiro Tonan Hospital, Hokkaido, Japan

Keisuke Koeda Iwate Medical College, Morioka, Japan

Jun Kumakiri Juntendo University, Tokyo, Japan

Geoffrey J. Lane Juntendo University, Tokyo, Japan

David Lomanto National University Singapore, Singapore, Singapore

Carlos Rodriguez Luppi University Autonomous of Barcelona, Barcelona, Spain

Rami E. Lutfi University of Illinois at Chicago, Chicago, IL, USA

Marcelo Martinez-Ferro Fundación Hospitalaria Private Children's Hospital, Buenos Aires, Argentina

Minoru Matsuda Nihon University, Tokyo, Japan

Gopal Menon University of California Irvine, Irvine, CA, USA

Yoav Mintz Hadassah Medical Center, Jerusalem, Israel

Takeyuki Misawa Jikei University, Kashiwa, Japan

Masaru Mizuno Iwate Medical College, Morioka, Japan

Tsunekazu Mizushima Osaka University, Osaka, Japan

Julio Lopez Monclova University Autonomous of Barcelona, Barcelona, Spain

Salvador Morales-Conde Hospital Universitario Virgen del Rocío, Sevilla, Spain

Masaki Mori Osaka University, Osaka, Japan

Toshiyuki Mori Kyorin University, Tokyo, Japan

Kunihiko Nagakari Juntendo University Urayasu Hospital, Urayasu, Japan

Takeshi Naitoh Tohoku University, Sendai, Japan

Toshirou Nishida Osaka Police Hospital, Osaka, Japan

Junichi Nishimura Osaka University, Osaka, Japan

Hiroyuki Nitta Iwate Medical College, Morioka, Japan

Kikuo Nutahara Kyorin University, Tokyo, Japan

Toru Obuchi Iwate Medical College, Morioka, Japan

Hideki Ohdan Hiroshima Hiramatsu Hospital, Hiroshima, Japan

Yasutomo Ojima Hiroshima Municipal Hospital, Hiroshima, Japan

Masazumi Okajima Hiroshima Municipal Hospital, Hiroshima, Japan

Manabu Okawada Juntendo University, Tokyo, Japan

Takatsugu Okegawa Kyorin University, Tokyo, Japan

Shunichi Okushiba Tonan Hospital, Hokkaido, Japan

Takeshi Omori Osaka Police Hospital, Osaka, Japan

Koki Otsuka Iwate Medical College, Morioka, Japan

Chinnusamy Palanivelu GEM Hospital, Coimbatore, India

Alessio Pigazzi University of California Irvine, Irvine, CA, USA

Dana Portenier Duke University Medical Center, Durham, NC, USA

Abhay Rane East Surrey Hospital, Redhill Surrey, UK

Alan A. Saber Colombia University, New York, NY, USA

Angie A. Saber Rutgers University, New Brunswick, NJ, USA

Jason M. Saber Pace University, New York, NY, USA

Juichiro Saito Juntendo University, Tokyo, Japan

Akira Sasaki Iwate Medical College, Morioka, Japan

Yosuke Seki Yotsuya Medical Cube, Tokyo, Japan

Palanisamy Senthilnathan GEM Hospital, Coimbatore, India

Kazunori Shibao University of Occupational and Environmental Health, Kitakyusyu, Japan

Noam Shussman Hadassah Medical Center, Jerusalem, Israel

James Skinovsky Positivo University Hospital, Curitiba, Brazil

María Socas Hospital Universitario Virgen del Rocío, Sevilla, Spain

Lawrence E. Tabone Duke University Medical Center, Durham, NC, USA

Roberto M. Tacchino Catholic University of Sacred Heart, Rome, Italy

Nobumi Tagaya Dokkyo University, Koshigaya, Japan

Hiroko Tina Tajima Tajima and Associates, Tokyo, Japan

Tadatoshi Takayama Nihon University, Tokyo, Japan

Satoru Takeda Juntendo University, Tokyo, Japan

Ichiro Takemasa Osaka University, Osaka, Japan

Minoru Tanabe Tokyo Medical and Dental University, Tokyo, Japan

Takashi Tanida Medical Topia Soka, Saitama, Japan

Eduardo M. Targarona University Autonomous of Barcelona, Barcelona, Spain

Hirotaka Tashiro Hiroshima Hiramatsu Hospital, Hiroshima, Japan

Manuel Trias University Autonomous of Barcelona, Barcelona, Spain

Fernanda Keiko Tsumanuma Red Cross University Hospital, Curitiba, Brazil

Kazunori Uchida Hiroshima Hiramatsu Hospital, Hiroshima, Japan

Mamoru Uemura Osaka University, Osaka, Japan

Yuki Ujihira Juntendo University, Tokyo, Japan

Akiko Umezawa Yotsuya Medical Cube, Tokyo, Japan

Anirudh Vij Bariatric and Metabolic International Surgery Centre, E-Da Hospital, Kaohsiung, Taiwan

Norihito Wada Keio University, Tokyo, Japan

Go Wakabayashi Iwate Medical College, Morioka, Japan

Koji Yamaguchi University of Occupational and Environmental Health, Kitakyusyu, Japan

Akio Yamaguchi Fukui University, Fukui, Japan

Hirofumi Yamamoto Osaka University, Osaka, Japan

Koji Yamashita Nippon Medical School, Tokyo, Japan

Atsuyuki Yamataka Juntendo University, Tokyo, Japan

Seiichiro Yoshikawa Juntendo University Urayasu Hospital, Urayasu, Japan

Masanori Yoshimitsu Department of Surgery, Hiroshima City Asa Hospital, Hiroshima, Japan

Monica T. Young University of California Irvine, Irvine, CA, USA

Chapter 1
History of Single-Port Laparoscopic Surgery

Shuji Kitashiro, Shunichi Okushiba, and Yo Kawarada

Abstract The practice of endoscopic surgery spread quickly around the world after an endoscopic cholecystectomy was performed in the late 1980s, and the number of organs to which endoscopic surgery is applied has increased steadily. Endoscopic treatment was actually introduced in the 1960s in the field of gynecology, and it was implemented in the form of single-port laparoscopic surgery (SPLS). The application of SPLS to many different organs is, however, something that began to emerge only a few years ago, and the recent rapid spread of SPLS is due largely to technological advances in endoscopic surgery over the past few years. The umbilical incision used in SPLS is subject to scar contraction; after surgery the scar shrinks so that it is almost unnoticeable. From a cosmetic perspective, the procedure offers greater advantage to patients than any other surgical method currently in general use. For surgeons, who are constantly required to reduce the cosmetic impact and implement minimally invasive approaches, SPLS is worthy of serious consideration. This chapter reviews the history of, and transitions in, SPLS, per the organ(s) to which it is applied.

Keywords Single-port laparoscopic surgery (SPLS) • History of single-port surgery • Single-port access (SPA)

1.1 Introduction

The practice of endoscopic surgery spread quickly around the world after an endoscopic cholecystectomy was performed in the late 1980s, and the number of organs to which endoscopic surgery can be applied has increased steadily. Endoscopic treatment was actually introduced in the 1960s in the field of gynecology, and it was implemented in the form of single-port laparoscopic surgery (SPLS). The application

S. Kitashiro (✉) • S. Okushiba • Y. Kawarada
Tonan Hospital, Kita 1, Nishi 6, Chuo-ku, Sapporo 060-0001, Japan
e-mail: kitasiro@cocoa.ocn.ne.jp

T. Mori and G. Dapri (eds.), *Reduced Port Laparoscopic Surgery*,
DOI 10.1007/978-4-431-54601-6_1, © Springer Japan 2014

1

of SPLS to many different organs emerged only a few years ago, and the recent rapid spread of single-port surgery is due largely to technological advances, over the past few years, in endoscopic surgery. This chapter reviews the history of, and transitions in, SPLS, per the organ(s) to which it is applied.

1.2   Transitions in SPLS

SPLS began in 1969, when Wheeless et al. [1] reported a successful tubal ligation via a 1-cm wound, through which carbon dioxide gas was introduced into the abdomen through an endoscope equipped with an eyepiece lens. In 1991, Pelosi et al. [2] reported the use of an endoscope with a working channel in performing a total hysterectomy, including removal of the fallopian tubes and ovaries. The same group also reported the first appendectomy achieved by this method [3]. Since then, endoscopes with working channels have become—and are still—widely used for SPLS. In 1997, Navara et al. [4] performed a single-port cholecystectomy, in which internal sutures were used for displaying the surgical field and for traction.

To maintain a good surgical view, Curcillo et al. [5] introduced, in 2007, a method by which straight grasping forceps can be used by direct puncture so that the surgical procedure does not rely on a single incision. In the following year, Cuesta et al. [6] used a Kirschner wire or a Mini Loop Retractor II™ (Covidien, New Haven, CT, USA) percutaneously, and Leroy et al. [7] subsequently reported a method of displaying the surgical view with the use of magnetic force for the tissue retraction.

Platforms changed over time. In 2007, Ates et al. [8] applied a 5-mm, 2-channel trocar (11-mm trocar, Applied Medical Resources Corp., Rancho Margarita, CA, USA) in SPLS. In the same year, the R-port was developed as a dedicated platform for SPLS, and the TriPort™ system (trademark pending, Advanced Surgical Concepts, Wicklow, Ireland), the Uni-X™ single laparoscopic port system (Pnavel Systems, Morganville, NJ, USA), and the SILS™ port (Covidien) followed as multi-channel ports.

The roticulator forceps that were made commercially available in 1991 (Roticulator Endo Grasp II™, Covidien) became popular once again for the use in SPLS due to their effectiveness in reducing "friction" in the surgical area, but in 2007, the multi-joint RealHand® (Novare Surgical Systems, Cupertino, CA, USA) forceps were developed, and in the following year, further improvements were seen in the prebent forceps (S-Portal Instruments, Karl Storz Endoskope, Tuttlingen, Germany). The addition of various energy devices to these platforms and forceps has meant that SPLS has gradually, SPLS has become applicable to an increasing number of organs.

1.3   Gallbladder

SPLS gallbladder surgery began in 1997, when Navara et al. [4] reported single-port endoscopic cholecystectomy. Two 10-mm trocars were inserted via the umbilical region, and three transabdominal sutures were used to retract the gallbladder and expose the triangle of Calot. The surgery was performed in 30 patients, taking an average of 123 min, with infection as the only complication in one case and no cases requiring opening of the abdomen.

In 2008, Cuesta et al. [6] reported ten cases in which two 5-mm trocars were inserted via an umbilical wound, and a Kirschner wire (φ1 mm) was inserted percutaneously, bent into a hook within the abdominal cavity, and used to pull the gallbladder. Average surgery time was 70 min. The gallbladder was perforated in three cases, but no infection was noted after surgery.

In 2008, Rao et al. [9] reported use of a dedicated SPLS port (R-port, Advanced Surgical Concepts), transabdominal stitches, and multi-joint forceps in 20 cases, three of which required the addition of a trocar.

Romanelli et al. [10, 11] reported performing cholecystectomies with the use of a dedicated SPLS port (TriPort, Advanced Surgical Concepts). Of 22 cases, one required the addition of a trocar.

Curcillo et al. [5, 12, 13] reported a method in which three 5-mm trocars were inserted from the umbilical region, and 5-mm forceps were directly inserted via the umbilical region to retract the gallbladder without the use of sutures. Subsequently, the same authors [13] reported 297 cases in which the umbilical incision measured 1.4–2 cm, the average surgical time was 71 min, and opening of the abdomen was required in only four cases.

1.4   Small Intestine and Colon

In 2007, Cobellis et al. [14] reported nine cases in which part of the intestinal tract was removed via a 10-mm wound in the umbilical region. The 10-mm wound facilitated both resection and reconstruction of the small intestine, and no case required hemostasis in the intestinal tract.

Single-port laparoscopic colectomy was reported by both Remzi et al. [15] and Bucher [16] in 2008. Remzi et al. [15] used a dedicated Uni-X™ (Pnavel Systems, NY USA) port to treat appendix polyps by means of right hemicolectomy. The wound measured 3.5-cm, and surgical time was 115 min. At the same time, Bucher et al. [16] carried out a right hemicolectomy using an endoscope with a working channel and transabdominal stitches. The incision was 3 cm, the surgery took 158 min, and reconstruction was carried out externally. Internal reconstruction was reported by Bucher et al. [17, 18] in a case of left colectomy. The incision was 2 cm, and the surgery took 213 min because it was performed concomitantly with cholecystectomy.

The reconstruction of the bowel was performed by a totally intracorporeal method [17, 18]. The anvil of the circular stapler was introduced in the abdominal cavity via the port wound. The anvil was then inserted in the bowel through an enterotomy near the anastomotic line in the segment to be resected. The central shaft of the anvil was exteriolized through a hole on the anti-mesenteric teniae. A linear stapler was applied to resect the specimen. The next steps were same as those of the standard double-stapling technique. Leroy et al. [7] reported using the magnetic force to retract the organ in a sigmoid colectomy. Access was established via a Triport™ (Advanced Surgical Concepts). A flexible scope inserted through the anus was utilized to insert the anvil. An external magnet was used to move the bowel intracororeally.

1.5   Stomach

In 2006, Kawahara et al. [19] reported performance of 22 single-site gastrostomies. After insertion of a single 10-mm trocar and introduction of an endoscope with a working channel, the abdominal cavity was observed, the anterior gastric wall was checked, and straight grasping forceps inserted via the working channel were used to pull out a part of the gastric wall via the trocar wound, after which a gastrostomy was created.

In 2008 Bucher et al. [20] reported performing a gastrojejunostomy in which three trocars (one 12-mm trocar and two 5-mm trocars) were inserted via a 2-cm incision in the umbilical area, and an abdominoscope with a working channel was used. Transabdominal sutures were used to lift the stomach and small intestine, and a linear stapler was used to attach the stomach and jejunum laterally, with the entry hole also being stapled and closed with the linear stapler. The surgery lasted 117 min.

Nissen surgery for GERD was reported by Hamzaogolu et al. [21] in 2010, with access gained via a SILS™ port (Covidien). The liver was retracted with the use of a Penrose drain 8-cm long and 1-cm wide, and it was lifted in a hammock fashion. Once the field of view of the esophagogastric junction was established, suturing was performed with SILS™Stitch (Covidien). The average surgical time was 190 min, and blood loss was 30 mL. Henckens et al. [22] reported partial gastric resection for gastrointestinal stromal tumor. A TriPort™ (Advanced Surgical Concepts) was inserted via a 2-cm incision in the umbilical area, and prototype multi-jointed forceps and a "gooseneck" videolaparoscope were used in the surgery, which took 140 min, and resulted in 10 mL blood loss. No post-surgical complications were reported, and the patient left the hospital 4 days after the surgery.

1.6   Appendix

Twenty-five cases of single-port appendectomy were reported in 1992 by Pelosi et al. [3]. In all cases, the appendix was mobilized with the use of a laparoscope with a working channel, and the appendix was resectioned externally. D'Alessio et al. [23] reported application of the same method in 116 cases, 22 (19 %) of which required the addition of a trocar, and 5 (4 %) of which required an abdominal incision. The average surgery time was 35 min. In 2007, Ates et al. [8] reported use of an 11-mm-diameter trocar with two 5-mm forceps openings in 35 cases of appendectomy.

A laparoscope with a working channel was used to dissect the area around the appendix and to pull out the mesoappendix percutaneously to create a field of view before internal ligation of the appendix root. The surgery took 38 min, and no post-operative complications were noted.

1.7 Liver

In 2010, Mantke et al. [24] performed fenestration surgery on a 9-cm diameter hepatic cyst by inserting a 10-mm trocar and two 5-mm trocars via a 2.5-cm umbilical incision. Cholecystectomy was performed at the same time, and the surgery took 64 min [24]. Patel et al. [25] reported performing a hepatic resection using TriPort™ (Advanced Surgical Concepts), also in 2010. Gaujoux et al. [26] reported single-port fenestration surgery in one case of hepatic cysts, single-port left lobe resection in three cases of metastatic liver tumor, and single-port wedge resection in one case of hepatocellular cancer. Access was obtained with a 40-mm Gelport™ (Applied Medical), and none of these cases required the addition of a trocar. Surgery took 55–140 min, blood loss ranged from 20 to 50 mL, and patients remained in the hospital for 2 days after surgery.

1.8 Spleen

The first two single-port splenectomies were performed by Barbaros et al. [27] in response to idiopathic thrombocytopenic purpura. The umbilical incision was 2 cm, into which three trocars were inserted, with surgery taking 110 min and 150 min, respectively. You et al. [28] reported one case of splenic injury and two of idiopathic thrombocytopenic purpura for which single-port splenectomy was carried out. A 3.5-cm incision was made in the lateral region along the left anterior axillary line, and an Alexis wound retractor (Applied Medical) was fixed and made airtight with the use of a glove, with four trocars (12, 10, 5, and 5-mm) inserted from the fingers of the glove. The field of view was extended with the use of a Snake retractor, and a linear stapler was applied to the splenic hilum. Surgery took 195 min in the first case due to injury to the stomach, but in the other two cases surgery took 125 min and 133 min, respectively.

1.9 Groin

The first single-port operation on an inguinal hernia was reported by Cugura et al. [29] in 2008. The surgical method was total extraperitoneal repair, with a 2.5-cm incision made below the umbilical area and three trocars (one 10-mm trocar and two 5-mm trocars) used, in an operation that took 90 min.

Surgery for transabdominal pre-peritoneal hernia was reported by Kroh et al. [30]. Surgery was implemented with a Uni-X™ (Pnavel Systems) and took 47 min.

1.10 Female Organs

A method involving the use of an endoscope with an eyepiece lens to introduce carbon dioxide gas through a 1-cm incision below the umbilical area for tubal ligation was reported by Wheeless et al. [1] in 1969. Three hundred sixty cases have since been reported, confirming the safety of the procedure [31].

In 1991, Pelosi et al. [2] reported performing total hysterectomy including bilateral salpingo-oophorectomy using an endoscope with a working channel.

In 2005, Ghezzi et al. [32] reported treatment of ten ectopic pregnancies for which three trocars were inserted via an umbilical incision to lift and resect the fallopian tubes.

1.11 Adrenal Gland, Kidney, Prostate

Single-port adrenalectomy was reported in 2008 by Castellucci et al. [33]. Three trocars were used for extirpation, via a 2-cm umbilical incision, of a left adrenal tumor measuring 4.5 cm.

Nephrectomy was reported by Rane et al. [34] in 2007 who used the R-port™ (Advanced Surgical Concepts) via a single port in the lateral region for retroperitoneal extirpation. The first nephrectomy performed via an umbilical port was reported by Desai et al. [35]. Gill et al. [36] reported four cases of single-port donor kidney removal for transplantation, in which the average surgical time was 210 min, blood loss was 50 mL, and the ischemic interval was 6.2 min. Total single-port extirpation of the prostate was reported in 2008 by Kaouk et al. [37]. The procedure was applied in four cases of prostate cancer. Surgery took an average of 285 min, and the average blood loss was 288 mL. The same authors subsequently reported single-port prostate extirpation performed with a Da Vinci robot [38].

1.12 Gastrointestinal Tract

In 2008, Nguyen et al. [39] reported single-port gastric banding surgery. A 4-cm incision was made between the xiphoid cartilage and the umbilical area, and a 15-mm trocar was inserted by which the band was inserted into the abdominal cavity. The 15-mm trocar was removed, and four 5-mm trocars were inserted to place and deploy the band. The surgery took 55 min. No difference was found in the time needed for surgery, the amount of blood lost, or complications between this surgery and 23 subsequent conventional endoscopic surgeries. Three cases of SPLS required the addition of a trocar [40].

In 2009, Saber et al. [41] reported six cases of single-port sleeve gastrectomy. The SILS™ port (Covidien) was positioned between the xiphoid cartilage and the umbilical area, and in three cases, the addition of a 5-mm trocar was required. Surgery took an average of 123 min. Saber et al. [42] also reported a Roux-en-Y gastric bypass performed through a SILS™ port (Covidien) in a patient with a BMI of 39 kg/m^2. The surgery took 133 min, and the patient left the hospital following day.

1.13 Conclusion

The umbilical incision used in SPLS is subject to scar contraction, and after surgery the scar shrinks so that it is nearly invisible. From the standpoint of cosmesis, the procedure offers greater advantages to patients than any other surgical method currently in general use. For surgeons, who are constantly required to reduce the cosmetic impact and implement minimally invasive approaches, SPLS is worthy of serious consideration. Various manufacturers of medical devices are in agreement with the admiration shown by surgeons and have started to work in this area. As this type of surgery extends its range with respect to various organs, surgical results from the period of introduction continue to improve, with many reports suggesting that the procedures are equivalent to conventional endoscopic techniques. Improvements continue in terms of development of new equipment and safe surgical techniques. Currently, however, SPLS remains in the introductory stage, and the number of cases in which it has been introduced is small. It is thought to be too early to objectively assess the safety, invasiveness, and reliability, and the efficacy of SPLS in various contexts must be seriously evaluated in the future.

References

1. Wheeless CR et al (1969) A rapid, inexpensive and effective method of surgical sterilization by laparoscopy. J Reprod Med 3(5):65–69
2. Pelosi MA et al (1991) Laparoscopic hysterectomy with bilateral salpingo-oophorectomy using a single umbilical puncture. N J Med 88:721–726
3. Pelosi MA et al (1992) Laparoscopic appendectomy using a single umbilical puncture (minilaparoscopy). J Reprod Med 37:588–594
4. Navarra G et al (1997) One-wound laparoscopic cholecystectomy. Br J Surg 84:695
5. Cucillo PG (2007) High dexterity instrumentation in laparoscopic surgery. Presented at SAGES in Las Vegas, NV, 22 April 2007
6. Cuesta MA et al (2008) The "invisible cholecystectomy": a transumbilical laparoscopic operation without a scar. Surg Endosc 22:1211–1213
7. Leroy J et al (2009) Single access laparoscopic sigmoidectomy as definitive surgical management of prior diverticulitis in a human patient. Arch Surg 144:173–179

8. Ates O et al (2007) Single-port laparoscopic appendectomy conducted intracorporeally with the aid of a transabdominal sling suture. J Pediatr Surg 42:1071–1074
9. Rao PP et al (2008) The feasibility of single port laparoscopic cholecystectomy: a pilot study of 20 cases. HPB (Oxford) 10(5):336–340
10. Romanelli JR et al (2008) Single port laparoscopic cholecystectomy with the TriPort system: a case report. Surg Innov 15(3):223–228
11. Romanelli JR et al (2010) Single-port laparoscopic cholecystectomy: initial experience. Surg Endosc 24(6):1374–1379
12. Podolsky ER et al (2009) Single port access (SPA) cholecystectomy: a completely transumbilical approach. J Laparoendosc Adv Surg Tech A 19(2):219–222
13. Curcillo PG et al (2010) Single-port-access (SPA) cholecystectomy a multi-institutional report of the first 297 cases. Surg Endosc 24(8):1854–1860. doi:10.1007/s00464-009-0856-x
14. Cobellis G et al (2007) One-trocar transumbilical laparoscopic-assisted management of Meckel's diverticulum in children. J Laparoendosc Adv Surg Tech A 17:238–241
15. Remzi FH et al (2008) Single-port laparoscopy in colorectal surgery. Colorectal Dis 10(8):823–826
16. Bucher P et al (2008) Single port access laparoscopic right hemicolectomy. Int J Colorectal Dis 23:1013–1016
17. Bucher P et al (2009) Single-port access radical left colectomy in humans. Dis Colon Rectum 52:1797–1802
18. Bucher P et al (2008) Totally intracorporeal laparoscopic colorectal anastomosis using circular stapler. Surg Endosc 22(5):1278–1282. doi:10.1007/s00464-007-9607-z
19. Kawahara H et al (2006) One-trocar laparoscopy-aided gastrostomy in handicapped children. J Pediatr Surg 41:2076–2080
20. Bucher P et al (2008) Transumbilical single-incision laparoscopic intracorporeal anastomosis for gastrojejunostomy: case report. Surg Endosc 23:1667–1670
21. Hamzaogolu I et al (2010) Transumbilical totally laparoscopic single-port Nissen fundoplication: a new method of liver retraction: the Istanbul technique. J Gastrointest Surg 14(6):1035–1039
22. Henckens T et al (2010) Laparoendoscopic single-site gastrectomy for a gastric GIST using double-bended instruments. J Laparoendosc Adv Surg Tech A 20(5):469–471
23. D'Alessio A et al (2002) One-trocar transumbilical laparoscopic-assisted appendectomy in children: our experience. Eur J Pediatr Surg 12:24–27
24. Mantke R et al (2010) Single-port liver cyst fenestration combined with single-port laparoscopic cholecystectomy using completely reusable instruments. Surg Laparosc Endosc Percutan Tech 20(1):e28–e30
25. Patel AG et al (2011) Single-incision laparoscopic left lateral segmentectomy of colorectal liver metastasis. Surg Endosc 25(2):649–650
26. Gaujoux S et al (2011) Single-incision laparoscopic liver resection. Surg Endosc 25(5):1489–1494
27. Barbaros U et al (2009) Single incision laparoscopic splenectomy: the first two cases. J Gastrointest Surg 13(8):1520–1523, Epub 2009 Apr 14
28. You YK et al (2010) Single-port laparoscopic splenectomy: the first three cases. Asian J Endosc Surg 3(1):33–35
29. Cugura JF et al (2008) First case of single incision laparoscopic surgery for totally extraperitoneal inguinal hernia repair. Acta Clin Croat 47(4):249–252
30. Kroh M et al (2009) Single-port, laparoscopic cholecystectomy and inguinal hernia repair: first clinical report of a new device. J Laparoendosc Adv Surg Tech A 19(2):215–217
31. Wheeless CR Jr et al (1973) Laparoscopic sterilization. Review of 3600 cases. Obstet Gynecol 42:303–306
32. Ghezzi F et al (2005) One-trocar salpingectomy for the treatment of tubal pregnancy: a 'marionette-like' technique. BJOG 112:1417–1419
33. Castellucci SA et al (2008) Single port access adrenalectomy. J Endourol 22(8):1573–1576

34. Rane A et al (2007) Clinical evaluation of a novel laparoscopic port (R-Port) and evolution of the single laparoscopic port procedure (SLiPP). J Endourol 21(Suppl 1):A22–A23
35. Desai MM et al (2008) Scarless single port transumbilical nephrectomy and pyeloplasty: first clinical report. BJU Int 101:83–88
36. Gill IS et al (2008) Single port transumbilical (E-NOTES) donor nephrectomy. J Urol 180(2):637–641
37. Kaouk JH et al (2008) Single-port laparoscopic radical prostatectomy. Urology 72(6):1190–1193
38. Kaouk JH et al (2009) Robotic single-port transumbilical surgery in humans: initial report. BJU Int 103(3):366–369, Epub 2008
39. Ninh T et al (2008) Single laparoscopic incision transabdominal (SLIT) surgery-adjustable gastric banding: a novel minimally invasive surgical approach. Obes Surg 18(12):1628–1631. doi:10.1007/s11695-008-9705-6
40. Ninh T et al (2010) Comparison study of conventional laparoscopic gastric banding versus laparoendoscopic single site gastric banding. Surg Obes Relat Dis 6(5):503–507
41. Saber AA et al (2009) Early experience with SILS port laparoscopic sleeve gastrectomy. Surg Laparosc Endosc Percutan Tech 19(6):428–430
42. Saber AA et al (2009) Single port access transumbilical laparoscopic Roux-en-Y gastric bypass using the SILS Port: first reported case. Surg Innov 16(4):343–347, Epub 2009 Dec 22

Chapter 2
Concept of Reduced Port Laparoscopic Surgery

Toshiyuki Mori

Abstract Since the first report of single-incision laparoscopic surgery (SLS) for gallbladder removal by Navarra in 1997, a number of approaches have been reported in the literature. Nevertheless, SLS failed to attract the wide attention of surgeons, because it violated a basic principle known as "triangular formation" resulting in a clashing problem between the scope and instruments. Surgical maneuver became technically demanding with these approaches. A new proposal for SLS with a new accessing device (SILS™ port (Covidien, New Haven, CT, USA)) and bendable forceps (Roticulator™ (Covidien)) was successful, and it reminded surgeons of the promise of SLS, and again proposed it as a viable next-generation surgical technique. Needle-scopic surgery was invented around the same time (1996) and evolved gradually. After the introduction of SLS, many surgeons took note of the pros and cons of SLS and needle-scopic surgery and that they are complementary to each other and the mixed use of the two techniques drastically mitigates the difficulty in SLS. Surgeons started using needle instruments as an active forceps. These approaches are collectively called reduced port laparoscopic surgery (RPLS). Robot and natural orifices translumenal endoscopic surgery (NOTES) devices have reportedly been used as tools of RPLS. The most appropriate combination of these tools would suggest the future shape of minimally invasive surgery.

Keywords Laparoscopic surgery • Single-incision surgery • Reduced port surgery

T. Mori (✉)
Kyorin University, 6-20-2 Shinkawa, Mitaka, Tokyo 181-8611, Japan
e-mail: mori@ks.kyorin-u.ac.jp

T. Mori and G. Dapri (eds.), *Reduced Port Laparoscopic Surgery*,
DOI 10.1007/978-4-431-54601-6_2, © Springer Japan 2014

2.1 Introduction

Although begun in the early 1900s, laparoscopy had limited applications. In 1986, a small CCD camera (small enough to be attached to the eye-piece of the laparoscope) was developed. This enabled all members of the surgical team to share the image of the surgical field inside the body cavity displayed on the monitor. In 1987, video-endoscopic cholecystectomy was first achieved by Mouret, and dramatic increase in adoption occurred in the late 1980s and early 1990s [1].

Since that time, laparoscopic surgery has then been applied to a variety of surgical fields. It became a less invasive alternative to the standard open wound procedures and accepted as standard care in many diseases.

Laparoscopic surgery was performed via accessing channel (port). Less destruction in the normal structure of the body wall was attributed to drastic reduction in surgical invasiveness [2]. Patients who underwent laparoscopic procedures experienced less pain, shorter hospital stay, and returned to normal activity much faster when compared to comparable open procedures. It did not take long for the pioneering surgeons to make further efforts to minimize the number and size of the port and the caliber of the devices with a belief that less destruction of the body wall would result in further reduction of surgical invasiveness [3]. Although it has been difficult to scientifically prove that these approaches could offer better outcomes to patients when compared to standard laparoscopic surgery, three port (even two port) surgery has been practiced in the pioneering centers, and reportedly been better or, at least, comparable to the standard laparoscopic procedures [4, 5]. One of the goals of these approaches is single incision laparoscopic surgery (SLS), in which the access to the body cavity is created via a small wound (i.e. the umbilicus). Dr. Navarra is usually credited with the first single incision laparoscopic cholecystectomy in humans [6]. Natural orifices translumenal endoscopic surgery (NOTES) has been thought of as the ultimate goal of these approaches [7, 8]. It can theoretically negate injury to the normal body wall, resulting in even further lessening of invasiveness. Nevertheless, NOTES is still considered as one of the future options of surgery, because of imperfect instrumentation and technical difficulty to date. Another approach to reduce body wall injury includes needle-scopic surgery, first advocated by Gagner in 1996 [9] and reported by Tanaka in 1997 [10], in which small caliber camera and instruments (<3 mm) are used. The resulting wound is just a puncture hole and almost invisible. Reduced port laparoscopic surgery (RPLS) is a relatively new term, first coined by Curcillo in 2010. Although the definition is still ambiguous, it is generally accepted to use the term 'reduced port surgery' to describe a condition where these approaches of minimally invasive surgery are in mixed use, as to reduce invasiveness of the procedure and provide good cosmetic results while maintaining visibility of the surgical field and permitting intuitive handling of the instruments, thus promoting patient safety.

2.2 Single-Incision Laparoscopic Surgery (SLS)

Since the first report of SLS by Navarra [6], a number of approaches have been reported in the literature [11–15]. It was in 2009 that SLS first gained wide acceptance by surgeons. In a seminar of the society of american gastrointestinal and endoscopic surgeons (SAGES), attendants voted for SLS to be the primary access method in a few years for relatively simple laparoscopic procedures (e.g. laparoscopic cholecystectomy for non-inflamed gallbladder). Many manufactures and venders of laparoscopic instruments have noticed the importance of the market for SLS, and have started providing new tools and gadgets (even without scientific verification). Some of the instruments that seemed already obsolete or less functional in standard laparoscopic surgery have been revived for use in SLS [16].

2.3 Characteristics of SLS

Laparoscopic surgery is generally more technically demanding when compared to the comparable open wound surgery. Visual perception is limited for two-dimensional display of the surgical field in laparoscopic surgery. Long and leveraged instruments make surgical maneuvers awkward. Loss of tactile and kinesthetic sensation in laparoscopic surgery further adds difficulty in recognition of surgical anatomy. Use of multiple instruments sometimes resulted in "sword fighting" between the scope and instruments. To cope with these problems, basic principles should always be adhered to reduce difficulty in surgical maneuvers and thus to promote patient safety. Among these principles, co-axial set-up and triangular formation of the instrument are most important. Co-axial set-up means that the monitor, surgical field, camera port, and the operator are ideally placed in a line (Fig. 2.1). Triangular formation is a principle of port placement for the operator, in which instruments from both sides make an angle of 30–60° to the line (axis) mentioned above (Fig. 2.2). With this set-up, the gap between visual perception and surgical exertion can be minimized (eye-hand coordination), avoiding mutual interference of the scope and instruments [17, 18].

In SLS, the ports for scope and instruments are placed in a restricted area, the angles between the scope and instruments are less than 10° at the surgical site. The principle of triangular formation is violated, which imposes problems that are not usual in standard laparoscopic surgery.

The shaft of the instruments and the scope interfere with each other ("sword fighting"). In standard laparoscopic surgery, the length of the instruments is uniformly 33–35 cm. This fact adds clashing problems, in which the handles of instruments interfere with each other outside the abdomen. The relatively large housing of regular ports also clash. In addition, the light guide in a rigid angled scope and the camera head further complicate this clashing problem. Furthermore, the shaft of the instruments tends to eclipse the surgical field for this narrow angle, making it difficult to see the exact place where the force and energy is applied (Fig. 2.3) [16].

Fig. 2.1 Co-axial setup.
Monitor, surgical field,
camera port, and the operator
are ideally placed in a line

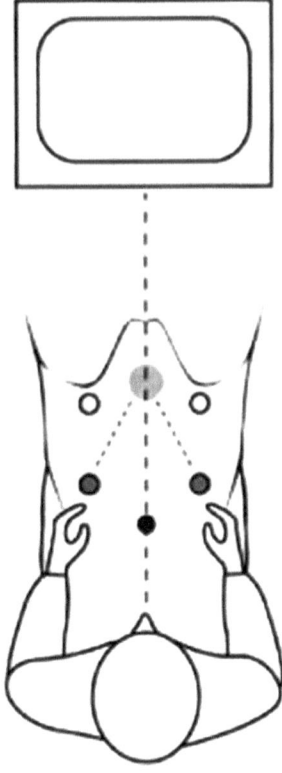

Fig. 2.2 Triangular
formation. Instruments from
both sides should make an
angle of 30° to 60° to the line
(*axis*) mentioned above

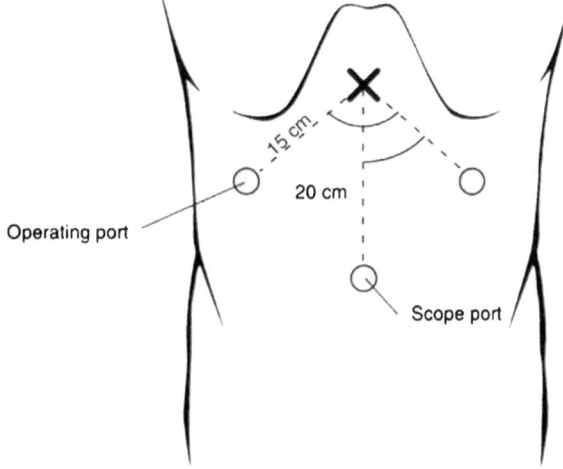

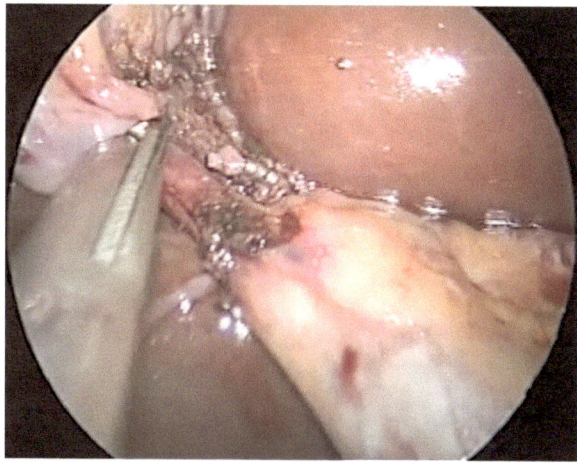

Fig. 2.3 Eclipse of the surgical field. Because of the narrow angle between the scope and instrument, the shaft of the instrument tends to eclipse the surgical site where the force and energy is applied

2.4 Instrumentation and Techniques in SLS

Regardless of the names, including SILS™ (Single-Incision Laparoscopic Surgery, Covidien http://www.covidien.com/), LESS™ (Laparo-Endoscopic Single-Site surgery, Olympus http://www.olympusamerica.com/LESS/, http://www. advancedsurgical.ie/), SSL™ (Single Site Laparoscopy J&J http://www.jnj.com/ connect/), and S-Portal™ (Karl Storz Endoskope, http://www.karlstorz.com/cps/ rde/xchg/karlstorz-en/hs.xsl/146.htm), the underlying concept is almost identical, restoration of triangular formation while avoiding clash and "sword fighting." In order to restore triangular formation, two basic techniques have been employed, first placing the operating ports at a good distance of separation from one another, and second using curved, angulated, or articulated instruments. The first technique is commonly referred to as the parallel technique, and the second one as the cross hand technique (Figs. 2.4 and 2.5). In clinical settings, these techniques are often in mixed use. Tissue retraction is a key step of operation for good exposure of the surgical field with some tension to apply force and energy to the surgical site. In standard laparoscopic surgery, the assisting forceps is inserted through an independent port to achieve this. In SLS, additional instruments from the same wound further complicate the clashing problem. Sutures are introduced in the abdominal cavity from a different site and the tissue is pierced, and then the sutures are retrieved through the abdominal wall. By pulling the thread outside, the tissue is retracted. Although some surgeons advocate this technique, it is cumbersome and sometimes causes bile spillage in laparoscopic cholecystectomy. Gadgets that measure 1.6–3 mm in caliber, including pre-tied loop, wire snare, and a needle grasper can be independently

Fig. 2.4 Parallel Technique
(Boxing Style). In parallel
technique, the operating ports
are placed at a distance of
1.5–2.5 cm away from the
scope port

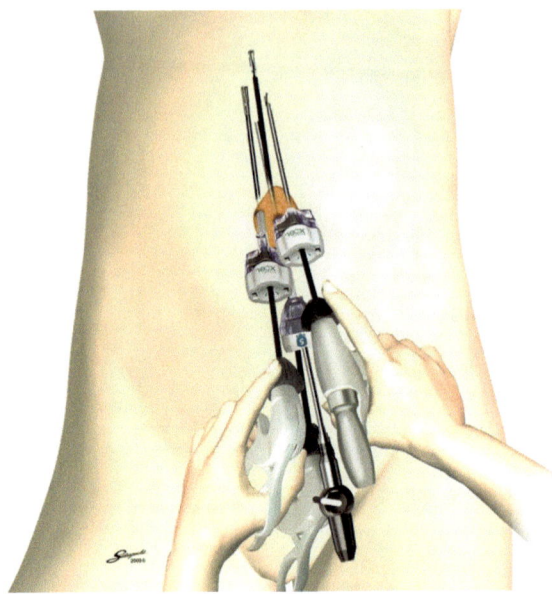

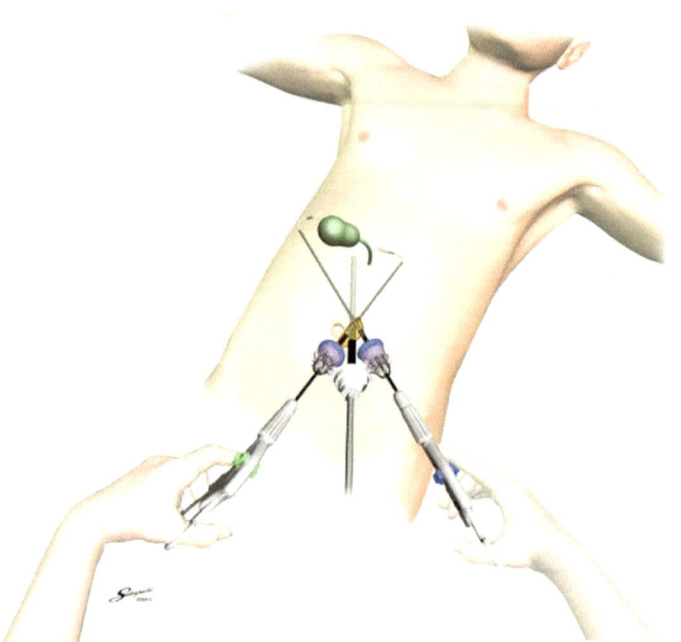

Fig. 2.5 Cross Hand Technique. In the cross hand technique, the shafts of the instrument cross at
some point and the instrument that approaches the surgical site from the left-side is manipulated
by the right hand

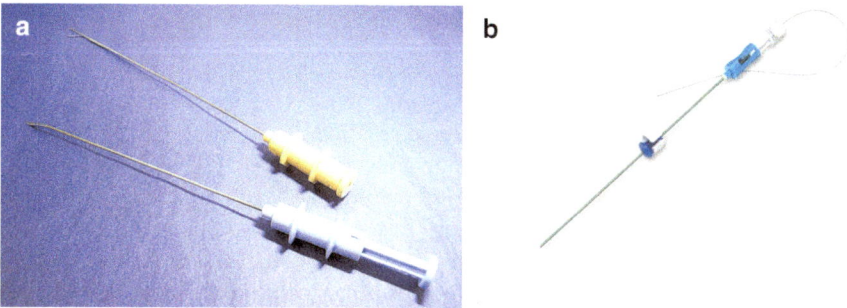

Fig. 2.6 Gadgets for Tissue Retraction. (**a**) Riza-Ribe Needle and GraNee Needle (M-Med). (**b**) Mini loop retractor (Covidien)

inserted elsewhere as in standard laparoscopic operations and used for tissue retraction (Fig. 2.6). The use of additional instruments adds confusion to the terminology of SLS, because these techniques leave an additional wound, even though small and in name, scarless. The purists of SLS demanded that these techniques requiring another wound should be distinguished from the pure one, resulting in further confusion of the terminology including with one additional port surgery, single plus one port laparoscopic surgery, or two-port laparoscopic surgery [19–21].

2.5 Needle-Scopic Surgery

Although the term needle-scopic surgery was first used in 1996 by Mathias [22], Tanaka in 1997 is usually credited with the first report of needle-scopic cholecystectomy in humans [10]. This report was followed by a number of clinical reports from various fields of surgery [23–25]. The merits of needle-scopic surgery included its cosmetic advantage over standard laparoscopic surgery while keeping the operability of instruments. Several randomized control studies were conducted, but failed to prove the better outcome of needle-scopic cholecystectomy when compared to standard laparoscopic cholecystectomy in regard to postoperative pain, convalescence and recovery [26–28]. The disadvantages of needle-scopic surgery result from the small caliber of the scope and instruments. The image that needle-scope provides is unsatisfactory. The shaft of the forceps bends when force is applied, and the small jaws of instruments tend to bite the organs more easily than atraumatically-designed jaws of standard laparoscopic instruments.

In a meta-analysis by Sajid et al. [29], needle-scopic cholecystectomy was reportedly associated with longer operating time and higher conversion rate comparing to standard laparoscopic cholecystectomy. Although needle-scopic surgery has been routinely performed for relatively simple procedures in pioneering institutions, it failed to gain wide acceptance as a standard procedure to date.

2.6 Inception of Reduced Port Laparoscopic Surgery (RPLS)

In general, SLS is more technically demanding than standard laparoscopic surgery. In the beginning, indications suggested that it was limited to relatively simple operations. Many surgeons have noticed that the pros and cons that SLS and needle-scopic surgery bring are complementary to each other and the mixed use of two techniques drastically mitigate difficulties in SLS. Surgeons started using needle instruments as an active forceps [30]. These approaches are collectively called RPLS. Unleashed from the limitations of SLS, RPLS widened its indication to a variety of procedures, as is described in this book. Interestingly, the introduction of RPLS evoked the idea of hybrid use of other approaches of minimally invasive surgery, including robotic surgery and NOTES [31, 32]. The daVinci single-site platform (Intuitive Surgical Inc., Sunnyvale, CA, USA) is already on the market (Fig. 2.7), and endoscopic robot designed for NOTES was introduced through an access device of SLS. A flexible endoscope is also introduced through the single access device, and the endoscopic device through the working channel is used as a forceps in cooperation with standard instruments [33]. Assisting forceps were reportedly introduced through the port placed in the vagina, and the specimen was eventually retrieved via the vagina [34]. Various approaches to minimize invasiveness of surgery merge here in reduced port laparoscopic surgery. In the toolbox of RPLS, we have a wide variety of tools, including standard and needle-scopic instruments, robots, NOTES devices, and even the flexible endoscope and its various forceps (Fig. 2.8).

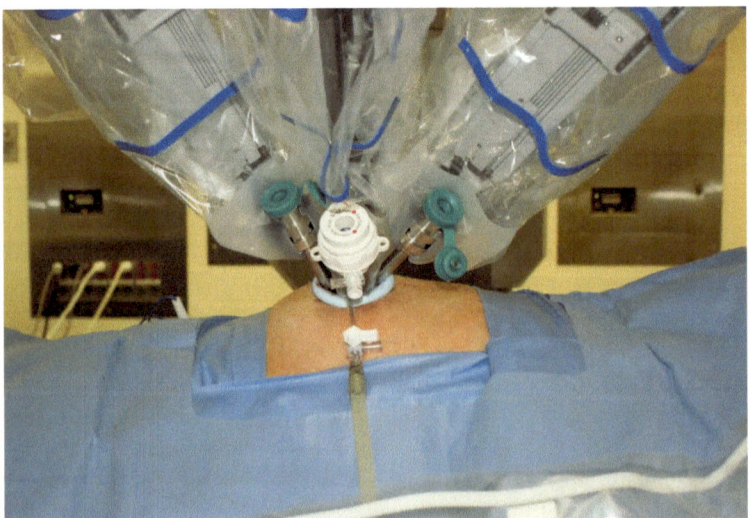

Fig. 2.7 Single Site daVinci (Intuitive). Single incision robotic surgery is already in clinical use

Fig. 2.8 NOTES device. NOTES device can also be used in reduced port laparoscopic surgery

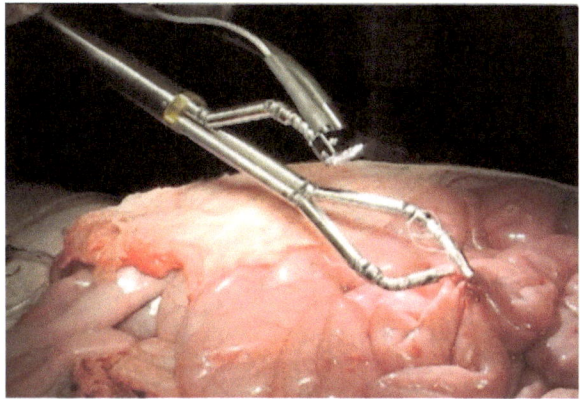

2.7 Future of Minimally Invasive Surgery

It is hardly possible to predict even the near future of minimally invasive surgery. Although technically feasible, RPLS is still in its infancy. The optimal combination of the hybrid use of a list of tools should be discussed from various points of view. The middle and long-term outcome of RPLS, especially for malignant diseases, should be extensively studied. One thing for sure is that patient preference would be a minimal wound. A short-as-possible convalescence and leave period is most desirable, as far as the selected treatment, RPLS, can give better or, at least comparable outcome to standard (laparoscopic) surgery. I believe that RPLS would be the mainstay of accessing method in minimally invasive surgery.

References

1. Polychronidis A, Laftsidis P, Bounovas A, Simopoulos C (2008) Twenty years of laparoscopic cholecystectomy: Philippe Mouret–March 17, 1987. JSLS 12(1):109–111
2. Cho JM, LaPorta AJ, Clark JR, Schofield MJ, Hammond SL, Mallory PL 2nd (1994) Response of serum cytokines in patients undergoing laparoscopic cholecystectomy. Surg Endosc 8:1380–1384
3. Matsuda T, Ogura K, Uchida J, Fujita I, Terachi T, Yoshida O (1995) Smaller ports result in shorter convalescence after laparoscopic varicocelectomy. J Urol 153:1175–1177
4. Sun S, Yang K, Gao M, He X, Tian J, Ma B (2009) Three-port versus four-port laparoscopic cholecystectomy: meta-analysis of randomized clinical trials. World J Surg 33:1904–1908
5. Poon CM, Chan KW, Lee DW, Chan KC, Ko CW, Cheung HY, Lee KW (2003) Two-port versus four-port laparoscopic cholecystectomy. Surg Endosc 17:1624–1627
6. Navarra G, Pozza E, Occhionorelli S, Carcoforo P, Donini I (1997) One-wound laparoscopic cholecystectomy. Br J Surg 84(5):695
7. Marescaux J, Dallemagne B, Perretta S, Wattiez A, Mutter D, Coumaros D (2007) Surgery without scars: report of transluminal cholecystectomy in a human being. Arch Surg 142:823–827

 8. Forgione A, Maggioni D, Sansonna F, Ferrari C, Di Lernia S, Citterio D, Magistro C, Frigerio
    L, Pugliese RJ (2008) Transvaginal endoscopic cholecystectomy in human beings: preliminary
    results. J Laparoendosc Adv Surg Tech A 18:345–351
 9. Gagner M, Garcia-Ruiz A (1998) Technical aspects of minimally invasive abdominal surgery
    performed with needlescopic instruments. Surg Laparosc Endosc 8(3):171–179
10. Tanaka J, Andoh H, Koyama K (1998) Minimally invasive needlescopic cholecystectomy.
    Surg Today 28(1):111–113
11. Podolsky ER, Curcillo PG 2nd (2010) Reduced-port surgery: preservation of the critical view
    in single-port-access cholecystectomy. Surg Endosc 24(12):3038–3043
12. Cuesta MA, Berends F, Veenhof AA (2008) The "invisible cholecystectomy": a transumbilical
    laparoscopic operation without a scar. Surg Endosc 22:1211–1213
13. Gumbs AA, Milone L, Sinha P, Bessler M (2009) Totally transumbilical laparoscopic
    cholecystectomy. J Gastrointest Surg 13(3):533–534
14. Hong TH, You YK, Lee KH (2009) Transumbilical single-port laparoscopic cholecystectomy:
    scarless cholecystectomy. Surg Endosc 23:1393–1397
15. Rivas H, Varela E, Scott D (2010) Single-incision laparoscopic cholecystectomy: initial evalu-
    ation of a large series of patients. Surg Endosc 24(6):1403–1412
16. Mori T, Aoki H, Sugiyama M, Atomi Y (2010) Instrumentation of single-access laparoscopic
    surgery. Asian J Endosc Surg 3:153–161
17. Bhoyrul S, Mori T, Way LW (1995) Principles of instrumentation. In: Way LW, Bhoyrul S,
    Mori T (eds) Fundamentals of laparoscopic surgery. Churchill Livingstone, New York, NY, pp
    13–78
18. Mori T, Bhoyrul S, Way LW (1995) Operative techniques. In: Way LW, Bhoyrul S, Mori T
    (eds) Fundamentals of laparoscopic surgery. Churchill Livingstone, New York, NY, pp 79–136
19. Gao Y, Xu DF, Liu YS, Cui XG, Che JP, Yao YC, Yin L (2011) Single plus one port laparo-
    scopic radical prostatectomy: a report of eight cases in one center. Chin Med J (Engl)
    124(10):1580–1582
20. Lim SW, Kim HJ, Kim CH, Huh JW, Kim YJ, Kim HR (2013) Umbilical incision laparoscopic
    colectomy with one additional port for colorectal cancer. Tech Coloproctol 17(2):193–199
21. Kikuchi I, Kumakiri J, Matsuoka S, Takeda S (2012) Learning curve of minimally invasive
    two-port laparoscopic myomectomy. JSLS 16(1):112–118
22. Mathias JM (1997) Needlescopic surgery is painless and scarless. OR Manager 13(11):24,
    26–27
23. Gill IS, Soble JJ, Sung GT, Winfield HN, Bravo EL, Novick AC (1998) Needlescopic adrenal-
    ectomy–the initial series: comparison with conventional laparoscopic adrenalectomy. Urology
    52(2):180–186
24. Tagaya N, Kita J, Kogure H, Kubota K (2001) Laparoscopic intragastric resection of gastric
    leiomyoma using needlescopic instruments. Case report. Surg Endosc 15(4):414
25. Mamazza J, Schlachta CM, Seshadri PA, Cadeddu MO, Poulin EC (2001) Needlescopic sur-
    gery. A logical evolution from conventional laparoscopic surgery. Surg Endosc
    15(10):1208–1212
26. Lee PC, Lai IR, Yu SC (2004) Minilaparoscopic (needlescopic) cholecystectomy: a study of
    1,011 cases. Surg Endosc 18(10):1480–1484
27. Franklin ME Jr, Jaramillo EJ, Glass JL, Treviño JM, Berghoff KR (2006) Needlescopic chole-
    cystectomy: lessons learned in 10 years of experience. JSLS 10(1):43–46
28. Tagaya N, Rokkaku K, Kubota K (2007) Needlescopic cholecystectomy versus needlescope-
    assisted laparoscopic cholecystectomy. Surg Laparosc Endosc Percutan Tech 17:375–379
29. Sajid MS, Khan MA, Ray K, Cheek E, Baig MK (2009) Needlescopic versus laparoscopic
    cholecystectomy: a meta-analysis. ANZ J Surg 79(6):437–442
30. Leroy J, Cahill RA, Peretta S, Marescaux J (2008) Single port sigmoidectomy in an experi-
    mental model with survival. Surg Innov 15:260–265

31. Autorino R, Kaouk JH, Stolzenburg JU, Gill IS, Mottrie A, Tewari A, Cadeddu JA (2013) Current status and future directions of robotic single-site surgery: a systematic review. Eur Urol 63(2):266–280
32. Noguera JF, Dolz C, Cuadrado A, Olea J, García J (2013) Flexible single-incision surgery: a fusion technique. Surg Innov 20(3):256–259
33. Abe N, Takeuchi H, Ohki A, Aoki H, Masaki T, Mori T, Sugiyama M (2012) Single-incision multiport laparoendoscopic surgery using a newly-developed short-type flexible endoscope: a combined procedure of flexible endoscopic and laparoscopic surgery. J Hepatobiliary Pancreat Sci 19(4):426–430
34. Navarra G, Currò G (2010) Trans-vaginally assisted single incision laparoscopic right hemicolectomy. ANZ J Surg 80(12):872–873

Chapter 3
Terminology

Takeshi Naitoh

Abstract A laparoscopic surgery through one skin incision by collecting all the ports to one incision is known as a single-port or a single-incision laparoscopic (SLS). Although many names and their acronyms have been proposed, a consensus name for this technique does not exist yet. Trans umbilical endoscopic surgery (TUES), embryonic natural orifices translumenal endoscopic surgery (E-NOTES) and natural orifices trans umbilical surgery (NOTUS) are terms derived from the natural orifices translumenal endoscopic surgery (NOTES) concept. Terms called single-port access (SPA) laparoscopic surgery, one port umbilical surgery (OPUS), single-port surgery (SPS), single-port laparoscopic surgery (SPLS), and single-port incisionless conventional equipment-utilizing surgery (SPICE) have also been used. Laparo-endoscopic single site surgery (LESS) was proposed by the United States multidisciplinary consortium. Needlescopic surgery is defined as a procedure using less than 3-mm laparoscopic instruments. Reduced port laparoscopic surgery (RPLS) is a concept that indicates a laparoscopic surgery aiming at both reducing the number of ports and reducing the diameter of the port. Therefore, both a SLS and a needlescopic surgery are considered to be included into the category of the RPLS.

Keywords Needlescopic surgery • Reduced port laparoscopic surgery • Single-port laparoscopic surgery

T. Naitoh (✉)
Department of Surgery, Graduate School of Medicine, Tohoku University,
1-1, Seiryo-machi, Aoba-ku, Sendai 980-8574, Japan
e-mail: naitot@surg1.med.tohoku.ac.jp

T. Mori and G. Dapri (eds.), *Reduced Port Laparoscopic Surgery*,
DOI 10.1007/978-4-431-54601-6_3, © Springer Japan 2014

23

3.1 Terminology of Single-Port Laparoscopic Surgery

Although more than 100 years have already passed since a surgeon in Dresden named Georg Kelling developed a "Coelioscope" in 1901, and Hans Christian Jacobaeus, a Swedish internist, applied a technique, named "Laparoscopy", when treating a patient suffering from abdominal tuberculosis in 1910 [1], the enthusiasm for minimally invasive surgery has not abated. Surgeons are still committed to reducing surgical stress and minimize scaring.

A laparoscopic surgery through one skin incision and performed by collecting all the ports to one incision, usually to the umbilical incision, is known as a single-port or a single-incision laparoscopic surgery (SLS). This technique was first described by Pelosi in 1992 and it was used for an appendectomy [2]. The surgery in which this technique is most frequently used is cholecystectomy. The first cholecystectomy with this technique was reported by Navarra in 1997 [3].

Although many names and their acronyms have been proposed, a consensus name for this technique does not exist yet. Pelosi et al. described their technique as single-puncture laparoscopic appendectomy, while Navarra titled their procedure, though it was different surgery, as one-wound laparoscopic cholecystectomy.

3.2 Acronyms of Single-Port Laparoscopic Surgery

In the literature, there are many acronyms used to express the single-port laparoscopic surgery. TUES stands for trans umbilical endoscopic surgery, which was first used by Zhu et al. [4]. This is rather similar technique to NOTES, which is natural orifices translumenal endoscopic surgery. E-NOTES [5–7], embryonic-NOTES and NOTUS [8], natural orifices trans umbilical surgery is also derived from the NOTES concept.

Likewise, terms called single-port access (SPA) laparoscopic surgery [9, 10], one port umbilical surgery (OPUS) [9], single-port surgery (SPS) [11], single-port laparoscopic surgery (SPLS) [12], and single-port incisionless conventional equipment-utilizing surgery (SPICE) [13] has also been used to explain this surgery.

In July 2008, a multidisciplinary consortium of surgeons from the United States concluded that the term, laparo-endoscopic single site surgery (LESS) conveys the broad philosophical and practical aspects of this technique. Besides, they created the laparo-endoscopic single-site surgery consortium for assessment and research (LESSCAR), which is a similar consortium to the natural orifice surgery consortium for assessment and research (NOSCAR) for the field of NOTES [14].

SILS™ is the acronym for single-incision laparoscopic surgery, and it is the trademark of Covidien Inc. (New Haven, CT, USA), while Ethicon Inc. (Cincinnati, OH, USA) proposed the term SSL, single site laparoscopic surgery [15] (Table 3.1).

Table 3.1 Terminology and acronyms of single port laparoscopic surgery

Trans umbilical endoscopic surgery (TUES)
Natural orifice trans umbilical surgery (NOTUS)
Embryonic natural orifice translumenal endoscopic surgery (E-NOTES)
Single port access (SPA) surgery
One port umbilical surgery (OPUS)
Single port surgery (SPS)
Single port laparoscopic surgery (SPLS)
Single port incisionless conventional equipment-utilizing surgery (SPICES)
Laparo endoscopic single-site surgery (LESS)
Single incision laparoscopic surgery (SLS)
Single site laparoscopic (SSL) Surgery

3.3 Definition of Needlescopic Surgery

The needlescope or minilaparoscope was first utilized for diagnostic purposes. Therapeutic procedures using needlescopic instruments began in the mid 1990s. Gagner et al. described the technical aspects of needlescopic cholecystectomy, splenectomy, appendectomy, inguinal herniorrhaphy, adrenalectomy, and fundoplication [16]. Needlescopic surgery is defined as a procedure using less than 3-mm laparoscopic instruments.

3.4 Terminology of Reduced Port Laparoscopic Surgery

Reduced port laparoscopic surgery (RPLS) is a recent concept that indicates a laparoscopic surgery aiming at both reducing the number of ports and reducing the diameter of the port. Reducing the number of ports means not only reducing the number of ports inserted to the abdominal cavity, but reducing the number of skin incision by collecting a couple of ports to one incision [17, 18]. Currently, a single-incision or single-port laparoscopic surgery is therefore considered to be included into the category of RPLS. Besides, the needlescopic surgery or minilaparoscopic surgery is also considered as a part of RPLS.

References

1. Litynski GS (1996) Highlights in the history of laparoscopy. Barbara Bernert Verlag, Frankfurt, pp 3–33
2. Pelosi MA, Pelosi MA 3rd (1992) Laparoscopic appendectomy using a single umbilical puncture (minilaparoscopy). J Reprod Med 37(7):588–594

3. Navarra G, Pozza E, Occhionorelli S et al (1997) One-wound laparoscopic cholecystectomy. Br J Surg 84(5):695
4. Zhu JF (2007) Scarless endoscopic surgery: NOTES or TUES. Surg Endosc 21(10):1898–1899
5. Gill IS, Canes D, Aron M et al (2008) Single-port transumbilical (E-NOTES) donor nephrectomy. J Urol 180:637–641
6. Canes D, Desai MM, Aron M et al (2008) Transumbilical single-port surgery: evolution and current status. Eur Urol 54(5):1020–1029
7. Desai MM, Stein R, Rao P et al (2009) Embryonic natural orifice transumbilical endoscopic surgery (E-NOTES) for advanced reconstruction: initial experience. Urology 73(1):182–187
8. Nguyen NT, Reavis KM, Hinojosa MW, Smith BR, Wilson SE (2009) Laparoscopic transumbilical cholecystectomy without visible abdominal scars. J Gastrointest Surg 13(6):1125–1128
9. Rané A, Rao P, Rao P (2008) Single-port-access nephrectomy and other laparoscopic urologic procedures using a novel laparoscopic port (R-port). Urology 72(2):260–263
10. Bucher P, Pugin F, Morel P (2008) Single port access laparoscopic right hemicolectomy. Int J Colorectal Dis 23(10):1013–1016
11. Hayashi M, Asakuma M, Komeda K et al (2010) Effectiveness of a surgical glove port for single port surgery. World J Surg 34(10):2487–2489
12. Remzi FH, Kirat HT, Kaouk JH et al (2008) Single-port laparoscopy in colorectal surgery. Colorectal Dis 10(8):823–826
13. Akgür FM, Olguner M, Hakgüder G et al (2010) Appendectomy conducted with single port incisionless-intracorporeal conventional equipment-endoscopic surgery. J Pediatr Surg 45(5):1061–1063
14. Gill IS, Advincula AP, Aron M et al (2010) Consensus statement of the consortium for laparo-endoscopic single-site surgery. Surg Endosc 24(4):762–768
15. Romanelli JR, Earle DB (2009) Single-port laparoscopic surgery: an overview. Surg Endosc 23(7):1419–1427
16. Gagner M, Garcia-Ruiz A (1998) Technical aspects of minimally invasive abdominal surgery performed with needlescopic instruments. Surg Laparosc Endosc 8(3):171–179
17. Podolsky ER, St John-Dillon L, King SA, Curcillo PG 2nd (2010) Reduced port surgery: an economical, ecological, educational, and efficient approach to development of single port access surgery. Surg Technol Int 20:41–46
18. Curcillo PG 2nd, Podolsky ER, King SA (2011) The road to reduced port surgery: from single big incisions to single small incisions, and beyond. World J Surg 35(7):1526–1531

Chapter 4
Pros and Cons

Akira Sasaki, Hiroyuki Nitta, Koki Otsuka, Toru Obuchi, Shigeaki Baba, Keisuke Koeda, Masaru Mizuno, and Go Wakabayashi

Abstract Recently, single-port laparoscopic surgery (SPLS) has seen renewed interest and has developed as an extension of the standard laparoscopic minimally invasive procedures. SPLS has the potential to provide patients with improved cosmesis, decreased pain, and higher satisfaction for with having only a single-wound. SPLS obviates the need to place ports externally for triangulation, thus allowing for the creation of a small, solitary portal of entry into the abdomen. However, many laparoscopic surgeons have already tried, and found, the technique challenging. Additionally, questions remain regarding the safety of the procedure, real benefits, and the ideal patient population for these new techniques. Recently, reports of a reduced port laparoscopic surgery (RPLS), a hybrid operation of SPLS and conventional laparoscopic surgery, are increasing because of the better-feasibility and safety than SPLS. We believe that standardization of RPLS will increase its adoption, decrease intraoperative complications, and improve the efficiency and safety of this approach. Further studies are necessary to identify clearly the risks and real benefits of this new approach.

Keywords Laparoendoscopic single-site surgery (LESS) • Laparoscopy • Reduced port laparoscopic surgery • Single-port laparoscopic surgery

A. Sasaki (✉) • H. Nitta • K. Otsuka • T. Obuchi • S. Baba
K. Koeda • M. Mizuno • G. Wakabayashi
Department of Surgery, Iwate Medical University School of Medicine,
19-1 Uchimaru, Morioka 020-8505, Japan
e-mail: sakira@iwate-med.ac.jp

T. Mori and G. Dapri (eds.), *Reduced Port Laparoscopic Surgery*,
DOI 10.1007/978-4-431-54601-6_4, © Springer Japan 2014

4.1 Introduction

Conventional multiport laparoscopic surgery (MPLS) using a laparoscopy is the standard of care for many abdominal operations. The benefits of MPLS over open surgery include decreased pain, shorter hospital stays, and an earlier return to normal activity. With the advent of natural orifice translumenal endoscopic surgery (NOTES) and the acknowledged limitations of the current technology, single-port laparoscopic surgery (SPLS) or laparoendoscopic single site surgery has emerged as a viable and more widely applicable minimally invasive technique [1]. In SPLS through the umbilicus, the scar was almost completely hidden within the umbilicus. SPLS allows for significant wound cosmesis and has even been termed "invisible surgery" (Fig. 4.1) or "embryonic natural orifice transumbilical endoscopic surgery (E-NOTES)" [2, 3].

Single-port laparoscopic cholecystectomy was first attempted in the 1990s [4, 5]; however, it has not enjoyed widespread use to date. Recently, SPLS has experienced renewed interest and has developed as an extension of the standard laparoscopic, minimally invasive procedures. SPLS has the potential to provide patients with improved cosmesis, decreased pain, and higher satisfaction with having a single-wound [6–11]. SPLS obviates the need to space ports externally for triangulation, thus allowing for the creation of a small, solitary portal of entry into the abdomen. However, many laparoscopic surgeons have already tried, and found, the technique challenging. Additionally, questions remain regarding the safety of the procedure, real benefits, and the ideal patient population for these new techniques.

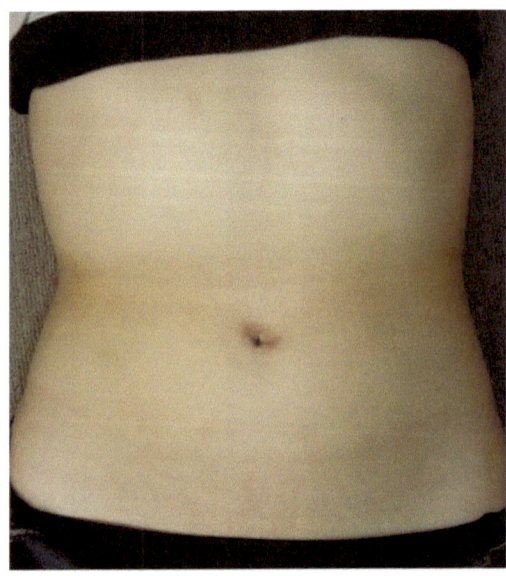

Fig. 4.1 Postoperative photograph of patient's abdomen at 6 months after single-port laparoscopic adrenalectomy. The patient has had excellent cosmetic results at postoperative follow-up

Recently, reports of a reduced port laparoscopic surgery (RPLS), a hybrid operation of SPLS and conventional laparoscopic surgery, are increasing because of the better feasibility and safety than SPLS [12–15]. In this chapter, we will summarize the pros and cons of RPLS.

4.2 Indications and Contraindications

Although the benefits of SPLS over conventional MPLS have not been clearly elucidated, worldwide use of the technique is constantly increasing. Currently, the feasibility of SPLS or RPLS has been demonstrated in a clinical setting for almost every type of gastroenterological surgery. At experienced laparoscopic centers, results equivalent to those of conventional MPLS have been documented for many SPLS or RPLS procedures, including general, gastroenterological, urologic, gynecologic, and other abdominally-related surgeries [16–22].

The indications, contraindications, and preoperative preparation for SPLS and RPLS are almost identical to those for MPLS. SPLS is a challenging operation for even experienced laparoscopic surgeons. The newer SPLS procedure may someday be equally efficacious and feasible as MPLS in high-volume centers [23]. However, patients with risk factors such as previous abdominal surgery, history of severe or on-going inflammation, and obesity were thought to have a higher incidence of conversion to MPLS or open surgery [24].

From our own experience, cholecystectomy for non-inflamed gallbladder, partial gastrectomy for gastric gastrointestinal stromal tumors (GISTs) located anterior or on the greater curvature, appendectomy, or inguinal hernia repair were the ideal indications for SPLS when compared to MPLS [6]. Alternatively, adrenalectomy [10, 25, 26], the Heller–Dor procedure [8], Nissen fundoplication [27, 28], liver resection [29, 30], and colectomy [31–33] were indications for RPLS and were equally feasible for experienced laparoscopic surgeons in terms of perioperative and postoperative parameters compared with MPLS. Splenectomy for patients with splenomegaly remains challenging, even for laparoscopic surgeons in high-volume centers [34, 35]. The major problems were spleen retraction and the control of excessive bleeding. Additionally, obese patients may not always be suitable candidates for the SPLS technique.

4.3 Knack of Surgical Technique

Access to the abdominal cavity in SPLS and RPLS should follow accepted standards for safe entry, including avoidance and recognition of complications. The introduction of new instruments, access devices, or new techniques should be done with caution and under a study protocol. Prior to its use, any new instrument or device should be proven safe to the fullest extent possible. Adequate training

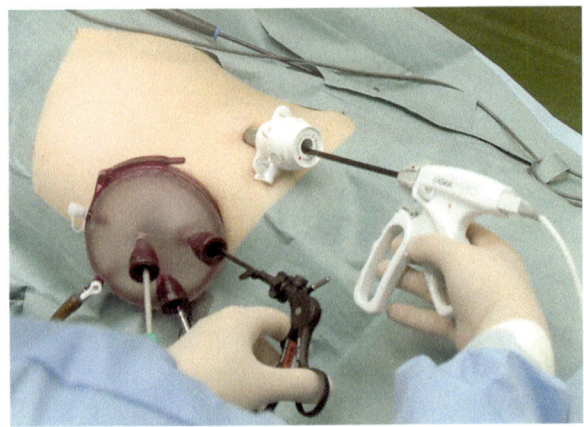

Fig. 4.2 Reduced port laparoscopic splenectomy. The patient was placed in the right semilateral position. GelPoint (Applied Medical, Rancho Santa Margarita, CA, USA) and 12 mm port were used for patient with splenomegaly

should also be provided. During initial procedures, a low threshold for using additional ports should be maintained so as not to jeopardize a safe dissection and result [23].

Access into the peritoneal cavity to achieve SPLS or RPLS has not been standardized. We believe that a multichannel port is advantageous, and we support this approach over multiple ports through a single-incision. A multichannel port is beneficial in that it minimizes air leaks, promotes safe insertions, enables insertion of curved instruments, provides a wider insertion point for instruments, and has better triangulation. Based on our experience, a reduced port approach using the multichannel port, plus one puncture or port, also makes it possible to triangulate even with standard instruments to ensure immediate control of any bleeding site, if necessary (Fig. 4.2).

Needlescopic-assisted SPLS is a variation of SPLS. In advanced SPLS, we typically use a multichannel port and an additional "needle-like" 2–3 mm instrument (Figs. 4.3 and 4.4). Needlescopic instruments reduce the main limitation of SPLS, that is, the lack of instrument triangulation. Their assistance can prevent a conversion of the procedure to a conventional MPLS when failure to progress is noted. Moreover, they can significantly reduce operating time. Additionally, needlescopic-assisted SPLS could be considered as an approach that diminishes the steep learning curve of pure SPLS, as it resembles conventional MPLS. Needlescopic assistance does not negate at all the cosmetic outcome, which is still considered the main advantage of SPLS over MPLS.

4.4   Tips and Tricks

Many important benefits of laparoscopic surgery result from preserving the integrity of the abdominal wall, including decreased operative trauma and complications, and improved cosmesis. For many operations, several attempts have been made to

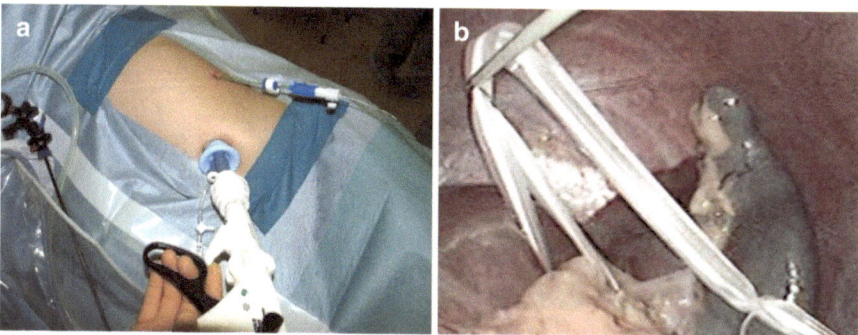

Fig. 4.3 Needlescopic-assisted single-port laparoscopic splenectomy. (**a**) The patient was placed in the right semilateral position. SILS™ port (Covidien, New Haven, CT, USA) and mini-loop retractor (Covidien) were used for idiopathic thrombocytopenic purpura. (**b**) The spleen was gently lifted up using a loop-shaped 4-mm Penrose drain, with traction supplied by a mini-loop retractor inserted from below the costal margin on the left midclavicular line

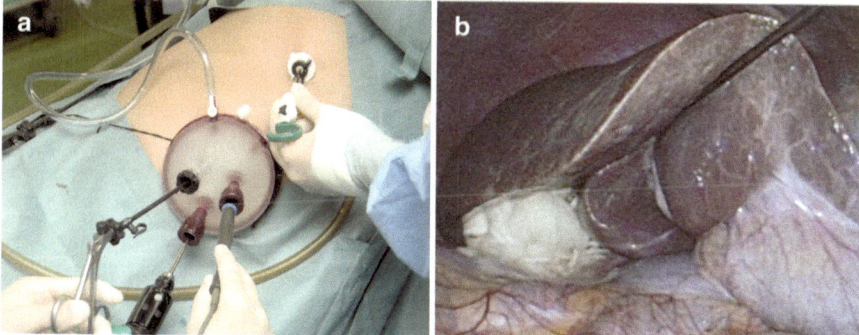

Fig. 4.4 Needlescopic-assisted single-port laparoscopic right adrenalectomy. (**a**) The patient was placed in the left semilateral position. GelPoint and MiniLap (Stryker, Kalamazoo, MI, USA) were used for primary aldosteronism. (**b**) The right liver lobe was evaluated using a MiniLap and small gauze, providing good visualization of the operative field surrounding the right adrenal gland

reduce operative trauma further by decreasing the number and size of the ports used in the procedure. The use of three ports instead of four, and the use of needlescopic instruments, is definitely a step in this direction. The use of a flexible scope, an articulating instrument, and a needlescopic instrument, along with standardization of the procedure, greatly reduces the "learning curve" for the procedure. Based on our experience, surgeons became familiar with both the technique and visualization of single-port laparoscopic cholecystectomy after about 20 cases. Other investigators have reported a similar learning curve in operating times for initial cases when single-port laparoscopic access was used [24, 36]. However, one of the concerns with SPLS and RPLS is that they are inherently one-operating-surgeon techniques. This may have a negative impact on resident education and the training of future surgeons. A formal course with collaborative learning, video simulations, "hands on" education with instrumentation, and in-operating room reservation would shorten the learning curve for new adopters.

In SPLS or RPLS, the control of bleeding is as important as it is in MPLS. Excessive bleeding must be dealt with and controlled immediately. While conversion may immediately lead to a conversion to an MPLS or open procedure, this is not a necessity. Controlling bleeding with a gauze compression or a grasper provides temporary control. Surgeons should not extend the damage by indiscriminately applying clips.

4.5 Recommendations for RPLS

RPLS is a safe and technically feasible procedure for patients with diseases of a general, gastroenterological, urologic or gynecologic fields. RPLS also offers cosmetic benefits and the potential for postoperative pain reduction. However, inexperienced surgeons performing SPLS should understand that the use of needlescopic instruments does not negate the cosmetic results for difficult cases. Additionally, obese patients may not always be suitable candidates for pure SPLS techniques. We should consider needlescopic-assisted SPLS as a valuable tool to employ whenever organ retraction or instrument triangulation for suturing is necessary.

Although safety should be the primary goal for any surgical intervention, cosmesis should not be overlooked as an overall secondary goal of patients [37]. Two important factors to consider in the future may be careful patient selection and recognition of the limitations of RPLS. Further studies are necessary to identify clearly the risks and real benefits of this new approach.

References

1. Ross S, Rosemurgy A, Albrink M et al (2012) Consensus statement of the consortium for LESS cholecystectomy. Surg Endosc 26:2711–2716
2. Cuesta MA, Berends F, Veenhof AA (2008) The "invisible cholecystectomy": a transumbilical laparoscopic operation without a scar. Surg Endosc 22:1211–1213
3. Canes D, Desai MM, Aron M et al (2008) Transumbilical single-port surgery: evolution and current status. Eur Urol 54:1020–1029
4. Paganini A, Lomonto D, Navordino M (1995) One port laparoscopic cholecystectomy in selected patients. Third International Congress on New Technology in Surgery, Luxemburg
5. Navarra G, Pozza E, Occhionorelli S et al (1997) One-wound laparoscopic cholecystectomy. Br J Surg 84:695
6. Sasaki A, Koeda K, Obuchi T et al (2009) Tailored laparoscopic resection for suspected gastric gastrointestinal stromal tumors. Surgery 147:516–520
7. Sasaki A, Koeda K, Nakajima J et al (2011) Single-incision laparoscopic gastric resection for submucosal tumors: report of three cases. Surg Today 41:133–136

8. Oyama K, Sasaki A, Chiba T et al (2011) Single-incision laparoscopic splenectomy for idiopathic thrombocytopenic purpura. Surg Today 41:1091–1094

9. Nakajima J, Sasaki A, Obuchi T et al (2011) Single-incision laparoscopic Heller myotomy and Dor fundoplication for achalasia: report of a case. Surg Today 41:1543–1547

10. Shimabu M, Sasaki A, Higa M et al (2011) Single-incision laparoscopic adrenalectomy for primary aldosteronism: report of a case. Surg Today 41:1306–1309

11. Kobayashi M, Mizuno M, Sasaki A et al (2011) Single-port laparoscopic Heller myotomy and Dor fundoplication: initial experience with a new approach for the treatment of pediatric achalasia. J Pediatr Surg 46:2200–2203

12. Monclova JL, Tagarona EM, Vidal P et al (2013) Single incision versus reduced port splenectomy–searching for the best alternative to conventional laparoscopic splenectomy. Surg Endosc 27:895–902

13. Kunisaki C, Ono HA, Oshima T et al (2012) Relevance of reduced-port laparoscopic distal gastrectomy for gastric cancer: a pilot study. Dig Surg 29:261–268

14. Costedio MM, Aytac E, Gorgun E et al (2012) Reduced port versus conventional laparoscopic total proctocolectomy and ileal J pouch-anal anastomosis. Surg Endosc 26:3495–3499

15. Kanehira E, Siozawa K, Kamei A et al (2012) Development of a novel multichannel port (X-Gate®) for reduced port surgery and its initial clinical results. Minim Invasive Ther Allied Technol 21:26–30

16. Frutos MD, Abrisqueta J, Lujan J et al (2013) Randomized prospective study to compare laparoscopic appendectomy versus umbilical single-incision appendectomy. Ann Surg 257:413–418

17. Bucher P, Pugin F, Buchs NC et al (2011) Randomized clinical trial of laparoendoscopic single-site versus conventional laparoscopic cholecystectomy. Br J Surg 98:1695–1702

18. Champagne BJ, Papaconstantinou HT, Parmar SS et al (2012) Single-incision versus standard multiport laparoscopic colectomy: a multicenter, case-controlled comparison. Ann Surg 255:66–69

19. Osbome AJ, Clancy R, Clark GW et al (2013) Single incision laparoscopic adjustable gastric band: technique, feasibility, safety and learning curve. Ann R Coll Surg Engl 95:131–133

20. Barth RN, Phelan MW, Goldschen L et al (2013) Single-port donor nephrectomy provides improved patient satisfaction and equivalent outcomes. Ann Surg 257:527–533

21. Greco F, Autorino R, Rha KH et al (2013) Laparoendoscopic single-site partial nephrectomy: a multi-institutional outcome analysis. Eur Urol 64:314–22. doi:10.1016/eururo.2013.01.025

22. Choi YS, Park JN, Oh YS et al (2013) Single-port vs. conventional multi-port access laproscopy-assisted vaginal hysterectomy: comparison of surgical outcomes and complications. Eur J Obstet Gynecol Reprod Biol 169:366–369. doi:10.1016/j.ejogrb.2013.03.026

23. Overby DW, Apelgren KN, Richardson W et al (2010) SAGES guidelines for the clinical application of laparoscopic biliary tract surgery. Surg Endosc 24:2368–2386

24. Tay CW, Shen L, Hartman M et al (2013) SILC for SILC: single-institution learning curve for single-incision laparoscopic cholecystectomy. Minim Invasive Surg. doi:10.1155/2013/381628

25. Sasaki A, Nitta H, Otsuka K et al (2013) Laparoendoscopic single site adrenalectomy: initial results of cosmetic satisfaction and the potential for postoperative pain reduction. BMC Urol 13:21

26. Sasaki A, Baba S, Obuchi T et al (2012) Single-port laparoscopic adrenalectomy for a right-sided aldosterone-producing adenoma: a case report. J Med Case Rep 18:208

27. Mizuno M, Kobatashi M, Sasaki A et al (2012) Early experience with single-incison laparoscopic Nissen fundoplication for gastroesophageal reflux disease in patients with mental retardation via a gastrostomy site incision: report of a case. Surg Today 41:601–604

28. Yilmaz H, Alptekin H (2012) Single-port laparoscopic Nissen fundoplication: a new method for retraction of the left lobe of the liver. Surg Laparosc Endosc Percutan Tech 22:e265–e266

29. Gaujoux S, Kingham TP, Jarnagin WR et al (2011) Single-incision laparoscopic liver resection. Surg Endosc 25:1489–1494

30. Parel AG, Belgaumkar AP, James J et al (2011) Video. Single-incision laparoscopic left lateral segmentectomy of colorectal liver metastasis. Surg Endosc 25:649–650

31. Takemasa I, Sekimoto M, Ikeda M et al (2010) Video. Transumbilical single-incision laparoscopic surgery for sigmoid colon cancer. Surg Endosc 24:2321
32. Haas EM, Nieto J, Ragupathi M et al (2012) Single-incision laparoscopic sigmoid resection: a technical video of a standardized approach. Surg Endosc 55:1179–1182
33. Makino T, Milsom JW, Lee SW et al (2012) Feasibility and safety of single-incision laparoscopic colectomy: a systematic review. Ann Surg 255:667–676
34. Targarona EM, Lima MB, Balaque C et al (2011) single-port splenectomy: current update and controversies. J Minim Access Surg 7:61–64
35. Misawa T, Sakamoto T, Ito R et al (2011) Single-incision laparoscopic splenectomy using the "tug-exposure technique" in adults: results of ten initial cases. Surg Endosc 25:3222–3227
36. Feinberg EJ, Agaba E, Feinberg ML et al (2012) Single-incision laparoscopic cholecystectomy learning curve experience seen in a single institution. Surg Laparosc Endosc Percutan Tech 22:114–117
37. Weibl P, Klingler HC, Klatte T et al (2010) Current limitations and perspective in single port surgery: pros and cons laparo-endoscopic single-site surgery (LESS) for renal surgery. Diagn Ther Endosc. doi:10.1155/2010/759431

Chapter 5
Access Device 1: Multiple Trocars Method

Hidenori Fujii

Abstract In this chapter, the Multiple Trocars Method will be explained using an Optical View Method.

A 2- to 2.5-cm vertical skin incision is made just above the umbilicus and the fascial defect is grasped with Kocher's clamp. After creation of the pneumoperitoneum by Veress needle, a 5 or 12 mm trocar suitable for optical viewing in which a direct vision camera is inserted via the fascial defect for optical viewing. Next, two trocars are inserted twisting without additional fascia incision. By using ports with different length, mutual interference of the port heads is easily avoidable. Since all of the devices can be inserted without additional fascia incision, as mentioned above, this method can minimize the injury of the insertion site. This method can be economical, because all of the devices used are reusable except the first optical viewing trocar.

For cholecystectomy for the non-inflamed gallbladder or small organs removal like appendectomy, an incision at the umbilicus can be very small. In this case, the procedure can be done by inserting two trocars from the umbilicus or using another thin forceps. Approximately 1- to 1.5-cm vertical incision is made from the center of the umbilicus to the cranial or caudal side, a concave of the navel is preserved. A camera trocar is inserted as described above. Only one working trocar is inserted from the umbilicus and a trocar for a thin forceps is inserted elsewhere. This particular procedure may be better cosmetically compared to the TANKO procedure.

Keywords Single-incision laparoscopic surgery (SLS) • Multiple trocars method • Optical view method

H. Fujii (✉)
Japanese Red Cross Fukui Hospita, 2-4-1 Tsukimi, Fukui 918-8501, Japan
e-mail: philadelphide@vesta.ocn.ne.jp

T. Mori and G. Dapri (eds.), *Reduced Port Laparoscopic Surgery*,
DOI 10.1007/978-4-431-54601-6_5, © Springer Japan 2014

5.1   Introduction

There are two approaches to single-incision laparoscopic surgery (SLS) via the umbilicus: the multiple trocar approach [1–3] and the multi-channel port approach [4–6]. In this chapter, the multiple trocar approach is explained.

With the multiple trocar approach, trocars are inserted directly into the peritoneal cavity through an umbilical incision made according to the number and size of the trocars needed. The first is an optical view trocar. This approach is not used for open laparoscopic surgery because there is a risk of pneumoperitoneum gas leakage.

5.2   Optical Insertion Technique

For performance of the so-called "TANKO surgery" which comes from the concept of reduced port laparoscopic surgery (RPLS), three (sometimes four) trocars are inserted via the umbilicus, one camera trocar and two working trocars. For insertion of three trocars, a 2- to 2.5-cm vertical skin incision is made just above the umbilicus, and the subcutaneous tissue is divided (and retracted) to widely (but minimally) expose the fascia. The subcutaneous tissue is dissected to confirm the fascial defect at the center of the umbilicus. The fascial defect is then grasped with Kocher clamp to elevate the anterior abdominal wall (Fig. 5.1a–c). A Veress needle is inserted into the fascial defect, angled vertically or toward the pelvis. Saline is then injected into the Veress needle with the stopcock closed. The saline should drip smoothly and quickly into the abdominal cavity when the stopcock is opened if the Veress needle is inserted correctly (saline test). Under the saline test, no bodily fluid or saline should be aspirated through the Veress needle. This step is used to confirm whether the Veress needle is correctly inserted into the abdominal cavity without damage to any organs. The abdominal cavity is insufflated with carbon dioxide, with the intra-abdominal pressure maintained at 7–8 mmHg. Total gas volume should be 1.5–3 L, depending on the patient's body size (Fig. 5.2a, b).

After creation of pneumoperitoneum, a 5-mm trocar suitable for optical viewing (Versaport Bladeless Optical Trocar or Xcel Trocar (Ethicon Johnson & Johnson,

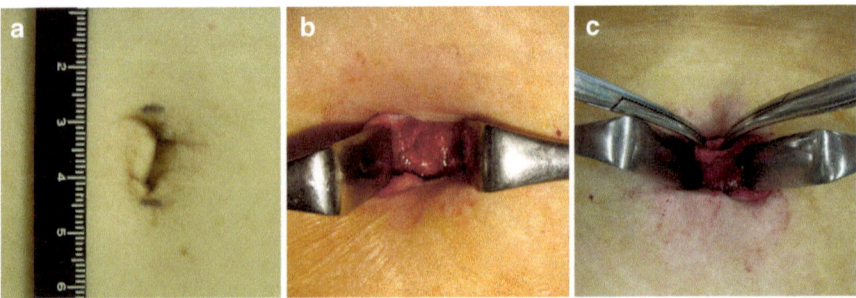

Fig. 5.1 An approximate 2–2.5-cm longitudinal incision is made from the center of the umbilicus (**a**). The fascial defect (**b**) is grasped with Kocher forceps (**c**)

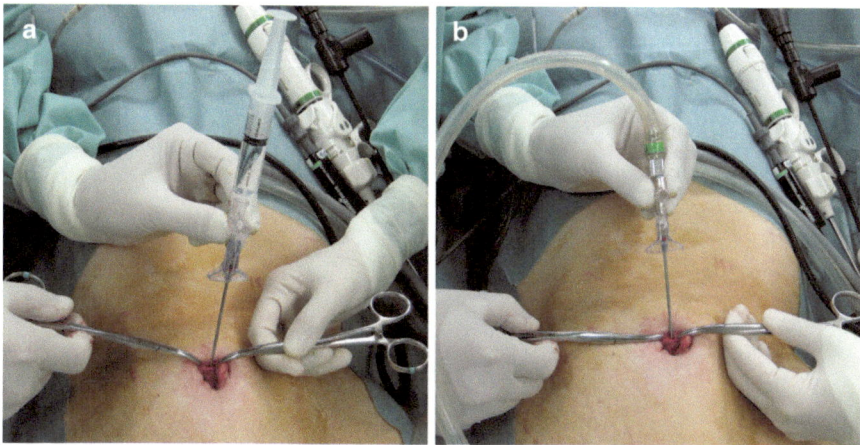

Fig. 5.2 An insufflation needle is inserted (**a**) for creation of pneumoperitoneum after a saline test (**b**)

Fig. 5.3 While the operator twists the optical trocar, the assistant stands to the patient's right and holds the laparoscope to prevent excess insertion force due to its weight

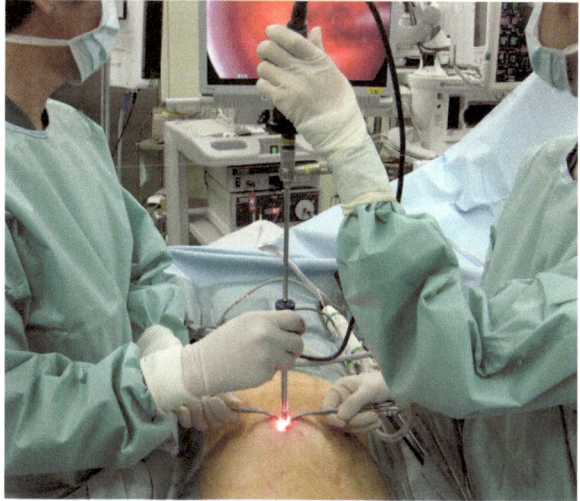

Cincinnati, OH, US), with a forward viewing scope (5 mm in diameter) is inserted via the fascial defect. If no 0-degree rigid scope is available, a 30-degree rigid scope can also be used. While the operator twists the trocar, an assistant holds the laparoscope to prevent excess insertion force due to its weight (Fig. 5.3). After assuring that the trocar is in the free abdominal cavity, the obturator is pulled out, and a Karl Storz Hopkins telescope (30°, 5.5 mm in diameter, 50 cm in length) is used with a high definition camera system. Because the scope is 50 cm in length, interference between the scope head and the forceps handles is prevented. During the operation, if a linear stapler is required, the 5-mm camera trocar is replaced with a 12-mm trocar (Fig. 5.4a–d). When forceps larger than 5 mm in diameter is needed, the same methodology is applied. However, for this procedure, opening the incision with

Fig. 5.4 View of the optical method: (**a**) edge of the fascial defect (*fascia*), (**b**) the fascia (*white layer*), and (**c**) fat (*yellow layer*); (**d**) 30-degree scope penetrates the peritoneum (*white*) and reaches the abdominal cavity

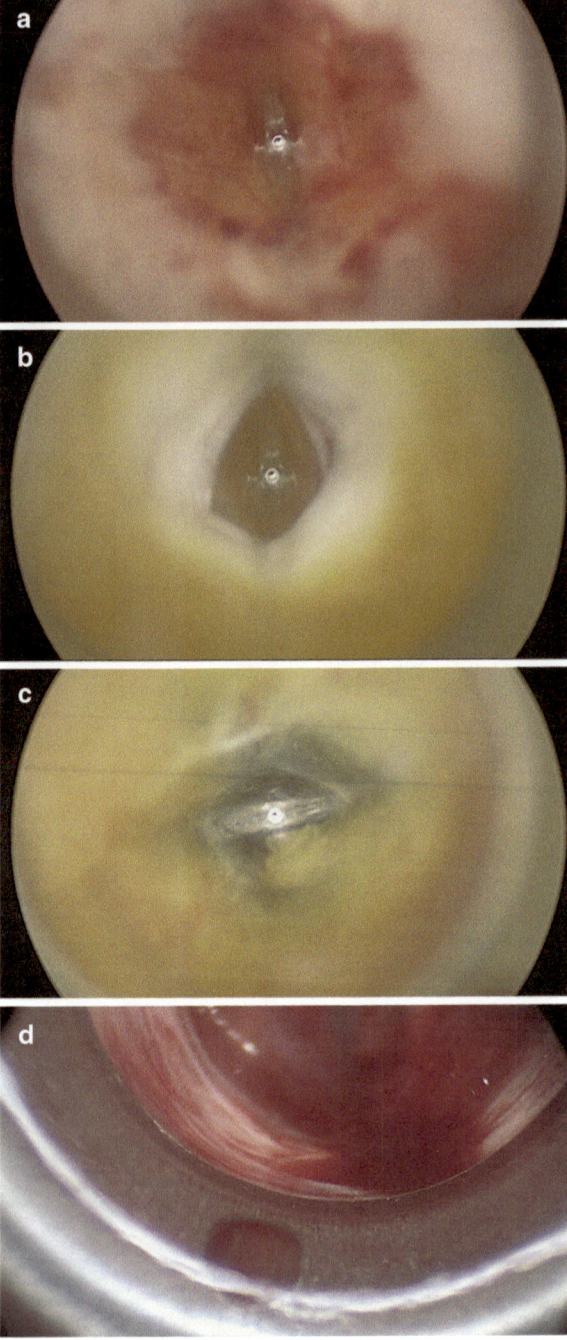

Kelly clamp or an additional skin incision is often required. Fascial incision is not usually required, and an unnecessary incision can lead to gas leakage.

Two trocars are then inserted. We normally use trocars of different lengths with a relatively small head, such as EndoTIP cannulas (both 6 mm in diameter), one 6 cm long and the other 10.5 cm long. These trocars are reusable and are thus economical. First an isosceles triangle centered on the line between the target organ as the vertex and the camera trocar insertion point is assumed, and the ports are inserted at the both ends of the incision corresponding to the angles at the base of the triangle. It is then possible to set the ports coaxially and to maximize the distance between them. Ports are inserted with a twisting motion, without any additional fascial incision. By using ports of different lengths, the port heads will be prevented from hitting each other. When the ports are inserted, the scope is replaced with a 50-cm 30-degree scope (Karl Storz-Endoskope, Tuttlingen, Germany). Use of a high definition system provides high quality viewing of the operation even though the scope is as small as 5 mm in diameter. The secret to success with this method is the best possible vertical insertion of both the camera trocar and the EndoTIP cannulas. When the devices are inserted obliquely, the procedure takes time because they slide along the abdominal wall. In addition, vertical insertion increases the safety of the procedure because insertion of the EndoTIP cannulas can be monitored through the transparent side wall of the camera trocar. Because all of the devices can be inserted without any additional fascial incision, this method minimizes injury at the insertion site. In addition, because the devices can be tightly inserted, there is no need for concern over leakage of the pneumoperitoneum gas (Fig. 5.5a–d).

Surgery is usually conducted with two working trocars, but if the surgery proves difficult, one more trocar can be used. For a pure TANKO surgery, forceps are inserted directly from an appropriate incision in the umbilicus, but it is possible for the pneumoperitoneum gas to leak. If a fourth trocar is needed, an additional incision may be needed. If the surgery is not a pure TANKO procedure, thin forceps may be used, as described below. 36- and 43-cm forceps are properly used according to the specific circumstances to avoid clashing of their handles. A 360-degree rotatable L-shape light cable is used in combination with a long scope to avoid interaction with the camera head. The correct combined use of the above-mentioned devices enables us to avoid interference between them. All of the devices used are reusable (Fig. 5.6a, b).

For some procedures, we can use another method. For particular organs, we also insert a working port toward the target organ, being conscious of the need for coaxial positioning. After directing the scope toward the target, a straight line is marked on the abdominal wall. Another line is assumed perpendicular to the straight line at the scope insertion point, a hook is inserted along the perpendicular line, and an EndoTIP cannula, as a working trocar, is inserted toward the hook. Thus, an isosceles triangle centered on the line of the camera heading toward the target is formed. This method secures sufficient distance from the port and allows coaxial positioning (Fig. 5.7a–c).

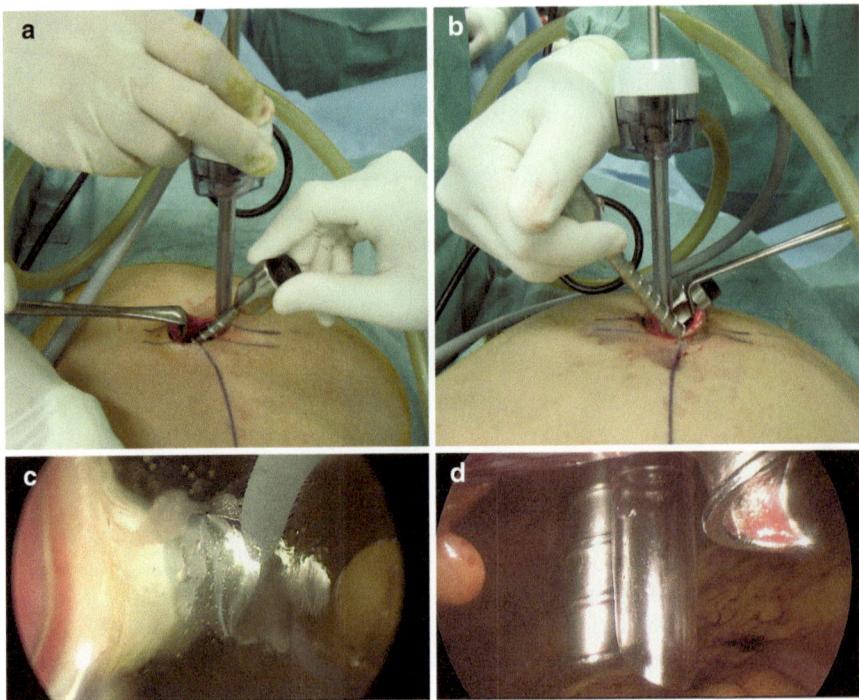

Fig. 5.5 (**a**, **b**) Endo TIP cannulas, 6.5 and 10.5 cm in length, are screwed in on both sides of the incision; (**c**) insertion of the EndoTIP cannulas is monitored through the transparent side wall of the camera trocar; (**d**) view of the umbilical site after trocar insertion

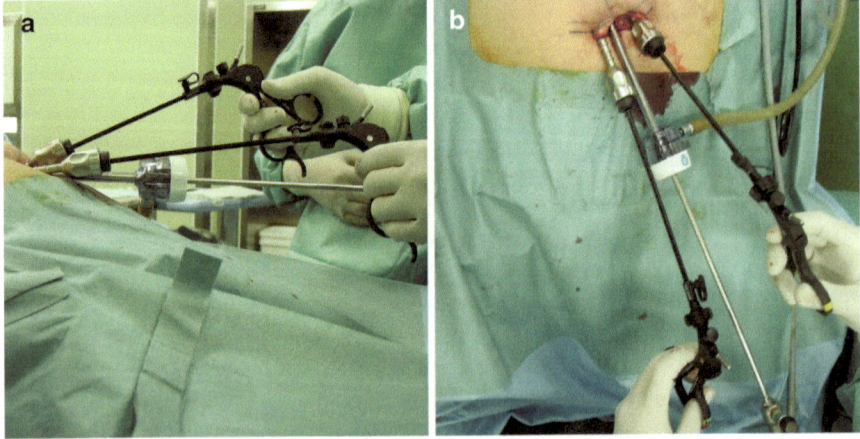

Fig. 5.6 Abdominal view after insertion of three umbilical ports. (**a**) The view from the top. (**b**) The view from the side. The 50-cm long scope and 36- and 43-cm forceps are properly used according to the particular circumstance to avoid interference between handles

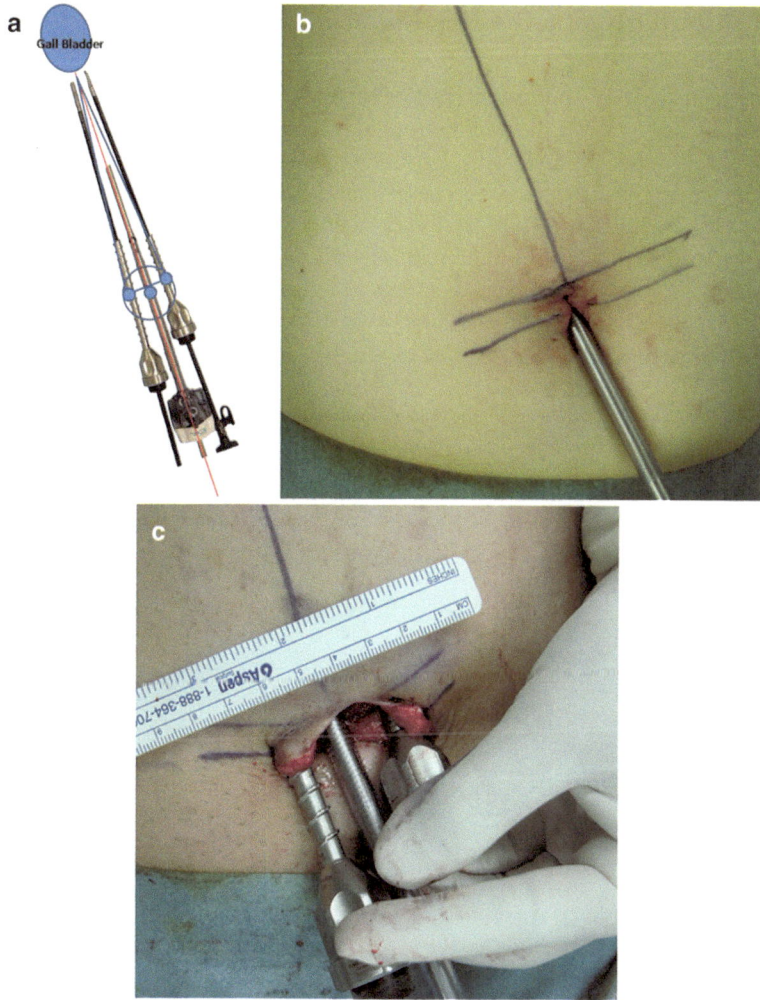

Fig. 5.7 (**a**) After insertion of the scope toward the target, a straight line is marked on the abdominal wall. Next, a line is assumed perpendicular to the straight line at the scope insertion point (**b**). An isosceles triangle centered on the line of the camera heading toward the target is thus formed. This method secures sufficient distance from the port and allows coaxial positioning (**c**)

Recent years have seen the development of very high quality thin forceps. From the standpoint of RPLS, TANKO is not the sole surgical ideal. For example, for cholecystectomy in cases without inflammation or for appendectomy, i.e., removal of a small organ, the incision at the umbilicus can be very small. In such cases, the procedure can be done by inserting two trocars from the umbilicus or by using thin forceps less than 3 mm in diameter.

5.3 Alternative Trocar Placement

A vertical incision of approximately 1 or 1.5 cm when a 12-mm trocar is required is made from the center of the umbilicus to the cranial or caudal side. The subcutaneous tissue is dissected to confirm the fascial defect at the center of the umbilicus. A camera trocar is inserted, as described above. Only one working trocar is inserted through the umbilicus (Fig. 5.8a–d). For cholecystectomy, the trocar is inserted from the patient's right side, and another trocar for thin forceps is inserted from the right side of the abdomen. For appendectomy, a working trocar is inserted from the patient's right side, and another trocar for thin forceps is inserted in the suprapubic region (Fig. 5.9a, b). Use of thin forceps allows for triangulation of the

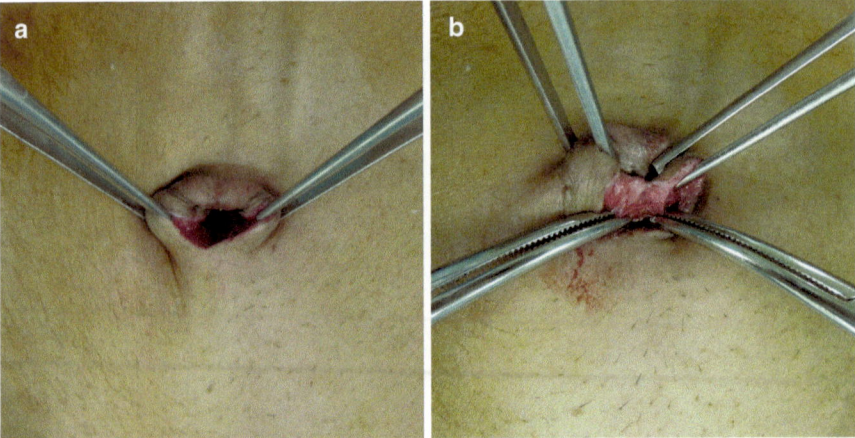

Fig. 5.8 An approximately 1-cm longitudinal incision is made from the center of the umbilicus to the cranial or caudal side (**a**). The fascial defect is grasped with Kocher forceps (**b**)

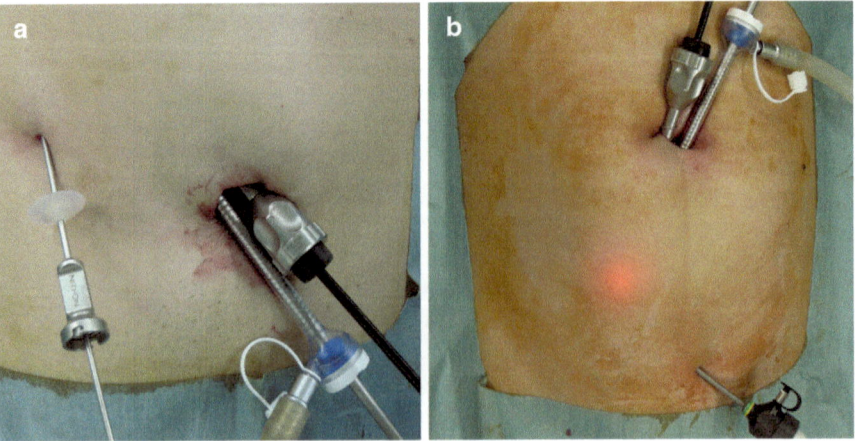

Fig. 5.9 Abdominal view after insertion of two umbilical ports and thin forceps for (**a**) cholecystectomy, (**b**) appendectomy

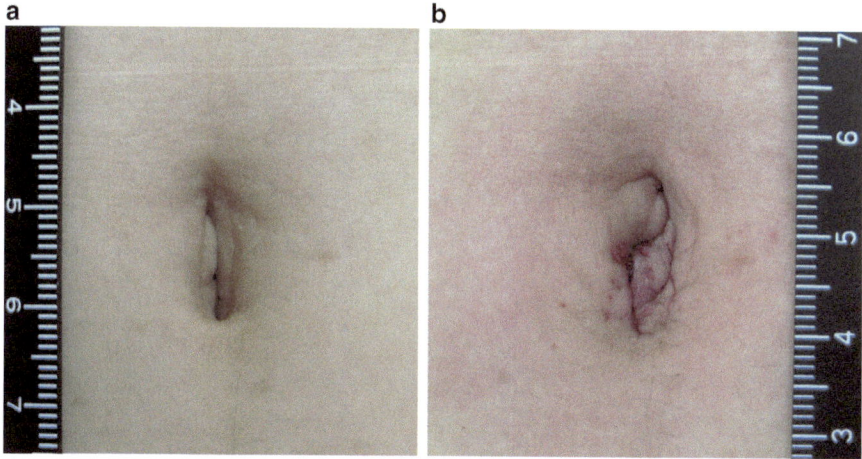

Fig. 5.10 The depression at the center of the umbilicus is preserved with this technique, as seen by comparing the umbilicus (**a**) just before surgery and (**b**) just after surgery

forceps, and maneuvering the forceps can be easier than from the umbilicus, as in TANKO. The incision for the thin forceps will be inconspicuous, and the umbilical incision will be hidden, so this particular procedure may be cosmetically better than the TANKO procedure (Fig. 5.10a, b).

5.4 Closure

The fascia where the EndoTIP cannula was inserted and the fascia at the umbilicus are closed with 2-0 absorbable interrupted sutures. The subcutaneous tissue is closed with buried 4-0 absorbable interrupted sutures. However, the EndoTIP cannula insertion site is hard to detect by palpation, so suturing this incision may be omitted.

References

1. Curcillo PG 2nd, Wu AS, Podolsky ER, Graybeal C, Katkhouda N, Saenz A, Dunham R, Fendley S, Neff M, Copper C, Bessler M, Gumbs AA, Norton M, Iannelli A, Mason R, Moazzez A, Cohen L, Mouhlas A, Poor A (2010) Single-port-access (SPA) cholecystectomy: a multi-institutional report of the first 297 cases. Surg Endosc 24:1854–1860
2. Feinberg EJ, Agaba E, Feinberg ML, Camacho D, Vemulapalli P (2012) Single-incision laparo-scopic cholecystectomy learning curve experience seen in a single institution. Surg Laparosc Endosc Percutan Tech 22:114–117

3. Oruc MT, Ugurlu MU, Boyacioglu Z (2012) Transumbilical multiple-port laparoscopic cholecystectomy using standard laparoscopic instruments. Minim Invasive Ther Allied Technol 21:423–428
4. Valverde A (2012) Single incision laparoscopic cholecystectomy using the SILS monotrocar. J Visc Surg 149:38–43
5. Kuon Lee S, You YK, Park JH, Kim HJ, Lee KK, Kim DG (2009) Single-port transumbilical laparoscopic cholecystectomy: a preliminary study in 37 patients with gallbladder disease. J Laparoendosc Adv Surg Tech A 19:495–499
6. Egi H, Okajima M, Hinoi T, Takakura Y, Kawaguchi Y, Shimomura M, Tokunaga M, Adachi T, Hattori M, Urushihara T, Itamoto T, Ohdan H (2012) Single-incision laparoscopic colectomy using the Gelport system for early colon cancer. Scand J Surg 101:16–20

Chapter 6
Access Device 2: Multi-Channel Port

Kazunori Shibao, Aiichiro Higure, and Koji Yamaguchi

Abstract Laparoendoscopic single-site (LESS) surgery and/or reduced port laparoscopic surgery (RPLS) is a new surgical modality that produces increased cosmetic benefits compared to conventional endoscopic surgery. A number of medical device companies have designed single-port devices to be placed through 15–25 mm open fascial incisions. This rapidly progressing technique is facilitated by developments and innovations in devices, allowing surgeons to perform a various LESS/RPLS procedures in safe with less stress. This chapter aims to summarize the characteristics of each multi-channel port devices, which is available at present for LESS/RPLS. A comprehensive electronic literature search was conducted in May 2013 using the Medline database to identify all publications relating to LESS/RPLS. Various multi-channel port devices are currently available for LESS/RPLS. Each port has advantages for application in specific disciplines. Further investigations will be needed in order to evaluate the efficacy and safety of multi-channel port devices in LESS/RPLS.

Keywords Port device • Reduced port laparoscopic surgery • Single-incision laparoscopic surgery (SLS) • Single-port laparoscopic surgery

6.1 Introduction to the Technique

Laparoendoscopic single-site (LESS) surgery and/or reduced port laparoscopic surgery (RPLS) is a new surgical modality that produces increased cosmetic benefits compared to conventional endoscopic surgery [1–3]. Since the initial report of

K. Shibao (✉) • A. Higure • K. Yamaguchi
Department of Surgery I, School of Medicine, University of Occupational and Environmental Health, 1-1 Iseigaoka, Yahatanishi-ku, Kitakyushu 807-8555, Japan
e-mail: shibao@med.uoeh-u.ac.jp

T. Mori and G. Dapri (eds.), *Reduced Port Laparoscopic Surgery*,
DOI 10.1007/978-4-431-54601-6_6, © Springer Japan 2014

single-port laparoscopic surgery, various surgical procedures have been performed [4–11]. However, LESS remains a challenge for the surgeon due to the lack of triangulation, the decreased working space and the risk of instruments clashing inherent to the use of a single-access. To facilitate the performance of these procedures, a number of medical device companies have designed multi-channel port devices that can be placed through an open 1.5- to 2-cm fascial incision. These devices have been designed either with multiple fixed low-profile ports or channels for instruments housed within the device or with a barrier that allows some degree of customization for the number and location of the ports. The aim of the present chapter is to describe the currently available multi-channel port devices for LESS and RPLS.

6.2 Indications and Contraindications

Since the induction of LESS, a wide variety of LESS procedures have been performed on many organs, including but not limited to the gallbladder, colon, small intestine, stomach, common bile duct, liver, pancreas, kidney, adrenal gland, ovary, and uterus [4–11]. Good indications for LESS are relatively simple laparoscopic procedures. Although, many surgeries that were once performed "laparoscopically" can be performed LESS/RPLS by skilled laparoscopic surgeon, surgeon should evaluate patient's safety and merit prior to their surgery. Any previous surgery can create scar tissue in the abdomen, especially around the umbilicus, making a LESS/RPLS procedure more technically difficult. Especially, the multiple trocar method is contraindication in patients who have an operative scar around the umbilicus. Since this method requires nearly blind trocar insertion to the abdominal cavity at the setup, the potential organ injury cannot be avoided because of adhesion. On the other hand, the multi-channel port method is not contraindication for the patient who has a past history of the abdominal surgery, because this method makes a small laparotomy in the umbilicus at the insertion of the multi-channel port device. As the abdominal cavity can be inspected by direct vision, adhesiolysis can be performed under the direct vision for ensuring the insertion space of the multi-channel port device.

6.3 Technique

The umbilicus is incised 1.5–2.5 cm long longitudinally. The length of incision is decided according to the patient's structure and depending on the procedure. The ligament beneath the umbilicus is sharply divided so that the fascial defect is clearly palpated. The fascial defect is extended to be approximately 2.5 cm in length by cutting the fascia longitudinally to both caudal and cephalic direction.

The peritoneum is sharply opened to enter the abdominal cavity. If there are local adhesions, they can be dissected by finger or sharply under the direct vision. A multi-channel port device can be introduced through this access.

The multi-channel port method involves the use of a singular access device that permits the ingress of three or four instruments through a single opening in the umbilicus. Starting in 2008 with the single-use TriPort system (Advanced Surgical Concepts, Wicklow, Ireland), there are many multi-channel port devices options for transumbilical laparoscopy currently available [12]. These are the TriPort+™/ QuadPort+™ (Olympus, Center Valley, PA, USA), the SILS™ Port (Covidien, Mansfield, MA, USA), GelPOINT™/GelPOINT Mini (Applied Medical, Rancho Santa Margarita, CA, USA), ENDOCONE®/X-Cone/S-PORT® (Karl Storz-Endoskope, Tuttlingen, Germany), Octo™ Port (Dalim Surgnet, Seoul, South Korea), SPIDER™ (TransEnterix, Durham, NC, USA), E•Z Access™ and E•Z Access Oval type (Hakko, Tokyo, Japan), x-GATE® (Sumitomo Bakelite, Tokyo, Japan), Free Access (TOP, Tokyo, Japan). All the devices' characteristics are summarized in the Table 6.1 and all available devices are exposed in Table 6.1. This unbiased pro–con listing is meant to inform the potential user and not to dissuade the usage of any one device.

6.3.1 TriPort+™ and QuadPort+™

The TriPort™ (Olympus) was the first available access system approved by the US Food and Drug Administration (FDA). Since Rane et al. [12] reported the first clinical use of the TriPort, it has been used in such common operations as single incision cholecystectomy but also more complex operations as adrenalectomy, hemicolectomy, distal pancreatic resection and finally in bariatric surgery [13, 14]. Recently, the next generation of their products, which named as TriPort+™ and QuadPort+™ are unveiled [15]. The TriPort+™ has four channels, allowing up to one 10-mm and three 5-mm instruments, while the QuadPort+™ has five lumens, permitting up to one 15-mm, one 12-mm, one 10-mm and two 5-mm instruments. The TriPort+™ is designed for standard laparoscopic surgeries, whilst the QuadPort+™ is constructed for more complicated types of surgical procedure that require large amounts of tissue to be removed and employ up to four instruments. Each channel has the duckbill/lipseal valve which allow for the smooth introduction and removal of instruments while maintaining pneumoperitoneum. Flexible instrument ports enhance access to the surgical site and accommodate different types and sizes of laparoscopic instruments: straight, curved and articulating. Reducer caps at the larger ports allow the insertion of 5-mm instruments without loss of pneumoperitoneum. The retraction sleeve provides wound protection and helps streamline specimen removal. It is self-adjusting to different incision length (TriPort+™/TriPort15: 12–25-mm, QuadPort+™: 20–60-mm) and abdominal wall thicknesses (up to 100-mm).

Table 6.1 Multi-channel ports available for reduced-port surgery

Feature	TriPort15™/TriPort+™/QuadPort+™ Olympus	SILS™ Port Covidien	GelPOINT™/GelPOINT™ Mini Applied medical	ENDOCONE®/X-Cone/S-PORT® Karl Storz	OCTO™ Port Dalim SurgNET	SPIDER™ TransEnterix	E·Z Access™/E·Z Access™ Oval Hakko	x-GATE® Sumitomo Bakelite	Free Access TOP
Incision length	10–60 mm	15–20 mm	15–70 mm	15–35 mm	15–50 mm	18 mm	15–50 mm	20–40 mm	15–70 mm
Channel type	Fixed trocar placement	Fixed trocar placement	Free trocar placement	Fixed trocar placement	Fixed trocar placement	Fixed trocar placement	Free trocar placement	Fixed trocar placement	Semi-free trocar placement
Number of channels	3/4/5	3	1–4	5/8	1–4	4	1–4	4	1–4
Channel size	5, 10, 12, and 15 mm	5 and 12 mm	10 and 12 mm (pre-packaged)	5 and 12.5 mm/5 and 15 mm	5, 10, and 12 mm	5 mm	Not limited	5 and 12 mm	Not limited
Maximum abdominal wall thickness	100 mm	50 mm	150 mm	30 mm/10 mm	70 mm	Not described	80 mm	55 mm	150 mm
Wound protection	Yes	No	Yes	Yes	Yes	No	Yes	Yes	Yes
Specimen removal	Easy	Difficult	Easy	Easy	Easy	Difficult	Easy	Easy	Easy
Rotatability	Easy	Stiff	Stiff	Stiff	Easy	Easy	Easy	None	Stiff

Some negative aspects of the TriPort+™/QuadPort+™ were encountered. One was the "chimney effect", where the pneumoperitoneum was leaking along the space between the port's sleeve and the wound. Moreover, retraction system is complicated with multiple steps including cinching of the sleeve attachment of two retainer clips, and removal of excess sleeve. Also, the sheath can easily be torn, which may result in a need to replace the device. These devices require crossing of curved or roticulating instruments.

6.3.2   SILS™ Port

The SILS™ Port (Covidien) is a blue flexible soft-foam port that conforms to the patient's abdominal wall to maintain pneumoperitoneum. The soft-foam minimizes abdominal bruising and provides stability/support to hand instruments. But no wound protection is brought to this port device. Although it recommends that the port is lubricated and inserted using a large Kelly clamp through a 20 mm incision, slightly larger fascial incision needed to accommodate port in most cases. It includes three cannula access channels, which can accommodate three 5-mm cannulas or two 5-mm cannulas and one 12-mm cannula. It's possible, but may not be easy to use 12-mm cannula because of relatively narrow trocar separation (1.5-mm). Using this device, crossing of roticulating or curved instruments is required. In obese patients, use of this port is difficult due to its foam design. Since Fader et al. [16] reported the first clinical use of the SILS™ Port, it has been used in such common operations as single incision cholecystectomy but also more complex operations as adrenalectomy, hemicolectomy, distal pancreatic resection and finally in bariatric surgery [17–22].

Burgos et al. [23] described their initial experience with the SILS™ Port in performing laparoscopic prostatectomy. They compared their experience with their previous experience with the TriPort (Olympus) and noted that the SILS™ Port was easier to place, had less leakage of pneumoperitoneum. Conversely, Brown-Clerk indicated the SILS™ Port's difficult insertion and lack of abdominal wall adjustability [24].

6.3.3   GelPOINT™ and GelPOINT Mini

The GelPOINT™ system (Applied Medical) consists of the Alexis® wound retractor, GelSeal cap, and 10 or 12-mm self-retaining trocars. The Alexis® wound retractor includes a distal and proximal ring that can accommodate a 1.5–7-cm (GelPOINT™) and 1.5–3-cm incisions (GelPOINT Mini), and a wide range of abdominal wall thicknesses. Trocars can be positioned anywhere within the GelSeal cap. This facilitates triangulation of standard instruments and provides additional procedural and instrumentation flexibility. Removable GelSeal cap streamlines specimen removal.

GelSeal cap bows outward during insufflation providing a flexible fulcrum for improved instrument articulation, but cannot provide stability/support to instruments. Use of this port in obese patients is restrictive secondary to the increased abdominal wall thickness. Endoscopic staplers can insert with included 12-mm trocar. There are many clinical reports using GelPOINT™ [25–28].

6.3.4 ENDOCONE®, X-Cone and S-PORT®

The ENDOCONE® (Karl Storz-Endoskope) system is manufactured from stainless steel with a design that facilitates both insertion and retention within the anterior abdominal wall. Additionally the system includes coaxially curved instruments designed to facilitate triangulation, provide traction and counter-traction during dissection of tissue planes and maximize their range of motion within the operating space.

X-CONE (Karl Storz-Endoskope) is a reusable metallic conical structure consisting of two half cones, to which a plastic cap is attached which have four instrument ports and an insufflation port [29]. The port insertion through a mini-laparotomy is quick and easy. They allow the insertion of curved or straight 3-mm to 12.5-mm (X-Cone) and up to 15-mm (ENDOCONE®) instruments. However, significant leakage and restricted mobility have been reported [30, 31].

S-PORT® (Karl Storz-Endoskope) is a modular system which is developed to improve these issues. It consists of the basic ring, upper part ring, and the wound protector. The upper part ring is compatible with the sealing caps of X-CONE and ENDOCONE®. Other merit of the S-PORT® is reusable except for the wound protector and simple recovery of resected tissue.

6.3.5 OCTO™ Port

The OCTO™ Port (Dalim Surgnet) consists of an inferior base plate that sits under the skin edge in the peritoneum, an external disc with self retractor, and a detachable port cap. It is capable of holding one to four working channels. The cap is easy to remove, thus allowing easy specimen extraction. The 360° port cap rotation during the surgery enables the surgeon to change the location of ports. The cannulas are of different heights, which reduce external clashing of instruments. The silicone cover cap supplies a flexible fulcrum for improved instrument articulation, while cannot provide stability/support to instruments. This port device requires crossing of curved or roticulating instruments [32].

6.3.6 The Single Port Instrument Delivery Extended Reach (SPIDER™)

The SPIDER™ (TransEnterix) consists of a retractable sheath, two laterally placed instrument delivery tubes that can operate in three dimensions, and two rigid channels. It is designed to allow multiple flexible instruments to be manipulated through a single cannula. Surgeons who use the SPIDER Surgical System benefit from single site triangulation with true left and true right control over flexible, articulating instruments. One of the demerits of the SPIDER™ is the cost. It costs $875.00 for main unit and $40-$95 for each instruments. It also provides articulation of instruments, which is useful, yet may limit retraction of tissues and torque due to force dissipation. Furthermore, the SPIDER™ flexible or rigid 5-mm ports are not large enough to allow for ≥10-mm Hem-o-lok clip application or a laparoscopic stapler. Moreover, no wound protection is ensured at the specimen retrieval with this device [33].

6.3.7 E•Z Access™ and E•Z Access Oval Type

The E•Z Access™ (Hakko) is made from a silicone-rubber cap and designed to be applied to an existing incision margin protector (LAPPROTECTOR) [34–36]. Trocars can be positioned anywhere within the cap, providing additional procedural flexibility and stability/support to hand instruments. Three size variations are currently available in E•Z Access™ (round type). Each of them is applied depending on the length of the skin incision (1.5–5 cm) in various LESS/RPLS procedures.

E•Z Access Oval type, which is one of the product lines of E•Z Access, is designed exclusively for use with the LAP PROTECTOR™ Oval type device [37].

The LAP PROTECTOR™ Oval type device has an oval-shaped flexible shape-memory frame, which allows abdominal wound openings to be expanded in the long axis direction.

This oval-shaped device was developed to utilize umbilical incisions in more efficient ways to ensure wider trocar separation. Actually, this device can maintain 35-mm of trocar separation with 25-mm umbilical incisions. A wide trocar separation distance decreases conflicts of instruments or clushing during surgery and makes RPLS surgery easier and safer to perform even with conventional straight laparoscopic instruments. The adjustment of device rotation during surgery enables surgeon to maintain wider trocar separation. Removable cap allows smooth specimen removal and re-pneumoperitoneum. This product is difficult to use with large abdominal wall, but longer sleeve variations are available (up to 70-mm).

6.3.8   x-GATE®

x-GATE® (Sumitomo Bakelite) is disassembled into two parts; the main unit and the converter [38]. The main unit attached to the abdominal wall is composed of two rings and a barrel with four belts connecting these rings. Pulling the four belts evenly slides the inner ring closer to the outer ring, while the belts expand the abdominal wall wound. Eventually, the abdominal wall is wedged between the inner and outer rings. In addition, as the belt forces the abdominal wall wound to open from the inside, resulting in the strong fixation of the main unit to the abdominal wall and in the expansion of the parietal incision.

The converter attached to the main unit has four channels (3×5-mm, 1×12-mm). An endoscopic stapling device can be inserted into the larger channel. The distance between the centers of the main channels ranges from 29 to 31-mm, which is relatively long distance among currently available port devices. It decreases conflicts of instruments or clushing during surgery. Furthermore, removable converter allows specimen removal easily. Since this device has a fixed channel, channel setting limitation may be a problem to adopt various procedures.

6.3.9   Free Access

The Free access (TOP) is made from a silicone membrane cap and designed to be applied to the Alexis® wound retractor. This cap has many cross-slits which are arranged in a matrix on a top of the cap for the trocar insertion. Trocars can be positioned in any cross-slits within the cap. This cross-slits minimize air leakage and facilitates triangulation of standard instruments. Removable cap streamlines specimen retrieval. The demerit of this device is easy to detach the cap accidentally during the surgery. Moreover, as the prepackaged 5-mm trocar has no valve, air leakage is the problem.

6.3.10   Surgical Glove Port

This homemade access port consists of an Alexis® wound (Applied Medical) retractor and a surgical glove. After insertion of the wound retractor into the abdomen, a non-powdered surgical glove is fixed to the outer ring of the wound retractor through which two or three 5-mm slim trocars are inserted via the finger tips. Trocars are fixed with a tie and a rubber band. The merit of this access port is the cost and increased flexibility in terms of the number and size of trocars. On the contrary the disadvantage of this method is unstability of instruments because of no instrument fulcrum [39, 40].

6.4 Tips and Tricks

Common problems of LESS/RPLS comparing to multitrocar laparoscopy are the lack of triangulation intracorporally, conflicts among the instruments (clashing), and insufficient surgical views (in-line viewing). To solve or reduce these problems, two approaches are currently introduced to LESS/RPLS with multi-channel port devices. One is to use bent, flexible, or articulating instruments and the other is to maintain wider trocar separation using small incision in an efficient way. Former approach is adopted in TriPort+™/QuadPort+™ (Olympus), the SILS™ Port (Covidien), GelPOINT™/GelPOINT Mini (Applied Medical), ENDOCONE®, X-Cone, S-PORT® (Karl Storz-Endoskope), Octo™ Port (Dalim Surgnet), and Free Access (TOP). Although most of these devices require the crossing hand to manipulate the instruments, SPIDER™ (TransEnterix) and ENDOCONE® do not need to cross hands. The later approach is relatively new concept and adopted in E•Z Access Oval type (Hakko) and x-GATE® (Sumitomo Bakelite). Umbilical small laparotomy is retracted with oval type basement device (E•Z Access Oval type) or four belts (x-GATE®). Eventually, the abdominal wall is opened in an efficient way and resulting in maintaining wider trocar separation. Crossing hands with bent, articulating instruments do not need with this approach, while a bit larger incision may need comparing to former approach.

The extra costs are another concern in multi-channel method. The universal acceptance of this method and its success hinges on whether the safety, efficacy, efficiency, and cost justify its use over multitrocar laparoscopy.

6.5 Recommendations from the Author

Regarding the choice of the mutichannel port device, it continues to be a matter of debate. At present the surgeon chooses the type of single-port device according to his personal preference. Table 6.1 summarized all the devices' characteristics and pros/cons.

Ross et al. reported the consensus statement of the consortium for LESS in cholecystectomy [41]. They did not mentioned which access port is superior over others, but described their standardized approach that surgeons with laparoscopic skills can follow with the prospect of quick mastery [15, 42, 43]. They recommended LESS four or three-trocar approach using multi-channel port with a bent grasper or articulating/roticulating grasper.

Thomas et al. [44] described the specific advantages and disadvantages of the multi-channel port devices. They commented that a rigid shaft like with the X-Cone (Karl Storz-Endoskope) leads in comparison to the flexible ports to a tighter fit in the abdominal wall, but the mobility of the instruments shafts is more restricted. In contrast, a very flexible approach as the TriPort (Olympus) makes the introduction easier but may lead to slight dislocation and corresponding gas loss. Schill et al. [45]

compared in a trainer box model the laparoscopic skills performance between four kinds of multi-channel port devices: GelPOINT™ (Applied Medical), SILS™ Port (Covidien), SSL Access System (Ethicon, Cincinnati, OH, USA), and TriPort (Olympus). They found no significant difference with task performance times among these multi-channel port devices.

Furthermore, Brown-Clerk et al. [24] also conducted a study to compare the three multi-channel ports (SILS™ Port, TriPort, and GelPOINT™) in a simulating box and concluded that the GelPOINT™ appears to be the easiest system for novices to use. Among the three devices the GelPOINT™ is the only one in which the users have freedom to select the points to insert the trocars at and could have a wider distance between the channels compared to the other two devices, which have a fixed distance (approximately 1.5-cm) between the channels [25]. There is a possibility that this accounted for the better results the GelPOINT™ demonstrated. In this point of view, E•Z Access Oval type (Hakko) and x-GATE (Sumitomo Bakelite) which can keep wider trocar separation comparing to other multi-channel port devices may contribute to overcome the difficulties in LESS/RPLS [37, 38].

As for the channel size exchange from 5-mm to 12-mm for a complex procedures, some devices can be exchanged to different size of trocar during the surgery (SILS™ Port, GelPOINT™ and GelPOINT Mini, E•Z Access™ and E•Z Access Oval type, and Free Access), other devices have a channel size converter (TriPort15™, TriPort+™, and QuadPort+™, and Octo™ Port). With respect to the specimen retrieval and wound protection, as most of the Multi-channel port device (TriPort15™, TriPort+™, QuadPort+™, ENDOCONE®, X-Cone, S-PORT®, Octo™ Port, GelPOINT™, GelPOINT Mini, E•Z Access™, E•Z Access Oval type, x-GATE®, and Free Access) has their removable top/basement system, specimen removal/re-pneumoperitoneum is much easier and the wound is protected.

6.6   Conclusions

This chapter summarized advantages and disadvantages of multi-channel port devices that are currently available for LESS/RPLS. The development of multi-channel port devices is still in the beginning. As with any new technology further development of instruments and surgical skills will be needed in order to make RPLS with multi-channel port devices easier and safer.

References

1. Gill IS, Advincula AP, Aron M et al (2010) Consensus statement of the consortium for laparo-endoscopic singlesite surgery. Surg Endosc 24:762–768
2. Markar SR, Karthikesalingam A, Thrumurthy S et al (2011) Single-incision laparoscopic surgery (SILS) vs. conventional multiport cholecystectomy: systematic review and meta-analysis. Surg Endosc 26:1205–1213

3. Garg P, Thakur JD, Garg M et al (2012) Single-incision laparoscopic cholecystectomy vs. conventional laparoscopic cholecystectomy: a meta-analysis of randomized controlled trials. J Gastrointest Surg 16:1618–1628
4. Navarra G, Pozza E, Occhionorelli S et al (1997) One-wound laparoscopic cholecystectomy. Br J Surg 684:695
5. Curcillo PG 2nd, Wu AS, Podolsky ER et al (2010) Single-port-access (SPA) cholecystectomy: a multi-institutional report of the first 297 cases. Surg Endosc 24:1854–1860
6. Pfluke JM, Parker M, Stauffer JA et al (2011) Laparoscopic surgery performed through a single incision: a systematic review of the current literature. J Am Coll Surg 212:113–118
7. Greaves N, Nicholson J (2011) Single incision laparoscopic surgery in general surgery: a review. Ann R Coll Surg Engl 93:437–440
8. Romanelli JR, Earle DB (2009) Single-port laparoscopic surgery: an overview. Surg Endosc 23:1419–1427
9. Rao PP, Rao PP, Bhagwat S (2011) Single-incision laparoscopic surgery – current status and controversies. J Min Acc Surg 7:6–16
10. Khanna R, White MA, Autorino R et al (2011) Selection of a port for use in laparoendoscopic single-site surgery. Curr Urol Rep 12:94–99
11. Jung YW, Kim YT, Lee DW et al (2010) The feasibility of scarless single-port transumbilical total laparoscopic hysterectomy: initial clinical experience. Surg Endosc 24:1686–1692
12. Rane A, Rao P, Rao P (2008) Single-port-access nephrectomy and other laparoscopic urologic procedures using a novel lapa- roscopic port (R-port). Urology 72:260–263
13. Romanelli JR, Mark L, Omotosho PA et al (2008) Single port laparoscopic cholecystectomy with the TriPort system: a case report. Surg Innov 15:223–228
14. Rao PP, Bhagwat SM, Rane A et al (2008) The feasibility of single-port laparoscopic cholecystectomy: a pilot study of 20 cases. HPB Oxford 10:336–340
15. Kia M, Lee C, Martinez J et al (2011) Single port cholecystectomy: the pathway back to a standardized technique. Surg Laparosc Endosc Percutan Tech 21:314–317
16. Fader AN, Escobar PF (2009) Laparoendoscopic single-site surgery (LESS) in gynecologic oncology: technique and initial report. Gynecol Oncol 114:157–161
17. Romanelli JR, Roshek TB 3rd, Lynn DC et al (2010) Single-port laparoscopic cholecystectomy: initial experience. Surg Endosc 24:1374–1379
18. Saber AA, El-Ghazaly TH (2009) Early experience with single incision transumbilical laparoscopic adjustable gastric banding using the SILS Port. Int J Surg 7:456–459
19. Saber AA, El-Ghazaly TH (2009) Early experience with SILS port laparoscopic sleeve gastrectomy. Surg Laparosc Endosc Percutan Tech 19:428–430
20. Ramos-Valadez DI, Patel CB, Ragupathi M (2010) Single-incision laparoscopic right hemicolectomy: safety and feasibility in a series of consecutive cases. Surg Endosc 24:2613–2616
21. Tunca F, Senyurek YG, Terzioglu T et al (2010) Single-incision laparoscopic left adrenalectomy. Surg Laparosc Endosc Percutan Tech 20:291–294
22. Barbaros U, Sümer A, Demirel T et al (2010) Single incision laparoscopic pancreas resection for pancreatic metastasis of renal cell carcinoma. JSLS 14:566–570
23. Burgos JB, Flores JA, de La Vega JS et al (2010) Early experience in laparoscopic radical prostatectomy using the laparoscopic device for umbilical access. Aetas Urol Esp 34:495–499
24. Brown-Clerk B, de Laveaga AE, LaGrange CA et al (2011) Laparoendoscopic single-site (LESS) surgery versus conventional laparoscopic surgery: comparison of surgical port performance in a surgical simulator with novices. Surg Endosc 25:2210–2218
25. Merchant AM, Cook MW, White BC, Davis SS et al (2009) Transumbilical Gelport access technique for performing single incision laparoscopic surgery (SILS). J Gastrointest Surg 13:159–162
26. Petrotos AC, Molinelli BM (2009) Single-Incision Multiport Laparoendoscopic (SIMPLE) cholecystectomy. Surg Endosc 23:2631–2634
27. Gimenez E, Leeser DB, Wysock JS et al (2010) Laparoendoscopic single site live donor nephrectomy: initial experience. J Urol 184:2049–2053

28. Borowski DW, Kanakala V, Agarwal AK et al (2011) Single-port access laparoscopic reversal of Hartmann operation. Dis Colon Rectum 54:1053–1056
29. Krajinovic K, Pelz J, Germer CT et al (2010) Single-port laparoscopic cholecystectomy with the x-cone: a feasibility study in 9 pigs. Surg Innov 18:39–43
30. Autorino R, Kim FJ, Rane A et al (2011) Low-cost reusable instrumentation for laparoendo-scopic single-site nephrectomy: assessment in a Porcine model. J Endourology 25:19–24
31. Mereu L, Angioni S, Melis GB et al (2010) Single Access Laparoscopy for Adnexal Pathologies using a Novel Reusable Port and Curved Instruments. Int J Gyn Obst 109:78–80
32. Kim BS, Kim KC, Choi YB (2012) A comparison between single-incision and conventional laparoscopic cholecystectomy. Laparoendosc Adv Surg Tech A 22:443–447
33. Leveillee RJ, Castle SM, Gorin MA et al (2011) Initial experience with laparoendoscopic single-site simple nephrectomy using the TransEnterix SPIDER surgical system: assessing feasibility and safety. J Endourol 25:923–925
34. Takagi T, Nakase Y, Fukumoto K et al (2011) Development of an access instrument for single-incision laparoscopic surgery. J Soc Endo Surg 16:375–380
35. Inufusa H, Ueda K, Kawabe T et al (2000) New wound protector for Laparoscopic colorectal surgery. J Soc Endo Surg 5:361–363
36. Nakagoe T, Sawai T, Tsuji T et al (2001) Minilaparotomy wound edge protector (LAP PROTECTOR): a new device. Surg Today 31:850–852
37. Shibao K, Takagi T, Higure A et al (2013) A newly developed oval-shaped port device (E•Z ACCESS Oval type) for use in reduced port surgery: initial clinical experiences with cholecys-tectomy. Surg Tech Int 23:75–79
38. Kanehira E, Siozawa K, Kamei A et al (2012) Development of a novel Multi-channel port (x-Gate®) for reduced port surgery and its initial clinical results. Min Inv Ther Allied Tech 21:26–30
39. Leroy J, Costantino F, Cahill RA et al (2010) Fully laparoscopic colorectal anastomosis involv-ing percutaneous endoluminal colonic anvil control (PECAC). Surg Innov 17:79–84
40. Uematsu D, Akiyama G, Matsuura M et al (2010) Single-access laparoscopic colectomy with a novel multiport device in sigmoid colectomy for colon cancer. Dis Colon Rectum 53:496–501
41. Ross S, Rosemurgy A, Albrink M et al (2012) Consensus statement of the consortium for LESS cholecystectomy. Surg Endosc 26:2711–2716
42. Hernandez JM, Ross SB, Albrink M et al (2009) Laparoendoscopic single site cholecystec-tomy: the first 100 patients. Am Surg 75:681–685
43. Hodgett SE, Hernandez JM, Morton CA et al (2009) Laparoendoscopic single site (LESS) cholecystectomy. J Gastrointest Surg 13:188–192
44. Thomas C (2012) Single port laparoscopic surgery, advances in laparoscopic surgery, InTech. Available from: http://www.intechopen.com/books/advances-in-laparoscopic-surgery/single-port-laparoscopic-surgery
45. Schill MR, Esteban Varela J et al (2011) Comparison of laparoscopic skills performance between single-site access (SSA) devices and an independent-port SSA approach. Surg Endosc 26:714–721

Chapter 7
Video-Endoscopes and Instruments

Minoru Matsuda, Ken Hagiwara, and Tadatoshi Takayama

Abstract In reduced port laparoscopic surgery (RPLS), insertion of the scope and instruments through the same port can cause interference. It is, thus, important to select theories and instruments that will minimize this interference. This chapter describes the scopes and devices that are currently available for use in RPLS (the development of a variety of new devices is also anticipated). Without a full understanding of these devices, surgeons in the field will be unable to perform RPLS safely and effectively. Sufficient preclinical training is strongly recommended before any of these devices are used clinically.

Keywords Instrument • Reduced port laparoscopic surgery • Single-port laparoscopic surgery • Sword fighting

7.1 Introduction

Reports in the literature include single-port laparoscopic surgery (SPLS) as one of several procedures within conventional laparoscopic surgery (CLS) [1, 2]. However, until recently SPLS has not been widely practiced. This has been due in part to the lack of suitable instruments, and in part because the procedures themselves were not yet mature. The first reports of natural orifice translumenal endoscopic surgery (NOTES) [3] produced a surge of interest in minimally invasive procedures with reduced scarring. With the associated development of instruments and the maturation of techniques, SPLS is coming into wide use. However, the procedural

M. Matsuda (✉) • K. Hagiwara • T. Takayama
Division of Digestive Surgery, Nihon University School of Medicine, Tokyo, Japan
e-mail: matsuda.minoru@nihon-u.ac.jp

T. Mori and G. Dapri (eds.), *Reduced Port Laparoscopic Surgery*,
DOI 10.1007/978-4-431-54601-6_7, © Springer Japan 2014

57

difficulties associated with SPLS have caused many surgeons to review their options and to consider the intermediate step of simply reducing the number of CLS ports and using slimmer forceps for what is known as reduced port laparoscopic surgery (RPLS). Although generally speaking SPLS would be the final objective in practicing RPLS, exclusive reliance on SPLS can be particularly challenging in some cases of malignant or benign disease. For a surgeon who has mastered SPLS procedures, the use of RPLS should not be considered as a "step down" but rather as an additional option: SPLS + 1 port or SPLS + 2 ports, as needed.

For these procedures, the introduction of both the scope and instruments through a single incision can result in interference. It is important to select theories and instruments that will even slightly minimize such interference.

In this section, we discuss the scopes and devices that are currently available for use in RPLS.

7.2   Characteristics of RPLS

RPLS refers to laparoscopic surgery procedures in which the scope and operating forceps are inserted through a single-port. The visual field is no different than that for CLS. However, the forceps vectors differ from those in CLS (Fig. 7.1), being tangential to the scope. Also, because the forceps are introduced through the navel, the distance from the abdominal wall to the target tissue is greater than for CLS.

When the left and right forceps are inserted through the same port, the angle between the forceps is reduced to less than 10° at the surgical site [4] and the principle of triangulation, established in CLS, is violated. As a result, when traction

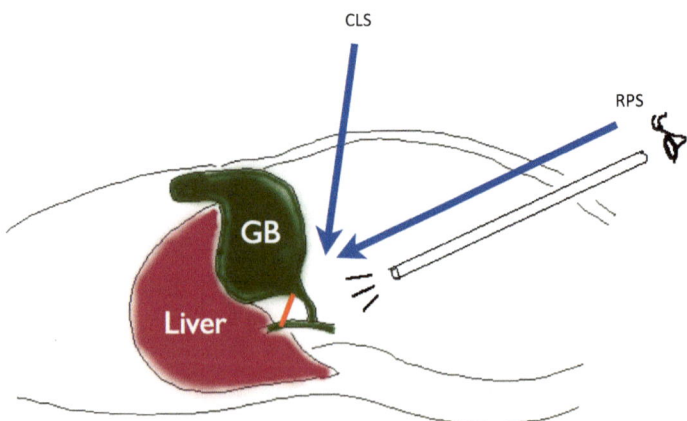

Fig. 7.1 Vector of forceps movement in laparoscopic cholecystectomy. In RPLS, the forceps are in coaxial becomes with the scope. (*CLS* conventional laparoscopic surgery, *RPLS* reduced port laparoscopic surgery)

Fig. 7.2 Clashing: clashing occurs because the forceps and scope are located within a limited space

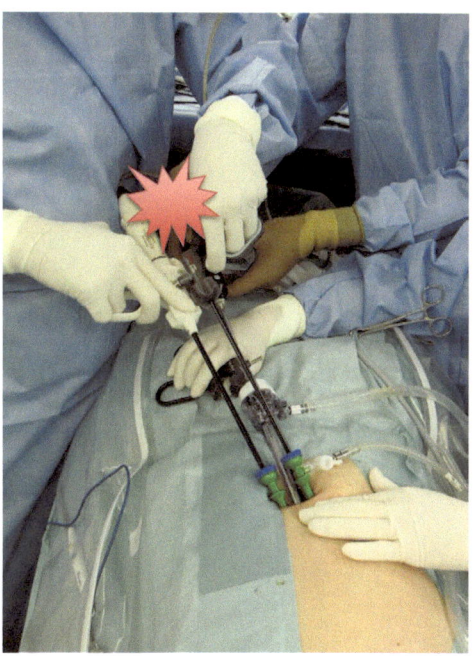

must be applied to tissue, the forceps are usually manipulated in a cephalad to caudal or anterior to posterior direction. Use of these instruments in SPLS can also result in interference between the handles and unwanted contact within the abdominal cavity, termed "clashing" and "sword fighting." Interference is also commonly seen between scope and ultrasonically activated device (USAD), vessel sealing system (VSD), and/or irrigation and suction device (Fig. 7.2).

7.3 Techniques for Avoiding Clashing and Sword Fighting

RPLS requires considerable adjustment to avoid interference when a multi-channel access device is inserted through the limited area of the navel. Here are some important points to remember.

7.3.1 Scopes

CLS commonly uses a rigid scope angled at 30° or 45°. The standard scope is approximately 30 cm in length and has an eyepiece attached to a camera head and light guide cable. The light guide cable is ordinarily positioned perpendicular to the

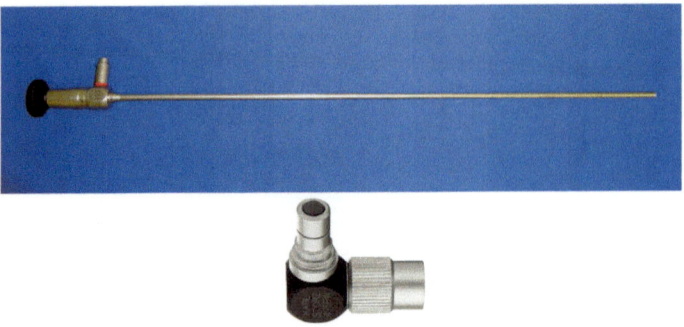

Fig. 7.3 A 50-cm long, 5-mm rigid scope and 90° light adapter (Karl Storz-Endoscope)

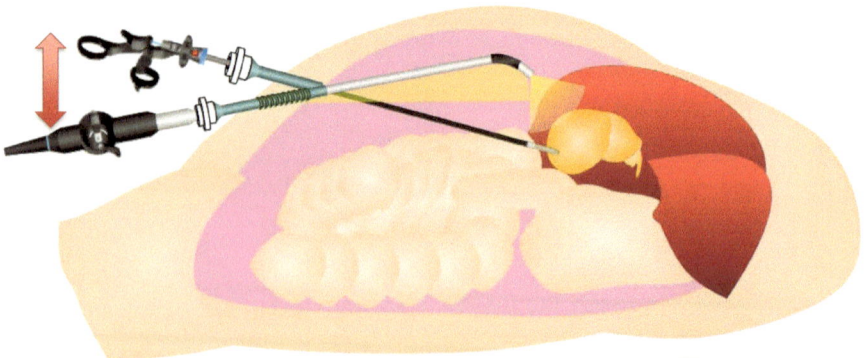

Fig. 7.4 The flexible scope can be used to establish a suitable distance between the forceps and the handheld scope

scope. In RPLS, the light guide cable and camera head can interfere with the operating forceps, making it difficult to maintain a clear visual field.

Use of a longer scope is one option for reducing interference between the scope and forceps. Recently, scopes for bariatric surgery have come onto the market, including a 45-cm scope from Stryker Corporation (Kalamazoo, MI, USA) and a 50-cm scope from Karl Storz-Endoscope (Tuttlingen, Germany) (Fig. 7.3). With these scopes, the camera head and light guide cable can be moved away from the hand that operates the forceps, reducing interference.

In particular, the light guide cable can interfere with forceps manipulation. This is because the cable is positioned perpendicular to the scope. Such interference can be avoided by using a light adapter angled at 90° (Fig. 7.4).

The use of a flexible scope requires less space between the hand operating the scope and the hand operating the forceps. The Olympus LTF-S19-5 (Olympus Medical Systems Co., Tokyo, Japan) is a flexible hi-vision scope 5.4-mm in diameter (Fig. 7.5) that maintains a clear visual field while reducing clashing.

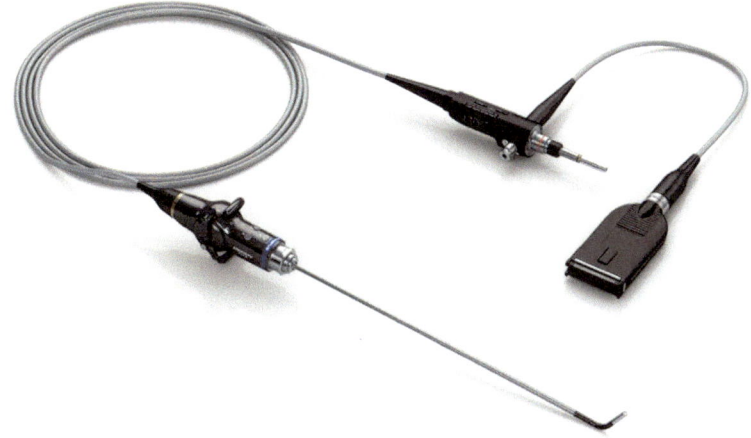

Fig. 7.5 LTF-S19-5 deflectable videoscope (Olympus). The tip of the scope can be moved 200° in four directions and the CCD/ light-guide cables are arranged in one line

Fig. 7.6 Trocar housing clashes are prevented by (**a**) use of different sleeve lengths (cx. 5-, 10- and 15-cm) and (**b**) use of small housings (low-profile trocars)

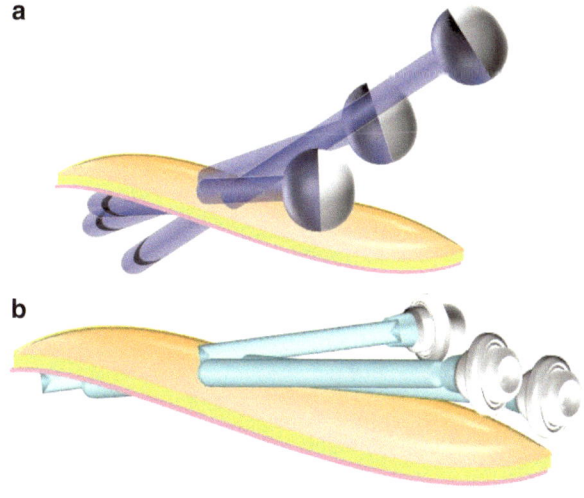

7.3.2 Trocars

Two or more trocars can be inserted directly through a single incision in the abdominal wall (multiple trocar approach). This permits the effective use of conventional tools in SPLS. However, only limited space is available for trocar positioning. The use of three to four conventional trocars can result in clashing of their housings, which interferes with accurate forceps manipulation. Such clashing can be avoided if we vary the trocar length (Fig. 7.6a). By using three trocars of different lengths (5-, 10-, and 15-cm), clashing can be reduced or eliminated.

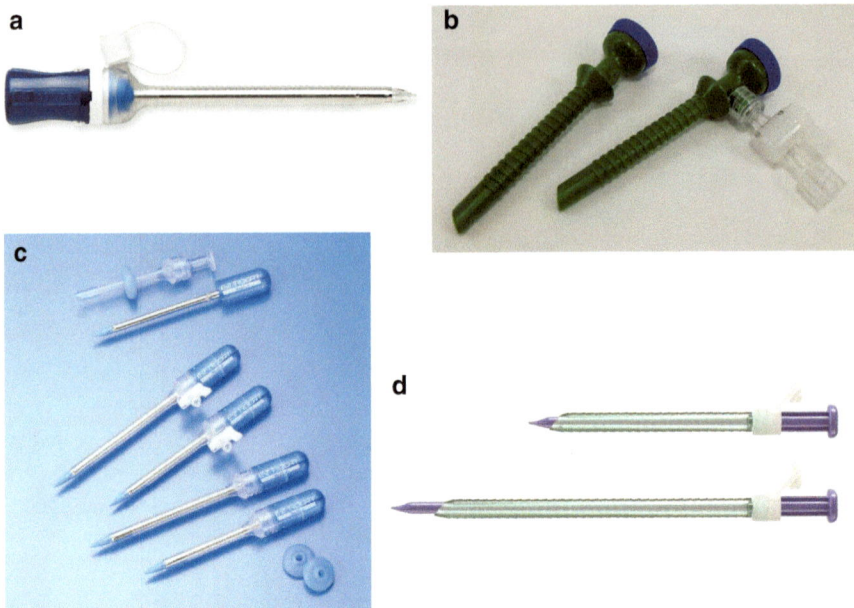

Fig. 7.7 Low-profile trocars. (**a**) Versaport Bladeless Optical Trocar (Covidien). (**b**) Linaport (LINA Medical). (**c**) E•Z Trocar Smart Insertion II (Hakko). (**d**) Slender port (TOP)

Another approach is to use trocars with smaller housings. These "low-profile" trocars also effectively reduce clashing (Fig. 7.6b). A number of brands are currently on the market (Fig. 7.7).

7.3.3   Access Ports

The multi-trocar approach can make it difficult to consistently insert the trocars in the appropriate positions, and it is subject to differences among surgeons. In addition, the location of the inner tip is difficult to confirm upon insertion of a second and third trocar. The use of a multi-channel port, in comparison to the multi-trocar approach, facilitates easier insertion of instruments developed for SPLS. Ordinarily, the port is inserted through a 2- to 4-cm skin incision.

Ports currently on the market are shown in Fig. 7.8. These include gel-based membrane devices that permit free positioning of dedicated trocars (GelPoint® (Applied Medical Resources Corporation, Rancho Santa Margarita, CA, USA)), devices with dedicated fixed channels for scopes and forceps (X-CONE® and ENDOCONE® (Karl Storz-Endoskope); TriPort and QuadPort (Advanced Surgical Concepts, Wicklow, Ireland); OCTO™ Port (Dalim Surgnet, Seoul, Korea); SILS™ Port (Covidien, New Haven, CT, USA); X-Gate (Ethicon Endosurgery, Cincinnati,

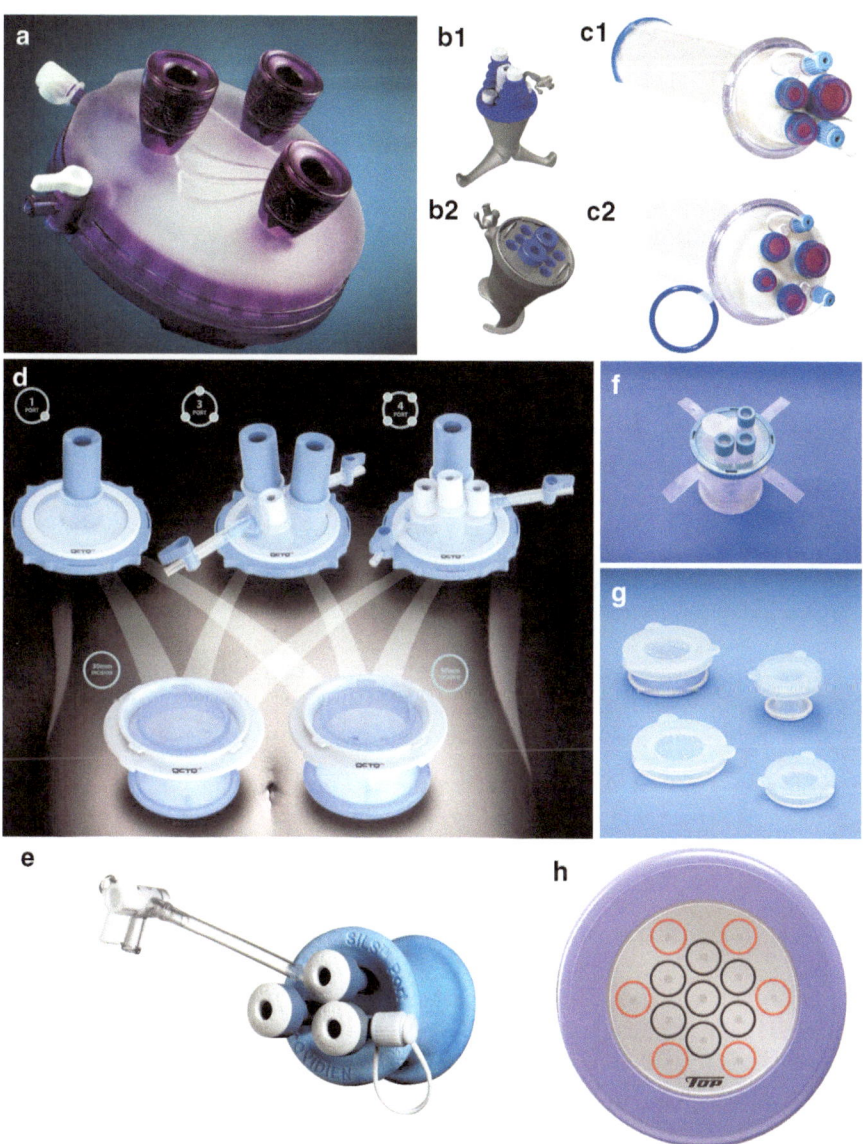

Fig. 7.8 Access devices. (**a**) GelPont (Applied Medical). (**b1**) X-CONE, (**b2**) ENDOCONE (Karl Storz-Endoscope). (**c1**) TriPort, (**c2**) QuadPort (Advanced Surgical Concepts). (**d**) OCTO Port (Dalim Surgnet). (**e**) SILS™ Port (Covidien). (**f**) X-Gate (Ethicon Endo-Surgery). (**g**) E•Z Access (Hakko). (**h**) Free Access (TOP)

OH, USA), and devices that use silicone membranes to permit the insertion of conventional trocars (E•Z Access (Hakko, Nagano, Japan); Free access (TOP Co., Tokyo, Japan). Please note that operating procedures can vary with respect to different devices, so caution is advised.

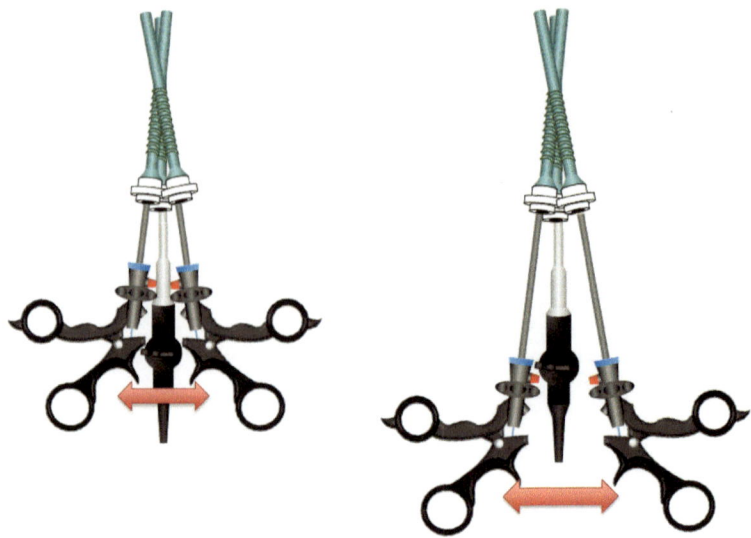

Fig. 7.9 Length of the forceps and distance between the hands. The distance between the hands increases when long forceps are used

7.3.4 Instruments for RPLS

RPLS allows greater distance between the two operating forceps, so clashing is reduced. However, with small incisions it can be difficult to maintain forceps spacing. A number of devices are currently available to prevent clashing.

7.3.4.1 Long Instruments

Ordinary forceps are 36-cm in length. Longer forceps allow greater distance between the hands and reduce clashing, even when the angle between the instruments is small (Fig. 7.9). A number of companies currently market 5-mm forceps with a 43-cm shaft. The forceps angle decreases for deeper surgical sites that are farther from the abdominal wall. Long-shaft forceps are particularly useful under these conditions. Powered devices can also be involved in instrument clashing. The Sonosurg® USAD (Olympus) has a shaft length of 45-cm, which is useful in avoiding such clashing (Fig. 7.10).

7.3.4.2 Articulated Instruments

Articulated forceps have been used in CLS to change the tip vector. Covidien has improved this forceps design for use with SPLS (Fig. 7.11a). These forceps [SILS™ articulating hand instruments (Covidien)] provide maximum articulation of 85° and

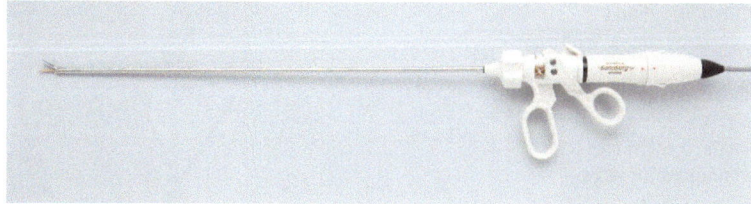

Fig. 7.10 The Sonosurg instrument is 45-cm long

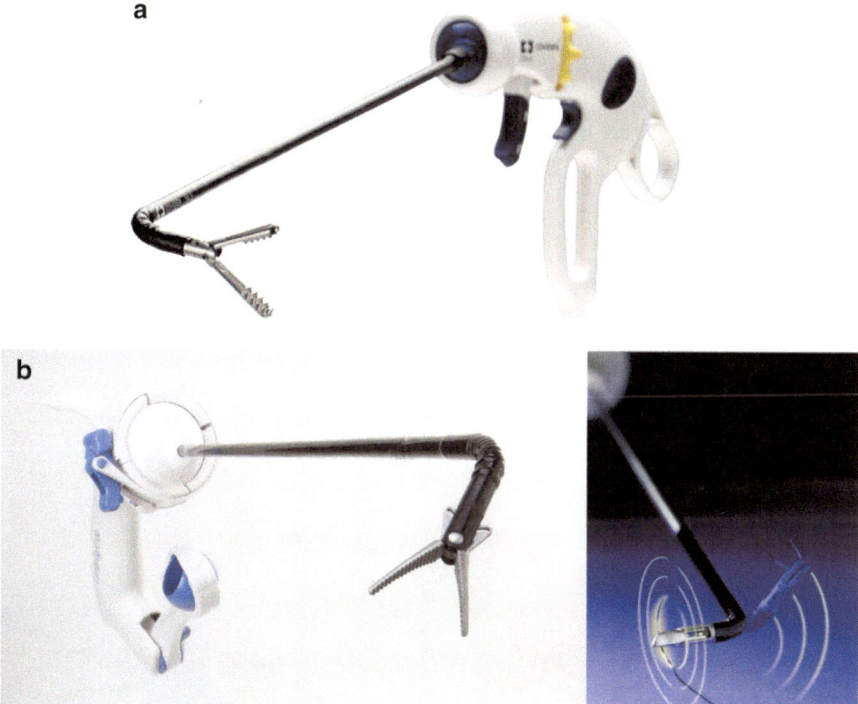

Fig. 7.11 Articulated forceps. (**a**) SILS™ articulating hand instruments (Covidien). (**b**) Autonomy Laparo-Angle instruments (Cambridge Endoscopic Devices)

can be fixed at any desired angle. The tip can be rotated 360°. The shafts are available in two lengths: 36- and 42-cm. With the cross-hand technique recommended by Covidien, the shafts of the instruments cross within the body. This eliminates instrument clashing, but the left-hand forceps perform operations that were conventionally done by the right hand, so training and practice are required (Fig. 7.12). Articulated forceps can also be used effectively with the parallel technique. Considerable clashing can be avoided by the use of articulated forceps for one of the grasping forceps (Fig. 7.13).

Fig. 7.12 Cross-hand technique (Covidien). With this technique, the instruments do not clash; however, practice is required because the forceps are applied to opposite sides

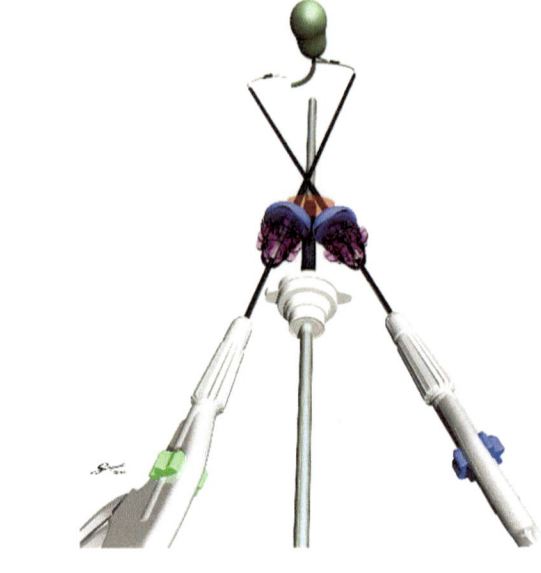

Fig. 7.13 Articulating forceps. Articulating forceps can be used to prevent handle clashing at hand when instruments are used in parallel

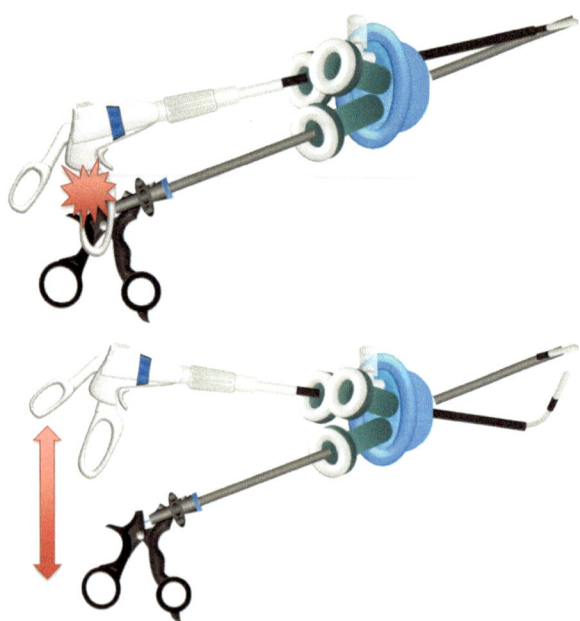

Suturing is also more challenging in SPLS than in CLS. The SILS™ Stitch (Covidien, Fig. 7.14) has a curved tip, which facilitates suture placement. The Autonomy™ Laparo-Angle™ Instruments (Cambridge Endoscopic Devices Inc., Framingham MA, USA) include articulated forceps (Fig. 7.11b) that can also be useful in suturing.

Fig. 7.14 SILS™ Stitch
(Covidien). Suturing and
ligation are relatively easy
with the bendable tip

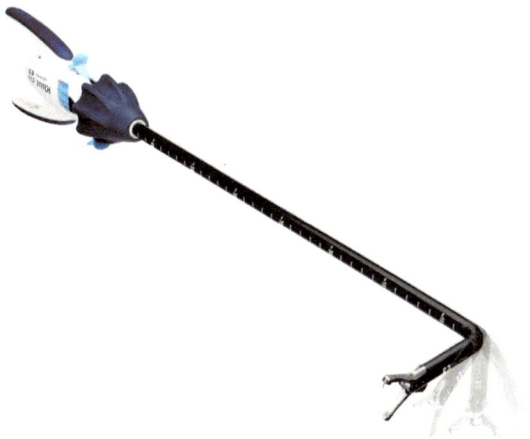

Fig. 7.15 Bending
instrument (S-Portal, Karl
Storz-Endoscope). Bending
forceps are designed to avoid
clashing and restore
triangulation

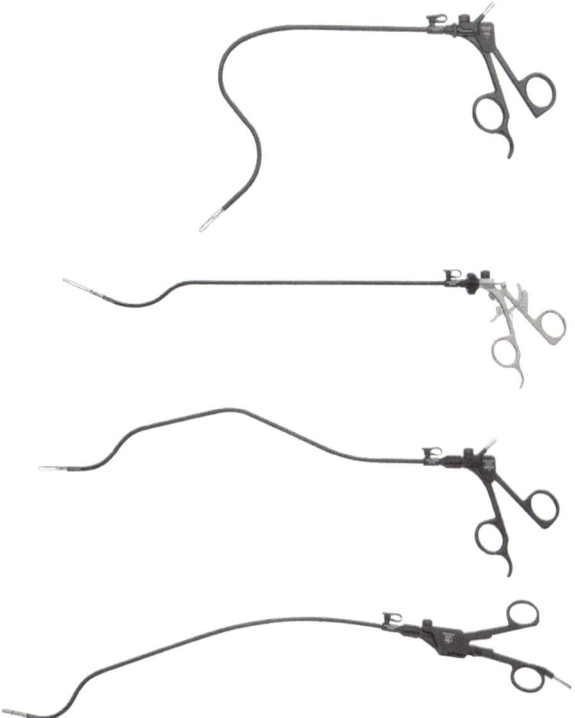

7.3.4.3   Bending Instruments

Bending forceps (S-Portal (Karl Storz-Endoskope) Fig. 7.15) are designed to change
the vector at the forceps tip and prevent handle clashing. They allow triangulation
even if little space is available between the forceps. However, they cannot be

Fig. 7.16 MIT port (Create Medic). Bending forceps can be inserted through this flexible trocar

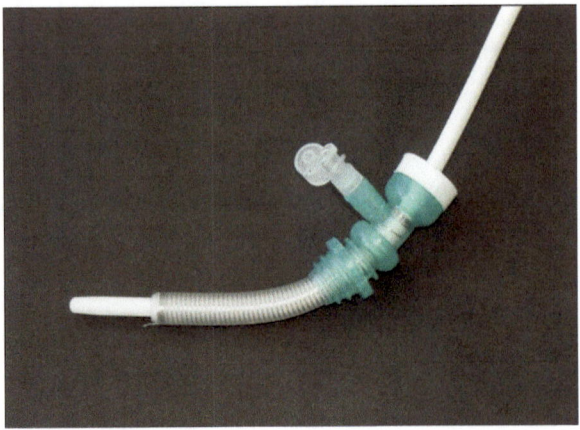

inserted into conventional trocars. Bending forceps must be used with a flexible trocar (MIT port (Create Medic Co. Ltd., Yokohama, Japan) Fig. 7.16) or a dedicated multi-channel port (ENDOCONE® (Karl Storz-Endoskope) Fig. 7.8b2). Although some special techniques are required for forceps insertion and manipulation, these instruments can provide operability equivalent to that achieved in CLS.

7.3.4.4 Needle Devices

Needle devices play an important role in RPLS. Slender forceps and other instruments used to assist in grasping tissue are commercially available. The Mini Loop Retractor II (Covidien) has a diameter of 2.2-mm. It can be inserted directly through the skin, and tissue can be grasped with the wire loop (Fig. 7.17a). Tissue can be retracted to provide a clear visual field. The MiniLap (Stryker) is a similar device that comes with four different types of forceps jaws to facilitate tissue grasping (Fig. 7.17b).

Small forceps (diameter, 3.5 mm or less) are now widely available. Because a thinner shaft is also weaker, shafts are generally limited to no more than 30-cm in length. However, the BJ Needle forceps (NITI-ON, Chiba, Japan) shaft is 2.1-mm in diameter and 33-cm in length, and is quite strong like the DAPRI trocarless grasping forceps (Karl Storz-Endoscope) with a shaft of 1.8-mm diameter and length of 25-cm. The 3-mm ClikLine® forceps (Karl Storz-Endoscope) shaft is 36-cm in length, and when used with the CARVALHO trocar (Karl Storz-Endoscope), is as strong as 5-mm forceps. These forceps can be used not only through an ancillary trocar for SPLS, but also as conventional grasping forceps and dissecting forceps.

7.3.4.5 Anchoring System for RPLS

The EndoGrab™ (Virtual Ports Ltd., Caesaera, Israel) and the Cinch Organ Retractor (Aesculap, B Braun Melsungen AG, Melsungen, Germany; Fig. 7.18) enable tissue retraction within the body cavity without the continued use of a

Fig. 7.17 Needle instruments. (**a**) Mini Loop Retractor II (Covidien). (**b**) Mini Lap (Stryker)

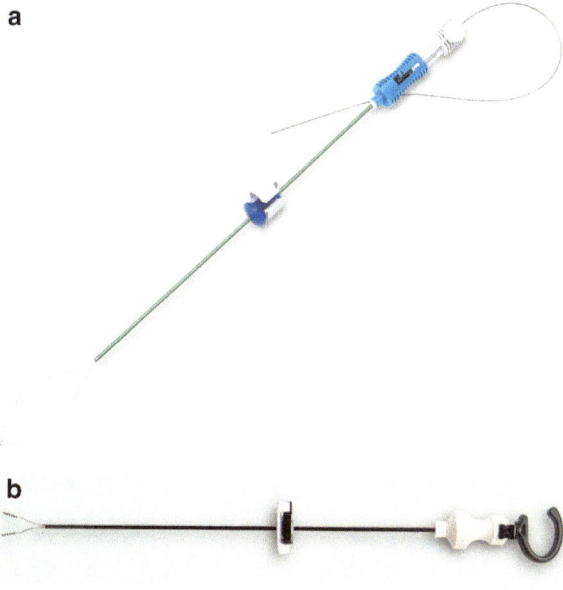

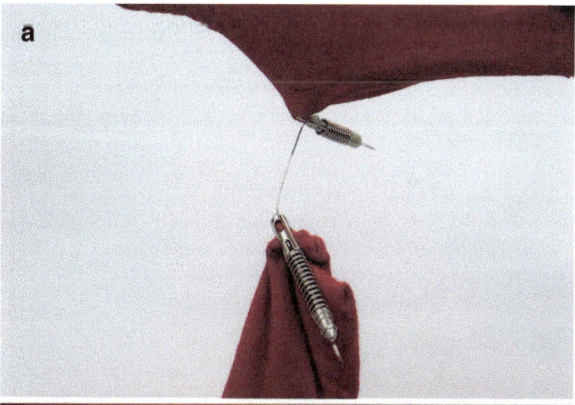

Fig. 7.18 Anchoring system for RPLS. (**a**) EndoGrab (Virtual Ports). (**b**) Cinch Organ Retractor (Aesculap)

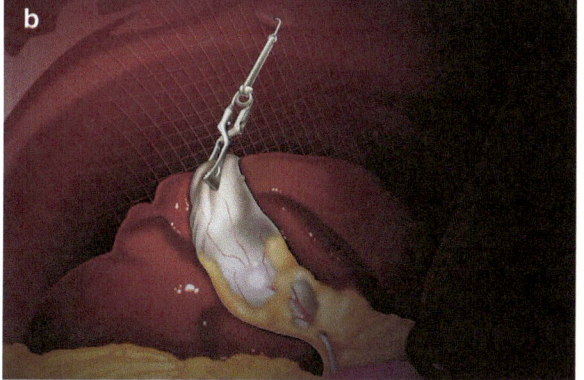

port. These devices make it possible to grasp and retract tissue by anchoring the hook directly to the peritoneum. No additional port is required. These devices are highly useful for RPLS, but training and practice are required for successful manipulation.

7.4 Conclusion

We anticipate the emergence of a number of new devices in the near future, some of which will involve the use of robotics [5]. Without a full understanding of these devices, surgeons in the field will be unable to perform RPLS safely and effectively. Sufficient preclinical training is strongly recommended before any of these new devices is used clinically.

References

1. Navarra G, Pozza E, Occhionorelli S et al (1996) One-wound laparoscopic cholecystectomy. Br J Surg 84:695
2. Tagaya N, Kita J, Takagi K et al (1998) Experience with three-port laparoscopic cholecystectomy. J Hepatobiliary Pancreat Surg 5:309–311
3. Kalloo AN, Singh VK, Jagannath SB et al (2004) Flexible transgastric peritoneoscopy: a novel approach to diagnostic and therapeutic interventions in the peritoneal cavity. Gastrointest Endosc 60:114–117
4. Mori T, Aoki H, Sugiyama M et al (2010) Instrumentation in single-access laparoscopic surgery. Asian J Endosc Surg 3:153–161
5. Joseph RA, Goh AC, Cuevas SP et al (2010) "Chopstick" surgery: a novel technique improves surgeon performance and eliminates arm collision in robotic single-incision laparoscopic surgery. Surg Endosc 24:1331–1335

Chapter 8
Needlescopic Devices and Pre-bent Forceps

Nobumi Tagaya

Abstract Reduced port laparoscopic surgery (RPLS) has recently been introduced into the laparoscopic arena as a result of efforts to find a method that is truly minimally invasive. RPLS is associated with limited tissue trauma and improved cosmetic outcomes. However, it is also associated with a high incidence of conversion to conventional laparoscopic or open surgery. Convenient and miniaturized surgical tools are thus necessary for good outcomes in patients undergoing RPLS. Here, we describe the tools that are available for surgeons who wish to minimize surgical trauma and provide optimal cosmesis during RPLS including single-access laparoscopic surgery and needlescopic surgery. RPLS has been further refined with the introduction of needlescopic devices and pre-bent forceps. The main purpose of these devices is three-fold: minimal invasion, nearly invisible scarring, and optimum post-surgical quality of life. To ensure such outcomes, we find it necessary to improve our own skills and understand the characteristics of each needlescopic device and pre-bent forceps.

Keywords Curved reusable instruments • Needlescopic device • Needlescopic surgery • Pre-bent forceps • Reduced port laparoscopic surgery

8.1 Introduction

Laparoscopic surgery has evolved over the past two decades. Laparoscopic surgeons have provided minimally invasive therapies while improving their own skills and developing special surgical instruments. Laparoscopic instruments themselves have been improved and updated year by year. Patients have benefitted from both

N. Tagaya (✉)
Department of Surgery, Dokkyo Medical University Koshigaya Hospital,
2-1-50 Minamikoshigaya, Koshigaya, Saitama 343-8555, Japan
e-mail: tagaya@dokkyomed.ac.jp

T. Mori and G. Dapri (eds.), *Reduced Port Laparoscopic Surgery*,
DOI 10.1007/978-4-431-54601-6_8, © Springer Japan 2014

minimal surgical invasion and minimal postoperative discomfort. Reduced port laparoscopic surgery (RPLS) was recently introduced into the laparoscopic arena as a result of efforts to develop an approach that is truly minimally invasive. Although reducing the size of the laparoscopic ports and instruments has, for patients, resulted in decreased tissue trauma and improved cosmetic outcomes, RPLS has proved to be relatively stressful for surgeons performing the procedures and resulted in a high incidence of conversion to conventional laparoscopic or open surgery. The surgeons increased stress is the result of a number of factors, including a narrow operative field, reduced light transmission and image quality, blurred vision with the use of electrocautery, increased difficulty in manipulating the instruments due to their increased flexibility, particularly in the presence of fibrosis or inflammation, and the learning curve associated with proficient use of the instruments. Convenient and miniaturized surgical tools are thus necessary for good outcomes in patients undergoing RPLS. Here, we describe the tools that are available for surgeons who are considering minimizing surgical trauma and providing improved cosmesis during RPLS including single-access laparoscopic surgery (SALS) and needlescopic surgery [1–3].

8.2 Surgical Tools

8.2.1 Optics (Fig. 8.1)

A significant obstacle to needlescopic surgery is the limited visualization achieved with 3-mm and smaller laparoscopes. Minilaparoscopes are available from Olympus Medical Systems Co. (Tokyo, Japan), Aesculap (Tuttlingen, Germany), Karl Storz-Endoskope (Tuttlingen, Germany), and Stryker (Kalamazoo, MI, USA) [1].

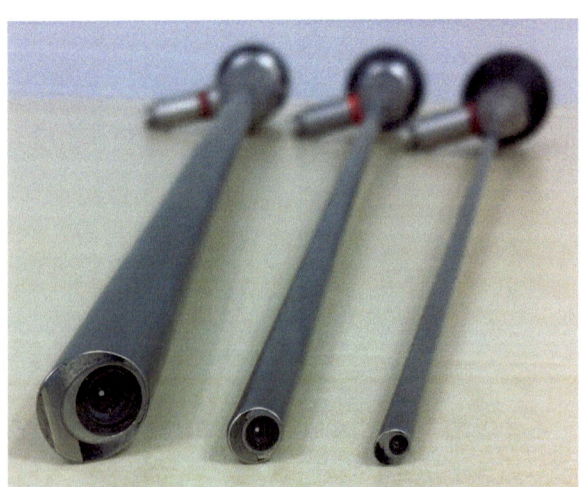

Fig. 8.1 Differences between 2-, 5- and 10-mm optics

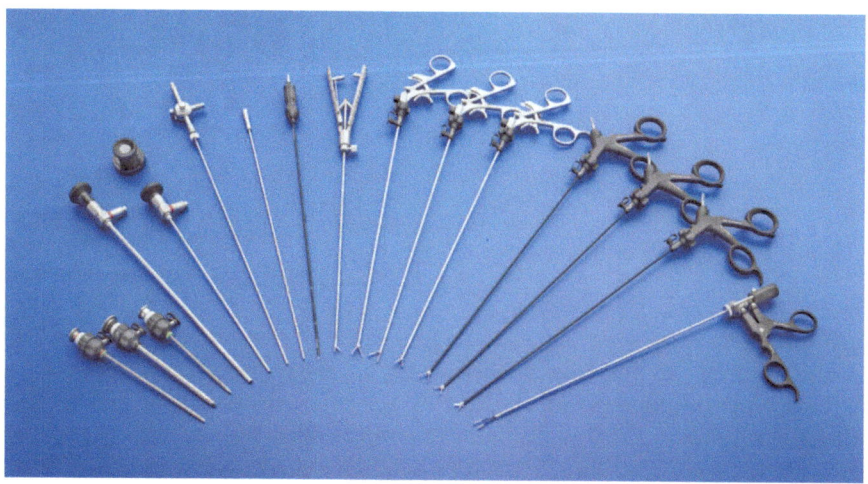

Fig. 8.2 The 3-mm minilaparoscopy system (Karl Storz-Endoskope)

The Stryker Ideal Eyes™ line includes a 2.9-mm pediatric scope, 20-cm in length. Karl Storz-Endoskope offers two 30-degree laparoscopes, a 2.4-mm scope and a 3.3-mm scope, 18 and 25 cm in length, respectively. Aesculap has 2- and 2.5-mm, 0-degree laparoscopes, 22 and 30 cm, long respectively. Because of the limited optics and limited available laparoscopes, many needlescopic procedures are performed with a fairly large umbilical port, which accommodates a larger laparoscope and offers better visualization. For procedures such as cholecystectomy, a needlescopic umbilical port site would most likely require enlargement for extraction of the gallbladder.

8.2.2 Laparoscopic Instruments

Currently several minilaparoscopic instrument sets are commercially available: the MiniSite™ disposable instrument set manufactured by Covidien (New Haven, CT, USA), the 3-mm minilaparoscopy set from Karl Storz-Endoskope, and a similar set of instruments from Stryker [1].

The MiniSite™ MiniShears™ (Covidien) 2-mm instrument with unipolar cautery is applicable to a variety of endoscopic procedures for mobilization and transection of tissue. This instrument has a 2-mm diameter insulated shaft that is approximately 33 cm in length, it is designed for introduction and use through the MiniPort™ (Covidien) introducer sleeve. The scissors blade has a cutting edge approximately 5.9 mm in length, and the maximum blade opening is 5.9 mm.

The 3-mm minilaparoscopy instrument set manufactured by Karl Storz-Endoskope (Fig. 8.2) is a completely reusable set of instruments 36 cm long. A full complement of instruments is available including graspers, dissectors, scissors,

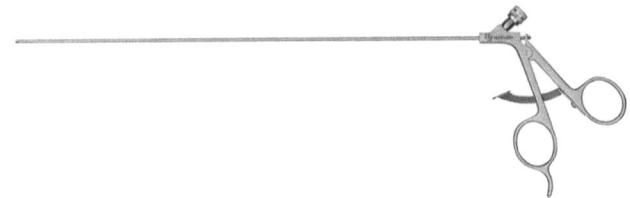

Fig. 8.3 BJ needle (NITI-ON)

electrocautery, suction device, and needle holders for intracorporeal suturing. The major advantage of this set is that it is made up of the longest currently available needlescopic instruments, which are thus versatile and can accommodate thick abdominal walls as well as operations in which relatively long instruments are needed. In addition to these 3-mm-diameter, 36-cm-long instruments, Karl Storz-Endoskope offers shorter 3-mm instruments (20 and 30 cm in length) as well as a line of 2-mm instruments in lengths of 20 cm and 30 cm instruments, but that set is available only in 20-cm lengths.

The Sovereign® mini-instrument set (Aesculap) is another set designed for mini-laparoscopy. These instruments are actually 3.5 mm in diameter, which by strict definition does not make them needlescopic. They are available in lengths of 20 and 29 cm. The set of Soverign® mini-instruments (Aesculap) work through a reusable trocar system and includes graspers, scissors, dissectors, and needle holders. Although this line does not fall under the definition of needlescopic surgery devices, it includes small-diameter instruments that are introduced through a 4-mm trocar. In comparison to a 5-mm instrument setup, such small instruments and trocar should reduce abdominal wall trauma. This is an example of compromising size for strength. These instruments are more rigid than the 2-mm instruments, making them particularly suitable for operations that require strong instruments, yet they still decrease abdominal wall trauma.

A new-generation 2-mm instrument called BJ Needle (NITI-ON Co., Ltd., Chiba, Japan) (Fig. 8.3) was recently introduced. This new instrument, in comparison to first-generation 2-mm instruments, allows more rigid grasping with less bending of the instrument shaft. The shaft is a 2.1 mm in diameter. We anticipate that the outcomes achieved with such instruments, in terms of operation time and the surgeon's stress level, will be similar to those achieved with 3-mm instruments.

Endo Relief forceps (Hope Denshi Co., Ltd., Chiba, Japan) (Fig. 8.4), which is used to grasp and retract the organs, consist of a 2.4-mm shaft and a 5-mm head, and the two parts are joined intraoperatively. To join the two parts, a 5-mm port and a 2/3-mm port are needed, because a 2/3-mm shaft is connected to the 5-mm head after incorporation of the shaft guide, the 2.4-mm shaft is moved from inside to outside the abdominal cavity through the 2/3-mm port. Manipulation of this device is similar to that of 5-mm instruments except for the easy bending of the shaft. The head cannot be easily changed during the operation.

Fig. 8.4 Endo Relief (Hope Densi)

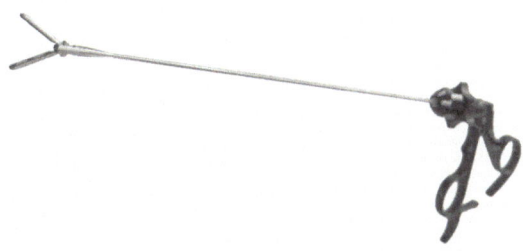

Fig. 8.5 The Mini-loop system (Stryker)

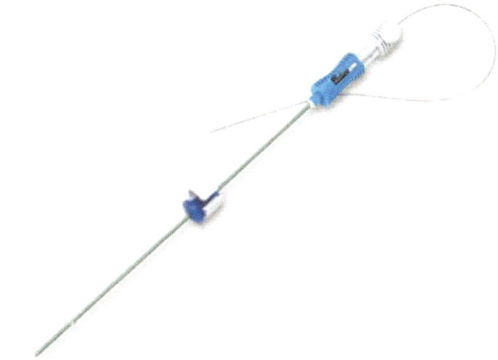

8.2.3 Trocar-Less Instruments

Mini-loop retractor II and Endo Surgi Retractor (Covidien) (Fig. 8.5) have two functions, direct insertion into the abdominal cavity and loop retraction of the internal organs. The shafts of both instruments are 2.2 mm in diameter and 200 mm in length, and both have a stopper that can be fixed at any desired position. These devices provide for hands-free retraction.

MiniLap instruments from Stryker are disposable instruments with a 2.3-mm outer diameter and a unique access insertion needle. The MiniLap system (Stryker) allows for percutaneous introduction without a trocar in even the thickest of abdominal walls, and it comprises several types of instruments including graspers and electrosurgical probes.

Riza-Ribe Needle (R-Med, Inc., Oregon, OH, USA) was initially used for the closure of port-induced fascial defects. GraNee Needle (R-Med, Inc.) is a 16-gauge grasper and needle for single use. It is used for transferring a ligature during laparoscopic procedures. It can be inserted at multiple sites with minimal penetration trauma. These needles are used for tissue retraction during laparoscopic surgery.

Fig. 8.6 Mini Step
(Covidien)

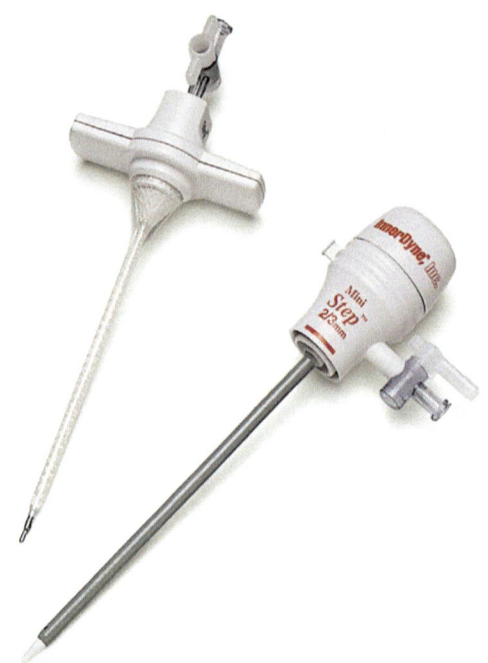

Karl Storz-Endoskope recently produced the DAPRI trocarless grasping forceps of 1.8 mm in diameter and 25 cm in length which can be inserted through the same hole created before by a classic Veress needle.

8.2.4 Trocar

The Karl Storz-Endoskope cannula and trocar system is the most traditional type of trocar. It consists of a rigid cannula that is introduced with a metal conical tip trocar and has silicone leaflet valves to help maintain pneumoperitoneum. The Karl Storz-Endoskope system has 10- and 15-cm reusable trocars. The longer trocar may add stability for cases in which relatively thick abdominal walls are encountered. The Aesculap trocar system is rigid, is available in 6- and 11-cm lengths, and is inserted with a conical sharp or blunt tip metal trocar.

The MiniPort™ (Covidien) 2-mm introducer system is a single-use introducer. A circular adjustable stopper located on the sleeve of the MiniPort™ allows for adjustment of depth in the cavity.

Mini Step produced by Covidien (Fig. 8.6) is a 2/3 mm disposable port for insertion of needlescopic or miniaturized instruments of less than 3.5 mm in diameter.

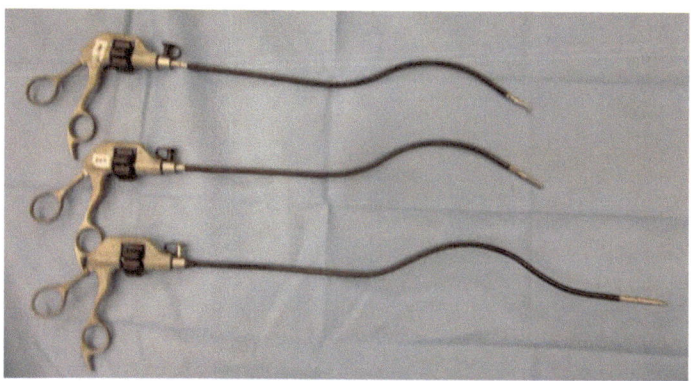

Fig. 8.7 YGT and AT forceps (Adachi)

8.2.5 Pre-bent Forceps

YAMAGATA (YGT) and ADACHI-TANKO (AT) forceps (Adachi Industry Co., Ltd., Gifu, Japan) (Fig. 8.7) are curved and reusable and designed for use during SALS. These devices are 5 mm in diameter, 47.5-cm and 65-cm in length, and they provide more direct pressure to target organs with adequate articulation. The tip can rotate 360° around its axis. These forceps can be used without a trocar in the setting of SALS performed by the glove port technique: however, a flexible trocar is useful for easy exchange of several curved devices. A flexible trocar is available for use with MIT™ port (Create Medic Co., Yokohama, Japan).

Curved instruments (Olympus) that rotate but do not reticulate are available. Thus the angle of curvature is fixed, which may be useful when additional rigidity is needed.

Curved and reusable forceps according to DAPRI (Karl Storz-Endoskope) (Fig. 8.8) are designed to be inserted into the abdomen through the umbilicus without trocars. The curved grasping forceps is advanced through a separate window, 5 mm outside the purse-string suture, and the other instruments (coagulating hook, scissors, suction device) are introduced on the other side of the grasper, alongside the 11-mm trocar and inside the purse-string suture.

8.3 Comments

Needlescopic devices and techniques are now being re-revaluated in view of the rapid development of SALS. However, several unresolved issues remain to be worked out before these devices can be used routinely. With the currently available technology, needlescopic devices have limitations related to surgical optics and manipulability. The needlescope is hampered by poor illumination, poor resolution,

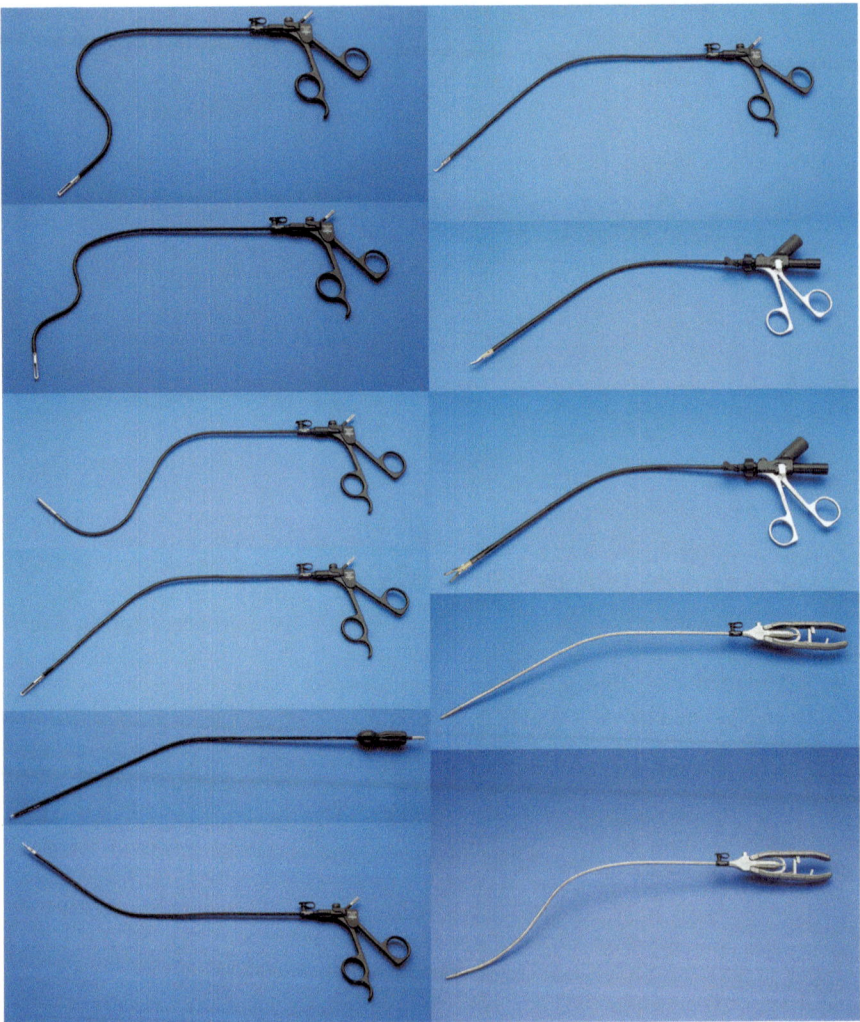

Fig. 8.8 Curved and reusable instruments according to DAPRI (Karl Storz-Endoskope)

and lack of clarity because of the optical limitations of the rod lens. Moreover, tiny laparoscopic devices are not as sturdy and manipulable as larger instruments. Furthermore, we must consider the increased risk of tissue damage during dissection performed with the pointed ends of fine graspers. These issues can prolong the operation time, increase the risk of perioperative complications, and increase the surgeon's stress level.

However, there are several advantages in performing needlescopic procedures. A tiny skin incision leaving an undetectable scar is cosmetically advantageous, and it requires no skin closure, thus reducing costs. Furthermore, access to the peritoneal cavity via needlescopic ports is relatively easy, reduces the risk of hernia-tion and port-related injury to both the abdominal wall and intra-abdominal organs, and minimizes the possibility of wound infection. Furthermore, the cost of needle-scopic ports themselves in a disposable setting is approximately 27.5 % lower than that of standard ports.

Two-millimeter needlescopic devices are employed in various surgical fields [2]. However, 3-mm instruments are much more versatile and resilient, allowing perfor-mance of a wide variety of procedures, and they can be used in patients with an inflamed or thickened gallbladder wall because they have good rigidity, facilitate easy division and dissection of a curved jaw is used, and provide sufficient suction and irrigation. Therefore, 3-mm instruments are more useful than 2-mm instruments for completion of needlescopic procedures. However, new generation instruments of less than 3-mm (BJ Needle (NITON) and EndoRelief (Hope Denshi) have been introduced. In comparison to standard 2-mm instruments, these devices allow more rigid grasping with less bending of the instrument shaft. The outcomes achieved with such devices, in terms of operation time and the stress experienced by the sur-geon, are similar to outcomes achieved with 3-mm instruments.

However, the outcomes of needlescopic procedures are greatly dependent on the skill of the individual surgeon. Therefore, new surgeons or surgical residents should not begin to learn laparoscopic surgery using needlescopic devices. The manipula-tion of needlescopic instruments is appreciably different from that of standard 5-mm or 10-mm devices. If surgeons do not bear this in mind, patients could be put at increased risk.

The curved and reusable instruments must be inserted in one of two ways through the umbilicus [3]. One method is to introduce the instrument alongside the 11-mm trocar and inside the purse-string suture without a trocar. The other is to insert it through the flexible trocar from the umbilicus. The purse-string is adjusted to main-tain a tight seal during the procedure, avoiding leakage of the pneumoperitoneum gas, and it is opened when the smoke issuing from the cautery must be evacuated or when the instruments need to be changed. Although flexible trocars are disposable and designed for single use, the exchange of several devices is less stressful than manipulations involving the flexible trocar and results in maintaining a better opera-tive field. The curved instruments avoid conflict between the surgeon's non-dominant hand and the laparoscope inside the abdomen as well as conflict between the surgeon's hand and the scope assistant's hand outside the abdomen.

8.4 Conclusion

RPLS has been further developed with the introduction of needlescopic devices and pre-bent forceps. The chief benefits of using these devices are minimal invasiveness, invisible scars, and optimum quality of life after surgery. To obtain these outcomes, it is necessary for us to improve our own skills and understand the characteristics of each needlescopic device and pre-bent forceps.

References

1. Krpata DM, Ponsky TA (2013) Needlescopic surgery: what's in the toolbox? Surg Endosc 27:1040–1044
2. Tagaya N, Kubota K (2012) Re-evaluation of needlescopic surgery. Surg Endosc 26:137–143
3. Dapri G (2014) Single-incision laparoscopy: a review of the indications, techniques and results after more than 700 procedures. Asian J Endosc Surg 7:102–116

Chapter 9
Different Tools

Noam Shussman and Yoav Mintz

Abstract In recent years, efforts to reduce post-operative pain, to lower wound related morbidities and to improve cosmetic outcomes have led to the development of single-port laparoscopic surgery (SPLS). This technique, however, is not straightforward. The technical complexity of the procedure results in a significant learning curve, which increases operating room time and mandates specialized equipment.

This chapter reviews the various tools, which have been developed and are aimed at overcoming the technical pitfalls of SPLS. Different access devices, cameras, retraction methods and operative instruments can be used in SPLS. Some are commercially available and some are now being used in clinical studies. Some tools were developed especially for SPLS after understanding the special needs for this approach and some are improvisations or adjustments of previously accepted instruments for standard laparoscopic surgery to the novel concept of SPLS. This chapter does not list all of the available instruments on the market, but rather serves as an overview of the principles that should guide surgeons in choosing the tools for SPLS. Optimization of the view, providing with adequate organ retraction and achieving triangulation should be the basis of the surgeon's decision when choosing which tools to use for performing SPLS.

Keywords Exposure • Field of view • Maneuverability • Retraction • Single-port laparoscopic surgery (SPLS) • Triangulation

N. Shussman (✉) • Y. Mintz
Department of General Surgery, Hadassah Medical Center,
PO. B. 12000, Jerusalem, Israel
e-mail: Noams@hadassah.org.il

T. Mori and G. Dapri (eds.), *Reduced Port Laparoscopic Surgery*,
DOI 10.1007/978-4-431-54601-6_9, © Springer Japan 2014

9.1 Introduction

Since being introduced more than three decades ago, laparoscopic surgery has become progressively accepted. For some procedures, the laparoscopic approach has become the standard of care. The classic example for such a procedure is laparoscopic cholecystectomy [1–4], and following the acceptance of this procedure more operations followed like adrenalectomy, Nissen fundoplication, Heller myotomy, splenectomy, appendectomy and more. In recent years, surgeons are faced with the challenge of accomplishing the requisite tasks of the same surgical procedure through smaller incisions and an ever-reducing number of ports, in an effort to reduce post-operative pain and morbidities such as wound infection and trocar site hernias. This challenge is being sought for further enhancing the cosmetic results as well. Initial attempts to perform surgery through a lower number of ports or with reduced diameter trocars ("needle-scopic surgery") [5–9] have since been superseded by even less invasive, more innovative techniques namely: single-port laparoscopic surgery (SPLS) and Natural Orifice Transluminal Endoscopic Surgery (NOTES) [10–13].

SPLS is an attractive technique due to the above-mentioned potential benefits of superior cosmetic results and the potential to reduce the rate of wound related complications (infection, hematoma, hernia, etc.). Another possible potential benefit is the reduction of postoperative pain. This technique, however, is not straightforward. The technical complexity of the procedure results in a significant learning curve, which increases operating room time and mandates specialized equipment.

The primary technical obstacles that make SPLS challenging include [14]:

- collision of instruments both within and outside the abdomen as a result of their common entry point ("sword fighting")
- inadequate triangulation and hence decreased maneuverability
- compromised field of view due to obstruction by the working instruments entering the common channel and inability to position the camera correctly for an adequate view
- inadequate exposure and retraction.

Due to these reasons, opponents of SPLS have concerns regarding the safety of this surgical approach. Proponents of SPLS, on the other hand, claim that it is purely an issue of employing dedicated instruments and mastering the learning curve of the techniques for maintaining the same high level of safety.

This chapter will review the various tools, which have been developed and are aimed at overcoming the pitfalls of SPLS. It was not the authors' intention to list here all the countless instruments available on the market for SPLS. Rather, this chapter is aimed at being an overview of the principles that can guide surgeons to choose the tools for SPLS.

9.2   Access Devices

The access device is the key component that can facilitate the SPLS technique. The intrinsic complexity of SPLS includes inadequate triangulation, compromised field of view, inadequate exposure and instrument collision. These can be simplified using a well-designed access port. Such a device should have the following characteristics:

- it should be small in order to minimize the skin and fascial incisions thereby reduce incision related morbidity and improve cosmetic outcomes
- it should be secured to the abdominal wall in order to provide an optimal airtight seal to prevent CO_2 leakage
- it has to enable the passage of a sufficient number of instruments into the abdominal cavity and allow some freedom of their motion without causing movement of the other tools.

Various methods to access the peritoneal cavity have been developed and described in a pursuit to achieve such an optimal access device. Some of these methods are improvised while others were developed as dedicated access devices for SPLS. The most common access methods and devices are described herein.

9.2.1   Multiple Ports Through a Single-Incision

A simplistic way of accessing the abdominal cavity through a single skin incision is to position several independent trocars through a single incision. Five millimeter low profile trocars (Fig. 9.1) have a better maneuverability than standard trocars and allow for a relatively independent movement for each one of the instruments with only some resultant movement of the other instruments [14]. In 2010, the

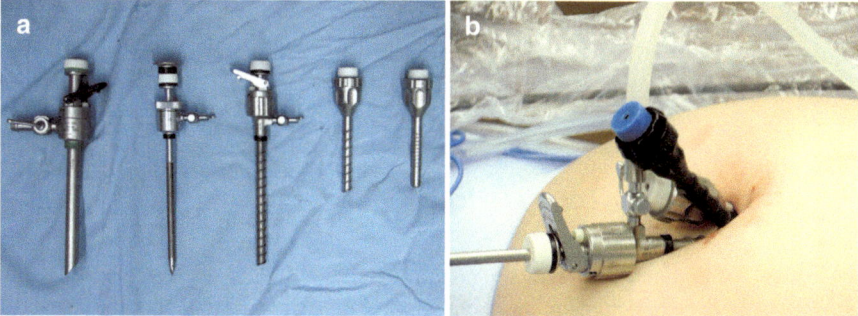

Fig. 9.1 (**a**) 5-mm low profile trocars (Karl Storz-Endoscope). The use of low profile trocars enables improved avoidance of instrument collision and better maneuverability. (**b**) Three low profile trocars inserted through a single 18-mm skin incision during a SPLS cholecystectomy. Note staged insertion of the trocars into the abdominal wall to minimize their collision with one another

consortium for Laparo-Endoscopic Single-Site (LESS) surgery has published a consensus statement which stated "the use of three standard laparoscopic trocars through a single skin incision (with multiple facial puncture sites) can provide the independence of movement necessary for LESS surgery" [15]. The length of the skin incision when using three 5-mm trocars should not be greater than 2-cm hence the incision is kept small. This method, however, may result in a sub-optimal maneuverability of the trocars resulting in a limited independent movement of each instrument, especially if non low profile trocars are being used. There is also a potential for a CO_2 leakage during the procedure if the trocars are not independently secured to the fascia, which might result in a challenge maintaining pneumoperitoneum. If organ removal is necessary, enlargement of the fascial incision takes place usually at the end of the procedure.

9.2.2 Improvised Access Device: The Glove Port

Several studies have reported an improvised technique to access the abdominal cavity through a single incision, with the application of a surgical glove. Hayashi et al. and Livraghi et al. reported on a series of SPLS (mainly cholecystectomies and appendectomies) using a standard wound protector covered with a surgical glove with several small incisions made on the tips of the glove-fingers to induce pneumoperitoneum and to create working channels for the laparoscopic instruments [16, 17]. The authors described this technique as having multiple advantages: easy to use, simply accommodated to the abdominal wall even in overweight patients, allows simultaneous passage of a maximum of 5-mm instruments and allows a wide axis of movements and hence minimizes instrument collision. The low cost of the application of this technique is mentioned as a potential advantage as well. Eumatsu et al. as well as Ishida et al. applied a similar technique for SPLS colectomies and concluded it is safe and feasible [18, 19].

Although the glove port technique may be safe and feasible, in the era of standartization and strict FDA control of medical devices, this technique may be used only in countries free from FDA/CE mark device approvals.

9.2.3 Dedicated Access Devices

A variety of dedicated access devices are available. These devices offer different solutions to the challenges mentioned above. Some are reusable, but most are disposable and thus increase the overall OR cost.

The SILS™ port (Covidien, New Haven, CT, USA) is a disposable access port. It has a firm foam-like consistancy and is inserted through a 2-cm fascial incision. The port adjusts to the wound edges and retracts the abdominal wall to provide an airtight seal. Through this port 5/12-mm trocars and instruments can be passed into the peritoneal cavity (Fig. 9.2).

Fig. 9.2 SILS™ port
(Covidien)

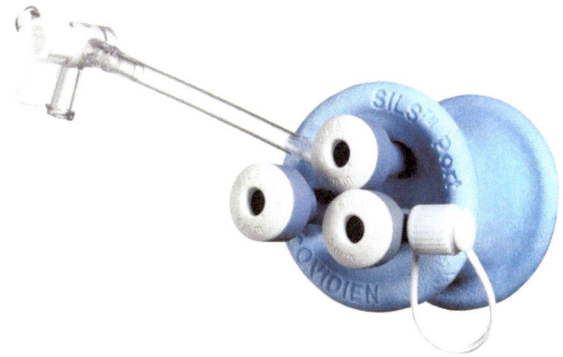

Fig. 9.3 GelPOINT® access
device (Applied Medical)

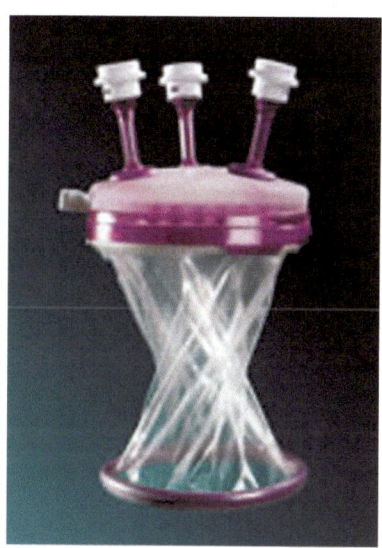

The GelPOINT® (Applied Medical, Rancho Santa Margarita, CA, USA) has a disposable gel platform connecting to an adjustable polyethilene sheath which has an inner and external rings (Fig. 9.3). This sheath serves also as a standard wound protector while extracting organs. The gel platform enables insertion of several dedicated or standard trocars wide apart from each other lowering the incidence of instrument collision.

The Triport® and Quadport® (Advanced Surgical Concepts, Wicklow, Ireland) are disposable devices. Both have a similar adjustable plastic sleeve which is inserted through a 2-cm fascial incision using a special introducer. The sleeve is then connected to an external cap with different configurations of several valves allowing passage of rigid and curved instruments into the abdominal cavity (Fig. 9.4).

The X-Cone™ (Karl Storz-Endoscope, Tuttlingen, Germany) is a rigid reusable port, which consists of two metallic parts and a reusable silicone cap (Fig. 9.5). The port is assembled following the positioning of both metallic parts through the

Fig. 9.4 Quadport® acces
device (Advanced Surgical
Concepts)

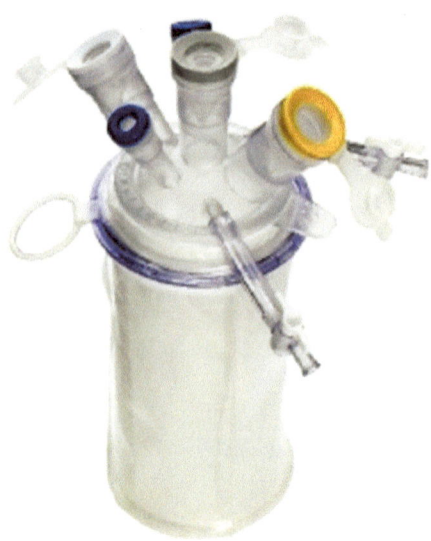

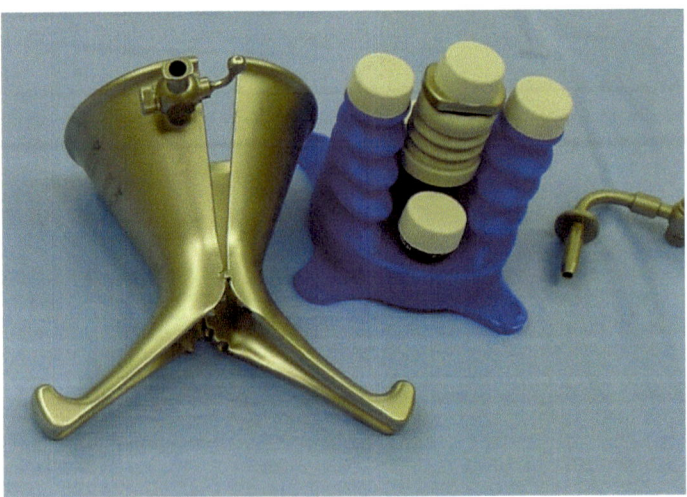

Fig. 9.5 X-Cone™ (Karl Storz-Endoscope), a reusable SPLS access device

incision, thereby creating an air tight seal and maintaining constant fascial incision
length. The silicone cap contains three flexible ports enabling the passage of rigid and
curved instruments, and two more ports, which have no profile height to reduce the
space occupied by the ports. In total the port offers introduction of five instruments.
The special rigid hourglass configuration facilitates the use of curved instruments to
achieve adequate retraction and triangulation.

Fig. 9.6 Single site laparoscopy access system (Ethicon)

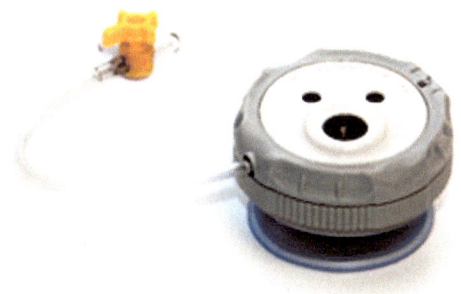

The Single Site Laparoscopy Access System (Ethicon Endosurgery Inc., Cincinnati, OH, USA) is a disposable port. It has a plastic sheath in various sizes that is inserted through the incision using a dedicated introducer. A unique rigid cap is then connected to the external ring of the sheath, which has three entry ports (Fig. 9.6). These ports are the seal mechanisms only without any tubing or trocars thereby maximizing the space offered for instruments and motion around the cap.

Several other devices are on the market like the ENDOCONE™ (Karl Storz-Endoscope), the S-Port® (Karl Storz-Endoscope), the X-Gate (Ethicon) and more. Most have similar designs with minor changes that differentiate them.

9.3 Cameras

As mentioned above, the view is compromised in SPLS, due to the common point of entry of instruments and camera into the abdominal cavity. The passage of instruments within the camera's visual field obscures the surgical field and creates a challenge. Excellent coordination and communication between the surgeon and the camera operator is crucial to the success of SPLS, but sometimes it is not enough. The consortium for LESS surgery has stated in their consensus statement that "the surgeon should be able to visualize structures from differing perspectives, preferably offline from the axis of the instruments" [15]. In an attempt to overcome the challenge of a compromised view, different cameras and endoscopes were evaluated.

9.3.1 Rigid Laparoscope

The rigid laparoscope is the most commonly used endoscope for SPLS, as in any other laparoscopic surgery. The use of a 30 degree laparoscope is highly recommended if a rigid laparoscope is being used, this is due to its ability to deviate from the axis of the instruments while viewing the surgical field [14, 20].

Standard telescopes are 30 cm in length, and this might exacerbate the challenge of instruments' "sword fighting", especially outside the abdomen. This issue might be somewhat alleviated with the use of bariatric length telescopes. Longer laparoscopes can make it possible for the camera operator to hold the laparoscope further back and to leave the space closer to the access device for the surgeon to operate the instruments. Another deviation from the standard technical operation of the laparoscope is the light cord assembly. Traditionally the light cord attaches to the laparoscope at a right angle, which makes the laparoscope three-dimensionally space occupying. Assembling the light cord via a 90-degree angle connector will make the light cord and camera parallel, thus adding free space near the access device and enhancing the surgeon's maneuverability to operate the surgical instruments.

9.3.2   Flexible Endoscope

Palanivelu et al. [21] were the first to describe the feasibility of flexible endoscope for performing single-port cholecystectomy in human patients. They used the endoscope's working channels to pass instruments which assisted in the procedure. Soon after, more reports were published about a series of SPLS in both porcine models and in humans [11, 14, 22–23].

While definitely improving the compromised view of SPLS (due to both its ability to overlook the surgical field from multiple different angles and its inherent irrigation system), the use of a flexible endoscope has disadvantages as well. The lack of rigidity causes the endoscopes shaft to surender to the forces of gravity and hence often times the angle of view achieved is from down-up instead of the standard view. Most surgeons do not have experience with the flexible endoscope (gastroscope) and operating with this tool in the abdominal cavity is a new challenge that needs to be mastered. Another problematic issue is the limited availability of this device in the OR and the need for collaboration and cordination with gastroenterologists.

9.3.3   Modified Laparoscopes

Several modifications for the "classic" rigid laparoscopes have been developed. These modifications attempt to provide improvements for the viewing capabilities.

Two examples for such modifications are the EndoCAMeleon™ (Karl Storz-Endoscope), a 10-mm rigid non articulating scope with adjustable viewing angle of 0° to 120° and the IDEAL EYES HD™ Articulating Laparoscope (Stryker, Kalamazoo, MI, USA), a 10-mm scope equipped with an articulating tip with an angle range of up to 100° of flexion in all directions.

One study evaluated the efficacy of semi-rigid laparoscopes used in extreme angles (to view the anterior pelvis trans-vaginally) [24]. The conclusion was that

Fig. 9.7 A miniature camera anchored to a laparoscopic articulating instrument has the ability to supply additional angles for optimizing the view during SPLS

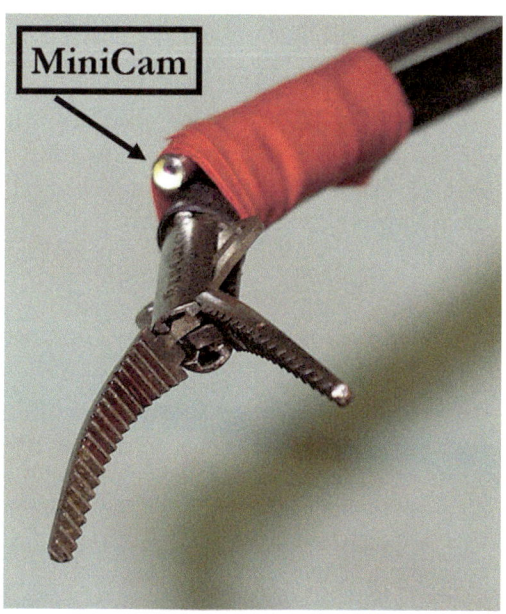

there was no obvious advantage gained by using the new laparoscopes. Another study has evaluated the Storz EndoCAMeleon™, the Olympus EndoEye™ and the Stryker IdealEye™. These articulating laparoscopes were compared using standard industry testing protocols for image resolution, distortion and color reproducibility and were concluded with conflicting results [25]. Their use, nevertheless has been shown to be feasible in several case series [26–29].

Articulating laparoscopes are important tools in SPLS, however they are still not the ideal solution for acquiring the best imaging necessary. Several experimental cameras aimed toward achieving better viewing angles in SPLS are being developed. One experimental method of achieving enhanced visualization in SPLS, either as the primary camera or as an adjunct is the use of a miniature camera anchored to a laparoscopic articulating instrument (Fig. 9.7). This camera is still under development and holds the promise of having the ability to acquire additional angles of view during SPLS [30].

9.4 Retraction

One of the basic requirements of any kind of surgery is retraction. Retraction enables the surgical field to be visible to the surgeons in both open and laparoscopic surgery and enhances surgical dissection. As procedures become less invasive, adequate retraction must often be sacrificed, as ports designated for retraction are invariably the first to be waived. Nevertheless, surgeons must find ways to provide adequate retraction even though they use a reduced number of ports. Inadequate retraction undoubtedly serves as an obstacle when performing SPLS, especially when the anatomy encountered is less than "textbook" [31]. Aside from its inevitable prolongation of operative time, inadequate retraction can potentially convert a technically straightforward case into a complex ordeal, lead to the conversion of a single-port surgical procedure to conventional laparoscopy or open surgery, and eventually increase morbidity. As such, the achievement of optimal retraction without additional ports is an everlasting pursuit.

9.4.1 Trans-Abdominal Stay Sutures and Endoloops

One commonly employed method of retraction in SPLS is trans-abdominal stay sutures [32]. The sutures can be placed through the dissected organ (e.g. through the fundus of the gallbladder in cholecystectomy) using a straight Keith needle and then externalized trans-abdominal to allow continuous extracorporeal manipulation. This method allows for continuous external manipulation of the target organ while leaving a negligible mark where the needle passed through the skin. Some surgeons perform a variation of this method whereby the needle enters and exits the abdomen in two different locations (e.g. enters at the subxiphoid region, is sutured to the Hartman's pouch and exits in the right lower quadrant) thereby enabling a "marionette" effect of external manipulation.

The major limitation of the trans-abdominal stay suture method of retraction is the potential perforation and leakage of gastrointestinal content into the peritoneal cavity; hence it is limited to surgeries which involve retraction of organs to be removed, e.g. cholecystectomy. Another drawback of this method is its restricted retraction capability, with a fixed anchoring point, which makes repositioning during surgery impossible.

Trans-abdominal endoloops have also been used to achieve gallbladder retraction during SPLS cholecystectomy [31, 33]. The endoloop is introduced trans-abdominally into the peritoneal cavity and is attached to the gallbladder, which is then retracted to the anterior abdominal wall. Endoloops are safer to use then stay sutures in the manner that they have less of a potential for a perforation or leak, given that they do not pierce the tissue. Nevertheless, their retraction capability is sub-optimal.

9.4.2 Magnetic Anchoring and Guidance System (MAGS)

Magnetic Anchoring and Guidance System (MAGS) employs intra-abdominal magnetically-anchored instruments to perform trocar-sparing laparoscopic surgery. MAGS uses 2 internal neodymium-iron-boron magnetic platforms introduced into the abdomen through a 12-mm trocar. The internal platforms are magnetically anchored to external anchors on the patient's skin, capable of manipulating and

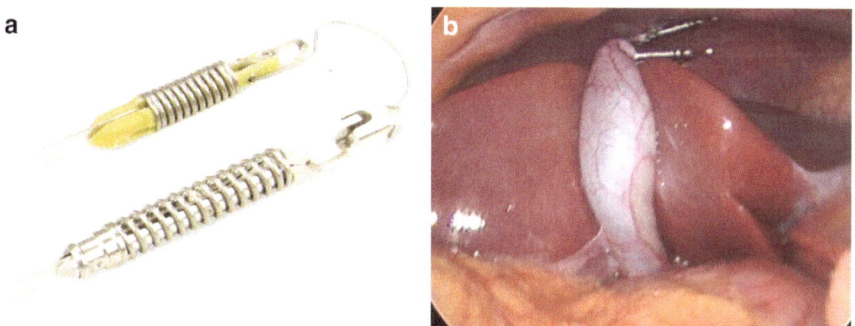

Fig. 9.8 (**a**) Endograb™ (Virtual Ports). The use of endo-retractors optimizes retraction and exposure capability including changing retraction angles during the operation. (**b**) Gallbladder retraction achieved with the device

stabilizing these platforms [34]. The internal magnetic platforms allow for a non-traumatic elevation and retraction of organs like the liver and spleen. A modification of the MAGS retraction system was described using magnet-conjugated clips, which were placed along the inferior edge of the liver and were used to accomplish retraction [35]. MAGS platform has recently also been described to operate surgical instruments and this way to enhance triangulation [36, 37]. Nevertheless, studies with the MAGS have only been performed on animal models and cadavers. The main technical pitfall of the MAGS system (in addition to its cost) is the exponential decrease in magnetic coupling strength as a function of distance (i.e. abdominal wall thickness). Hence, a tissue thickness greater than 15-mm does not allow use of the magnetic anchoring system [34].

9.4.3 Internal Retractors

The decreased ability to achieve optimal retraction in SPLS has led to the development of newly designed internal retractors. These devices are introduced to the abdominal cavity via the SPLS access system and anchor the target organ to the abdominal wall. An example for such a retractor is the EndoGrab™ (Virtual Ports Ltd., Caesaera, Israel) (Fig. 9.8) [14, 31]. This is an internally-anchored retracting device which can be introduced into the abdomen through a 5-mm port. Once deployed, one of the two grasping ends is attached to the target organ and the other is then anchored to the abdominal wall. Internal retractors can be anchored in different places within the abdominal cavity, including under the diaphragm without concern of entering the thoracic cavity. In addition, their position can be repeatedly adjusted throughout surgery in order to allow for a dynamic retraction, just like in open surgery. The ability of internal retractors to accomplish complete anterior-superior retraction of the gallbladder fundus was shown to be a distinct advantage over other methods [31].

9.5 Instruments

Traditional laparoscopic instruments are straight and rigid. The mobility of straight instruments is limited and when a few straight instruments are inserted through a common entry point in the abdominal wall, their maneuverability is lacking. In addition, in these circumstances triangulation of the instruments and camera towards the surgical field is limited as well, which turns even a simple surgical procedure into a technically demanding ordeal. This problem is even more prominent if the single-port access device is bulky and long [20]. Many efforts have been made to develop instruments that would simplify the technical challenge and would achieve triangulation, mainly curved and articulating instruments. Even though the use of straight laparoscopic instruments comes with technical difficulty, all laparoscopic instruments can still be used for SPLS. The main pros for the use of straight ("conventional") laparoscopic instruments is the reduced cost associated with their use by eliminating the need to buy new instruments, and the elimination of a learning curve for the use of a new type of instruments [38]. Some studies have shown the feasibility and safety of large series of SPLS using standard laparoscopic instruments [38, 39].

9.5.1 Articulating Instruments

Articulating (also called "roticulating" or "wristed") instruments are ones with maneuverability at their tip that can be controlled with movement of the surgeon's wrist. Some of them allow locking of the articulation at the desired angle as well as 360° rotation of the tip (which when combined with the tip's angulation creates a three-dimensional tip movement). The use of articulating instruments facilitates triangulation towards the surgical field and hence enhances the view and dissection capability (Fig. 9.9).

Many articulated instruments are available on the market. The authors' main experience is with RealHand™ articulating instruments (Novare Surgical, Cupertino, CA, USA) (Fig. 9.10) [14]. Other brands include SILS™ Hand Instruments (Covidien), Autonomy™ Laparo-Angle™ instruments (Cambridge Endo®, Framingham, MA, USA) and EnTouch® handles and AEM® articulating laparoscopic instrument (Encision Inc, Boulder, CO, USA).

The main advantage of articulating instruments are the ability to create instrument triangulation and a very particulate dissection capability. The disadvantage is the need for a learning curve for their operation, which is complex especially due to the fact that handling the instruments is not intuitive and adds a third dimension of movement while operating with a two dimensional view. Also, best retraction and triangulation is achieved while crossing the handles (i.e. the surgeon's right hand controls the instrument which approaches the surgical field from the left and vice versa) (Fig. 9.9).

Fig. 9.9 Illustration of the need for triangulation, and the way to achieve it in SPLS surgery. Articulating instruments use enhances triangulation hence improving the view

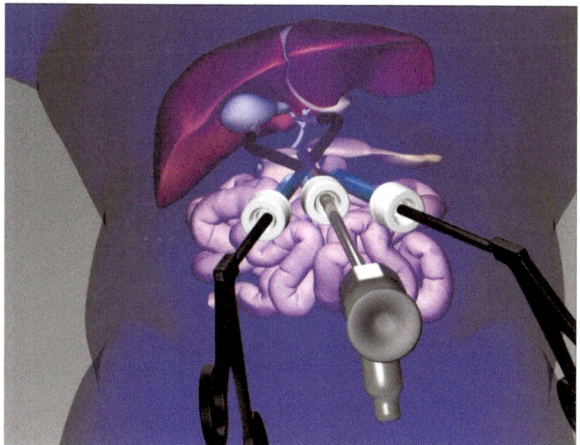

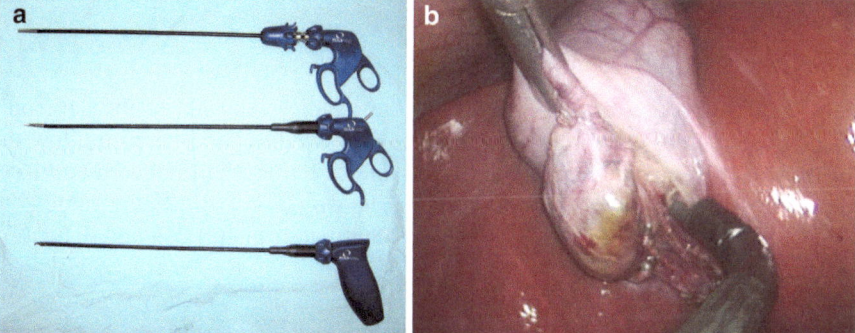

Fig. 9.10 (**a**) RealHand™ (Novare) articulating laparoscopic instruments. (**b**) Dissection of the gallbladder from its fossa by an articulating hook during single-port cholecystectomy. The use of articulating instruments enables local triangulation, enhances dissection capability and improves the view

The more complex operation of the articulating devices was demonstrated by Tuncel et al. which compared the success of medical students in completing standardized laparoscopic suturing tasks with a standard versus an articulating needle driver [40].

Sodergren et al., on the other hand, have shown no difference in the learning curve when using straight or curved laparoscopic instruments when performing simple laparoscopic tasks [41]. The only significant factor they found related to a quicker learning curve was the subjects' prior exposure to multiport laparoscopy, with a quicker improvement of the single-port technique in subjects who were multiport laparoscopic proficient.

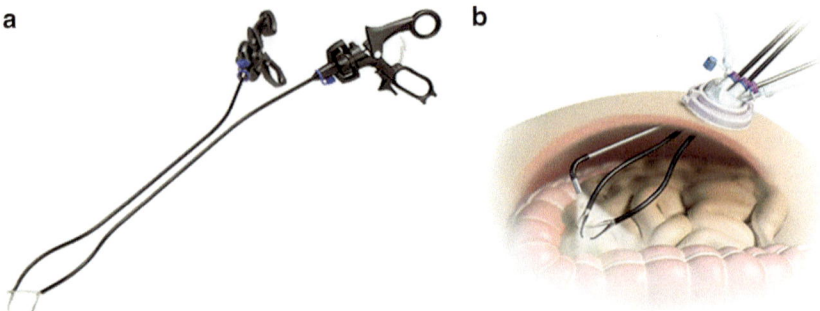

Fig. 9.11 (**a**) HiQ™ LS curved laparoscopic instruments (Olympus). (**b**) The instruments' curves result in their tip and handle having the same axis, which gives the surgeon the feeling of using virtual trocars with triangulation as in traditional laparoscopy without crossing hands

9.5.2   Curved Instruments

The use of curved instruments situates the handles (and hence the surgeon's hands) apart from each other. Instruments with double curvings also allow the instrument tip and handle to come in the same direction, as in standard multiport laparoscopy. This technique is intuitive in the way that it allows the surgeon to work without crossing handles and hence facilitate triangulation and dissection (Fig. 9.11).

As in articulating instruments, there is also a large variety of curved instruments available on the market. An example is "S-PORTAL® Instruments acc. to LEROY" (Karl Storz-Endoskope) which have four curves, resulting in the instrument tip and handle having the same axis ("coaxial instruments"), which is reported by the manufacturer as giving the surgeon the feeling of using virtual multiport laparoscopy with triangulation without crossing hands. Another example is HiQ™ LS curved instruments (Olympus, Tokyo, Japan) (Fig. 9.11).

Manukyan et al. have shown ergonomic superiority of curved over straight instruments in a prospective study on multiport laparoscopic sigmoid resections [42]. Stolzenberg et al. compared curved (single-port), articulating (single-port) and straight (multiport) instruments both in basic laparoscopic simulator and in an animal lab and showed superiority of the curved instruments over articulating instruments with decreased operative time in both the simulator and in the animal model. In that manner they found that using curved instruments via a single-port is comparable to the use of straight instruments via multiport laparoscopy [43]. Rimonda et al. showed the superiority of curved coaxial instruments over straight instruments in the rate of task performance in a laparoscopic single-port lab simulation performed by surgical residents [44]. Botden et al. evaluated box trainer task performance of experienced (>50 laparoscopic procedures) surgeons and compared

Fig. 9.12 A flexible CO_2 laser tool (Lumenis®, Yokneam, Israel) delivers thermal energy to porcine small bowel mesentery, causing division and coagulation of the mesentery. Conventional thermal energy devices are rigid, hence they do not enhance triangulation in SPLS

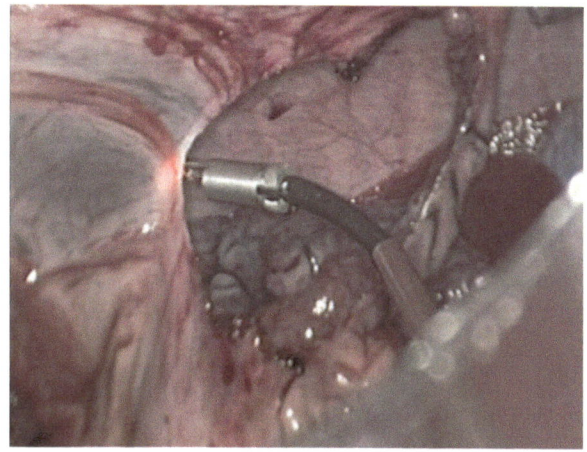

standard laparoscopy, SPLS with straight crossed instruments and SPLS with curved instruments. Their results, however, showed faster task performance with both standard laparoscopy and single-port crossed instruments than with single-port curved instruments. Fourteen out of the fifteen participants preferred standard laparoscopy over SPLS [45]. To date, the evidence for the superiority of one of the types of instruments over the others is lacking.

9.5.3   Instruments for Hemostasis

As in any laparoscopic surgery, energy devices are crucial. Obviously, standard laparoscopic thermal energy devices can be used in SPLS as well as in standard laparoscopy. Current technologies are based on either ultrasonic energy like the Harmonic™ (Ethicon) and the Sonicision™ (Covidien) or bipolar coagulation (e.g. LigaSure™ (Covidien) and Enseal™ (Ethicon)). The problem with these standard energy delivering devices is their inability to articulate in order to enhance triangulation which is a crucial element in making SPLS "user friendly" as mentioned above.

In 2009 Ogura et al. reported the development of a small ultrasonically-activated transducer attached to the tip of an articulating device [46]. They reported that the device offered both coagulation and dissection performance similar to that of conventional instruments in a porcine model. Unfortunately, no follow up studies with this device were reported in humans.

Recently a novel technology to deliver thermal energy via a flexible laparoscopic instrument has been developed: it features CO_2 laser energy transmitted through a specialized flexible optical fiber [47, 48]. This technology was tested in animal models and is reported to provide excellent hemostasis and to cause minimal collateral tissue damage [48] (Fig. 9.12). Human studies are currently under way mainly using robotic articulating devices.

Fig. 9.13 The SPIDER®
Surgical System
(TransEnterix), a minimally
invasive surgical device that
includes an access device and
a combination of two
articulating instruments and
one straight instrument for
retraction

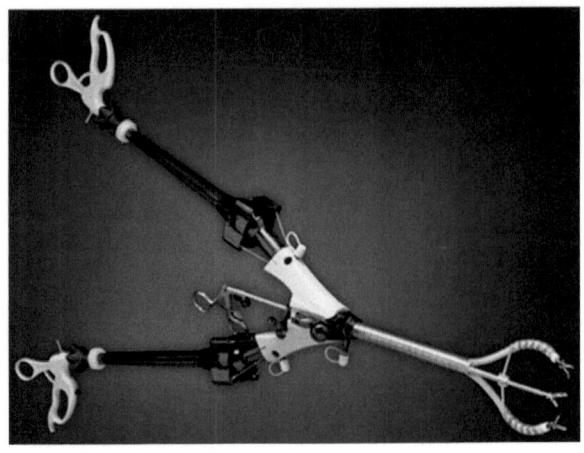

9.5.4 Combined Dedicated Systems

The SPIDER® (Single-port Instrument Delivery Extended Reach) Surgical System
(TransEnterix Inc., Durham, NC, USA) is a minimally invasive surgical device that
includes an access device and a combination of two articulating instruments and one
straight instrument for retraction (Fig. 9.13). It is claimed that it is able to achieve
intra-abdominal triangulation via a single site and to offer true left and true right
motion with flexible, articulating instruments. Recent feasibility studies in animal
models and one case report in a human have shown the feasibility and safety of its use
[49–51]. The most recent study noted difficulty in achieving optimal retraction with
the system [50]. No comparative studies to other systems were performed up to date.

9.6 Summary

Many different access devices, cameras, retraction methods and operative instruments are available for use and can be used in SPLS. Some of these are commercially available and some are still experimental. Some are dedicated tools which
were developed especially for SPLS and some are improvisations or adjustments of
previously accepted instruments for standard laparoscopic surgery to the novel concept of SPLS. Maintaining the principles of optimizing the view, supplying adequate retraction, and achieving triangulation should be at the basis of the surgeon's
selection of which tools to use when performing SPLS.

References

1. Cameron JL, Gadacz TR (1991) Laparoscopic cholecystectomy. Ann Surg 213:1–2
2. Gadacz TR, Talamini MA, Lillemoe KD, Yeo CJ (1990) Laparoscopic cholecystectomy. Surg
   Clin North Am 70:1249–1262

3. Cuschier A, Terblanche J (1990) Laparoscopic cholecystectomy: evolution, not revolution. Surg Endosc 4:125–126

4. Phillips E, Daykhovsky L, Carroll B, Gershman A, Grundfest WS (1990) Laparoscopic cholecystectomy: instrumentation and technique. J Laparoendosc Surg 1:3–15

5. Tagaya N, Kita J, Takagi K, Imada T, Ishikawa K, Kogure H, Ohyama O (1998) Experience with three-port laparoscopic cholecystectomy. J Hepatobiliary Pancreat Surg 5:309–311

6. Reardon PR, Kamelgard JI, Applebaum B, Rossman L, Brunicardi FC (1999) Feasibility of laparoscopic cholecystectomy with miniaturized instrumentation in 50 consecutive cases. World J Surg 23:128–132

7. Leung KF, Lee KW, Cheung TY, Leung LC, Lau KW (1996) Laparoscopic cholecystectomy: two-port technique. Endoscopy 28:505–507

8. Kagaya T (2001) Laparoscopic cholecystectomy via two ports, using the "Twin-Port" system. J Hepatobiliary Pancreat Surg 8:76–80

9. Ngoi SS, Goh P, Kok K, Kum CK, Cheah WK (1999) Needlescopic or minisite cholecystectomy. Surg Endosc 13(3):303–305

10. Tacchino R, Greco F, Matera D (2009) Single-incision laparoscopic cholecystectomy: surgery without a visible scar. Surg Endosc 23(4):896–899

11. Elazary R, Khalaileh A, Zamir G, Har-Lev M, Almogy G, Rivkind AI, Mintz Y (2009) Single-trocar cholecystectomy using a flexible endoscope and articulating laparoscopic instruments: a bridge to NOTES or the final form? Surg Endosc 23(5):969–972

12. Rolanda C, Lima E, Pego JM et al (2007) Third-generation cholecystectomy by natural orifices: transgastric and transvesical combined approach. Gastrointest Endosc 65:111–117

13. Mintz Y, Horgan S, Cullen J, Ramamoorthy S, Chock A, Savu MK, Easter DW, Talamini MA (2007) NOTES: the hybrid technique. J Laparoendosc Adv Surg Tech A 17:402–406

14. Shussman N, Schlager A, Elazary R, Khalaileh A, Keidar A, Talamini M, Horgan S, Rivkind AI, Mintz Y (2011) Single-incision laparoscopic cholecystectomy: lessons learned for success. Surg Endosc 25(2):404–407

15. Gill IS, Advincula AP, Aron M, Caddedu J, Canes D, Curcillo PG 2nd, Desai MM, Evanko JC, Falcone T, Fazio V, Gettman M, Gumbs AA, Haber GP, Kaouk JH, Kim F, King SA, Ponsky J, Remzi F, Rivas H, Rosemurgy A, Ross S, Schauer P, Sotelo R, Speranza J, Sweeney J, Teixeira J (2010) Consensus statement of the consortium for laparoendoscopic single-site surgery. Surg Endosc 24(4):762–768

16. Hayashi M, Asakuma M, Komeda K, Miyamoto Y, Hirokawa F, Tanigawa N (2010) Effectiveness of a surgical glove port for single port surgery. World J Surg 34(10):2487–2489

17. Livraghi L, Berselli M, Bianchi V, Latham L, Farassino L, Cocozza E (2012) Glove technique in single-port access laparoscopic surgery: results of an initial experience. Minim Invasive Surg 2012:415430

18. Uematsu D, Akiyama G, Matsuura M, Hotta K (2010) Single-access laparoscopic colectomy with a novel multiport device in sigmoid colectomy for colon cancer. Dis Colon Rectum 53(4):496–501

19. Ishida H, Okada N, Ishibashi K, Ohsawa T, Kumamoto K, Haga N (2011) Single-incision laparoscopic-assisted surgery for colon cancer via a periumbilical approach using a surgical glove: initial experience with 9 cases. Int J Surg 9(2):150–154

20. Dhumane PW, Diana M, Leroy J, Marescaux J (2011) Minimally invasive single-site surgery for the digestive system: a technological review. J Minim Access Surg 7(1):40–51

21. Palanivelu C, Rajan PS, Rangarajan M, Parthasarathi R, Senthilnathan P, Praveenraj P (2008) Transumbilical flexible endoscopic cholecystectomy in humans: first feasibility study using a hybrid technique. Endoscopy 40(5):428–431

22. Binenbaum SJ, Teixeira JA, Forrester GJ, Harvey EJ, Afthinos J, Kim GJ, Koshy N, McGinty J, Belsley SJ, Todd GJ (2009) Single-incision laparoscopic cholecystectomy using a flexible endoscope. Arch Surg 144(8):734–738

23. Noguera J, Tejada S, Tortajada C, Sánchez A, Muñoz J (2013) Prospective, randomized clinical trial comparing the use of a single-port device with that of a flexible endoscope with no other device for transumbilical cholecystectomy: LLATZER-FSIS pilot study. Surg Endosc 27(11):4284–4290

24. Hackethal A, Ionesi-Pasacica J, Eskef K, Oehmke F, Münstedt K, Tinneberg HR (2011) Transvaginal NOTES with semi-rigid and rigid endoscopes that allow adjustable viewing angles. Arch Gynecol Obstet 283(1):131–132

25. Goldsmith ZG, Astroza GM, Wang AJ, Simmons WN, Iqbal MW, Lipkin ME, Preminger GM, Ferrandino MN (2012) Optical performance comparison of deflectable laparoscopes for lapa-roendoscopic single-site surgery. J Endourol 26(10):1340–1345

26. Misawa T, Sakamoto T, Ito R, Shiba H, Gocho T, Wakiyama S, Ishida Y, Yanaga K (2011) Single-incision laparoscopic splenectomy using the "tug-exposure technique" in adults: results of ten initial cases. Surg Endosc 25(10):3222–3227

27. Gocho T, Misawa T, Suzuki F, Ito R, Shiba H, Futagawa Y, Wakiyama S, Ishida Y, Yanaga K (2013) Single-incision laparoscopic surgery for giant hepatic cyst. Asian J Endosc Surg 6(3):237–240

28. Kumakiri J, Kikuchi I, Kitade M, Matsuoka S, Tokita S, Takeda S (2010) Linear salpingotomy with suturing by single incision laparoscopic surgery for tubal ectopic pregnancy. Acta Obstet Gynecol Scand 89(12):1604–1607

29. Zhang G, Liu S, Yu W, Wang L, Liu N, Li F, Hu S (2011) Gasless laparoendoscopic single-site surgery with abdominal-wall lift in general surgery: initial experience. Surg Endosc 25(1): 298–304

30. Abu Gazala M, Shussman N, Abu Gazala S, Schlager A, Elazary R, Ponomernco O, Khalaila A, Rivkind AI, Mintz Y (2012) Miniature camera for enhanced visualization for single-port surgery and NOTES. J Laparoendosc Adv Surg Tech A 22(10):984–988

31. Schlager A, Khalaileh A, Shussman N, Elazary R, Keidar A, Pikarsky AJ, Ben-Shushan A, Shibolet O, Horgan S, Talamini M, Zamir G, Rivkind AI, Mintz Y (2010) Providing more through less: current methods of retraction in SIMIS and NOTES cholecystectomy. Surg Endosc 24(7):1542–1546

32. Solomon D, Bell RL, Duffy AJ, Roberts KE (2010) Single-port cholecystectomy: small scar, short learning curve. Surg Endosc 24(12):2954–2957

33. Uras C, Boler DE (2013) Endoloop retraction technique in single-port laparoscopic cholecys-tectomy: experience in 27 patients. J Laparoendosc Adv Surg Tech A 23(6):545–548

34. Park S, Bergs RA, Eberhart R, Baker L, Fernandez R, Cadeddu JA (2007) Trocar-less instru-mentation for laparoscopy: magnetic positioning of intra-abdominal camera and retractor. Ann Surg 245(3):379–384

35. Ryou M, Thompson CC (2009) Magnetic retraction in natural-orifice transluminal endoscopic surgery (NOTES): addressing the problem of traction and countertraction. Endoscopy 41(2): 143–148

36. Joseph RA, Salas NA, Donovan MA, Reardon PR, Bass BL, Dunkin BJ (2012) Single-site laparoscopic (SSL) cholecystectomy in human cadavers using a novel percutaneous instru-ment platform and a magnetic anchoring and guidance system (MAGS): reestablishing the "critical view". Surg Endosc 26(1):149–153

37. Arain NA, Cadeddu JA, Hogg DC, Bergs R, Fernandez R, Scott DJ (2012) Magnetically anchored cautery dissector improves triangulation, depth perception, and workload during single-site laparoscopic cholecystectomy. J Gastrointest Surg 16(9):1807–1813

38. Podolsky ER, Curcillo PG (2010) Single port access (SPA) surgery: a 24-month experience. J Gastrointest Surg 14(5):759–767

39. Tsai YC, Lin VC, Chung SD, Ho CH, Jaw FS, Tai HC (2012) Ergonomic and geometric tricks of laparoendoscopic single-site surgery (LESS) by using conventional laparoscopic instru-ments. Surg Endosc 26(9):2671–2677

40. Tuncel A, Lucas S, Bensalah K, Zeltser IS, Jenkins A, Saeedi O, Park S, Cadeddu JA (2008) A randomized comparison of conventional vs articulating laparoscopic needle-drivers for per-forming standardized suturing tasks by laparoscopy-naive subjects. BJU Int 101(6):727–730

41. Sodergren M, McGregor C, Farne HA, Cao J, Lv Z, Purkayastha S, Athanasiou T, Darzi A, Paraskeva P (2013) A randomised comparative study evaluating learning curves of novices in a basic single-incision laparoscopic surgery task. J Gastrointest Surg 17(3):569–575

42. Manukyan GA, Waseda M, Inaki N, Torres Bermudez JR, Gacek IA, Rudinski A, Buess GF (2007) Ergonomics with the use of curved versus straight laparoscopic graspers during recto-sigmoid resection: results of a multiprofile comparative study. Surg Endosc 21(7):1079–1089
43. Stolzenburg JU, Kallidonis P, Oh MA, Ghulam N, Do M, Haefner T, Dietel A, Till H, Sakellaropoulos G, Liatsikos EN (2010) Comparative assessment of laparoscopic single-site surgery instruments to conventional laparoscopic in laboratory setting. J Endourol 24(2): 239–245
44. Rimonda R, Tang B, Brown SI, Cuschieri A (2012) Comparison of endoscopic task performance with crossed versus uncrossed straight and curved instruments through a single port. Surg Endosc 26(12):3605–3611
45. Botden S, Strijkers R, Fransen S, Stassen L, Bouvy N (2011) The use of curved vs. straight instruments in single port access surgery, on standardized box trainer tasks. Surg Endosc 25(8):2703–2710
46. Ogura G, Nakamura R, Muragaki Y, Hashizume M, Iseki H (2009) Development of an articulating ultrasonically activated device for laparoscopic surgery. Surg Endosc 23(9):2138–2142
47. Cheetham PJ, Truesdale MD, Lee DJ, Landman JM, Badani KK (2010) Use of a flexible carbon dioxide laser fiber for precise dissection of the neurovascular bundle during robot-assisted laparoscopic prostatectomy. J Endourol 24(7):1091–1096
48. Gofrit ON, Khalaileh A, Ponomarenko O, Abu-Gazala M, Lewinsky RM, Elazary R, Shussman N, Shalhav A, Mintz Y (2012) Laparoscopic partial nephrectomy using a flexible CO_2 laser fiber. JSLS 16(4):588–591
49. Pryor AD, Tushar JR, DiBernardo LR (2010) Single-port cholecystectomy with the TransEnterix SPIDER: simple and safe. Surg Endosc 24(4):917–923
50. Kim SD, Landman J, Sung GT (2013) Laparoendoscopic single-site surgery with the second-generation single port instrument delivery extended reach surgical system in a porcine model. Korean J Urol 54(5):327–332
51. Leveillee RJ, Castle SM, Gorin MA, Salas N, Gorbatiy V (2011) Initial experience with laparoendoscopic single-site simple nephrectomy using the TransEnterix SPIDER surgical system: assessing feasibility and safety. J Endourol 25(6):923–925

Chapter 10
Technical Considerations

Masazumi Okajima, Yasutomo Ojima, and Masanori Yoshimitsu

Abstract In this paper we describe the basic techniques for a single-port laparoscopic surgery. The surgical techniques are classified into the multiple trocar method and the multi-channel port method because of access port differences. They are also classified as well according to technique, e.g., the parallel technique, cross technique, and cross hand technique. Forceps manipulation is different in each technique, therefore, it is important for surgeons to understand the characteristics of these methods. An appropriate method should be chosen on the specific situation to render surgical maneuver to be easily performed.

Keywords Cross hand technique • Cross technique • Multi-channel port method • Multiple trocar method • Parallel technique

10.1 Introduction

It is important to understand the difference between single-port laparoscopic surgery (SPLS) and conventional laparoscopic surgery when considering a SPLS. Trocars should be placed in consideration to forceps selection and its manipulation. In a SPLS, there are a great number of limitations with respect to surgical manipulation because multiple devices are inserted almost coaxially within a single small incision, and thus, the devices or surgeon's hands can interfere with each other (Fig. 10.1). It is vital to exercise ingenuity regarding the approach and the manipulation of the forceps to overcome this limitation.

M. Okajima (✉) • Y. Ojima
Department of Surgery, Hiroshima City Hospital,
7-33 Motomachi, Naka-ku, Hiroshima 730-8518, Japan
e-mail: mokajima@hiroshima-u.ac.jp

M. Yoshimitsu
Department of Surgery, Hiroshima City Asa Hospital, Hiroshima, Japan

T. Mori and G. Dapri (eds.), *Reduced Port Laparoscopic Surgery*,
DOI 10.1007/978-4-431-54601-6_10, © Springer Japan 2014

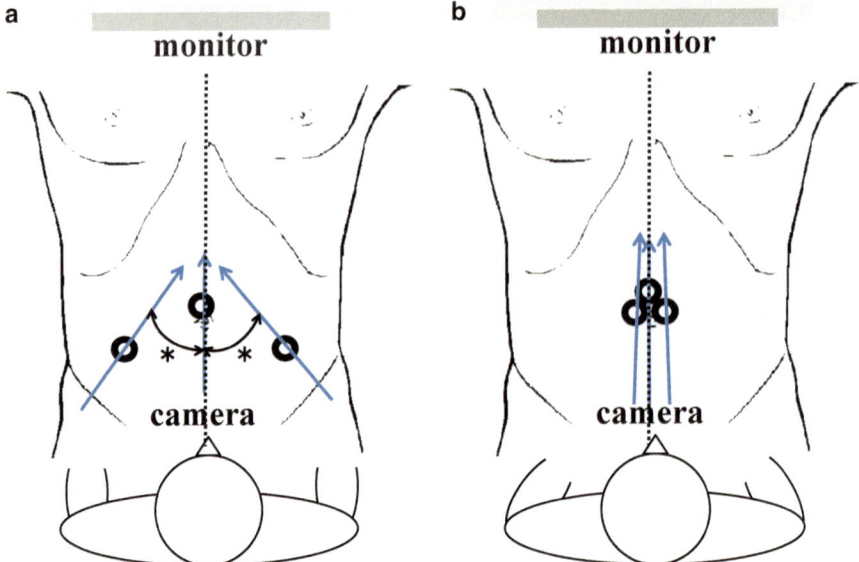

Fig. 10.1 The difference between conventional laparoscopic surgery (**a**) and SPLS (**b**)

10.2 Types and Characteristics of Access Ports

Usually, a trans-navel approach is chosen. This approach consists of a method that uses a platform exclusively applied in a SPLS and has several trocars inserted into a single incision.

10.2.1 Multiple Trocar Method (Fig. 10.2) [1]

This method requires the gathering of multiple trocars that are used in conventional laparoscopic surgery in a limited space within the umbilical region. Several trocars are inserted into one skin incision. For the forceps used exclusively for tissue retraction, direct puncture insertion can also be performed. Direct insertion of the forceps is of great help to avoid interference of trocar head. On the other hand, this causes difficulty in replacing the forceps, and manipulation of the forceps is encumbered. In addition, occurrence of tissue damage should be in consideration. Usually, a common surgical method is to insert about three 5-mm trocars into the umbilical region. If trocars with large heads are used, they may interfere with one another. To avoid this issue, it is better to use a trocar with a small head or to arrange trocars of differing lengths. Once a 2-cm incision in the umbilical region and then an incision in the region between the umbilical fossa and beneath the skin is made, a space of about 2.5 to 3 cm can be obtained. With this approach, a distance of 3 cm or more

Fig. 10.2 Multiple trocar
method

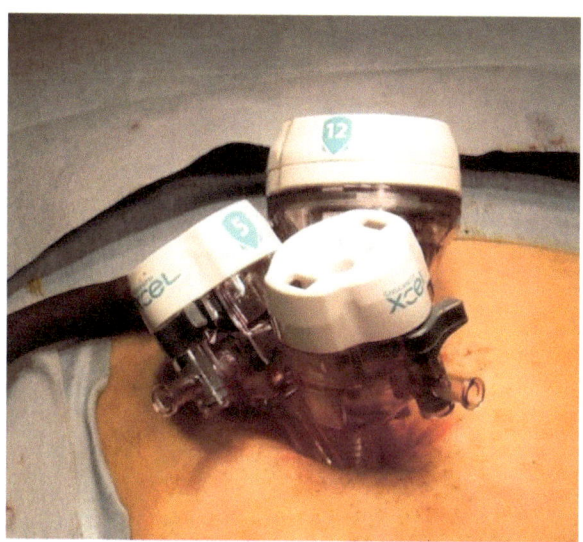

between two forceps can be ensured. Moreover, if the incision is extended to about 2.5 cm, the distance between the two forceps could be 3 cm or more. Therefore, it becomes possible to operate via laparoscopy and have a feeling similar to that of performing a conventional operation. On the other hand, if the incision is too small and excessive stress is applied to the skin, the tissue could sustain injury, and wound healing could be delayed. Hence, an incision with some margin should be made. Moreover, if resection of an organ is required, it might be necessary to incise the fascia more. In that case, attention is required because if the fascial closure were performed too securely, a complicating hernia could occur.

Because a major advantage of the multiple trocar method is the greater flexibility and configurability of the distance between the two forceps, we can also use a conventional trocar or forceps; that is to say, SPLS can be performed without using special equipment. For a multiple organ resection, attention is required because a trocar positional change can be difficult once the trocar is inserted. It is difficult to always insert a trocar in the same position for various cases. Individual differences among surgeons are likely to occur. In addition, upon insertion of the first trocar, it is necessary to use the optical view trocar or to make a small incision. Moreover, manipulation proficiency is required to insert the second and third trocars safely because positional confirmation of the trocar tip is difficult.

10.2.2 Multi-Channel Port Method (Fig. 10.3) [2]

The advantages of the multi-channel port method are in opposition to those of the multiple trocar method. With this method, insertion and indwelling are easy, and

Fig. 10.3 Multi-channel port method

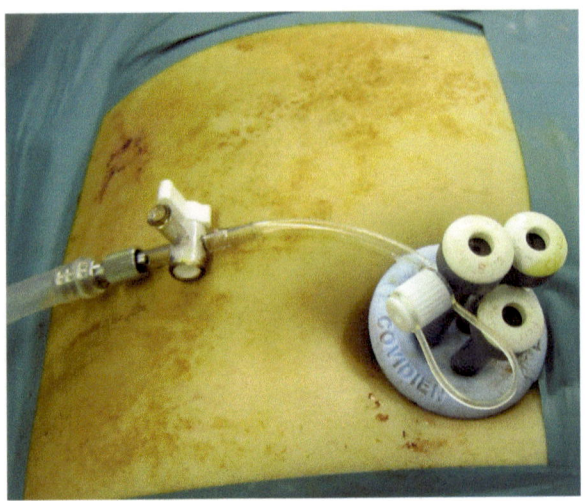

experience has shown that there is little negative impact. Moreover, it can be performed safely because the port in this method is kept in place after a fasciotomy has been performed appropriately. The indwelling of the second and third trocars is also easy. However, the distance between the two forceps is generally smaller than that of the multiple trocar method, as the trocars are arranged at a given distance. On the other hand, this method becomes effective for surgeries such as a multiple organ resection or large intestine surgery because we can move each channel position by turning a trocar's port.

10.3 Classification of Basic Surgical Techniques

In a SPLS, a device having the smallest possible diameter is desirable to reduce interference between the devices. The basic surgical techniques are classified as follows. However, these classifications can be further broken into two types, depending on whether a surgeon uses a straight-type or flexure-type device. We will describe the techniques with the different characteristics of forceps to be considered.

10.3.1 Parallel Technique (Fig. 10.4)

In the parallel technique, a surgeon performs a surgical technique while holding two straight-type devices in both hands. As for the implementation of the parallel technique, it is similar to that of the conventional laparoscopic surgery in that a surgeon

Fig. 10.4 Parallel technique

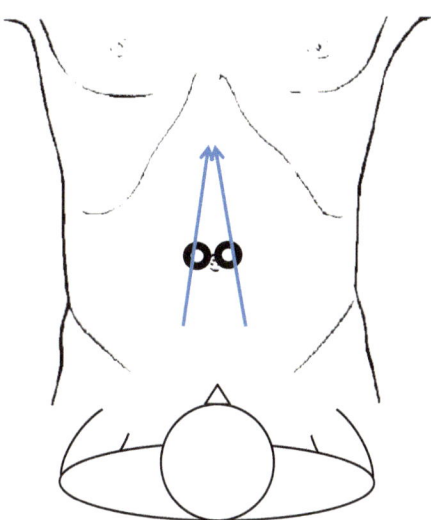

holds an electro-cautery and a dissecting forceps in the dominant hand, as well as a holding forceps in the non-dominant hand to display the operation field. Therefore, this technique is easy to introduce. However, as the distance between the trocars in the umbilical region becomes smaller, the devices overlap coaxially, and their movements interfere with each other making surgical techniques difficult. In the multiple trocar method, the distance between the two trocars can be expanded to 3–4 cm, a distance that is suitable for the parallel technique. Because the distance between the two trocars is less than 3 cm in the multi-channel port method, there are only a limited number of surgical techniques that can be applied in the parallel technique because the devices may collide with one another.

10.3.2 Cross Technique (Fig. 10.5)

In this technique, a triangular formation can be re-established with the intersection of the forceps. Surgeons must become accustomed to the fact that the right and left sides on a monitor are the reverse of the surgeon's right and left hands actually being used.

As for the right and left tips of a forceps, they can be gradually detached at the intersecting point. Therefore, it is easier to use bent forceps. With this technique, the best triangular formation is obtained if the forceps has both tips bent. However, using such a forceps is technically difficult. This is because even if a retention forceps is bent, its manipulation is relatively easy; however, if those apparatuses are used for incision or dissection and are also bent, the difficulty of the manipulation increases. Therefore, it is appropriate to use only (exclusively?) a curved forceps among the surgical instruments used in this clinical setting.

Fig. 10.5 Cross technique
using bent forceps

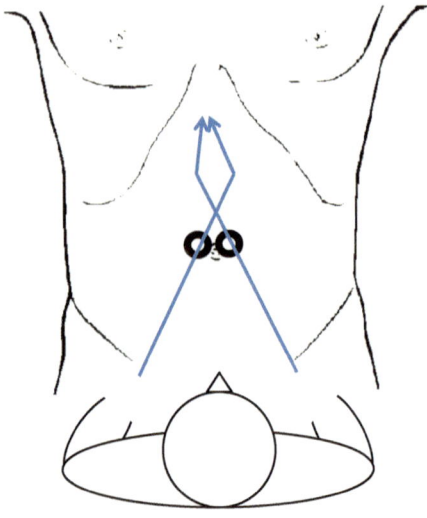

Fig. 10.6 Cross hand
technique

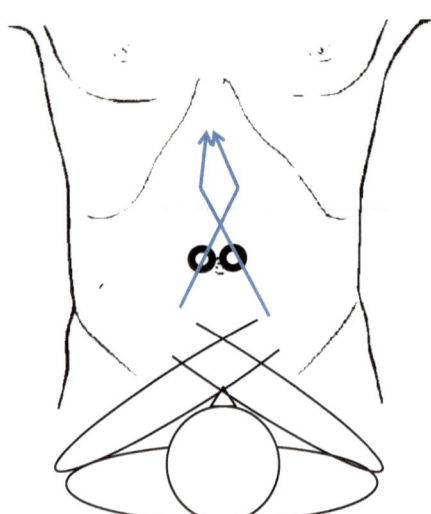

10.3.3   *Cross Hand Technique (Fig. 10.6)*

A technique to correct the left–right reversal on a monitor is the cross technique.
In clinical settings, surgeons rarely prefer this technique. As a result of this reversal,
the forceps sometimes move in a direction different to the surgeon's intention. The
above-mentioned techniques can also be applicable to the parallel technique and the
cross technique. It is important to understand that these three techniques have their
own property and character. Before the clinical application of SPLS, surgeons

should be trained for ingenuity of these techniques. In clinical settings, it is absurd to be a fundamentalist of a specific technique. As techniques differ by situations, surgeons should be prepared to apply the best technique described above or combine applicable techniques.

In this section, we described the basic concept of techniques in performing a SPLS. It is also true that each procedure needs to be discussed more in detail not only for incision or dissection, but for tissue retraction or tissue approximation. More detailed information regarding techniques for each procedure may be described in the following chapters.

References

1. Curcillo PG et al (2010) Single Port Access (SPATM) cholecystectomy: a multi-institutional report of the first 297 cases. Surg Endosc 24:1854–60
2. Rivas H et al (2010) Single-incision laparoscopic cholecystectomy: a surgeon's initial experience with 56 consecutive cases, and review of the literature. J Gastrointest Surg 14:506–10

Chapter 11
Suturing and Knot-Tying Technique

Kazunori Uchida, Hirotaka Tashiro, and Hideki Ohdan

Abstract Suturing in endoscopic surgery is greatly influenced by the set-up of the forceps. For the so-called "TANKO procedure" which comes from the concept of reduced port laparoscopic surgery (RPLS), the distance from forceps to the other is very small and the angle of the forceps becomes very narrow. In order to suture in this situation, two ways of manipulation are necessary. One is the technique to manipulate the tip of the needle holder that controls suture materials and the other is the technique to control the hands of the operator who controls the needle holder. To control the hands is a technique common in RPLS, so in this chapter, the selection of a proper user-friendly needle holder (even when the distance between forceps is small) and suturing technique will be explained.

Keywords Knot-tying • Single-port laparoscopic surgery • Suturing

11.1 Introduction to the Technique

Suturing in endoscopic surgery is greatly influenced by the set-up of the ports. For the so-called "TANKO procedure" which comes from the concept of reduced port laparoscopic surgery (RPLS), the distance between forceps is very small and the angle of the forceps becomes very sharp. In order to suture in this situation, two ways of manipulation are necessary. One is the technique to manipulate the tip of the needle holder that controls suture materials and the other is the technique to control the hands of the operator who controls the needle holder. To control the

K. Uchida (✉) • H. Tashiro • H. Ohdan
Department of Gastroenterological and Transplant Surgery, Applied Life Sciences
Institute of Biomedical and Health Sciences, Hiroshima University, Hiroshima, Japan
e-mail: uchidake@ms1.megaegg.ne.jp

T. Mori and G. Dapri (eds.), *Reduced Port Laparoscopic Surgery*,
DOI 10.1007/978-4-431-54601-6_11, © Springer Japan 2014

Fig. 11.1 Types of inline
handles

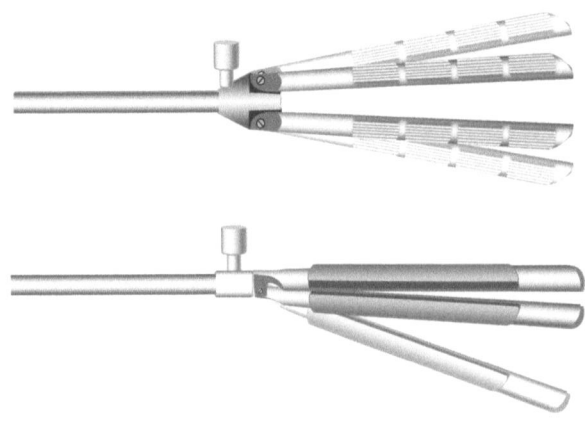

hands is a technique common in RPLS, so in this chapter, the selection of a proper
user-friendly needle holder (even when the distance of forceps is small) and suturing
technique will be explained.

11.2   Selection of the Needle Holder

Most needle holders have a straight handle called an in-line handle. The handle is in
this particular shape in order to operate the forceps and to permit rotation to make
loops for suturing easier. There are two types of inline handles: a double-action type
and a single-action type (Fig. 11.1). For TANKO, it is better to use one with a com-
pact handle to avoid clashing of the handles. The double-action type opens up to the
both sides, so they can easily cause interference with the other forceps. On the other
hand, the single-action type opens up only in one direction, so the possibility of
interference decreases. Moreover, it can be used even in a narrower space (Fig. 11.2).
The parts of the single action type may clash, but this can be avoided by removing
the screw cap (plug) (Fig. 11.3).

To approximate the tissue, it is absolutely necessary to grasp the tissue by an
assistant forceps with rotating mechanism. Otherwise, even with the single-action
type, depending upon how you open the handle, the handles may easily interfere
with each other. In order to avoid this, it is also helpful to use a needle holder that
has a rotation knob (Fig. 11.4). It is recommended to use a diamond type jaw surface, not a serrated type, which can provide with a good grip. It is of key importance
to use the needle driver and assisting forceps of different length to avoid interference of the handles (Fig. 11.5). The handle grip needs a little "twist", too. If one
holds an in-line type handle with a palm grip, the operator's hands interfere with
each other, so it is better to hold it with a pencil grip (Fig. 11.6).

Fig. 11.2 Clashing of handles

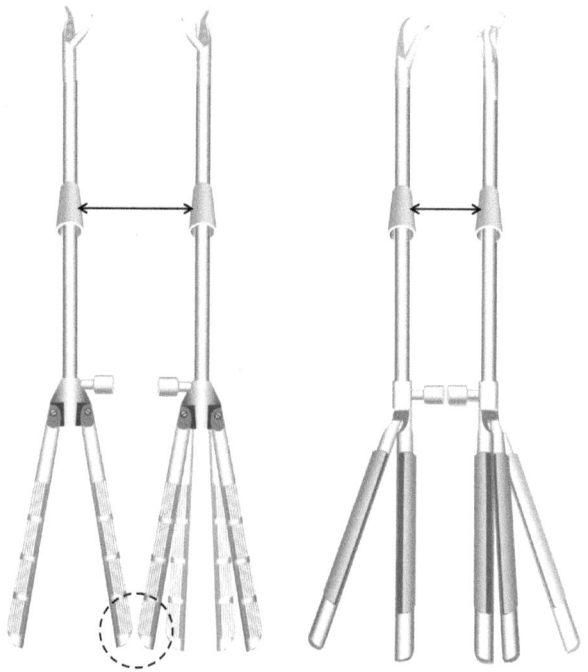

Fig. 11.3 Screw off

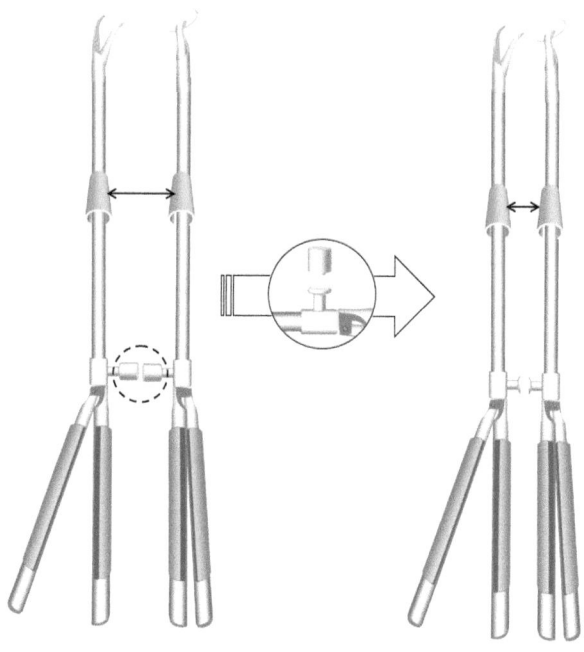

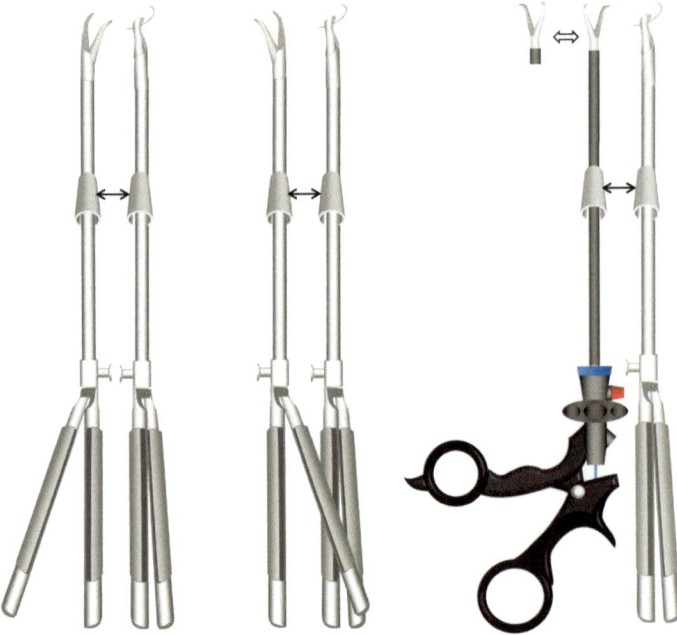

Fig. 11.4 The handle interference

Fig. 11.5 Change the length of forceps

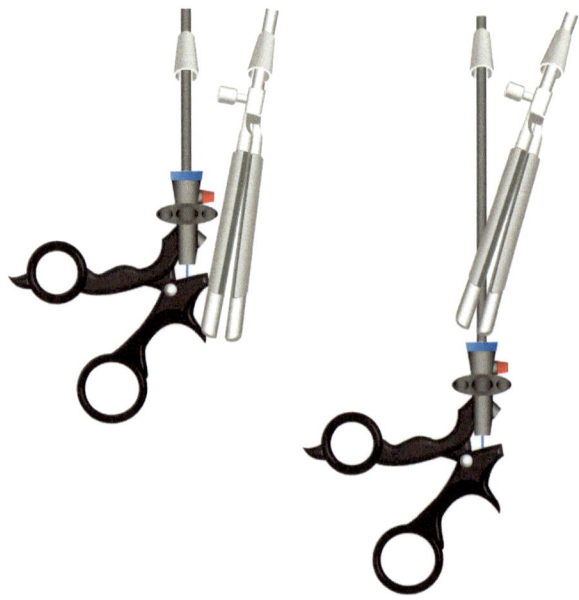

Fig. 11.6 Palm grip and
pencil grip

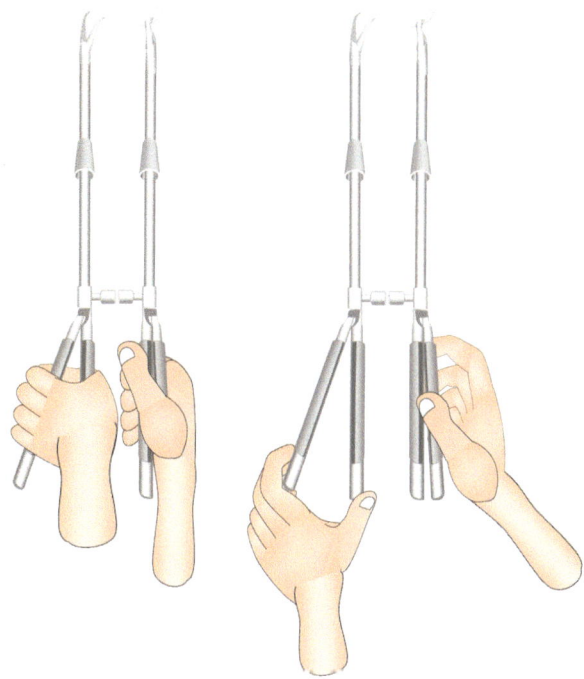

  In conclusion, at present, for needle holders, the Szabo-Berci needle holder or
the Snowden-Pencer needle holder with a rotation knob are both considered very
useful.

11.3 Knot-Tying Technique in Reduced Port
Laparoscopic Surgery

In general, the use of two needle holders makes knot tying easier. We will describe
our "thumb's up technique" [1] which can even be done with almost parallel needle
holders as shown in the illustration.

  1. Make "C loop" (Fig. 11.7a)
     Make a C loop first. The important point here is how you hold the long tail with
     the right needle holder. By turning the suture toward the needle holder, catching
     the thread becomes easier.
  2. Open the jaw (Fig. 11.7b)
     Open the jaw of the left needle holder. This is the "thumb's up" technique.
  3. Hook the suture (Fig. 11.7c)
     By moving the needle holder forward, hook the suture on the back of the jaw.
  4. Coiling the suture (Fig. 11.7d)
     Usually, for knot tying, one would twist the suture around the forceps, but for
     this particular suturing, turn the left needle holder to the left and coil the thread.

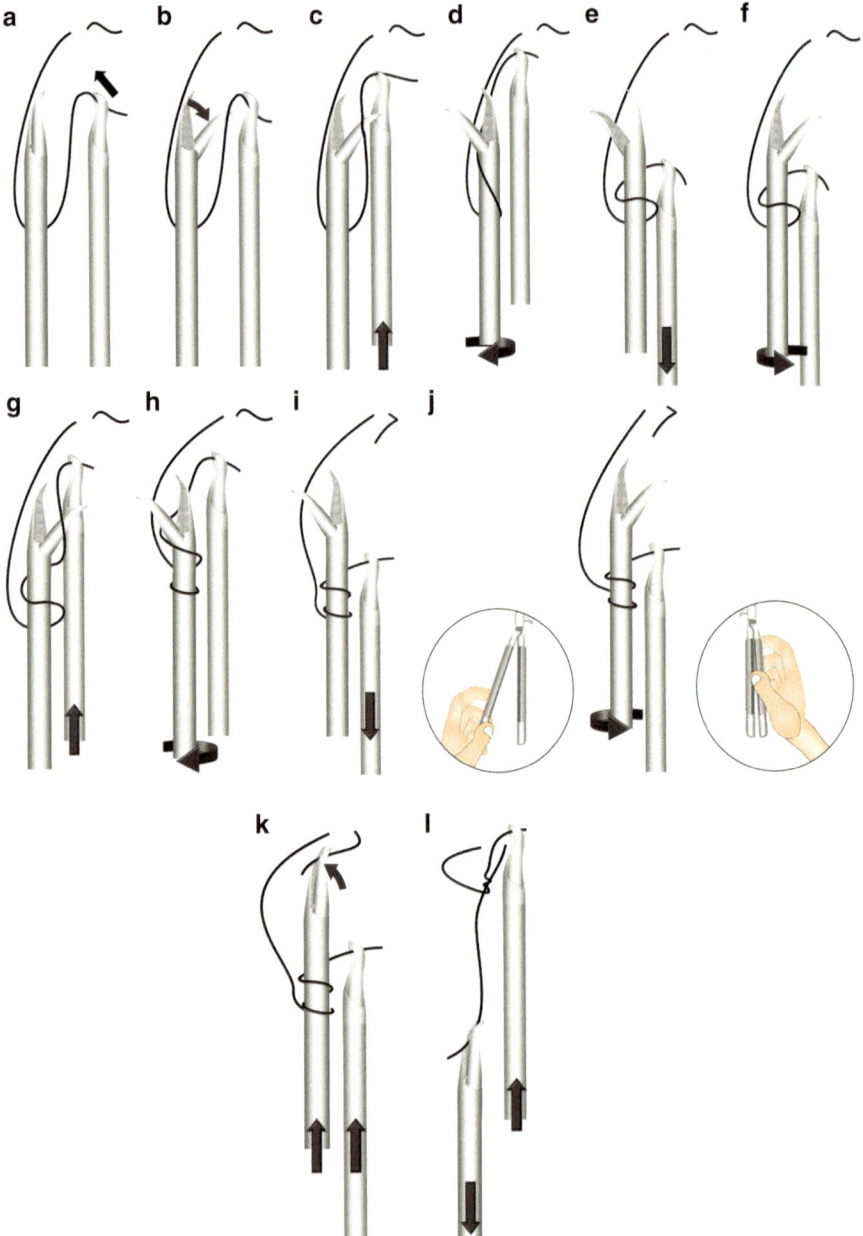

Fig. 11.7 (**a**) Make "C loop" (**b**) Open the jaw (**c**) Hook the suture (**d**) Coiling the suture (**e**) Completion of the loop (**f**) Completion of the half hitch knot (**g**) Surgeon's knot (**h**) Coiling the suture again (**i**) Completion of the double loop (**j**) Keep "thumb's up" (**k**) Completion of the Surgeon's knot (**l**) Making a complete knot

5. Completion of the Loop (Fig. 11.7e)

   Make a loop by trying not to touch the lower part of the left needle holder and pull the thread with the right needle holder. By turning the left one to the point where you can see the back of the holder, the long tail will go smoothly behind the left needle holder.

6. Completion of the Half Hitch Knot (Fig. 11.7f)

   Turn the left needle holder to the right and pick up the short tail to complete the half hitch knot

7. Surgeon's knot (Fig. 11.7g)

   By repeating a set of above suturing technique, a surgeon's knot is easily completed.

8. Coiling the suture Again (Fig. 11.7h)

   By turning the left needle holder to the left, coiling the suture is done.

9. Completion of the Double Loop (Fig. 11.7i)

   By pulling the right needle holder, a double loop can be made on the left needle holder.

10. Keep "Thumb's Up" (Fig. 11.7j)

   During the procedure, the jaw of the left needle holder needs to be open all the time. By doing so, slackening of the loop and potential escape can be avoided. Also, interference of the holder's hands can be lessened.

11. Completion of the Surgeon's Knot (Fig. 11.7k)

   By picking up the short tail, the Surgeon's knot is completed.

12. Making a Complete Knot (Fig. 11.7l)

   Almost all procedures are done by moving the forceps back and forth. By doing so, interference of the forceps can be avoided and suturing can be accomplished.

Reference

1. Uchida K, Haruta N, Okajima M, Matsuda M, Yamamoto M (2005) The keys to the new laparoscopic world Thumbs up! knot and Tornado knot. Surg Endosc 19(6):859, Multimedia article

Chapter 12
Single-Incision Robotic Surgery

Gopal Menon, Monica T. Young, and Alessio Pigazzi

Abstract Robotic surgery represents the latest advance in minimally invasive techniques. Single-incision robot-assisted surgery is the ultimate robotic surgery technology and has received enthusiastic acceptance in field of gallbladder surgery. However, apart from improved cosmesis, its reported benefits are thus far not widely known. Its application is limited largely to cholecystectomy, but it is gradually being applied to other procedures. As the results of further studies surface, a clearer picture of the role of reduced-port robotic surgery will emerge.

Keywords Access port • Cholecystectomy • Colectomy • da Vinci surgical system • Single-incision robotics

12.1 Introduction

12.1.1 Overview

Robotic surgery represents a relatively new and exciting stage in the development of minimally invasive surgical techniques. The last quarter of a century has seen the rapid growth of robotic surgery from a tentative concept to an established modality in medical practice. The benefits of robotic surgery over conventional laparoscopic surgery remain controversial. However, recent reports in the United States and other countries show a trend toward an increasing use of robotics in various procedures. Single-incision robotic surgery is the latest development in the robotic surgery armamentarium and has been hailed by many enthusiasts as the answer to the difficulties encountered during single-access laparoscopic procedures.

G. Menon (✉) • M.T. Young • A. Pigazzi
Department of Surgery, University of California Irvine, Orange, CA, USA
e-mail: gopal@genebrew.com; mtyoung@uci.edu; apigazzi@uci.edu

T. Mori and G. Dapri (eds.), *Reduced Port Laparoscopic Surgery*,
DOI 10.1007/978-4-431-54601-6_12, © Springer Japan 2014

12.1.2 History

The term "robot," when used to describe a current robotic surgical system, is a misnomer of sorts. A robot is technically defined as "a machine capable of carrying out a complex series of actions automatically, especially one programmable by a computer." Surgical robots are fully automated yet incapable of independent movement or decision-making. They rely on a "master–slave" interaction, with the robot (slave) mimicking movements of the surgeon (master).

The Puma 560 is credited with being the first in a long line of surgical robots. In 1985, this machine was used to perform a CT-guided stereotactic brain biopsy with greater accuracy and precision than previously achieved. The FDA approved the first robot, christened ROBODOC, for surgical use in 1990. In the years that followed, the range of robotic procedures expanded quickly. Urologic, gynecologic, and cardiothoracic surgeons pioneered the robotic surgery movement. The first transurethral robotic prostatectomy was performed in 1992. In 1998, the first robot-assisted coronary artery bypass graft surgery was performed. Urologists in particular embraced this new technology and made rapid strides in the surgical technique and in the scope of what could be accomplished.

In the general surgery arena, robotic techniques have been adopted more slowly. Several contributing factors have been proposed. Urological procedures are generally localized to the pelvis. General surgery procedures often involve more than one abdominal quadrant, making the use of a robot at times cumbersome, as it must be repositioned for each quadrant. The first general surgery procedure successfully completed robotically was a cholecystectomy, in the year 2000. A variety of additional procedures have been performed since. Three years later a fully robotic Whipple procedure was successfully completed. Currently, the most common robotic general surgery procedures are cholecystectomy via a single-incision platform, colorectal resection (especially total mesorectal excision), and some foregut surgeries. The 12 most frequently performed robotic general surgery procedures are given below.

1. Anti-reflux surgery
2. Adrenalectomy
3. Low anterior rectal resection
4. Proctocolectomy
5. Rectopexy
6. Hepatectomy
7. Gastrectomy
8. Splenectomy
9. Cholecystectomy
10. Donor nephrectomy
11. Gastric bypass
12. Heller myotomy

12.1.3   Advantages and Disadvantages

There are several stated advantages to robotic surgery over traditional laparoscopic surgery. Improved access to anatomically difficult locations is perhaps the most significant. This is particularly true for surgery involving the mediastinum and pelvis, where traditional laparoscopy is technically challenging due to space restrictions. Robotic assistance allows for superior three-dimensional visualization, improved dexterity provided by articulating instruments, improved ergonomics for the operating surgeon, and precise instrument control. Electronic mitigation of hand tremor allows for finer and more accurate dissection [10]. The latest generation of robots permits seven degrees of movement, mimicking the range of movement of the human wrist. All of these factors contribute to improved operative techniques and potentially improved surgical outcomes.

Despite the advantages, cost remains a serious concern. Robots are expensive, with costs running into millions of dollars for each robotic platform. The da Vinci platform (Intuitive Surgical, Sunnyvale, CA, USA) currently holds virtually the entire market share. Each robotic platform costs about two million dollars with a two hundred thousand dollar annual service contract. Is it worth the investment? In the climate of increasing austerity, is it a viable and, more importantly, justifiable option? These questions will remain unanswered until a substantial number of large-scale prospective studies are conducted to evaluate the clinical benefits of robotic surgery.

12.2   Indications and Contraindications

12.2.1   Indications

The use of robotic assistance in general surgery is increasing. Each year, newer, cutting edge procedures are performed. However, broad consensus on the best indications for robotic surgery has yet to be reached, and this is especially true for single-access robotic procedures.

The Society of American Gastroenterology and Endoscopic Surgery (SAGES) consensus statement on the indications for robotic surgery, single- and multiple-port surgeries included, recommends its use for the procedures listed below. This list is based on the results of studies looking at operative and post-operative outcomes for each of the procedures listed. No significant benefit was noted for other general surgery procedures.

1. Heller myotomy
2. Paraesophageal hernia repair
3. Gastric bypass
4. Gastric resection
5. Biliary reconstruction
6. Esophagectomy
7. Distal pancreatectomy
8. Rectal resection

Table 12.1 Reports published to date on single-site robotic general surgery

Investigators	Evidence type	Procedure	Number of patients	Access	Operation time (in minutes)
Ostrowitz et al. [1]	Prospective clinical series	Right hemicolectomy	3	SILS port	166
Romanelli et al. [2]	Case report	Cholecystectomy	1	Separate fascial incisions	156
Ragupathi et al. [3]	Clinical case report	Partial cecetomy	1	GelPort	120
Singh et al. [8]	Clinical case report	Right hemicolectomy	1	GelPort	179
Kroh et al. [5]	Prospective clinical series	Cholecystectomy	13	Glove technique	107
Wren and Curet [4]	Comparative study[a]	Cholecystectomy	10	da Vinci SSI	105.3
Morel et al. [6]	Prospective clinical series	Cholecystectomy	28	da Vinci SSI	80
Spinoglio et al. [9]	Comparative study[b]	Cholecystectomy	25	da Vinci SSI	62 [13]
Konstantinidis et al. [11]	Case series	Cholecystectomy	45	da Vinci SSI	84.5
Pietrabissa et al. [12]	Multicenter prospective case series	Cholecystectomy	100	da Vinci SSI	71

[a]Comparative study vs. standard laparoscopic cholecystectomy
[b]Comparative study vs. laparo-endoscopic single-site surgery

Very few studies have analyzed the impact, benefit, and outcomes of reduced-port or single-incision robotic surgery, and to date there have been no long-term prospective trials comparing reduced-port to multiport robotic procedures. Much of the work done thus far has pertained to cholecystectomy; thus, commenting at this time on the virtue of single-incision robotics in other fields would be premature. The studies published to date on single-site robotic general surgery are summarized in Table 12.1.

12.2.2 Outcomes

Outcomes gleaned from the literature seem to establish the safety of single-incision robotic surgery. Pietrabissa et al. reported a conversion rate of 2 % in a series of 100 cholecystectomies, with one conversion to multiport laparoscopy and the other to open surgery, both due to severe chronic inflammation. Minor complications encountered included gall bladder rupture (7 %) and bleeding (5 %). Konstantinidis et al. in a study of 45 patients who underwent cholecystectomy reported no conversion to open surgery, although additional port placement was required in three patients. Complication rates were similarto the study by Pietrabissa et al. and 40 of

Table 12.2 Physiologic changes associated with the Trendeleburg position

Physiologic variable	Position-induced change
Intracranial/intraocular pressure	Increase
Central venous pressure	Increase
Cardiac output	Decrease
Blood pressure	Increase
Venous return	Increase then decrease
Systemic vascular resistance	Decrease
Airway resistance	Increase

the patients were discharged within 24 h. Interestingly, the duration of surgery did not change significantly with increasing operative experience. The remaining studies were too small to draw meaningful conclusions regarding outcomes, but the feasibility of such procedures has been established.

12.2.3 Contraindications

Contraindications for single-incision robotic surgery are not dissimilar to those for conventional laparoscopic surgery or multiport robotic surgery. Robotic general surgery (abdominal procedures) are usually performed in the Trendelenburg or reverse Trendelenburg position; thus, the physiologic effects of a steep incline and pneumoperitoneum creation must be taken into account. The most important physiologic changes are listed in Table 12.2.

Due to the potential for risky physiologic changes, the following are considered relative contraindications for robotic surgery:

- History of cerebrovascular accident, intracranial aneurysm, elevated intracranial pressure, or glaucoma
- Severe chronic obstructive pulmonary disease, bullous emphysema, spontaneous pneumothorax, or diaphragmatic hernia

12.3 Description of the Technique

12.3.1 Basic Structure

The typical robot consists of the surgical console, a three-dimensional camera system, and a bedside cart equipped with robotic arms. Conventional robotic surgery uses four separate arms; one for the camera and the other three for the instruments. Slight variations exist between different generations of systems, but the principles remain the same. The locations of the ports vary according to the type of procedure being performed.

Single-port/single-site robotic surgery is a modification of the multiport approach and can be carried out in two ways. One method involves inserting three ports of the multiport robotic system through separate but closely placed incisions or through a

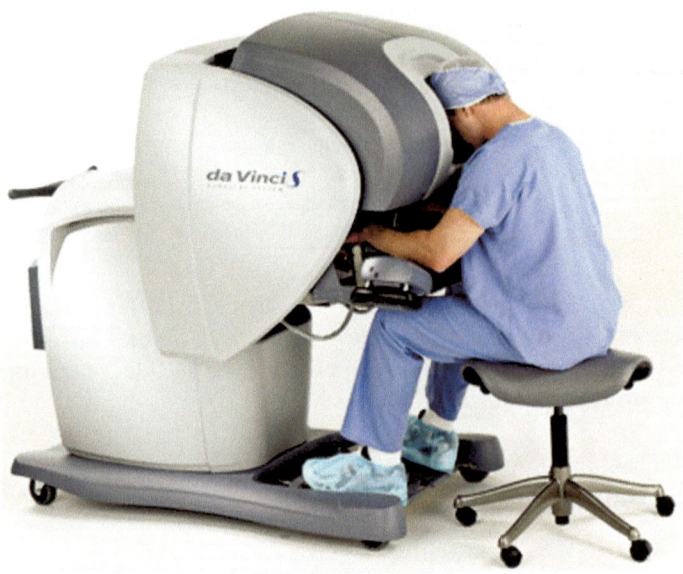

Fig. 12.1 The da Vinci robotic console

GelPort® device (Applied Medical, Rancho Santa Margarita, USA) or simply through the fingers of a standard surgical glove. A newer method takes advantage of a specially designed single-incision platform comprising a large silicone port with four channels and commonly placed in the umbilicus. The single-port robotic trocars and instruments differ in design from those of the conventional robotic system.

12.3.2 Individual Components

12.3.2.1 Console

The da Vinci console developed by Intuitive Surgical is currently the only commercially available robot. A number of robot alternatives are in various stages of development and are projected to enter the market within the next few years. The console shown in Fig. 12.1 may be housed at a remote location, but at most hospitals, the console is housed within the operating room itself.

The da Vinci console controls translate movements of both the hands and the wrists to the instruments inside the patient's body. A high-definition image, typically produced by two separate endoscopic camera lenses, allows stereoscopic, magnified vision.

12.3.2.2 Access Platform

Access platforms provide the conduit through which robotic components enter the body. The platform must form an airtight seal, preventing the escape of gas used for

Fig. 12.2 Typical access port

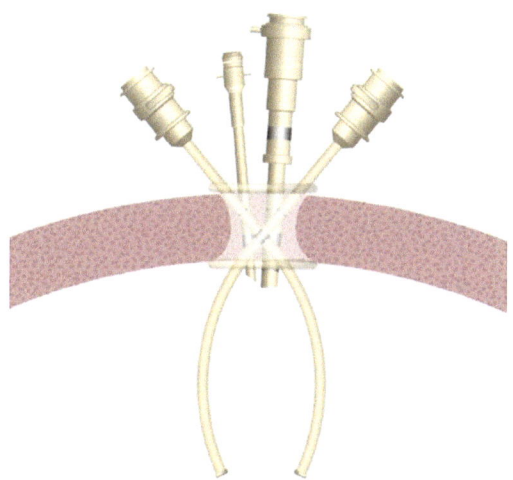

insufflation. Multiport robotic surgery uses devices similar to laparoscopic entry ports. With single-incision robotics, however, improvisation became necessary. Modified platforms include the "glove port," comprising a glove folded around an Alexis wound retractor (Applied Medical) for insertion of instruments through the finger holes; the "GelPort" (Applied Medical) into which the instruments are inserted directly; the "TriPort or QuadPort" (Olympus, Tokyo, Japan) multichannel ports with valves for instrument insertion [7]; the "SILS™ port" (Covidien, New Haven, CT, USA), which is made of one piece of elastopolymer that deforms with instrument placement; and the recent "da Vinci SSI" (Intuitive Surgical) a soft silicon port with four channels that accommodate instruments designed for single-incision procedures. Some surgeons have opted to insert instruments through multiple fascial incisions, thereby avoiding the need for a special device.

A typical access port and orientation of the instruments through the device are shown in Fig. 12.2.

12.3.2.3   Instruments

Single-incision robotic surgery requires specially designed instruments. To achieve instrument triangulation through a single access site, the ports are curved, so that the instruments meet at their tips. This allows for unobstructed movement of the robotic arms with respect to each other. The camera is positioned at the center of the curved arms, such that it does not interfere with movement. The instruments are flexible so that they can be easily inserted through the curved trocars.

Unlike standard robotic instruments, the single-site instruments do not articulate at the tip, losing some of the advantages of the increased robotic articulation commonly associated with the conventional robotic platform. As a result, movement is along straight lines, as in conventional laparoscopy. However, the curved working instruments allow for optimal triangulation, thus obviating some of the limitations associated with single-site laparoscopic surgery conflicts [4]. In addition, the system software ensures that even if the instruments cross inside the abdominal cavity, the actual control of the instruments at the console will remain with the appropriate hands without the surgeon being aware of any differences in comparison to multi-port robotic surgery.

A variety of semi-rigid instruments, such as hooks, scissors, graspers, needle drivers, and clip appliers, are available for the robotic platform. The optics consists of an 8.5-mm stereoscopic telescope in either a 0° or 30° configuration to be used according to the specifics of the case.

12.3.2.4   Patient-Side Cart

The patient-side cart consists of a scaffolding to which the robotic arms are attached. The robotic cart has four arms, one of which remains unused during single-incision robotic surgery (usually arm 3).

12.3.2.5   Assistance

The operating surgeon at the console requires assistance in manipulating tissues and in providing traction. The assistant uses a laparoscopic instrument through one of the ports. Several different methods are used to provide traction. They vary, depending on the location of the assistant's port. Occasionally, a marionette or transparietal technique is used whereby the tissues are suspended by sutures.

12.3.3   Procedure

The single-site port is inserted by first making a 2–3 cm incision at the desired fascial level. CO_2 is insufflated via a specific side valve, and the camera is then introduced to allow insertion of the curved port. The robotic curved trocars are inserted under direct vision. Because the curved trocars are longer than straight robotic trocars, care must be taken to avoid damage to surrounding structures and other organs during their insertion.

The robotic cart is brought in by a appropriate approach, and the camera and the arms are docked sequentially, resulting in the configuration shown in Fig. 12.3.

12.3.3.1   Cholecystectomy

The robotic cholecystectomy procedure follows the same principles as in other approaches. The assistant's port can be used to grasp the dome of the gallbladder,

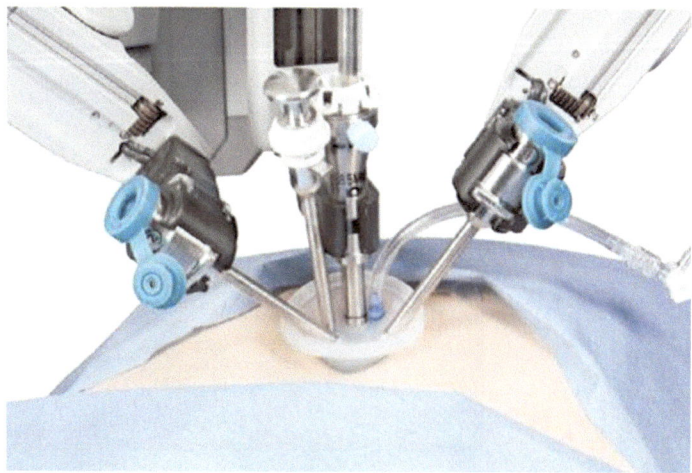

Fig. 12.3 Docked system

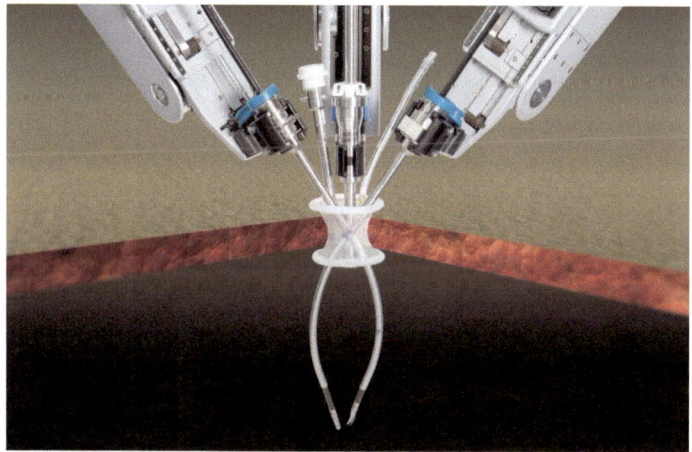

Fig. 12.4 Single-incision robotic cholecystectomy

thus elevating it cephalad. The hilum can be dissected with a hook or scissors manipulated by the surgeon's right hand and a grasper manipulated by the left hand, according to surgeon's preference. After identification of the cystic duct and artery, these structures can be clipped and divided (Fig. 12.4). The single-incision robotic system with its fluorescent "firefly" mode allows visualization of the biliary structures with the use of indocyanine green (ICG) and a special light source with a near infrared wavelength. This can be useful in cases in which the anatomy is unclear, in essence creating a fluorescent cholangiogram Fig. 12.5–12.9.

Fig. 12.5 Adhesiolysis

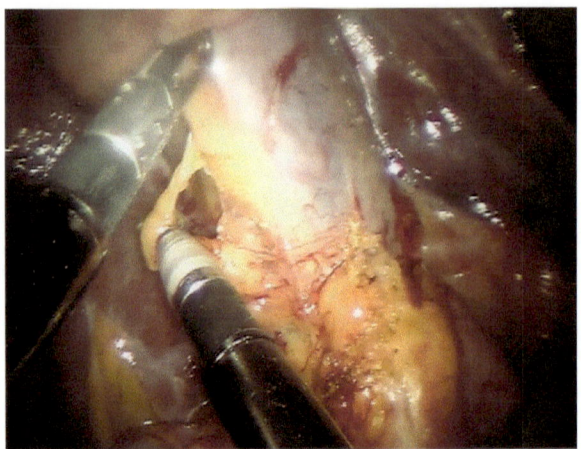

Fig. 12.6 Triangle
of Calot dissection

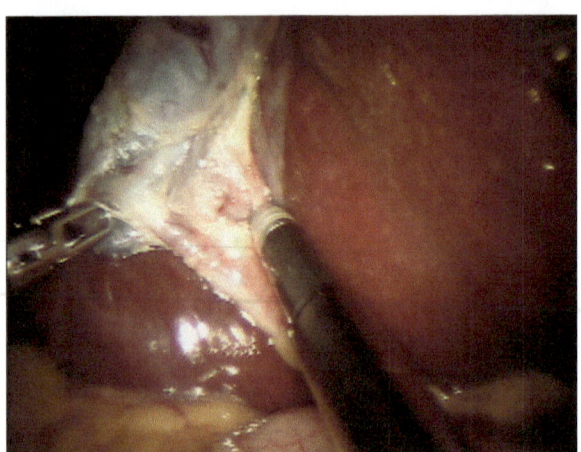

Fig. 12.7 Critical view
approach

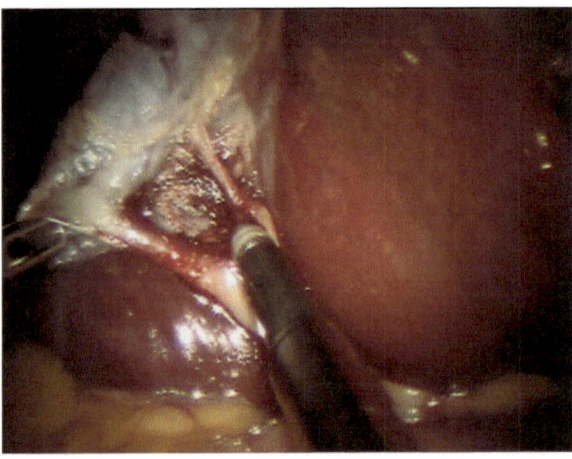

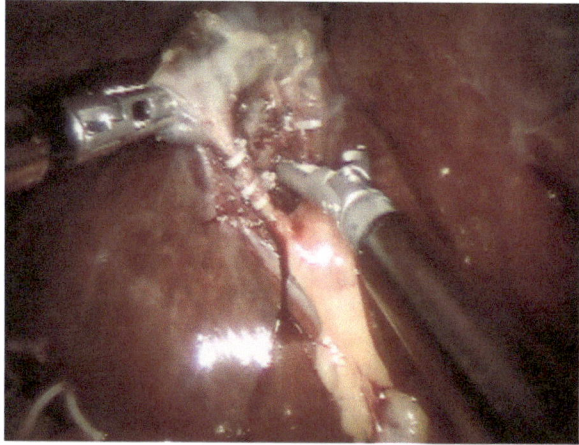

Fig. 12.8 Cystic duct and artery ligation

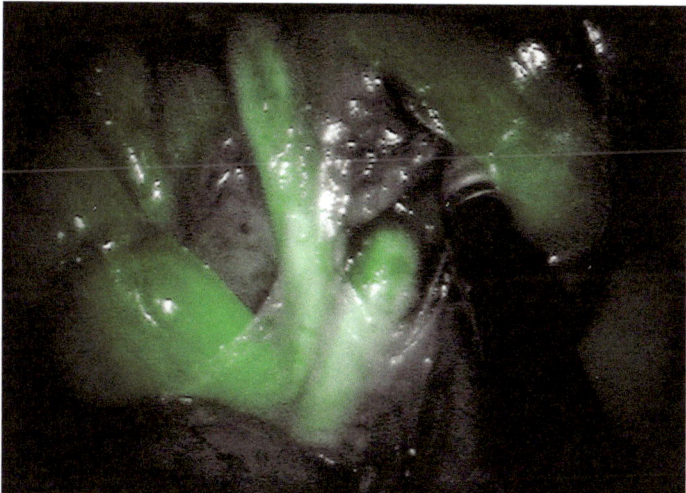

Fig. 12.9 'Firefly' mode fluorescence with Indocyanine green

12.3.3.2 Colectomy

Single-site robotic-assisted colectomy has been performed in a few centers with the use of a single-site platform or simply by using the glove or GelPort (Applied Medical) technique. Colectecomy is carried out in a medial-to-lateral or lateral-to-medial fashion, according to surgeon's preference. Tilting the table to the side opposite the lesion exposes the mesentery and assists in moving the small intestine out of the way. The surgeon at the console, and, using appropriate atraumatic robotic graspers, retracts the mesentery; because no vessel sealer device is available for the single-site platform designed for curved instruments, the vessels are divided by the assistant or clipped and divided by the operating surgeon. If the multiport arms are used in a single-site configuration, the operating surgeon can divide the vessels independently. Performing intracorporeal anastomosis in patients undergoing right colectomy is quite difficult under the single-incision approach. Thus, most surgeons exteriorize the bowel and perform extracorporeal anastomosis according to standard techniques. In sigmoid or low anterior resection, after division of the vessels and mobilization of the mesentery, the sigmoid or descending colon can be exteriorized through the single site; an anvil can be inserted into the proximal bowel, and anastomosis can be performed under robotic or laparoscopic visualization after re-insufflation of the abdominal cavity.

12.4 Tips and Tricks

As with every new procedure, appropriate patient selection is key to success, especially at the beginning of the single-access robotic experience. While single-incision robotic surgery offers certain advantages over use of a laparoscopic platform, the robotic platform poses unique challenges that can render the procedure equally arduous. Challenges include the lack of tactile feedback and the need to find or move instruments that are outside the visual field. Thus, the potential for complications and errors is ever present. Familiarity with the robotic system is key, and extensive practice with a simulator will be beneficial at any stage of training. Incisional hernia at the single-incision site is a known postoperative complication; therefore, closure of the fascia must be carried out in a very methodical manner. Despite this precaution, umbilical hernia will likely occur in a substantial number of obese patients. In our opinion, then, single-incision robotic surgery is contraindicated for individuals with a high body mass index.

12.5 Recommendations from the Author

Cholecystectomy is currently the only FDA-cleared application for the single-site robotic surgery platform. We suggest performing the procedure in cases of uncomplicated gallbladder disease, at least initially, before venturing into more difficult cases. Finally, given the increasing medicolegal scrutiny under which all robotic surgeons currently operate, we advise performing other single-site robotic procedures under an IRB protocol or at least after extensive and documented patient counseling.

References

1. Ostrowitz MB, Eschete D, Zemon H, DeNoto G (2009) Robotic-assisted single-incision right colectomy: early experience. Int J Med Robot 5(4):465–470
2. Romanelli JR, Roshek TB 3rd, Lynn DC, Earle DB (2010) Single-port laparoscopic cholecystectomy: initial experience. Surg Endosc 24(6):1374–1379
3. Ragupathi M, Ramos-Valadez DI, Pedraza R, Haas EM (2010) Robotic assisted single-incision laparoscopic partial cecectomy. Int J Med Robot 6(3):362–367
4. Wren SM, Curet MJ (2011) Single-port robotic cholecystectomy: results from a first human use clinical study of the new da Vinci single site surgical platform. Arch Surg 146(10): 1122–1127
5. Kroh M, El-Hayek K, Rosenblatt S et al (2011) First human surgery with a novel single-port robotic system: cholecystectomy using the da Vinci single-site platform. Surg Endosc 25(11): 3566–3573
6. Morel P, Hagen ME, Bucher P et al (2011) Robotic single-port cholecystectomy using a new platform: initial clinical experience. J Gastrointest Surg 15(12):2182–2186
7. Sugimoto M, Tanaka K, Matsuoka Y et al (2011) da Vinci robotic single incision cholecystectomy and hepatectomy using single-channel GelPort access. J Hepatobiliary Pancreat Sci 18(4):493–498
8. Singh J, Podolsky ER, Castellanos AE, Stein DE (2011) Optimizing single port surgery: a case report and review of technique in colon resection. Int J Med Robot 7(2):127–130
9. Spinoglio G, Lenti LM, Maglione V et al (2011) Single-site robotic cholecystectomy (SSRC) versus single-incision laparoscopic cholecystectomy (SILC): comparison of learning curves. First European experience. Surg Endosc 26(6):1648–1655
10. van der Schatte Olivier RH, van't Hullenaar CDP, Ruurda JP, Broeders IAMJ (2009) Ergonomics, user comfort, and performance in standard and robot-assisted laparoscopic surgery. Surg Endosc 23(6):1365–1371. doi:10.1007/s00464-008-0184-6, Published online 2008 October 15
11. Konstantinidis KM, Hirides P, Hirides S, Chrysocheris P, Georgiou M (2012) Cholecystectomy using a novel Single-site® robotic platform: early experience from 45 consecutive cases. Surg Endosc 26(9):2687–2694. doi:10.1007/s00464-012-2227-2, Epub 2012 Apr 5
12. Pietrabissa A, Sbrana F, Morelli L, Badessi F, Pugliese L, Vinci A, Klersy C, Spinoglio G (2012) Overcoming the challenges of single-incision cholecystectomy with robotic single-site technology. Arch Surg 147(8):709–714
13. Morel P, Buchs NC, Iranmanesh P, Pugin F, Buehler L, Azagury DE, Jung M, Volonte F, Hagen ME (2013) Robotic single-site cholecystectomy. J Hepatobiliary Pancreat Sci doi:10.1002/jhbp.36. Epub ahead of print

Chapter 13
The Umbilicus as the Access Site

Atsushi Iida and Akio Yamaguchi

Abstract The umbilicus is the scar that remains after the umbilical cord is removed from a newborn baby. As a simple structure without layers, the umbilicus is suitable as the surgical access window for entry into the peritoneal cavity as well as the site for tissue extraction. Reduced port laparoscopic surgery requires use of the umbilicus as the access site. There are some very important points to remember for reconstructing the umbilicus after surgery. A beautiful finish requires a beautiful incision. A vertically oriented umbilicus is commonly favored. To close the incision, the fascial wound and the floor of the umbilicus must be closed firmly to avoid incisional hernia. The umbilicus is a key aesthetic landmark. To avoid complications from the incision as well as patient dissatisfaction with the shape of the umbilicus after surgery, surgeons must understand the details of its anatomy and the fine points of reconstructing the umbilicus, giving proper attention to cosmesis.

Keywords Laparoscopic surgery • Single-port laparoscopic surgery • Umbilicus

13.1 Anatomy of the Umbilicus

The umbilicus is the scar that remains after the umbilical cord has been removed from a newborn baby. The umbilical cord itself contains the umbilical vessels, remnant allantois, and the remnant vitelline duct [1] (Fig. 13.1). The structure of the umbilicus is completely different from that of the abdominal wall, which comprises

A. Iida (✉) • A. Yamaguchi
First Department of Surgery, University of Fukui, 23-3 Shimoaizuki, Matsuoka, Eiheiji, Yoshida-gun, Fukui 910-1193, Japan
e-mail: axiida@u-fukui.ac.jp

T. Mori and G. Dapri (eds.), *Reduced Port Laparoscopic Surgery*,
DOI 10.1007/978-4-431-54601-6_13, © Springer Japan 2014

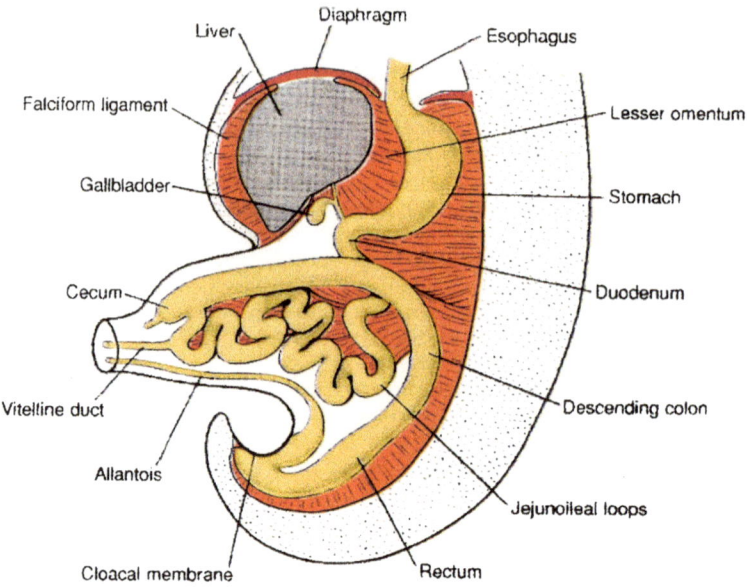

Fig. 13.1 Illustration of the human embryo at 8 weeks

Fig. 13.2 Computed
tomography image at the
level of the umbilicus. There
is no muscle layer or
subcutaneous fat layer at the
umbilicus

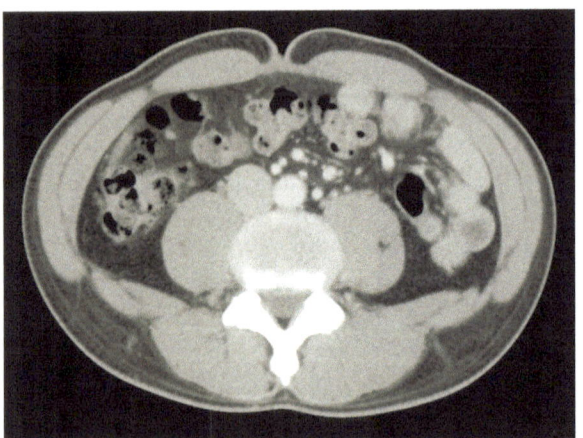

layers of muscle, fascia, skin, fat, and peritoneum. The structure of the umbilicus is simple. There are no layers. Rather, the umbilicus is made up of skin, scar tissue, and peritoneum at its center. The suitability of the umbilicus as an access window for entry into the peritoneal cavity is evident on a computed tomography scan (Fig. 13.2).

The deepest part of the umbilicus is the scar where the round ligament of the liver, the para-umbilical vein, and the urachus were once attached (Fig. 13.3).

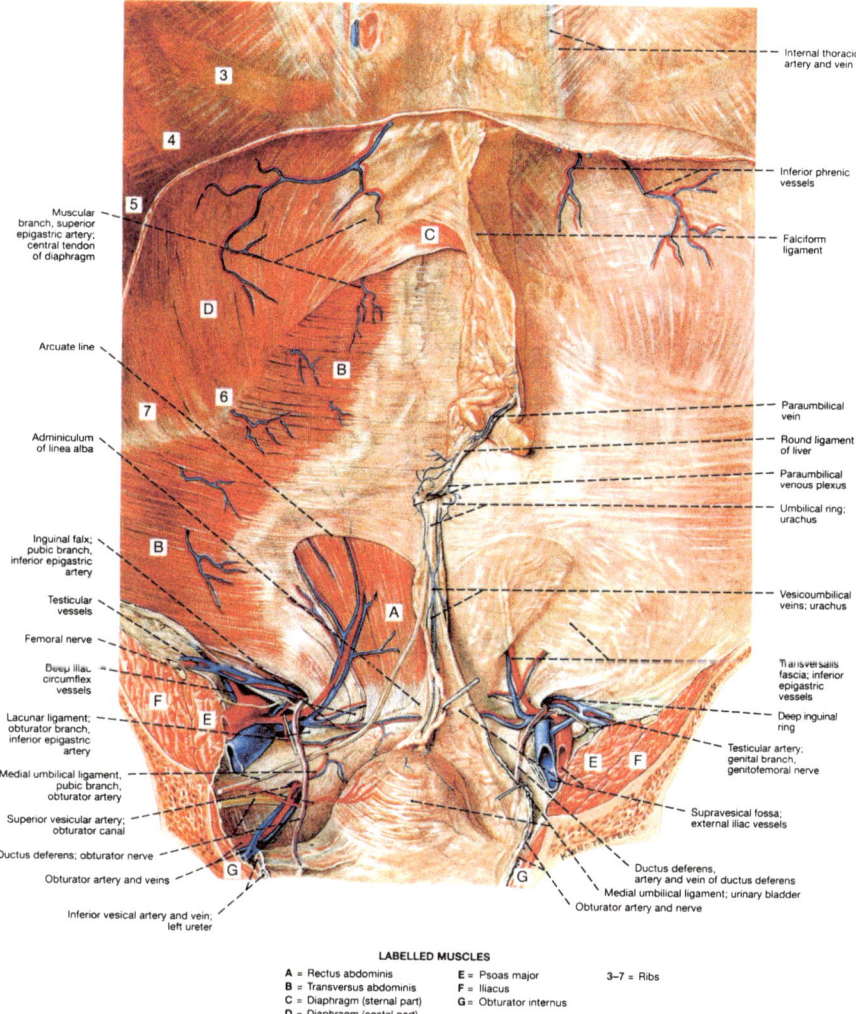

Fig. 13.3 The deep surface of the umbilicus is the scar where the round ligament of liver, the paraumbilical vein, and the urachus are attached

The fascia of the umbilical scar differs in structure from the linea alba, which is the site of fusion between the bilateral posterior layers of the rectus sheath [2–4].

The umbilicus, unique in shape, is also a key aesthetic landmark on the abdominal surface. The shape of the umbilicus varies from person to person. Most commonly, the umbilicus is either T-shaped or rounded. A crescent shape is common in obese persons, but the floor of even a crescent-shaped umbilicus is rounded, formed by the disk-shaped scar tissue.

13.2   Surgical Window to Access the Peritoneal Cavity

In conventional open surgery, laparotomy is performed without cutting out the umbilicus. Cutting the umbilicus has been avoided for very specific reasons: the risk of bleeding from umbilical vessels, the risk of surgical wound contamination and ensuing infection by bacteria harbored in the umbilicus, and the difficulty involved in reconstructing the umbilicus aesthetically. Laparoscopic surgery necessitates only small wounds for the trocars and a route for tissue extraction. Because of its anatomy, the umbilicus is the perfect candidate for a workable surgical access site. It meets the goal of reducing or eliminating the need for laparoscopic trocars and has made it easy for surgeons to improve outcomes [5] (Fig. 13.4).

13.3   Surgical Window for Tissue Extraction

Due to its anatomical structure, the umbilicus is a suitable gate for extraction of the resected specimen. When the umbilicus is cut out, the incision is approximately 2 cm; however, the surgeon can extract a specimen that is as large as 4 cm in diameter by withdrawing it through the umbilicus. The simple structure of the umbilicus lends elasticity, which in turn facilitates the removal of a large specimen (Fig. 13.5). The incision should be sized according to the size of the specimen.

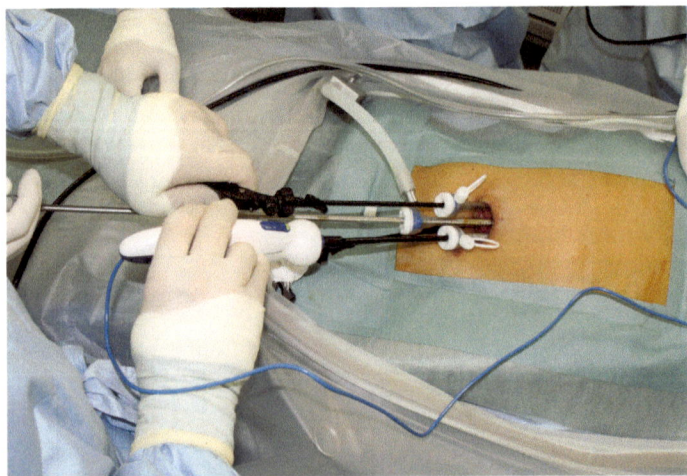

Fig. 13.4 The single-incision multi-trocar method applied to laparoscopic cholecystectomy. The operation is completed strictly through the umbilicus

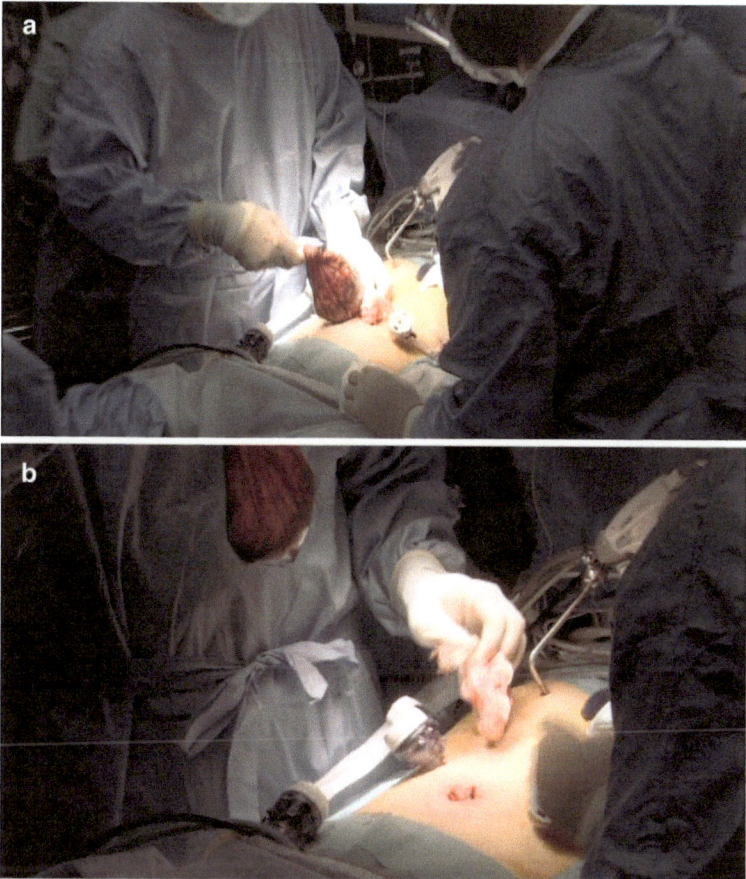

Fig. 13.5 The resected gastric specimen, together with dissected lymph nodes, is extracted through the umbilicus. The tissue is removed in a bag that, when packed, is 3–4 cm in diameter and pulled through the opened umbilicus

13.4 Methods for Single-Port Laparoscopic Surgery at the Umbilicus

There are two main single-port laparoscopic surgery (SPLS) methods: the single-incision multi-trocar method and the multi-channel port method [6]. The former is the original SPLS method. With this method, several trocars are placed in the same single incision. The advantages of this method are the ease of placing the trocars, the ease in manipulating the forceps even from the small single incision, and the fact that standard devices can be used. However, the single-incision multi-trocar method can be problematic. The procedure is not standardized, and proper placement of the trocars depends on the surgeon's experience and skill level [5, 7].

The other method, the multi-channel port method, has become the preferred and most commonly used approach. This method originated with the use of a surgical glove, leading to the development of the SILS™ port (Covidien, New Haven, CT, USA) as the first commercially available multi-channel port. The advantage of this method is its simplicity as a means of setting and fitting the window through the opened umbilicus. The multi-channel port makes it possible for every surgeon to set the trocars in a standard fashion, depending on the surgery that is to be performed. There are some disadvantages to using the multi-channel port, however. Because standard forceps cannot be manipulated from outside the window, the surgeon is often required to use bent or curved forceps [8, 9]. The recent development of a multi-channel port with dedicated forceps has provided for the performance of advanced laparoscopic surgeries.

13.5   Closure of the Opened Umbilicus

Closure of the opened umbilicus and umbilicoplasty are very important steps in SPLS. In terms of trauma to the abdominal wall, SPLS through the umbilicus is a real advantage for the patient, but when the surgeon cannot reconstruct a beautiful umbilicus, the patient is greatly disappointed by the outcome, having lost the aesthetic appeal of this abdominal landmark.

To reconstruct a beautiful umbilicus, there are some surgical principles to be adhered. When the incision is made in the umbilicus, the surgeon must imagine how to close and shape the wound, not simply how to use the wound for surgical access and instrumentation. A beautiful result requires a beautiful incision; thus, the surgeon's forethought and artistic skill become important.

An aesthetically pleasing umbilicus is difficult and even controversial to define. One yardstick is the shape of the navels of fashion models. Not only are fashion models attractive in body and face, but they tend to have a T-shaped or small rounded umbilicus. Craig et al. reported that the longitudinally oriented, small T-shaped navel is favored in the cosmetic evaluation of the umbilicus [10].

There are various ways of making the umbilical incision. Some surgeons make a vertical incision, whereas others make a curved, transverse, or zigzag incision. The vertical incision is currently the most popular umbilical incision. For purely cosmetic considerations, an incision within the scar at the base of the umbilicus is ideal, but we must remember that the length of the incision affects the performance of the surgery as well as the size of the specimen that can be extracted.

Thereafter, the fascial wound and the base of the umbilicus must be closed firmly to avoid incisional hernia. The umbilical vessels and the urachus must be surely ligated. Because the deep portion of the umbilicus is made up of both scar tissue and skin, the skin at that site must be trimmed to close the fascia. This is the most important step in reconstructing a beautiful umbilicus. After the wound is washed with saline to prevent infection, the skin should be closed with absorbable hairline sutures and include umbilicoplasty (Fig. 13.6).

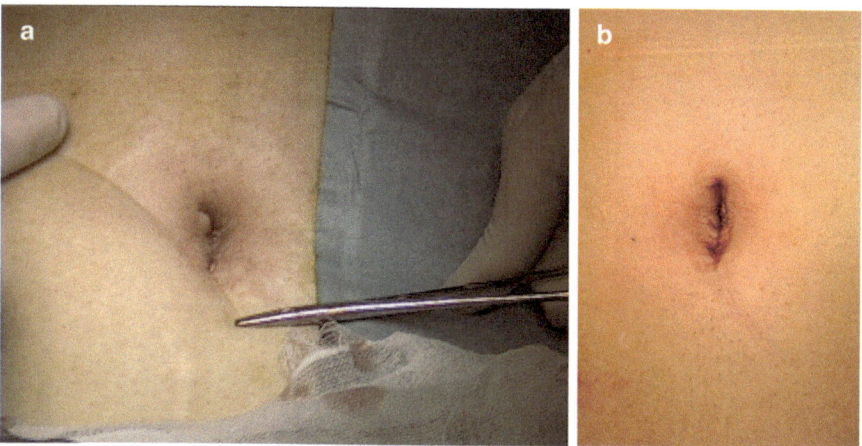

Fig. 13.6 Closure and reconstruction of the opened umbilicus. Vertical orientation of the umbilicus is favored for the reconstruction

The umbilicus is a very suitable gate for abdominal surgery. If we understand the anatomy of the umbilicus and how to properly use it, patients will be satisfied with the cosmetic results of the procedure and the skill of the surgeon. Of course, this is not without the performance of a skilled operative procedure within the abdominal cavity.

References

1. Sadler TW (2009) Langman's medical embryology, 11th edn. Lippincott Williams & Wilkins, Philadelphia, p 225
2. Clemente CD (1997) Anatomy: a regional atlas of the human body, 4th edn. Lippincott Williams & Wilkins, Philadelphia, pp 160–171
3. Fathi AH, Soltanian H, Saber AA (2012) Surgical anatomy and morphologic variations of umbilical structures. Am Surg 78:540–544
4. O'Dey DM, Akabogu C, Bozkurt OA et al (2010) Perforator vessel anatomy of the papilla umbilicalis: topography and importance for reconstructive abdominal wall surgery. Langenbecks Arch Surg 395:1121–1127
5. Iida A, Yamaguchi A (2009) Single port laparoscopic cholecystectomy through the minimum navel incision from the bottom to the lower edge. J Jpn Soc Endosc Surg 15:531–536
6. Yasuda K, Kitano S (2009) Single port surgery: review of the literature and our initial experience. Asian J Endosc Surg 2:29–35
7. Curcillo PG 2nd, Wu AS, Podolsky ER et al (2010) Single-port-access (SPA) cholecystectomy: a multi-institutional report of the first 297 cases. Surg Endosc 24:1854–1860
8. Rivas H, Varela E, Scott D (2010) Single-incision laparoscopic cholecystectomy: initial evaluation of a large series of patients. Surg Endosc 24:1403–1412
9. Kanehira E, Siozawa K, Kamei A, Tanida T (2012) Development of a novel multichannel port (x-Gate®) for reduced port surgery and its initial clinical results. Minim Invasive Ther Allied Technol 21:26–30
10. Craig SB, Faller MS, Puckett CI (2000) In search of the ideal female umbilicus. Plast Reconstr Surg 105:389–392

Chapter 14
Cholecystectomy

James Skinovsky, Marcus Vinícius Dantas De Campos Martins,
Francisco Almeida, and Fernanda Keiko Tsumanuma

Abstract In 1987, the practice of videosurgery in the hands of the French surgeons Mouret and Perissat began one of the greatest revolutions in the history of the art of surgery, comparable to such landmark advances as the discovery of anesthesia and development of antibiotic therapy. Minimally invasive surgery has reduced suffering, decreased metabolic changes, and sped up patient recovery, being welcomed quickly and enthusiastically in operating rooms around the world.

The steady improvement in optical systems as well as the instruments used in videosurgery has allowed increasingly complex operations to be performed by minimally invasive methods.

For more than 20 years, videosurgery has been the gold standard for treating gallstones. New surgical approaches have been proposed as substitutes or complements to traditional, i.e., conventional videolaparoscopy, such as NOTES (natural orifice transluminal endoscopic surgery), needlescopy, and surgery by single access or LESS (laparoendoscopic single-site surgery). NOTES remains in the experimental stages, while LESS is a step ahead and expected to soon see widespread use.

In this chapter, the techniques, indications, possible contraindications, and preliminary results of LESS cholecystectomy are discussed.

Keywords Videosurgery • Cholecystectomy • LESS

J. Skinovsky (✉)
Surgery Department, LapSurg International Institute of Endoscopic Surgery, Positivo University, Red Cross University Hospital, Curitiba - Brazil
e-mail: skinovsky@gmail.com

M.V.D. De Campos Martins
Surgery Department, Estacio de Sa University, Rio de Janeiro - Brazil

F. Almeida • F.K. Tsumanuma
Surgery Department, Red Cross University Hospital, Curitiba - Brazil

T. Mori and G. Dapri (eds.), *Reduced Port Laparoscopic Surgery*,
DOI 10.1007/978-4-431-54601-6_14, © Springer Japan 2014

14.1 LESS: The Evolution

Since the report of experiments conducted by Kalloo et al. [1, 2], which signaled a new approach to endoscopic surgery, now known as NOTES, several researchers around the globe have been examining new devices and instruments to support the method as well as other new approaches, attempting to clarify their viability and practical applications.

The NOTES approach, a current challenge that will ultimately affect the future of minimally invasive surgery, presents several problems that remain to be resolved; examples include difficult internal orientation, the need for innovative hence expensive equipment and instruments, as well as training stations and courses, the infectious potential, and the questionable capacity to close the hollow organs appropriately. The use of standard endoscopes is problematic because surgeons are not used to the inverted view given by these devices. Accordingly, several barriers must be overcome to allow for adequate development of transluminal surgery, transforming NOTES into a routine clinical and surgical reality.

The transumbilical path currently presents itself as the most acceptable approach because the view is similar to that of conventional videosurgery, and the use of flexible and/or articulated instruments allows a better degree of triangulation, facilitating the necessary surgical manipulations.

Wheelees is credited as being the first to use the principles of single-access surgery, performing laparoscopic tubal ligations in 1969 [3].

In 1997 Navarra et al. [4] described cholecystectomy performed through two 10 mm trocars, which were introduced via the umbilicus.

Single-access surgery entered a period of latency, reappearing in 2007, when Zhu published his early experience using the umbilicus as a single access passage to the peritoneal cavity. He referred to this new approach as transumbilical endoscopic surgery (TUES) [5].

In 2008, Zhu et al. [6] described new clinical applications of TUES: hepatic cyst fenestration (two cases), cholecystectomy (six cases), and appendectomy (nine cases). The surgeries were achieved with the use of one trocar with three working channels.

Also in 2008, Palanivelu et al. [7], practicing in India, published a paper describing eight transumbilical appendectomies achieved with a standard flexible endoscope. The authors considered the technique as a stepping stone to NOTES.

Since then, single-access surgery, now called LESS, has been performed for different procedures such as nephrectomy and pyeloplasty [8–10], adrenalectomy [11], right colectomy [12], sleeve gastrectomy [13, 14], adjustable gastric band [15], Roux-en-Y gastric bypass [16], gastrostomy [17], intracorporeal gastrojejunostomy [18], and splenectomy [19], among others.

Several different multichannel trocars have been developed by companies around the world, such as the SITRACC® device (Edlo, Brazil), the Single-Site Laparoscopic Access System® (Ethicon Endo-Surgery, Cincinnati, OH, USA), GelPOINT® (Applied Medical, Rancho Santa Margarita, CA, USA), the TriPort or R-Port® system (Advanced Surgical Concepts, Wicklow, Ireland), X-Cone® and Endocone®

Fig. 14.1 SITRACC® (Edlo)
multichannel platform

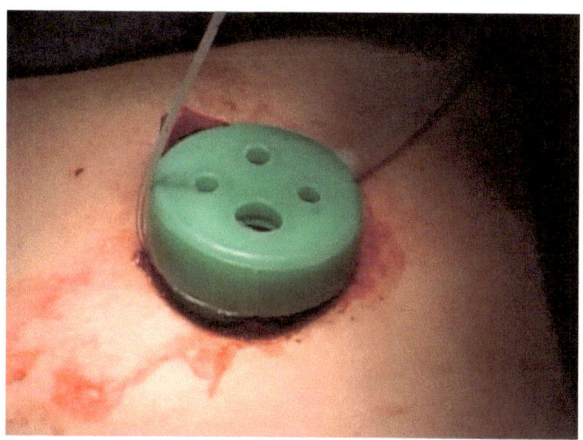

Fig. 14.2 (**a, b**) Articulated
distal extremity; prehension
forceps and hook for
coagulation

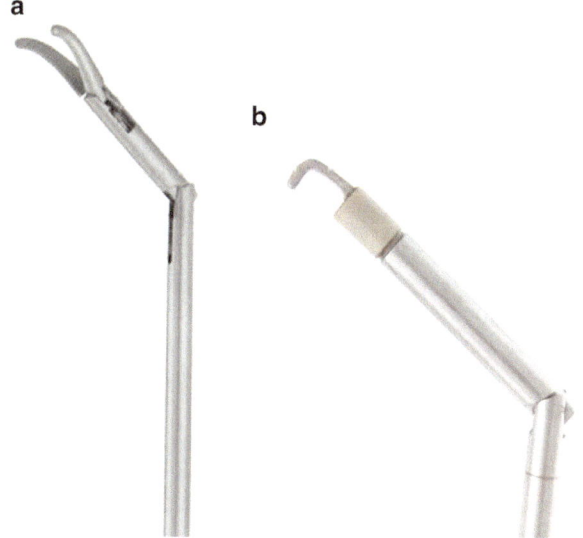

(Karl Storz-Endoskope, Tuttlingen, Germany), SILS™ (Covidien, New Haven, CT, USA), AirSeal® (SurgiQuest, Orange, CA, USA), and the SPIDER® system (TransEnterix, Durham, NC, USA) [20, 21], all of them assuming the use of a multichannel trocar and curved, flexible and/or articulated instruments.

Pioneering work in Brazil reported in 2007 issued in the development of a platform for single-access surgery, called SITRACC® (Single Trocar Access, Edlo, Porto Alegre, Brazil), consisting of a trocar with four working channels; flexible and/or articulated instruments were specially developed for this platform (Figs. 14.1, 14.2, and 14.3). With the technique studied in experimental animals, the first SITRACC® cholecystectomies performed in humans were reported in the following year [22, 23].

Fig. 14.3 Disposition of
internal and external
SITRACC® platform (Edlo)
and its curved/articulated
instruments

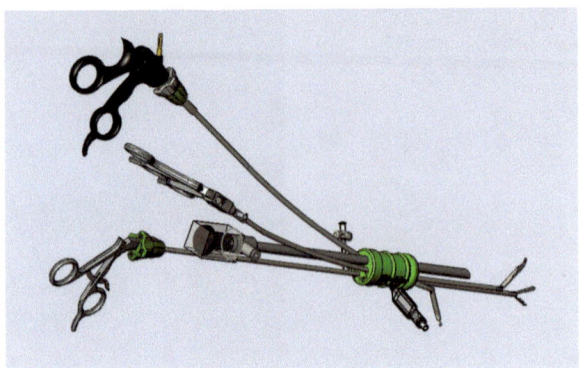

14.2   LESS Cholecystectomy: Technique

The SITRACC® platform (Edlo) consists of a multichannel trocar, with three 5-mm openings and one 10-mm opening, which can be changed to a 5-mm opening with the use of a reducer that is provided. Curved, articulated end, and flexible instruments have been specially created for this platform and approach. The use of 5-mm optics, with a minimum angle of 30°, is highly recommended.

The team positions are similar to those for conventional videolaparoscopic cholecystectomy, except the surgeon must stand more caudal to the patient, on the patient's left side. The camera person also stands on the left side (Fig. 14.4).

The multichannel trocar is introduced by the open technique through the umbilicus. It must be noted that better aesthetic results can be obtained with a completely perpendicular intra-umbilical incision. With such an incision, the surgical scar is fully hidden within the natural scar.

After introduction of the platform, the distal fixator balloon, which has a dual function (fixation in the abdominal wall and prevention of pneumoperitoneum leakage), must be inflated with approximately 15 mL of air; tension is registered and controlled externally (Fig. 14.5a, b). The entry portals of the platform must remain in the form of a cross, with the largest placed in the lower quadrant.

The first instrument introduced is the fully flexible grasper, which must grasp the bottom of the vesicle, pulling it toward the diaphragm and, at the same time, retract the liver to facilitate exposure of Calot's Triangle (Fig. 14.6).

The curved prehension forceps (which remain in the surgeon's left hand) are introduced through the left entry portal. These forceps must grasp the gallbladder infundibulum and, with lateral and anterior traction, adequately expose Calot's Triangle so that the cystic duct and artery are properly visualized.

The instruments for dissection/sectioning are then introduced under direct visualization, through the right entrance. These instruments, which may vary according to the circumstance and the surgical strategy, include the articulated hook, articulating dissector forceps, and curved scissors. It should be noted that, at certain times

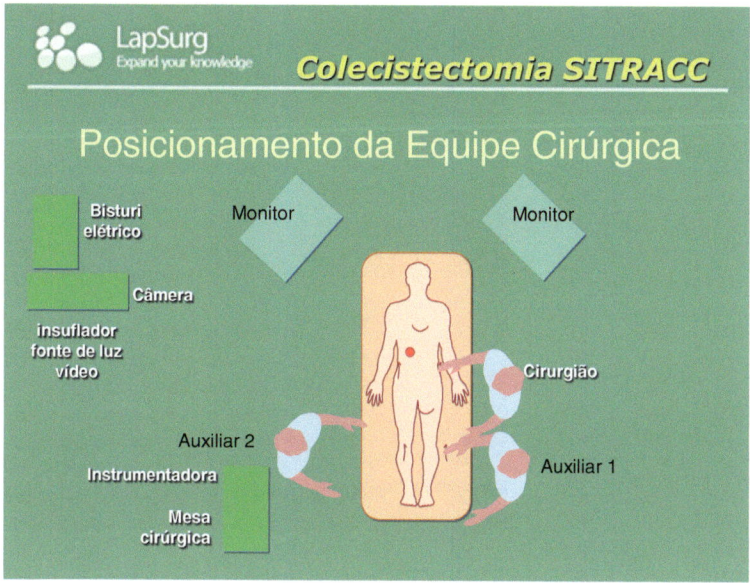

Fig. 14.4 Positioning of the surgical team

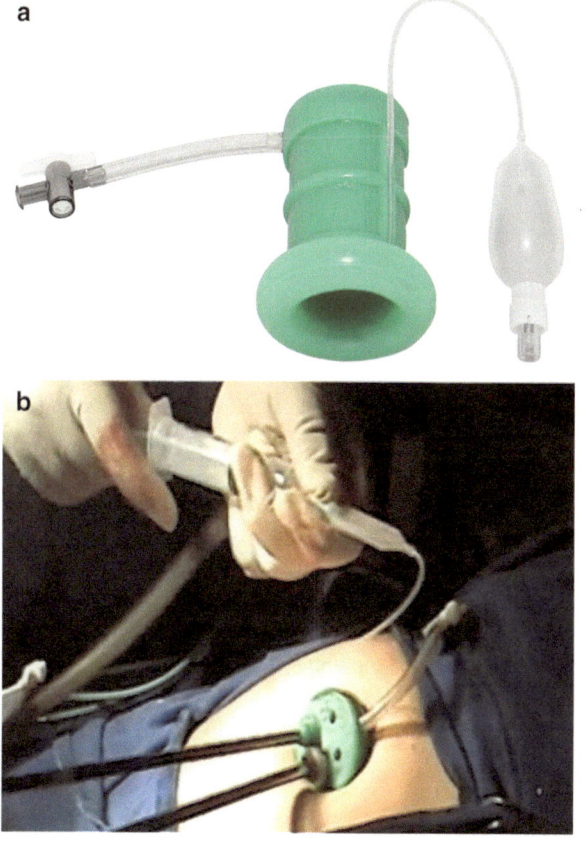

Fig. 14.5 (**a**) Platform with balloon (**b**) External insufflation of the balloon

Fig. 14.6 Totally flexible
grasper. Note the dual
function – to pull the
gallbladder and retract the
liver

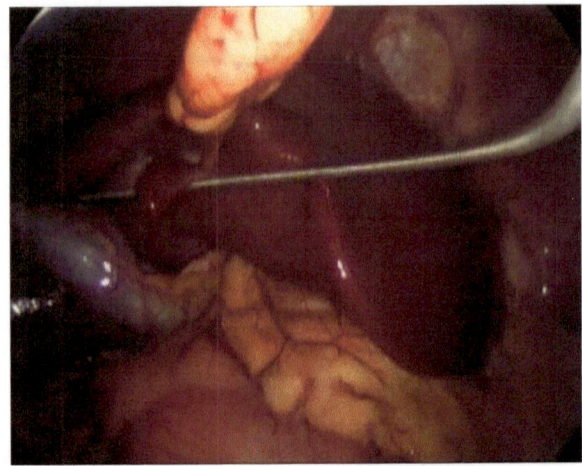

Fig. 14.7 Isolation of the
cystic duct by forceps for
articulated dissection

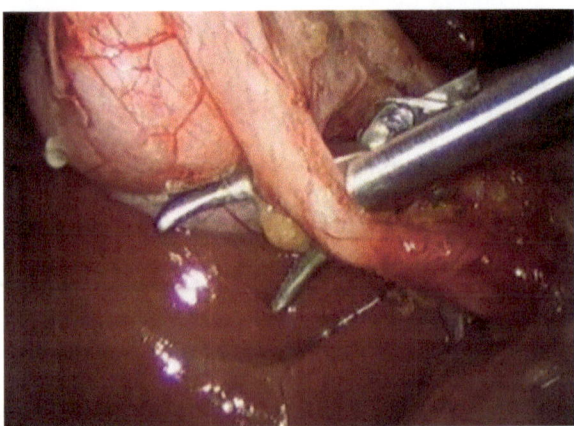

during the surgery, conventional rigid laparoscopic instruments may be needed. These can be used in a hybrid way, especially in cases of advanced inflammation and/or adhesion, because they provide greater strength for dissection.

The elements of the pedicle are then dissected and isolated, with movement facilitated by the distal articulation of the dissector instrument (Fig. 14.7). The cystic duct and pedicle vessels are then doubly clipped with 5-mm clips. If the cystic duct is particularly wide, a 10-mm clip applicator (LT400) can be used through the south entry portal. In this case, the reducer is removed, and the 5-mm optic is placed laterally. The curvature of the scissors helps greatly here (Fig. 14.8).

The gallbladder is then dissected from the liver bed by means of a coagulation hook with distal articulation (Fig. 14.9). This device allows adequate and ample movement for this step. After dissection of the gallbladder, hemostasis is established, and the organ is removed through the interior of the platform after the distal balloon is deflated (Fig. 14.10).

Fig. 14.8 Section of the
clipped cystic duct

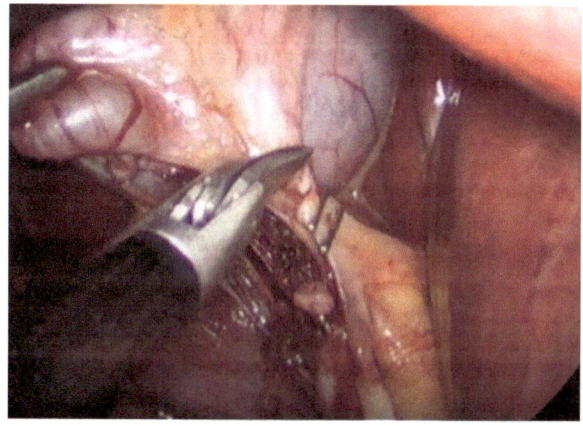

Fig. 14.9 Dissection of the
gallbladder by the articulating
hook

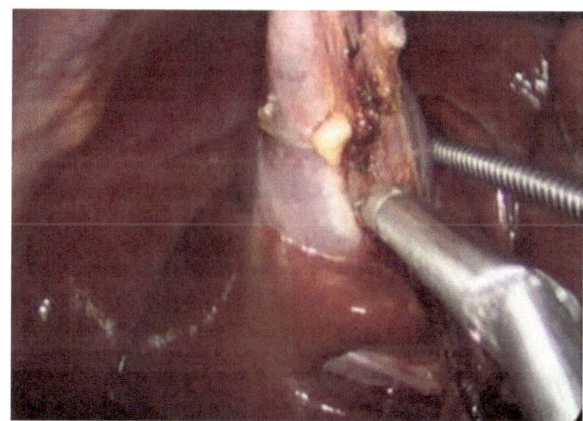

Fig. 14.10 Removal of the
gallbladder inside the
platform; the balloon is
deflated posteriorly

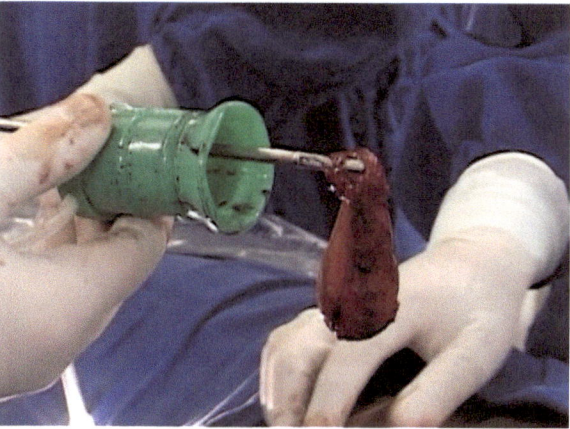

Fig. 14.11 Immediate
postoperative results

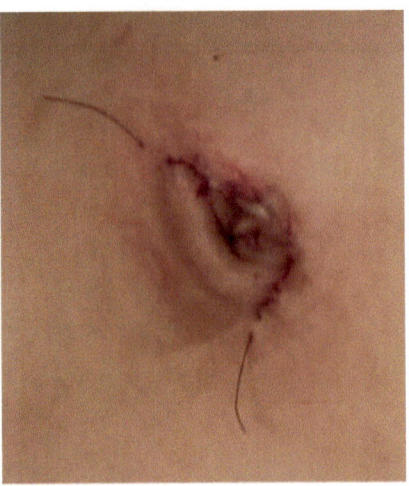

In difficult cases, it is possible to make use of a trocar of 5-mm or even 2-mm and positioned in the right hypochondrium to facilitate exposure of Calot's Triangle through traction at the bottom of the vesicle. When necessary, a Penrose drain can be inserted through the platform and removed via the same trocar.

The final scar measures about 20-mm (Fig. 14.11).

14.3 LESS Cholecystectomy: Results

A multicenter study [23] performed in 2008 and reported the next year, involved nine Brazilian surgery services in several cities and culminated in the performance of 81 LESS cholecystectomies. Ten surgeries required placement of an extra trocar in the right hypochondrium, due to technical difficulties. Three of the LESS procedures were converted to conventional videolaparoscopy.

Our personal experience with the LESS approach, using the SITRACC® platform, includes 172 cholecystectomies performed at the Red Cross Hospital/Positivo University, Curitiba, Brazil between October 2008 and June 2013, under approval of the institution's Ethics in Research Committee. All patients had symptomatic gallstones. Eight procedures required an additional portal of 5 mm in the right hypochondrium and, in four cases, full conversion to what we call conventional videolaparoscopy was required (all because of "difficult infundibulum"). There were no conversions to open surgery. The average operative time was 43 minutes, and all patients were released 24 hours after the surgery.

Post-operative complications were few. In one case, reoperation by means of conventional laparoscopy was necessary due to bleeding of the cystic artery within minutes after the procedure. In another case, a trocar-site hernia was found 11 months after the surgery.

14.4 Discussion

LESS maintains the principles of so-called scarless surgery, which leaves minimal or no scars. It also allows an operative view close to the view that the surgeon is already used to in regular laparoscopic procedures.

Due to the inherent difficulty of the method, there is a learning curve, and the team that proposes to perform LESS cholecystectomy must first attend preparatory courses and simulator training. Even surgeons experienced in the conventional laparoscopic approach will face initial difficulties with the peculiarities of the method: visualization is not always centered on the monitor, movements are restricted, the positions of the surgical team are different, and the manipulation of the instruments is particular. For this approach, a cohesive team that has worked together for a substantial amount of time is crucial to success.

Some challenges remain to be overcome before LESS can be considered a standard surgical reality. The triangulation capacity must be enhanced by the development of better articulated and curved instruments, allowing safer dissection movements. New lower caliber instruments and platforms are needed to increase ease of movement inside the abdominal cavity and decrease the surgical trauma.

The main difficulty to overcome arises from the need to work in a single axis of action, with the instruments disposed in parallel. The attempt to meet this challenge is represented by the above-mentioned development of flexible instruments and/or instruments articulated at their distal extremity, allowing for optimum albeit limited triangulation.

Internal movement of the instruments, even those adapted for LESS, is arduous, and it must be kept in mind that, when moving a single instrument, the whole tends to move in a single axis, requiring a team trained and experienced in the technique so that the visual field is not altered. The use of optics with angulation of at least $30°$ provides optimum visualization of the target tissue.

The training requires patience and time because, as shown, the procedure is not a simple variation of laparoscopy, and indeed, it is a new approach. Surgery workshops that provide practice in experimental animals as well as simulations are essential for good outcomes in human surgical settings.

The arrival of new tools and new and longer optics and use of output light source cables that can rotate $180°$ will facilitate the implementation of LESS and secure the ultimate popularity of this promising surgical method. We should remember that the LESS approach is part of the minimal-access surgery concept, and, in the event of need, nothing should prevent its use as a hybrid method, with, for example, elements of needlescopy and, in the near future, even a NOTES approach. The ultimate goal is a safely performed procedure, quick recovery, and satisfactory aesthetic results.

LESS cholecystectomy is feasible and safe in experienced hands. The operative time, after the learning curve, becomes similar to that of conventional laparoscopic surgery procedures. New studies in a large patient series are needed to compare this new approach to conventional endoscopic surgery procedures, especially with respect to metabolic response and the trocar hernia rate [24–26].

   LESS procedures must be considered part of an operative arsenal that includes
open surgery, endoscopic surgery, needlescopy, and eventually NOTES. Each
patient is unique, as is his illness. It is up to the surgeon to determine the best
approach in each particular case, with overall regard for the patient's safety and
optimum surgical and aesthetic results.

References

1. Kalloo AN, Sibgh VK, Jagannath SB, Niiyama H, Vaughn CA, Magee CA, Kantsevoy SV
   (2004) Flexible transgastric peritoneoscopy: a novel approach to diagnostic and therapeutic
   interventions. Gastrointest Endosc 60:114–117
2. Giday SA, Kantsevoy SV, Kalloo AN (2006) Principle and history of natural orifice translumenal endoscopic surgery (NOTES). Minim Invasive Ther Allied Technol 15:373–377
3. Wheeless CR (1969) A rapid, inexpensive and effective method of surgical sterilization by
   laparoscopy. J Reprod Med 3:65–69
4. Navarra G (1997) One-wound laparoscopic cholecystectomy. Br J Surg 84(5):695
5. Zhu JF (2007) Scarless endoscopic surgery: NOTES or TUES. Surg Endosc 21:1898–1899
6. Zhu JF, Hu H, Ma YZ, Xu MZ, Li F (2008) Transumbilical endoscopic surgery: a preliminary
   clinical report. Surg Endosc. http//www.springerlink.com/content. Accessed 2 Oct 2010
7. Palanivelu C, Rajan PS, Rangarajan M, Parthasarathi R, Senthilnathan P, Praveenraj P (2008)
   Transumbilical endoscopic appendectomy in humans: on the road to NOTES: a prospective
   study. J Laparoendosc Adv Surg Tech 18:579–582
8. Desai MM, Rao PP, Aron M, Haber GP, Desai M, Mishra S, Kaouk JH, Gill IS (2008) Scarless
   single port transumbilical nephrectomy and pyeloplasty: first clinical report. Br J Urol
   101:83–88
9. Kaouk JH, Haber GP, Goel RK (2008) Single-port laparoscopic surgery in urology: initial
   experience. Urology 71(1):3–6
10. Rané A, Rao P, Pr R (2008) Single-port-access nephrectomy and other laparoscopic urologic
    procedures using a novel laparoscopic port (R-Port). Urology 72:260–264
11. Castellucci SA, Curcillo PG, Ginsberg PC et al (2008) Single-port access adrenalectomy.
    J Endourol 22:1573–1576
12. Bucher P, Pugin F, Morel P (2008) Single port access laparoscopic right hemicolectomy. Int J
    Colorectal Dis 23:1013–1016
13. Saber AA, Elgamal MH, Itawi EA, Rao AJ (2008) Single incision laparoscopic sleeve gastrec-
    tomy (SILS): a novel technique. Obes Surg 18:1338–1342
14. Reavis KM, Hinojosa MW, Smith BR et al (2008) Single laparoscopic-incision transabdominal
    surgery sleeve gastrectomy. Obes Surg 18(11):1492–1494
15. Teixeira J, McGill K, Binenbaum S, Forrester G (2009) Laparoscopic single-site surgery for
    placement of na adjustable gastric band: initial experience. Surg Endosc 23:1409–1414
16. Saber AA, El-Ghazaly T, Minnick D (2009) Single port access transumbilical laparoscopic
    Roux-en-Y gastric bypass using the SILS port: first reported case. Surg Innov 16(4):343–347,
    http://sri.sagepub.com
17. Podolsky ER, Rottman SJ, Curcillo PG (2009) Single port access (SPA™) gastrostomy tube in
    patients unable to receive percutaneous endoscopic gastrostomy placement. Surg Endosc
    23:1142–1145
18. Bucher P, Pugin F, Morel P (2009) Transumbilical single-incision laparoscopic intracorporeal
    anastomosis for gastrojejunostomy: case report. Surg Endosc 23:1667–1670
19. Targarona EM, Balague C, Martinez C, Pallares L, Estalella L, Trias M (2009) Single-port
    access: a feasible alternative to conventional laparoscopic splenectomy. Surg Innov 16(4):
    348–352, http://sri.sagepub.com

20. Galvão Neto M, Ramos A, Campos J (2009) Single port laparoscopy access surgery. Tech Gastrointest Endosc 11(2):84–94
21. Romanelli JR, Earle DB (2009) Single-port laparoscopic surgery: an overview. Surg Endosc 23:1419–1427
22. Dantas MVDC, Skinovsky J, Coelho DE, Torres MF (2008) SITRACC – single trocar access: a new device for a new surgical approach. Bras J Vide Surg 1(2):60–63
23. Dantas MVDC, Skinovsky J, Coelho DE, Ramos A, Galvão Neto MP, Rodrigues J, de Carli L, Cavazolla LT, Campos J, Thuller F, Brunetti A (2009) Cholecystectomy by single trocar access – SITRACC: the first multicenter study. Surg Innov 16(4):313–316
24. Podolsky ER, Rottman SJ, Curcillo PG (2009) Single port access (SPA) cholecystectomy: two year follow-up. JSLS 13(4):528–535
25. Rasić Z, Schwarz D, Nesek VA, Zoricić I, Sever M, Rasić D, Lojo N (2010) Single incision laparoscopic cholecystectomy – a new advantage of gallbladder surgery. Coll Antropol 34(2):595–598
26. Skinovsky J, Dantas de Campos Martins MV, Chibata M, Cavalieri R, Tsumanuma F, Falcão D (2012) Comparison between single trocar access (SITRACC) cholecystectomy and conventional laparoscopic cholecystectomy – one year follow-up. Bras J Video Surg 5(1):3–8

Chapter 15
Cholecystectomy with Improved Retraction

Guillermo Domínguez and Marcelo Martinez-Ferro

Abstract The concept of Transumbilical Cholecystectomy with Magnetic Retraction (TCMR) is founded on reproducing classic laparoscopic surgery of the gallbladder, with an optimum vision and exposition of the triangle of Calot. Newly designed and already existing instruments and devices are deployed inside the abdominal cavity and used to perform surgical procedures. Thereafter, they are removed together with the surgical specimen through a single umbilical incision. Because TCMR is only performed with a single 12-mm trocar, it results in no visible scars and provides a superlative cosmesis and inferior pain scores in comparison to classic laparoscopy and other transumbilical approaches. The internal magnetic device replaces the use of graspers, needles or sutures and supplies the necessary retraction/countertraction force to enable sufficient triangulation. An external, larger and more powerful magnet placed over the abdominal wall controls it. Moreover, since it is not fixed at any level it can freely cruise the abdominal cavity according to the surgeon's need. Despite its few limitations and the need for further research, TCMR is a feasible and safe alternative to videosurgery and other transumbilical approaches. It is simple to learn and applicable in patients weighing more than 10 kg and a body mass index inferior to 40kg/m^2.

Keywords Magnetic retraction • Magnetic triangulation • Single-port cholecystectomy • Magnet assisted laparoscopic surgery

G. Domínguez (✉)
Department of General Surgery, Fundación Hospitalaria Private Children's Hospital, Crámer 4601, 3rd Floor, (C1429AKK), Ciudad Autónoma de Buenos Aires, Argentina

ImanLap Ltd Project, Crámer 4601, 3rd Floor, (C1429AKK), Ciudad Autónoma de Buenos Aires, Argentina
e-mail: info@imanlap.com

M. Martinez-Ferro
Department of Pediatric Surgery, Fundación Hospitalaria Private Children's Hospital, Crámer 4601, 3rd Floor, (C1429AKK), Ciudad Autónoma de Buenos Aires, Argentina
e-mail: martinezferro@fibertel.com.ar

T. Mori and G. Dapri (eds.), *Reduced Port Laparoscopic Surgery*,
DOI 10.1007/978-4-431-54601-6_15, © Springer Japan 2014

15.1 Introduction

Laparoscopic cholecystectomy has become the procedure of choice for the treatment of symptomatic stones and polyps in the gallbladder. The advantages of minimally invasive surgery have been widely accepted including shorter operation times, faster recoveries as well as decreased blood loss, scarring and pain [1–3]. In an effort to further minimize its invasiveness, surgeons have commenced operating on patients via a natural orifice or through a single transabdominal incision, generally umbilical, through which all instruments are introduced, either into a single specialized port or multiple small fascial incisions. Compared to laparoscopy, transumbilical surgery is associated to less parietal aggression, less risks of complications due to trocar incisions, inferior pain scores and improved patient cosmesis [4–6]. However, there are several technical complications that limit these practices including a safe access to the abdominal cavity, poor triangulation of the instruments and scope, instrument collisions and lack of maneuverability and reach [7].

Magnet-assisted laparoscopic surgery was developed in an effort to overcome the already mentioned shortcomings while reducing the number and size of trocars and incisions and the number of instruments and staff required in the operating room. It enables efficient multi-axial retraction, countertraction, mobilization and separation maneuvers just as if there were multiple access ports with opposite directions [8, 9]. The main objective is basically to create a safe and reproducible therapeutic option, so that patients can be treated even more gently and effectively though a single incision.

In 2005, one of the authors (GD) began with the design and development of the IMANLAP™ project (<<Iman>> stands for magnet in spanish and <<Lap>> is the abbreviation for Laparoscopy) to replace the use of graspers, needles or sutures commonly employed to retract an organ or tissue and sometimes associated to surgical trauma. In March 2007, GD performed the first laparoscopic single trocar cholecistectomy in Buenos Aires, Argentina. The surgery was completely assisted by IMANLAP™ technology. It was further registered at the argentine copyright registration office and a patent was requested in USA in August 2007 [10]. The following 40 consecutive cholecystectomies carried out in adults [11] and both authors pediatric experience with magnet-assisted laparoscopic surgery, have also been described [12] and shared with the scientific community.

The basic concept of this novel surgical modality is the use of a magnetic intracorporeal deployable device, the Internal Dominguez Magnetic Grasper internal magnetic grasp, composed by a spring-loaded alligator clamp linked to an 11.83-mm neodynium magnet coated with steel (Fig. 15.1) and guided by a larger, extracorporeal and powerful External Dominguez Magnetic Device external magnet (Fig. 15.2). The internal magnetic grasper is used to firmly grab and retract organs or tissues of up to 0.5 kg. By moving the external magnet (IMANLAP Ltd) in any direction, the internal magnetic grasper (IMANLAP Ltd) is displaced accordingly within the peritoneal cavity. The retracting magnetic force transmitted to the internal magnetic grasper is modulated by varying the distance between the external magnet and the abdominal wall.

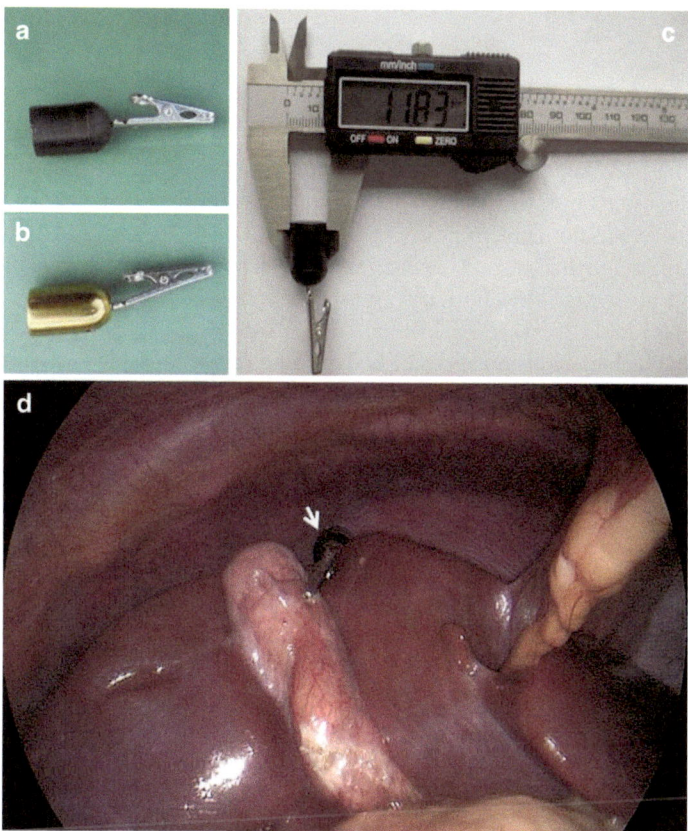

Fig. 15.1 The internal magnetic grasper (IMANLAP Ltd) can be (**a**) disposable or (**b**) reusable and is composed of a spring-loaded alligator clamp linked to an (**c**) 11.83-mm neodynium magnet. (**d**) The jaws of the alligator clamp (previously opened with the Thomas grasper™) are fastened tightly to the gallbladder's fundus (*arrow*). The gallbladder is tractioned cephalad and retracted over the liver edge towards the patient's right shoulder

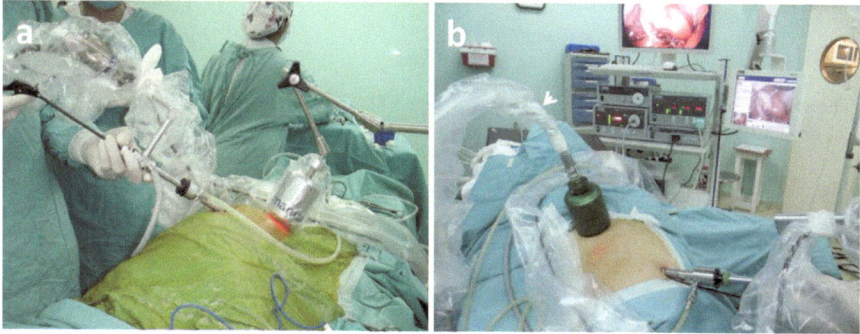

Fig. 15.2 (**a**) The external magnet (IMANLAP Ltd), coupled to its articulating self-retaining arm, is placed over the patient's abdominal wall. The laparoscope allows the surgeon to operate (take note of the 5-mm instrument inserted through the working channel) and drive the camera simultaneously (remember the camera headlight is coupled to a different and independent line). Visualization at the point of dissection can also be fixed this way (observe the red light below the external magnet) without the need for cumbersome roticulating instruments. (**b**) New version of the articulating self-retaining arm (*arrowhead*), which can be easily manipulated with one hand. It is more flexible and articulated

15.2   Instruments and Devices

Magnet-assisted laparoscopic surgery requires two sets of instruments and devices.

The first one comprises those *specifically designed* for magnet-assisted laparoscopic surgery as the Thomas grasper™ (IMANLAP Ltd, Buenos Aires, Argentina), the internal magnetic grasper, the external magnet, the Dominguez articulating self-retaining arm, and the Williams grasper™ (IMANLAP Ltd, Buenos Aires, Argentina) (Table 15.1).

The internal magnetic grasper (IMANLAP Ltd) can be reusable—environmentally friendly—or disposable (Fig. 15.1). By covering the intracorporeal magnet with biocompatible plastic, attractions between the instruments and the magnet are impeded. Moreover this material prevents the alligator clamp from transmitting electricity to the abdominal wall and enables the use of monopolar hook even in those cases in which the electrocautery device is leaning on the alligator clamp. This new version of

Table 15.1 Special instruments and devices for MALS (IMANLAP, Buenos Aires, Argentina)

Instrument	Brand	Description	Image
Internal dominguez magentic grasper internal magnetic grasper	IMANLAP Ltd, Buenos Aires, Argentina	It is a spring-loaded alligator clamp linked to an 11.83-mm neodynium magnet (5,000 Gauss or 0.5 Tesla) coated with steel. The newest versions are additionally coated with biocompatible plastic	
External dominguez magnetic device external magnet	IMANLAP Ltd, Buenos Aires, Argentina	Of major size and potency. It can be used solely or, as in the image, fixed to the Dominguez articulating self-retaining arm	
Thomas grasper™	IMANLAP Ltd, Buenos Aires, Argentina	Size: 5-mm × 50-cm. Made of austenitic surgical steel, which is unaffected by magnetic fields. It has two converging indented arms to handle, open, close and remove the internal magnetic grasper by its alligator clip. It allows its easy position and reposition within the body cavity	
Williams grasper™	IMANLAP Ltd, Buenos Aires, Argentina	Size: 5-mm × 50-cm. Curved, non-magnetic, roticulating and rigid grasper	

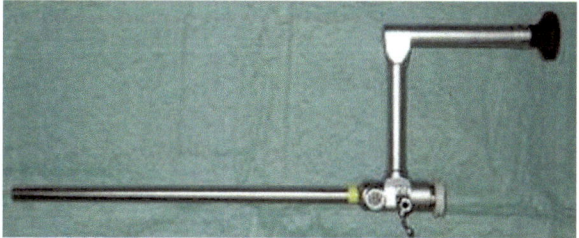

Fig. 15.3 10-mm, 27-cm, 0° laparoscope with a 6-mm working channel

the internal magnetic grasper ensures its sterilization with ethylene dioxide and is far more practical as there is no need to disassemble it for cleansing.

With the aim of achieving an effective surgical manipulation of the target organ, flexible control of its application point is essential. Fixation of the internal magnetic grasper (IMANLAP Ltd) was consequently improved by linking the alligator clamp to the magnet via a flexible connector. This results in softer retraction movements as the distance between the barycenter of the magnet and the application point is reduced.

The Thomas grasper™ (IMANLAP Ltd) handles the jaws of the alligator clamp intra-corporeally. It was specially designed to be unaffected by electromagnetic fields and with the necessary strength to open and close the alligator clamp. The force needed for these maneuvers is substantially greater than that required for any other routine endosurgical grasping action, what explains the reason why the internal magnetic grasper (IMANLAP Ltd) is held tightly at the application site and rarely becomes loose, being a safe and effective retraction tool. If by chance, the internal magnetic grasper is released, it can be rapid and easily managed with the Thomas grasper™ and attached where it corresponds.

The external magnet (IMANLAP Ltd) frees surgical assistants for other tasks and can enable the main surgeon to operate alone whenever coupled to the Dominguez articulating self-retaining arm fixed to the operating table. Since the external magnet can be easily engaged and disengaged from the arm, it is possible to use it manually when dynamic magnetic retraction is needed. However, when static magnetic retraction is required, the external magnet can always be re-engaged to the arm without difficulty (Fig. 15.2).

The second set comprises already existing instruments and devices as a single 12-mm trocar (any brand is suitable) to accommodate the 11.83-mm internal magnetic grasper (IMANLAP Ltd) or the SILS™ port (Covidien, New Haven, CT, USA) for operations requiring more extensive dissection or intraabdominal suturing. We recommend the use of a 10-mm, 27-cm, 0° laparoscope, with a 6-mm working channel (Karl Storz-Endoskope, Tuttlingen, Germany) because it allows surgeons to operate and drive the camera simultaneously (the camera headlight is coupled to a different and independent line) (Fig. 15.3). Commercially available 42-cm, 5-mm instruments (irrigation/aspiration devices, dissectors, graspers, scissors, forceps, harmonic scalpels, staplers, needle holders, etc), can be perfectly accommodated. The Thomas grasper™ (IMANLAP Ltd) and the 5-mm Hem-o-Lok clip applier (Weck Teleflex, Research Triangle Park, NC, USA) have been lengthened up to 45-cm, to enhance reach and to allow extra maneurability within the body cavity (Fig. 15.4). Regular transumbilical instruments with exaggerated curves or roticulating tips are impractical for magnet-assisted laparoscopic surgery because they transmit little torque and their movements are counteractive. We therefore prefer to use a 5-mm, gently curved non-roticulating grasper (Karl Storz-Endoskope).

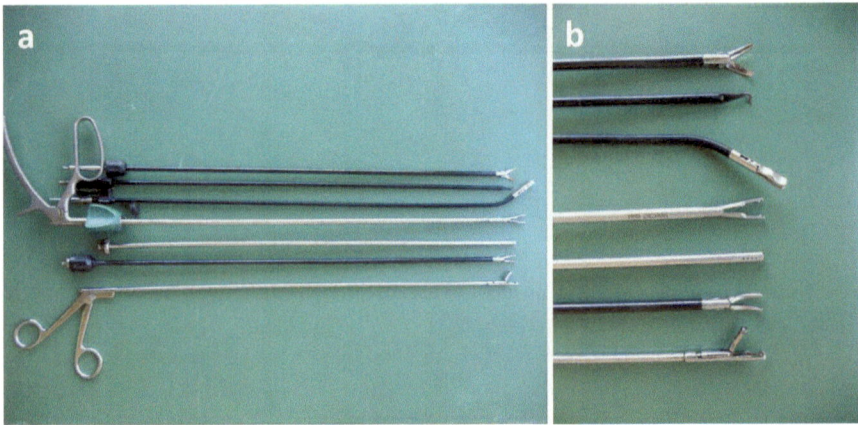

Fig. 15.4 (**a**) Instruments and devices required to perform a transumbilical cholecystectomy with magnetic retraction. (**b**) A closer view to their tips. From *left* to *right*: Thomas grasper™ (IMANLAP Ltd), dissector, irrigation/aspiration device, Hem-o-Lok clip applier (Weck Teleflex), gently curved non-roticulating grasper, monopolar hook, scissor

15.3 Contraindications

The absolute constrainments are pregnancy and pacemaker patients.
  The relative constrainments are:

- *Size of the patient:* in those patients weighing <10 kg magnet-assisted laparoscopic surgery is unrecommended, as the internal magnetic grasper (IMANLAP Ltd) diameter is 11.83-mm, what means that at least a 12-mm trocar is needed. This trocar size can be too large for small patients as neonates or nursing babies. Moreover, the small size of the body cavity difficults a safe and effective movement of instruments and magnetic devices.
- *Thickness of the abdominal wall:* for patients with a BMI >40 kg/m^2, magnet-assisted laparoscopic surgery is not suggested as the thickened abdominal wall provokes a loss of tractive and/or repelling force of the magnet. However in patients undergoing bariatric surgery they can be safely used with a larger and more powerful external magnet (IMANLAP Ltd).
- *Adhesions, distance from the abdominal wall and weight of the tractive organ:* can reduce the tractive force of the magnetic devices, though it is not necessarily a contraindication to magnet-assisted laparoscopic surgery.

15.4 Technique

Transumbilical Cholecystectomy with Magnetic Retraction, or in other words, magnet-assisted laparoscopic surgery of the gallbladder is founded on reproducing the classic laparoscopic cholecystectomy, with an optimum vision and exposition of the triangle of Calot. Before describing the technique, it must be pointed out that the technique can also be used as a complement in classic laparoscopic cholecystectomy since it clearly does not replace videosurgery but adds a surgical variant to the so called reduced port surgeries [11]. Additionally it makes possible the retraction of key structures without the need for needles, sutures and retractors permitting minimization of the number of access ports, incisions, and eventually staff.

General anesthesia is used in the same fashion as for a laparoscopic cholecystectomy. The patient's umbilicus is infiltrated with local anaesthesia (bupivacaine) to facilitate an equilibrated analgesia. A single 1.5-cm umbilical incision for a 12-mm port is performed. Even though in the beginning, we used to create the 12/14-mm Hg pneumoperitoneum using a Veress needle, we nowadays prefer the Hasson's technique, which is safe and recommendable since many years ago, and because it is the best alternative in those occasions in which a good exposition of the umbilical aponeurosis is indispensable for the extraction of surgical specimens.

15.5 TCMR with One Trocar and Assisted by Two internal magnetic grasper (IMANLAP Ltd)

The patient is placed in a reverse Trendenlenburg's position slightly rotated to the left. Initially the surgeon would stand up between the legs with the assistant aside and the scrub nurse opposite to the assistant (French position). Nowadays we use the American position with the monitor placed at the head of the operating table (Fig. 15.5).

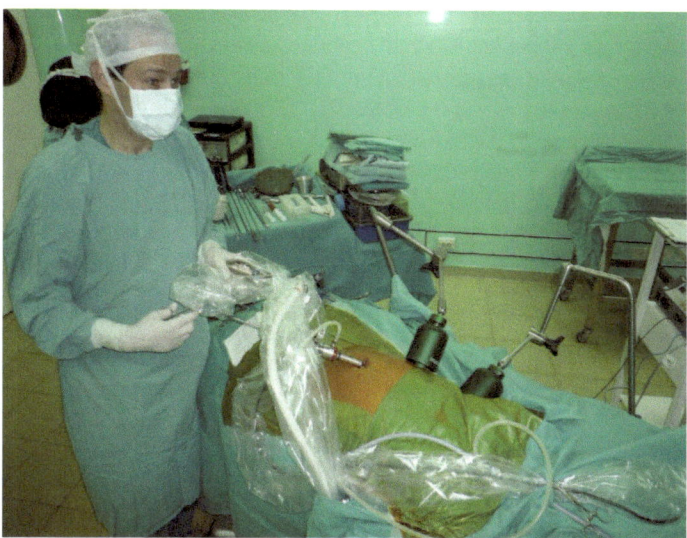

Fig. 15.5 Patient placed in the anti-Trendelenburg position and slightly rotated towards the *left*. The monitor (not seen in the picture) is placed at the head of the operating table. Transumbilical cholecystectomy with magnetic retraction permits operating on patients through one single incision, with one trocar and only one surgeon. Patients can therefore be operated on with less complications (as postoperative pain and wound infection), superlative cosmesis (scarless surgery) and inferior costs in comparison to other laparoscopic and transumbilical approaches

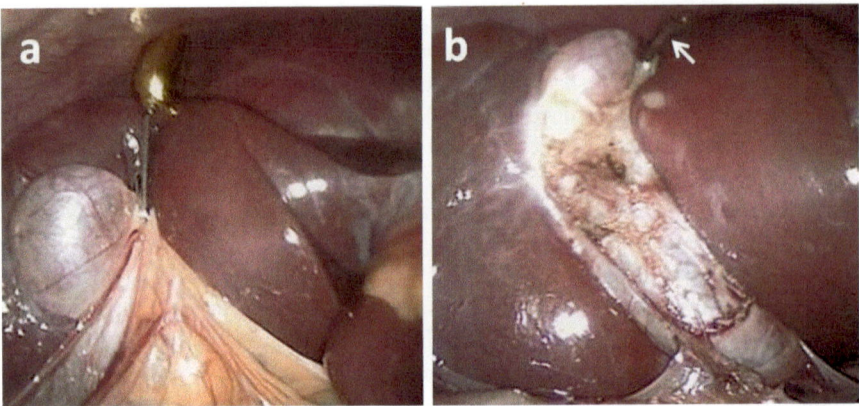

Fig. 15.6 The 1° internal magnetic grasper (IMANLAP Ltd) is used (**a**) to grasp the gallbladder and once the adhesions are released (**b**) to retract its fundus over the liver edge (*arrow*)

The approach is transumbilical in all patients. The umbilical stem is never removed to accomplish an excellent cosmetic result. The laparoscope is introduced through the 12-mm trocar. Once the first internal magnetic grasper (IMANLAP Ltd) is progressed into the abdominal cavity, it is manipulated under direct vision with the Thomas grasper™ (IMANLAP Ltd). The latter enables the surgeon to maneuver the alligator clamp (onward, from behind, laterally and from its tip) to further orient it towards the gallbladder whereas the magnet faces the parietal peritoneum.

The external magnet (IMANLAP Ltd) attached to the articulating self-retaining arm, is drawn near the patient's skin to generate a magnetic field across the abdominal wall that allows the mobilization of the internal magnetic grasper (IMANLAP Ltd) in all directions to suit the surgeon's need. The jaws of the alligator clamp are opened with the Thomas grasper™ (IMANLAP Ltd) and fastened tightly to the gallbladder's fundus or Hartmann's pouch. By moving the external magnet in the direction of the axilla, the liver is lifted cephalad exposing the gallbladder, which is retracted over the liver edge toward the patient's right shoulder (Fig. 15.6). By repositioning the external magnet on the abdominal wall, the intraabdominal magnet moves to provide further traction. Because the magnet is not fixed at any level, it can freely cruise around the peritoneal cavity, extending the surgeon's reach without the need for additional ports. Next, the laparoscope is removed and another internal magnetic grasper is inserted in the same way as the first one. This 2° internal magnetic grasper is placed in the infundibulum and managed by another external magnet to expose the triangle of Calot for its dissection (Fig. 15.7a) at first and for the cholecystectomy next (Fig. 15.7b, c).

Once the surgical field is exposed, each 5-mm diameter instrument can be passed through the laparoscope's 6-mm working channel for the cystic duct and vessels dissection, ligation and section, the cholangiography (whenever necessary), and the gallbladder dissection in the usual way that traditional laparoscopic cholecystectomy is performed. The cystic duct is sealed with a proximal medium sized Hem-o-lok polymer clip using the Hem-o-lock ligation applier, size M-L (Weck Teleflex) (Fig. 15.7a). The gallbladder is dissected at its base using an insulated hook. Finally, both internal magnetic grasper (IMANLAP Ltd) are released

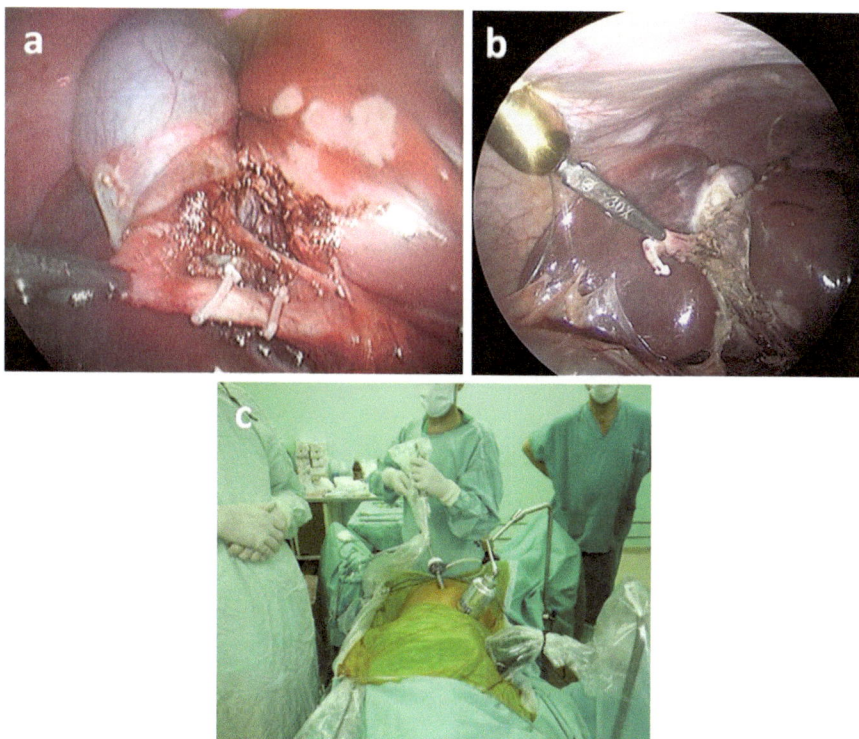

Fig. 15.7 The 2° internal magnetic grasper (IMANLAP Ltd) is placed in the infundibulum to expose the triangle of Calot as in (**a**). The cystic duct is sealed with proximal Hem-o-lok clips (Weck Teleflex). The gallbladder is dissected with an insulated hook. In (**b**) the 2° internal magnetic grasper is placed in the infundibulum and managed by a 2° external magnet (**c**) to complete the cholecystectomy

using the Thomas grasper™ (IMANLAP Ltd) and removed through the umbilical 12-mm trocar. The gallbladder is withdrawn under direct vision.

15.6 Transumbilical Cholecystectomy with Magnetic Retraction with One internal magnetic grasper: The Hybrid Method

The inconvenient of working with two internal magnetic grasper (IMANLAP Ltd) within the body cavity is the possibility of interactions produced between them. Despite this is infrequent when handled by experts, it can easily be solved by adding a leash to the 2° internal magnetic grasper (Fig. 15.8).

Another solution to this problem is the implementation of the non-magnetic curved Williams grasper™ to replace the 2° internal magnetic grasper (The Hybrid Method).

To carry out the surgeries, the same 12-mm trocar is used and the Williams grasper™ introduced parallel to the trocar (Fig. 15.9). This facilitates the election of the most adequate fixation site for the internal magnetic grasper. When the Williams grasper™

Fig. 15.8 A leash is added to the 2° internal magnetic grasper (IMANLAP Ltd) to prevent interactions produced between IDMGs. This is helpful when beginning with the practice of magnet-assisted laparoscopic surgery

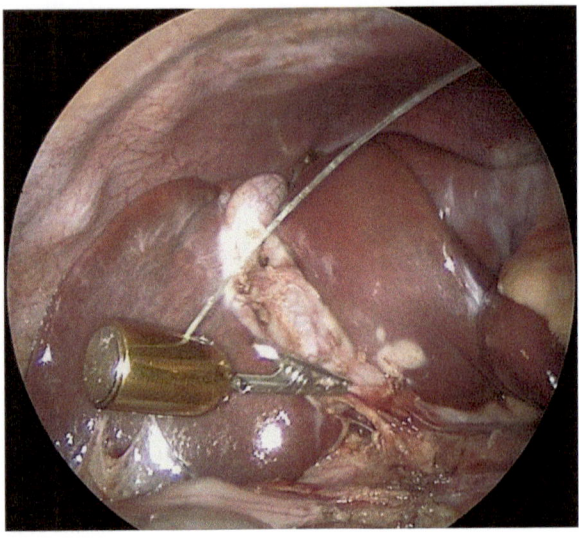

Fig. 15.9 The hybrid method: The Williams grasper™ (IMANLAP Ltd) introduced parallel to the trocar facilitates the election of the most adequate fixation site for the internal magnetic grasper (IMANLAP Ltd)

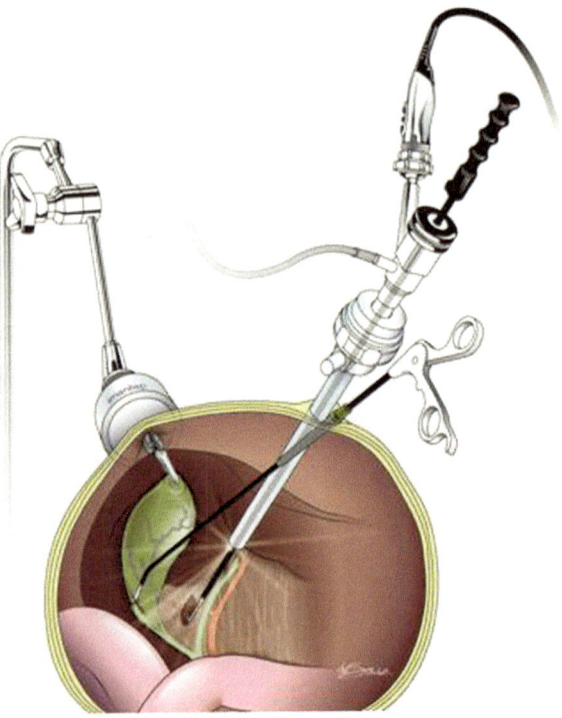

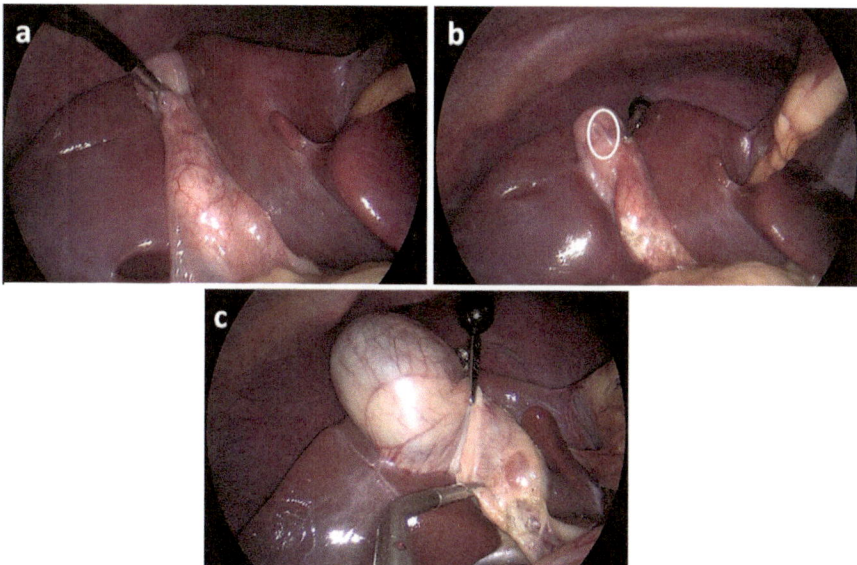

Fig. 15.10 (**a**) When the Williams grasper™ (IMANLAP Ltd) leaves an indentation (*circle*) in the gallbladder (**b**) the internal magnetic grasper (IMANLAP Ltd) can be anchoraged straightforwardly. (**c**) The Williams grasper™ and the internal magnetic grasper are grasping the gallbladder. Once the fundus is retracted, the Williams grasper™ is used to take control of the movements in the already formed bassinet

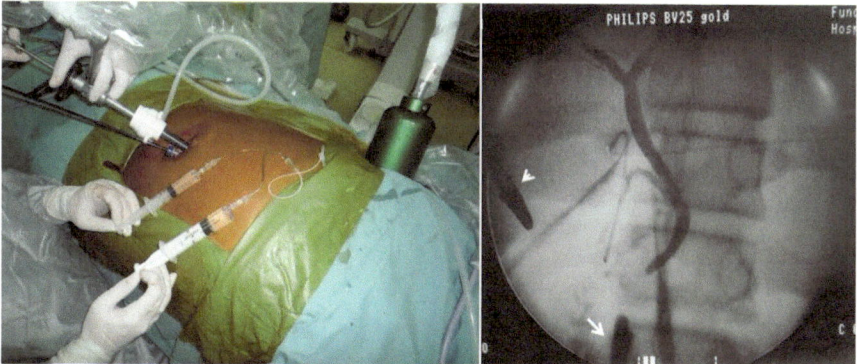

Fig. 15.11 Surgeon and assistant performing the cholangiography (*left*) and imaging of the bile duct (*right*). Take notice of the internal magnetic grasper (IMANLAP Ltd) (*arrow head*) and of the Williams grasper™ (IMANLAP Ltd) (*arrow*) inside the abdominal cavity

(IMANLAP Ltd) leaves an indentation in the gallbladder, the internal magnetic grasper can be anchoraged straightforwardly. Once the fundus is retracted over the liver edge, the non-magnetic curved grasper is used to take control of movements in the already formed bassinet (Fig. 15.10). Whenever necessary a colangiography can be done by performing the puncture in the right hipocondrium (Fig. 15.11). The rest of the procedure is as described anteriorly (Fig. 15.12). The pneumoperitoneum remained stable even during the fulfillment of extreme movements (Figs. 15.13, 15.14).

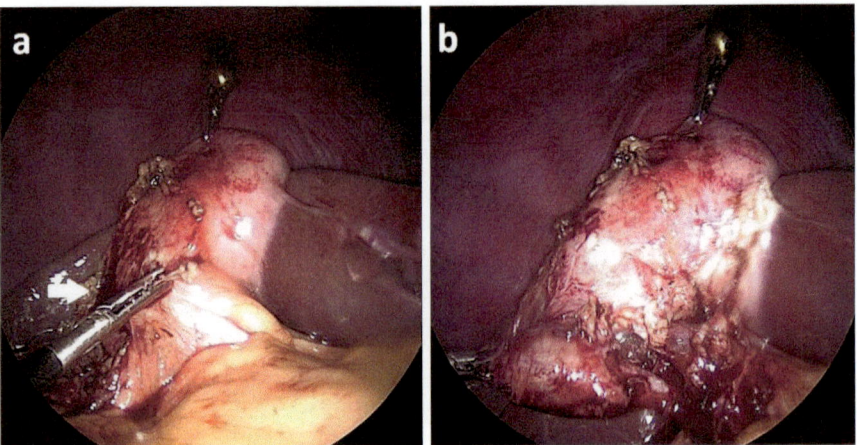

Fig. 15.12 The internal magnetic grasper (IMANLAP Ltd) retracts the fundus while the Williams grasper™ (IMANLAP Ltd) retracts the infundibulum (**a**) and releases the adhesions (**b**) to facilitate the dissection of the triangle of Calot

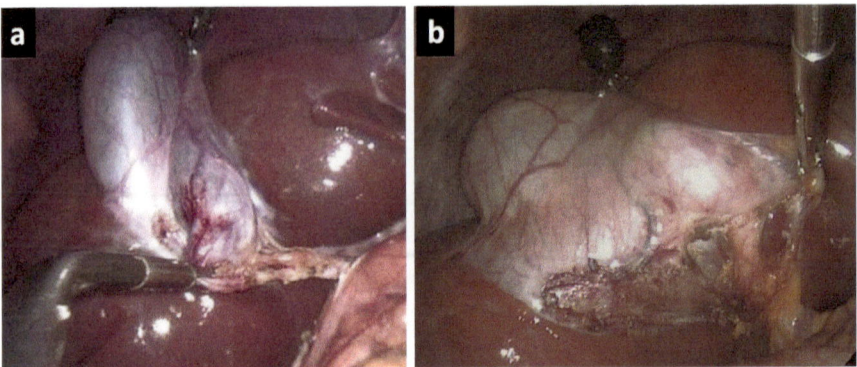

Fig. 15.13 (**a**) Exposition of the triangle of Calot after the dissection. The cystic duct and cystic artery are identified (flag technique) in (**b**) to be further clipped and cut

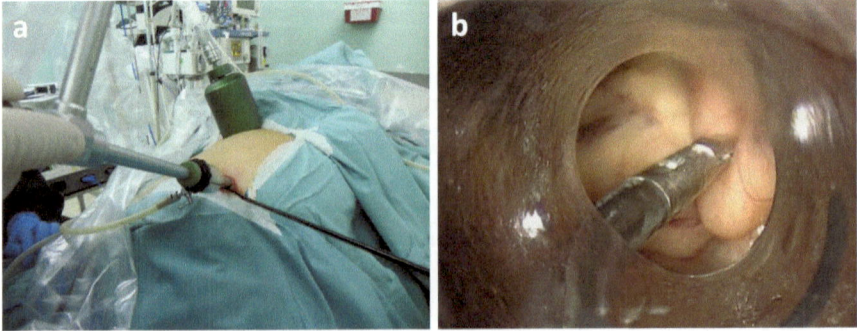

Fig. 15.14 (**a**) The non-magnetic curved grasper is inserted straightforwardly, parallel to the 12 mm trocar. The pneumoperitoneum remains stable even during the fulfillment of extreme movements. (**b**) The introduction of the Williams grasper™ (IMANLAP Ltd) can be observed by using a transparent trocar as the XCEL® trocar (Ethicon, Cincinnati, OH, USA)

15.7 Results

The results were very satisfactory for both procedures and for both programmed and urgent cholecystectomies (Table 15.2). All the cholecystectomies were completed exclusively with magnetic retraction, with no need to convert to open surgery. Even though a second additional port was required in three cases (0.76 %), the steps of multiport laparoscopy were successfully recreated and an optimal surgical view and working space, triangulation and ergonomics were attained in all cases.

The overall mean operation time was 54 min (range, 45–130 min) Intraoperative cholangiography resulted normal in all cases. There was a 1 % rate of minor intra-operative complications. In two cases, a small disruption of the gallbladder wall occurred and was solved with an alligator clamp (without magnets) that closed the hole. The operations continued as usual. In two of the first cases, the internal magnetic grasper (IMANLAP Ltd) fell in the abdominal cavity, and it was necessary to look for it with radioscopy. The new versions of the internal magnetic grasper for training surgeons have a leash that passes through the working port and enable their separation if they get entangled with each other. The recent biocompatible plastic they are covered with, additionally diminishes their probability of coupling.

There were no anesthetic complications related to the magnetic devices, such as changes in the pulse rate or the electrocardiographic monitoring. One adult patient had a metallic prosthesis in the dorso-lumbar backspin, but no interference with the magnetic devices was observed. Moreover, no interference between the magnetic devices and other devices and equipment in the operating room was detected.

One patient developed an infection at the site of the umbilical trocar insertion and received oral antibiotics for 1 week. No patient required opioid analgesia in the post-operative course.

Although not clinically studied, it was obvious in all cases that the postoperative pain was inferior in comparison to that reported after classic videosurgery. The hospital stay was the expected one for a laparoscopic cholecystectomy. In adults it was <24 h. The cosmetic results were superlative due to the use of one umbilical incision <15-mm. No scars were left even in pediatric patients. No biliar leakages were recorded. There were no re-operations or deaths. The time of follow-up time was 6 years (03-2007/03-2013).

Table 15.2 Results of cholecystectomies by magnet-assisted laparoscopic surgery

MALS	Case #	Mean operative time (min)	Conversion to open surgery; n=# (%)	Conversion to MIS with two trocars; n=# (%)	Reoperation; n=# (%)
Two IDMGs	138	60	0 (0)	2 (1.45)	0 (0)
Hybrid	207	50	0 (0)	1 (0.05)	0 (0)

15.8 Discussion

Laparoscopic surgery has outgrown conventional techniques thanks to endoscopic monitoring and specially designed instruments, which transmit the actions of the surgeon, as kinetic and static forces, to key structures with a good and safe exposition of the surgical field. Its main disadvantage compared with open surgery is the loss of tridimensional vision, but this has been rapidly compensated by an improved image and lightning quality, as well as professional training [1–3]. During the last few years, there have been various attempts to minimize the invasiveness of laparoscopic surgery including the development of needle-scopic instruments (with a diameter of < or = 3-mm) [13, 14], and the decrease in the size and number of access ports and instruments [4–6]. Several technical challenges have aroused, related principally to retraction and triangulation. Additionally, since both the instruments and laparoscope are introduced through the same incision and on the same axis, they often interfere with each other not only within the abdomen but also extra-abdominally, where attachments such as the camera light head, often impede movement.

Cholecystectomy is one of the most commonly performed transumbilical. In 1997 Navarra et al. described the first transumbilical cholecystectomy using transabdominal stay sutures on a Keith needle, secured externally using a clamp to allow for retraction of the gallbladder and infundibulum [15, 16]. Rawlings et al. proposed the addition of endoclips on each side of infundibular sutures to allow for extra external control in a "puppeteering" fashion [17]. Intracorporeal suture retraction has been described to eliminate the need to pass a needle through the abdominal wall [18]. Other authors [19, 20] recommend the use of an endoloop around the gallbladder fundus to replace any kind of sutures or the Endograb™ (Virtual Ports, Inc., Caesaera, Israel), a retraction system consisting of a reusable hand instrument (insertion tool) introduced via a 5-mm port and two disposable spring-loaded graspers (a gallbladder and an infundibular grasper) which are deployed in the abdominal cavity [19, 20]. The specific attachment points may be adjusted by simply opening the graspers and reattaching them to a different location. Last but not least, Horgan et al. have reported on the use of an extra-long RealHand™ grasper (Novare Inc., Cupertino, CA, USA) to perform a hybrid transvaginal cholecystectomy [5, 21]. The RealHand™ instrument is advanced transvaginally through a trocar and used to retract and manipulate the gallbladder. Other groups in Europe have depicted similar retraction strategies using extralong laparoscopic graspers placed transvaginally during NOTES cholecystectomy [22].

Even though numerous investigators have described the use of these techniques with good results, several potential drawbacks as bile spillage, tissue shearing, risk of bleeding from piercing blood vessels with either the needles or graspers, the fact the Keith needle is 6-cm in length and may be particularly awkward to manipulate, the difficulty to learn the procedure in some cases or the high cost of using the endoloop and the Endograb™ device.

Different other authors have accounted the use of magnets as retraction devices for less invasive gallbladder surgery. Cadeddu and Scott developed a magnetic anchoring and guidance system (MAGS) for endoscopic surgery [23, 24], consisting of a portable magnet placed intraabdominally and then coupled to an extracorporeal handheld neodymium magnet across the abdominal wall. MAGS instruments, which include a camera, tissue retractors, and monopolar cautery, are then controlled trans-abdominally, allowing for unrestricted intraabdominal movement and improvement in spatial orientation. The internal magnet can be attached to an 18-gauge percutaneous needle lock, anchoring the platform to permit the removal of the external magnet. Continuous instrument development and rapid prototyping have created more robust MAGS platforms while potentially obviating the need for laparoscopic assistance. Animal work to date has been promising with successful completion of a single-port nephrectomy as well as transvaginal NOTES cholecystectomy in both non-survival and survival porcine models [7]. Ryou and Thompson described the use of magnets attached to endoclips to elevate the liver for gallbladder retraction during transcolonic cholecystectomy in a porcine model [25]. They used several magnetic clips placed along the inferior edge of the liver and a very large external magnet to elevate the right anterior portion of the liver. This in turn provided good exposure of the gallbladder to facilitate dissection with flexible endoscopic instruments. After completion of the procedure, the clips were removed with apparently no major tissue trauma. Kume et al. presented a swine operation performed with a magnetic retraction system. One magnet was inserted into the peritoneal cavity and fixed to the gallbladder's fundus using an endovascular clip. The other one was located outside the abdominal wall to guide the intra-peritoneal magnet. They concluded the newly designed magnet-retracting forceps could transfer the electromagnetic force through the abdominal wall with good endoscopic view. The magnets enabled highly flexible retraction with variable angle, distance and location [26]. However they pointed out a series of drawbacks and limitations mainly that although neodymium represents an adequate material for efficient magnetic power, it is fragile and susceptible to corrosion. Multiple magnets would interfere with each other and their force could crush intra-peritoneal tissue. The magnetic interactions with a lot of magnetic materials contained in various surgical instruments would not only disturb smooth surgical procedures, but also generate unexpected motions that could not be controlled. The magnetic force could also affect the electro-magnetic function of human physiology and interact with electrical devices and equipment in the operating room.

Concerned by the potential tissue effects of magnet compression, Mashaud et al. examined abdominal wall tissue grossly and histologically after transumbilical cholecystectomy using a MAGS cautery dissector device in a porcine model [27]. They observed no histological evidence of tissue necrosis or damage of skin, muscle, or peritoneum. However, they highlighted insufficient coupling strength may be a problem. Magnetic coupling across the abdominal wall is exponentially related to the distance between magnets, with magnetic attraction decreasing dramatically as separation distance increases. In an ex vivo model investigating magnetic force decay, Best et al. found that static coupling was maintained to a maximum distance of 4.78-cm [28]. Milad et al. conducted an investigation in 138 women in which they measured abdominal wall thickness in the left upper quadrant and umbilicus after insufflation using a spinal needle during gynecologic laparoscopy [29]. They found that only 1.5 % of women with a BMI greater than 40 kg/m^2 had an abdominal wall thickness greater than 4 cm. While these data do not account for potential frictional forces, current data suggest that the MAGS platform should be suitable for a significant portion of the adult population undergoing procedures such as cholecystectomy.

The IMANLAP™ technology permits dynamic and flexible retraction and triangulation from different angles as if there were multiple trocars with opposite directions as well as enough instrument spacing to prevent collisions, in patients of all ages, whose BMI is inferior to 40 Kg/m^2. An electromagnetic field is generated by drawing the external magnet (IMANLAP Ltd) upon the abdominal wall. This allows magnetic devices to move unrestrictedly from the upper abdomen to the pelvis with no need for a new incision. The magnetic retraction forces depend on the distance between the internal magnetic grasper (IMANLAP Ltd) and the external magnet and the magnetic field strength of each, which in turn depend on the thickness of the abdominal wall [16, 17]. Therefore, regulation of the distance between magnetic devices enables regulation of magnetic retraction forces during the entire surgery. Since retraction is not confined by an access-port fixed to the abdominal wall, the operation turns out to be less invasive and surgical trauma is further decreased. Magnet-assisted laparoscopic surgery provides good visual access to the point of dissection too.

By performing a transumbilical cholecystectomy with magnetic retraction the use of tractor stitches, needles and hepatic separators can be avoided by firmly fixing the alligator clamp to key structures as the gallbladder's fundus and the infundibulum. Bile spillage, tissue shearing and the risk of bleeding from piercing blood vessels is thereby precluded.

Recent redesign of the IDMGs (IMANLAP Ltd) makes them easier to handle within the peritoneal cavity and yet more difficult to couple; however, if this happens, the IDMGs can be easily separated without intraoperatory complications as tissue damage or uncontrollable maneuvers. Alterations in physiological parameters resulting from the interaction of the magnetic devices with the patient, the anesthetic monitoring and the rest of the devices and equipment in the operating room were never noticed.

The internal magnetic grasper (IMANLAP Ltd) enhances intracorporeal instrument manipulation and facilitates comfortable operating movements. Surgical devices made of austenitic stainless steel which are unaffected by alterations in magnetic fields, are used to handle and take control of them.

In comparison to other transumbilical approaches, transumbilical cholecystectomy with magnetic retraction reduces the number of instruments and staff necessary, thereby lowering the costs. Since the number of incisions required is one, it leads to less postoperative pain, less risks of wound related complications and a superlative cosmesis (the surgical scar can generally be hidden within the umbilicus). Transumbilical cholecystectomy with magnetic retraction is environmentally friendly. X-rays or fluoroscopy can be carried out without inconveniencies. Hospital stay and operatory time are commensurate with traditional videosurgical results. The only current limitation is patient weight and BMI.

15.9   Tips, Tricks and Recommendations

1. Whenever the patient has voluminous breasts or breast prosthesis, these are displaced with hypoallergenic tape to avoid putting the external magnet (IMANLAP Ltd) over them and to decrease the distance between the magnetic devices. Extra efficient maneuvers are thereby enhanced.

2. If the gallbladder is distended or its wall is thickened as it occurs in many patients with cholecystitis, the organ can be punctured and evacuated, and then the alligator clamp is fixed to the puncture site to avoid biliary leakages.
3. The external magnet (IMANLAP Ltd) can be easily engaged and disengaged from the Dominguez articulating self-retaining arm, which is quite flexible, whenever dynamic magnetic retraction is needed. The external magnet is used manually then. Nonetheless, whenever static magnetic retraction is required, the external magnet can always be linked to the Dominguez articulating self-retaining arm without difficulty.
4. Even though it is believed that two magnets might interfere with each other and that their magnetic retraction force could eventually press and crush intra-peritoneal tissue, this is solved by adding a leash to the $2°$ internal magnetic grasper (IMANLAP Ltd) in order to facilitate their rapid separation in case they get entangled. Surgeons with experience in magnet-assisted laparoscopic surgery can further opt to employ the Williams™ grasper to replace the $2°$ internal magnetic grasper, at first through a 5 mm trans-aponeurotic trocar and later alone.
5. The interactions with magnetic materials contained in various surgical instruments is a big problem because they do not only disturb smooth surgical procedures, but can also generate unexpected and uncontrollable motions. This dangerous property was solved carefully by using the Thomas™ grasper (IMANLAP Ltd) which is made of austenitic surgical steel, unaffected by magnetic fields. It has two converging indented arms to handle, open, close and remove the internal magnetic grasper (IMANLAP Ltd) by its alligator clip. It basically allows the internal magnetic grasper to be easily positioned and repositioned within the body cavity thus avoiding any kind of magnetic interaction between instruments and devices. The biocompatible plastic of which the inner magnet is coated additionally reduces the probability of IDMGs entanglement.
6. Since magnetic fields can affect the electro-magnetic function of human physiology and interact with electrical devices in the operation room, the IDMGs (IMANLAP Ltd) are coated with martensitic surgical steel additionally covered by a biocompatible plastic to prevent this from happening.
7. By using the internal magnetic grasper (IMANLAP Ltd) a secure grabbing is warranted. The gallbladder's fundus and infundibulum are never released. No organ or tissue has ever been perforated. The Thomas grasper™ (IMANLAP Ltd) has been lengthened to further enhance reach and to allow extra maneurability within the body cavity.
8. Transumbilical instruments with exaggerated curves or roticulating tips are unrecommended because they transmit little torque and their movements are counteractive.

15.10 Conclusions

Magnet-assisted laparoscopic surgery is feasible and safe in hands of experienced laparoscopic surgeons. It reproduces classic laparoscopy through a single umbilical incision, resulting in no visible scars, a superlative cosmesis and lesser pain. The possibility to control the magnetic field provides enough strength for retraction and sufficient triangulation for adequate exposure of the surgical field. The technique is reproducible, easy to learn and applicable in pediatric, adolescent and adult patients.

References

1. Trondsen E, Reiertsen O, Andersen OK, Kjaersgaard P (1993) Laparoscopic and open chole-cystectomy. A prospective, randomized study. Eur J Surg 159:217–221
2. Berggren U, Gordh T, Grama D, Haglund U, Rastad J, Arvidsson D (1994) Laparoscopic ver-sus open cholecystectomy: hospitalization, sick leave, analgesia and trauma responses. Br J Surg 81:1362–1365
3. Kiviluoto T, Siren J, Luukkonen P, Kivilaakso E (1998) Randomised trial of laparoscopic versus open cholecystectomy for acute and gangrenous cholecystitis. Lancet 351:321–325
4. Ponsky TA, Diluciano J, Chwals W et al (2009) Early experience with single-port laparoscopic surgery in children. J Laparoendosc Adv Surg Tech A 19(4):551–553
5. Horgan S, Cullen JP, Talamini MA et al (2009) Natural orifice surgery: initial clinical experi-ence. Surg Endosc 23(7):1512–1518
6. Qiu Z, Sun J, Pu Y, Jiang T, Cao J, Wu W (2011) Learning curve of transumbilical single inci-sion laparoscopic cholecystectomy (SILS): a preliminary study of 80 selected patients with benign gallbladder diseases. World J Surg 35(9):2092–2101
7. Raman JD, Scott DJ, Cadeddu JA (2009) Role of magnetic anchors during laparoendoscopic single site surgery and NOTES. J Endourol 23(5):781–786
8. Padilla BE, Domínguez G, Millán C et al (2013) Initial experience with magnet-assisted single trocar appendectomy in children. J Laparoendosc Adv Surg Tech A 23(5):463–466
9. Morales-Conde S, Dominguez G, Cañete Gomez J, Socas M, Barranco A, García Moreno J, Padillo FJ (2013) Magnetic-assisted single-port sleeve gastrectomy. Surg Innov 20(4): NP9–NP11
10. Dominguez G (2007) Colecistectomía con un trocar asistida por imanes de neodimio. Reporte de un caso. Asociación Mexicana de TCMRugía Endoscópica AC 8(4):172–176
11. Dominguez G, Durand L, De Rosa J et al (2009) Retraction and triangulation with neodymium magnetic forceps for single-port laparoscopic cholecystectomy. Surg Endosc 23(7): 1660–1666
12. Padilla BE, Dominguez G, Millan C, Martinez-Ferro M (2011) The use of magnets with single-site umbilical laparoscopic surgery. Semin Pediatr Surg 20(4):224–231
13. Gagner M, Garcia-Ruiz A (1998) Technical aspects of minimally invasive abdominal surgery performed with needlescopic instruments. Surg Laparosc Endosc 8(3):171–179
14. Lee KW, Poon CM, Leung KF, Lee DW, Ko CW (2005) Two-port needlescopic cholecystec-tomy: prospective study of 100 cases. Hong Kong Med J 11(1):30–35
15. Navarra G, Pozza E, Occhionorelli S et al (1997) One wound laparoscopic cholecystectomy. Br J Surg 84:695
16. Ponsky T (2009) Single port laparoscopic cholecystectomy in adults and children: tools and techniques. J Am Coll Surg 209:e1–e6
17. Rawlings A, Hodgett S, Brunt M et al (2010) Single-incision laparoscopic cholecystectomy: initial experience with critical view of safety dissection and routine intraoperative cholangiog-raphy. J Am Coll Surg 211:1–7
18. Rivas H, Varela E, Scott D (2010) Single-incision laparoscopic cholecystectomy: initial evalu-ation of a large series of patients. Surg Endosc 24:1403–1412
19. Schlager A, Khalaileh A, Mintz Y et al (2009) Providing more through less: current methods of retraction in SIMIS and NOTES cholecystectomy. Surg Endosc 24:1542–1546

20. Shussman N, Schlager A, Mintz Y et al (2011) Single-incision laparoscopic cholecystectomy: lessons learned for success. Surg Endosc 25:404–407
21. Horgan S, Mintz Y (2009) NOTES: transvaginal cholecystectomy with assisting articulating instruments. Surg Endosc 23:1900
22. Zornig C, Mofid H, Emmermann A et al (2008) Scarless cholecystectomy with combined transvaginal and transumbilical approach in a series of 20 patients. Surg Endosc 22: 1427–1429
23. Park S, Bergs RA, Eberhart R, Baker L, Fernandez R, Cadeddu JA (2007) Trocar-less instrumentation for laparoscopy: magnetic positioning of intra-abdominal camera and retractor. Ann Surg 245(3):379–384
24. Scott DJ, Tang SJ, Fernandez R et al (2007) Completely transvaginal NOTES cholecystectomy using magnetically anchored instruments. Surg Endosc 21(12):2308–2316
25. Ryou M, Thompson C (2009) The use of magnets in natural ori fi ce transluminal endoscopic surgery (NOTES): addressing the problem of traction and countertraction. Endoscopy 41: 143–148
26. Kume M, Miyazawa H, Abe F, Iwasaki W et al (2008) A newly designed magnet-retracting forceps for laparoscopic cholecystectomy in a swine model. Minim Invasive Ther Allied Technol 17(4):251–254
27. Mashaud L, Kabbani W, Scott D et al (2011) Tissue compression analysis for magnetically anchored cautery dissector during single-site laparoscopic cholecystectomy. J Gastrointest Surg 15:902–907
28. Best S, Bergs R, Scott D et al (2011) Maximizing coupling strength of magnetically anchored surgical instruments: how thick can we go? Surg Endosc 25:153–159
29. Milad M, Terkildsen M (2002) The spinal needle test effectively measures abdominal wall thickness before cannula placement at laparoscopy. J Am Assoc Gynecol Laparosc 9:514 518

Chapter 16
Common Bile Duct Exploration

Akiko Umezawa

Abstract Treatment for common bile duct stones (CBDS) has been divided roughly into two different procedures, two-step and single step methods. In the two-step method, LC is performed after endoscopic treatment. The single-step method includes open or laparoscopic surgery in which common bile duct stones are removed during surgery. Single-step laparoscopic surgery, namely laparoscopic common bile duct exploration (LCBDE), is preferred because of the simplicity of treatment. Needlescopic LCBDE has two benefits. One is completion of treatment for CBDS during one time laparoscopic surgery, and the other is less invasiveness to the abdominal wall and resulting cosmetic improvement.

There are two kinds of approaches in LCBDE, according to the route of exploration: trans-cystic duct exploration (LTCE) and trans-choledochal exploration (LCHE).

Although there are limitations to the indication for needlescopic LTCE, it is feasible and should be the first line of treatment for CBDS. The benefits of this approach include not only the fact that it is non-invasive to the sphincter and does not injure the CBD wall, but also that it can offer a good cosmetic result. With LCHE as a redeeming approach, LCBDE with needle forceps is also feasible and offers good clinical outcomes in treatment for CBDS.

Keywords Choledocholithiasis • Common bile duct exploration • Common bile duct stone • Laparoscopic surgery • Needlescopic surgery

A. Umezawa (✉)
Minimally Invasive Surgery Center, Yotsuya Medical Cube,
7-7 Ni-bancho, Chiyoda-ku, Tokyo 102-0084, Japan
e-mail: umezawa@mcube.jp

T. Mori and G. Dapri (eds.), *Reduced Port Laparoscopic Surgery*,
DOI 10.1007/978-4-431-54601-6_16, © Springer Japan 2014

171

16.1   Introduction to the Technique

Laparoscopic cholecystectomy (LC) has been the most common procedure world-wide. Patients who undergo LC may have certain expectations for their surgery, such as safeness, minimal invasiveness, and cosmetic satisfaction. In an effort to fulfill those expectations, ports and instruments need to be as thin as possible while maintaining their maneuverability. The term "needlescopic" is for operations performed with laparoscopic instruments up to 3-mm in diameter, as introduced by Gagner and Garcia-Ruiz [1].

Common bile duct stone (CBDS) is one of the most common comorbidities in cholecystolithiasis and occurs in 10–15 % of the patients. It occurs more frequently in the elderly.

Treatment for CBDS has been divided roughly into two different methods, two-step and one-step methods. In the two-step method, LC is performed after endoscopic treatment (EST). The single step method includes open or laparoscopic surgery in which common bile duct stones are removed during surgery. The two-step method requires endoscopic treatment, which is time consuming, sometimes requiring several sessions. Residual choledochal stone is not a rare condition after the endoscopic removal.

In contrast, single step laparoscopic surgery, namely laparoscopic common bile duct exploration (LCBDE), is preferred because of the simplicity of treatment. There are two kinds of approaches in LCBDE according to the route of exploration: trans-cystic duct exploration (LTCE) and trans-choledochal exploration (LCHE).

Needlescopic LCBDE has two benefits. One is completion of treatment during one time laparoscopic surgery, and the other is less invasiveness to the abdominal wall and resulting cosmetic improvement.

16.2   Indications and Contraindications

Our indications of needlescopic LCBDE are as follows.

Generally, patients with eligibility for general anesthesia, no acute settings such as obstructive cholangitis, no severe inflammation as with Mirizzi's syndrome with biliobiliary fistula, and no recent previous abdominal operations are always suitable for LCBDE.

When the number of stones is 4 or less and within 8-mm in diameter, the case will be suitable for LTCE (Table 16.1). Other conditions and failure of LTCE are indications for LCHE.

Table 16.1 Indications of approach for common bile duct exploration

	LTCE	LCHE
Conditions of stones		
Number	≤ 4	$5<$
Size	<8 mm	8 mm$\leq$
Others		Unsuitable for LTCE

Although some say that the cases with recent previous abdominal operations should be excluded, but it is worth trying even after LC. Those with Mirizzi's syndrome, cicatrice change of Calot's triangle, confluence stone and atrophic gallbladder are not suitable for needlescopic LCBDE, but it may depend on the surgeon's skill.

16.3 Description of the Technique

16.3.1 Port Arrangement and Needle Equipment

LCBDE is usually performed with LC. Unless the patient has been proven suitable for LCHE preoperatively, indication of LCBDE should be decided during intraoperative cholangiography (IOC), according to the size and number of the stones. The port arrangement is identical to those in needlescopic-LC (N-LC), consisting of two punctures and two incisions (Fig. 16.1). The primary surgeon stands on the patient's left side, with the assistant on the patient's right. Initial entry into the abdomen is made via an open approach at the umbilicus. Typically, a 12-mm port is inserted at this location. Another incision is made below the left costal margin for the 5-mm port (OP). The puncture sites are below the right costal margin on the mid-clavicular line (MC) and on the right anterior axillary line of the navel level (AA). Two-millimeter forceps are inserted through these thin caliber ports (Fig. 16.2). We used 'BJ needle' (Niti-On Company, Tokyo, Japan) or 'Mini-Site' (Covidien, New Haven, CT, USA) as 2-mm forceps. These forceps can be inserted through the thin caliber trocar 'Mini-Port' (Covidien, New Haven, CT, USA) by puncture without

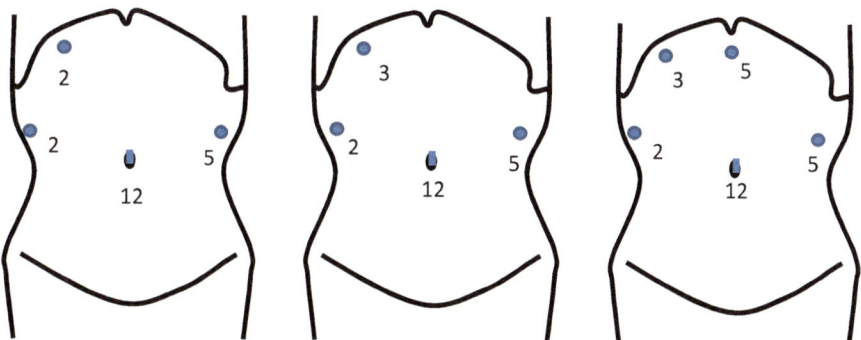

Fig. 16.1 Port arrangements. *Left*: Port arrangement for cholecystectomy. A 12-mm port is inserted via open approach at the umbilicus. A 5-mm port is below the left costal margin (OP). Two puncture sites with a 2-mm port are below the right costal margin on the mid-clavicular line (MC) and on the right anterior-axillary line of the navel level (AA). *Middle*: Arrangement for transcystic duct exploration. The MC port is changed to a 3-mm port for exploration. *Right*: In the arrangement for trans-choledochal exploration (LCHE), a 5-mm port is added at the subxiphoid level. When LCHE is clearly supposed to apply preoperatively, the MC port will be arranged as 3-mm

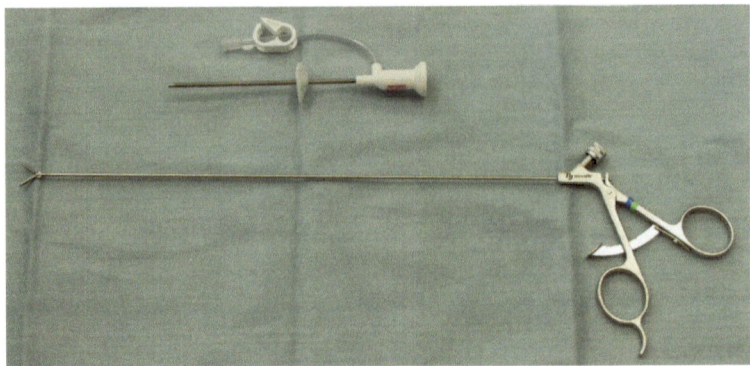

Fig. 16.2 Two-millimeter needle forceps and port

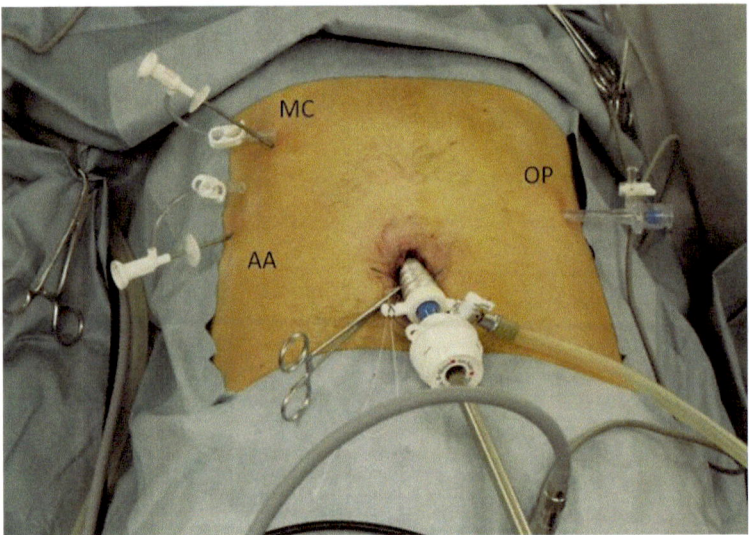

Fig. 16.3 Port set up for needlescopic cholecystectomy

incision. Because Mini-Site (Covidien) was discontinued, we have mainly used BJ needle (Niti-On) in recent years. Fig. 16.3 shows the set up for a N-LC. For both N-LC and LCBDE procedures, a 30°, 10-mm laparoscope is introduced through the umbilical port. The MC port is used for retracting and manipulating the gallbladder and the liver with a BJ needle (Niti-On) by the assistant. The primary surgeon uses the OP and the AA ports. A 5-mm titanium clip, a 5-mm energy device, such as electrical cautery and laparoscopic ultrasonic coagulating shears (LCS), or 5-mm scissors are introduced through the OP port. We routinely perform IOC using

Urographine (Bayer Yakuhin, Osaka, Japan) diluted with saline by 30 % with an introducing catheter via the MC. The catheter for IOC is LAP-13 (Ranfac, Avon, MA, USA), Cholagiocatheter TH type (Hakko-medical, Tokyo, Japan), or thin caliber (2-mm) feeding tube (atom tube, Atom Medical, Tokyo, Japan).

With the confirmation of CBDs with IOC, LCBDE is performed followed by cholecystectomy.

16.3.2 LTCE with Needle Forceps

Following IOC, the route of LCBDE is decided according to the condition of CBDs (Fig. 16.4). When the number of stones is 4 or less and within 8-mm in diameter, the case will be suitable for LTCE (Table 16.1).

At the beginning of LTCE, the MC port is changed to 3-mm for exploration, and the grasper through the AA port is fixed to hold the tail of the gallbladder (Fig. 16.1).

The atom tube from the MC port is cannulated in the cystic duct about 5-cm long. Then the guide wire (0.035-mm in diameter) is inserted into the common bile duct (CBD) through the atom tube, but not through it. The atom tube is removed, leaving the guide wire, and a 6Fr balloon catheter (Ascend AQ balloon catheter, Cook Japan, Tokyo, Japan) is then inserted over the guide wire. The balloon is gradually inflated until it reaches 6-mm in diameter with an atmospheric pressure of 13. After 4 min, the balloon is deflated and removed, leaving the guide wire, and a 2.8-mm cholangioscope (CHF-CB30S, Olympus, Tokyo, Japan) is inserted over the guide wire. Under the cholangioscope vision, the stones are removed via the cystic duct using 3.2Fr basket catheter (Fig. 16.5).

To end the exploration, a cholangiography is performed to confirm that there are no residual stones and that the contrast agent flows out to the duodenum freely (Fig. 16.6). Then the cystic duct is closed with clips, and cholecystectomy is performed in a routine manner. Generally, a biliary drainage tube is not necessary when performing LTCE.

16.3.3 LCHE with Needle Forceps

To perform LCHE, a 5-mm port is added at the subxiphoid level (SX) after cholangiography (Fig. 16.1). When LCHE is clearly indicated preoperatively, the ports are arranged as 2-mm for AA, 3-mm for MC and OP, and 5-mm for SX. The operator uses the MC and the SX ports from the beginning of the procedure. In this instance, OP is used for a needle driver.

After confirmation of CBDS with cholangiography, the cystic duct is temporarily closed with a clip or thread to avoid unnecessary bile spillage during operation. This clip is removed afterward to place a catheter for a completion cholangiography at

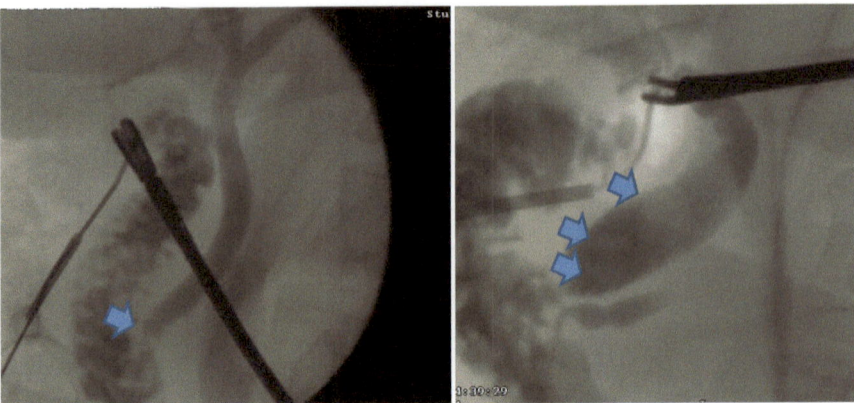

Fig. 16.4 Indications of approaches to common bile duct according to intraoperative cholangiography. *Left*: One small stone (*arrow*) is observed at the end of common bile duct. This is for transcystic duct exploration. *Right*: Stones more than 8-mm in diameter (*arrows*) are for the choledochal approach

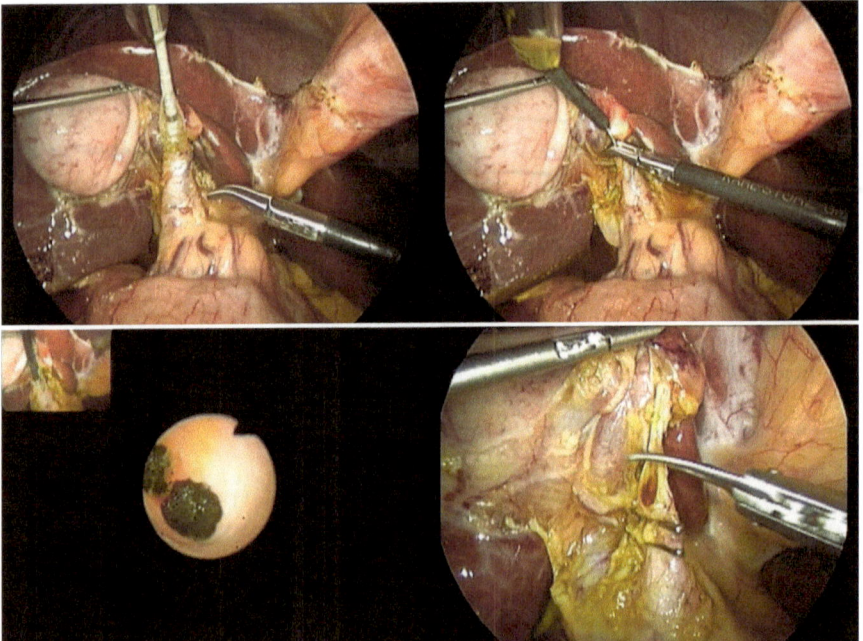

Fig. 16.5 Trans-cystic duct exploration. *Upper left*: A 6Fr balloon catheter is inserted via guide wire to cystic duct and inflated until 6 mm in diameter. *Upper right*: A 2.8-mm cholangioscope is inserted along with the guide wire. *Lower left*: Under the cholangioscope vision, a stone is removed via cystic duct using 3.2Fr basket catheter. *Lower right*: After exploration, the cystic duct is closed and cholecystectomy is performed in a routine manner

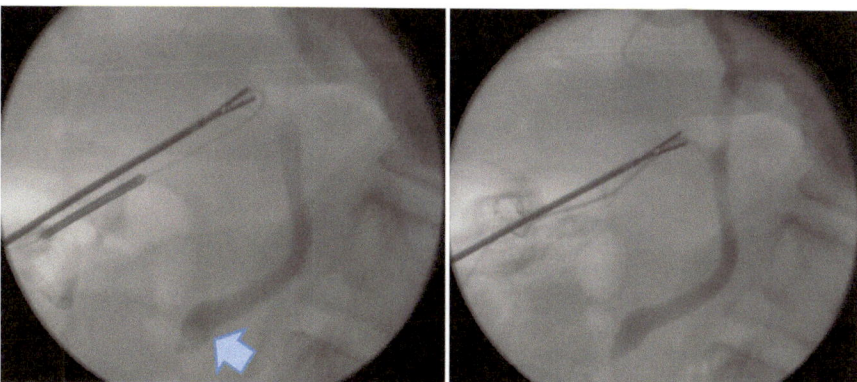

Fig. 16.6 Completion cholangiography. *Left*: Confirmation of a common bile duct stone (*arrow*) with intraoperative cholangiography. *Right*: At the end of exploration, completion cholangiography is performed to confirm there are no residual stones, and the contrast agent flows out to the duodenum freely

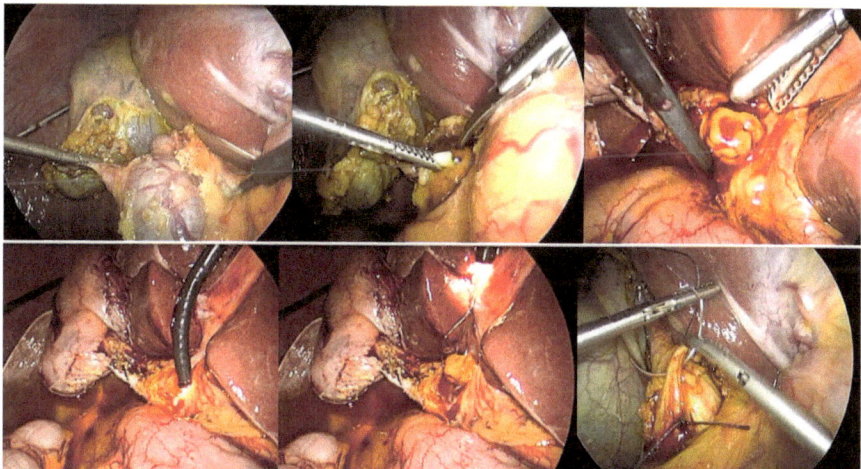

Fig. 16.7 Procedure of choledochal approach. *Upper left* to *middle*: The anterior surface of the common bile duct is exposed widely and cut with a scalpel. *Upper right*: A stone flows out from the opening spontaneously. *Lower left* to *middle*: A 4.9-mm cholangioscope is inserted through the opening to extract stones with a basket catheter. *Lower right*: The opening is closed with a running suture

the end of common bile duct exploration. Next, the anterior surface of the common bile duct is exposed widely, and cut with a scalpel or scissors through SX to a length long enough to remove the stones (Fig. 16.7).

There are several maneuvers to extract the stones. Useful methods include flushing the CBD or common hepatic duct (CHD) with saline using a thin caliber tube or

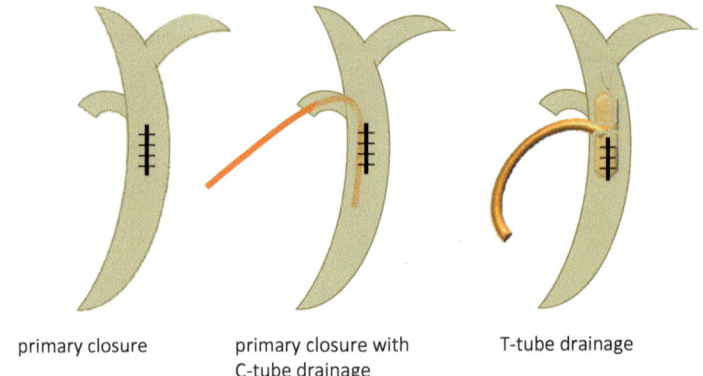

| primary closure | primary closure with C-tube drainage | T-tube drainage |

Fig. 16.8 Primary closure of the opening and drainages for choledochal exploration

irrigation cannula, using a Fogarty balloon catheter, or using a basket catheter with 4.9-mm cholangioscope (CHF-P20, Olympus, Tokyo, Japan) inserted through SX. SX, sometimes MC, is suitable to approach the opening since it is the nearest port. Two different procedures are usually used to close the opening after completing exploration: primary closure (with or without transcystic biliary drainage, C-tube drainage) or T-tube drainage (Fig. 16.8).

For primary closure, the opening is closed with one anchor stitch at the end, followed by a fine running suture using 4-0 or 5-0 absorbable thread. The 3- to 5-mm needle-driver inserted from OP and 2- to 3-mm from AA are suitable for suturing.

After closing the opening, a completion cholangiography is performed to confirm there are no residual stones, no leakage of contrast medium, and no stenosis of the suture line.

Bile duct drainage is placed, depending on the case. A C-tube might prevent postoperative bile leakage and allow for a postoperative cholangiography to check for bile duct stenosis or residual stones. It is also beneficial for the endoscopic treatment in the case of a residual stone. In 1–7 days after the operation, a cholangiography through the C-tube is performed to identify any residual stones or stenosis following the C-tube removal.

When a T-tube is required, it is inserted through the opening in the duct and placed on the cranial side. The arms of the T-tube are usually shortened to make the removal easy after the operation. The remaining opening below the catheter is closed with an absorbable interrupted suture (Fig. 16.9). The main stem of the T-tube is pulled out from the appropriate port site, usually SX or MC, after completing the cholecystectomy.

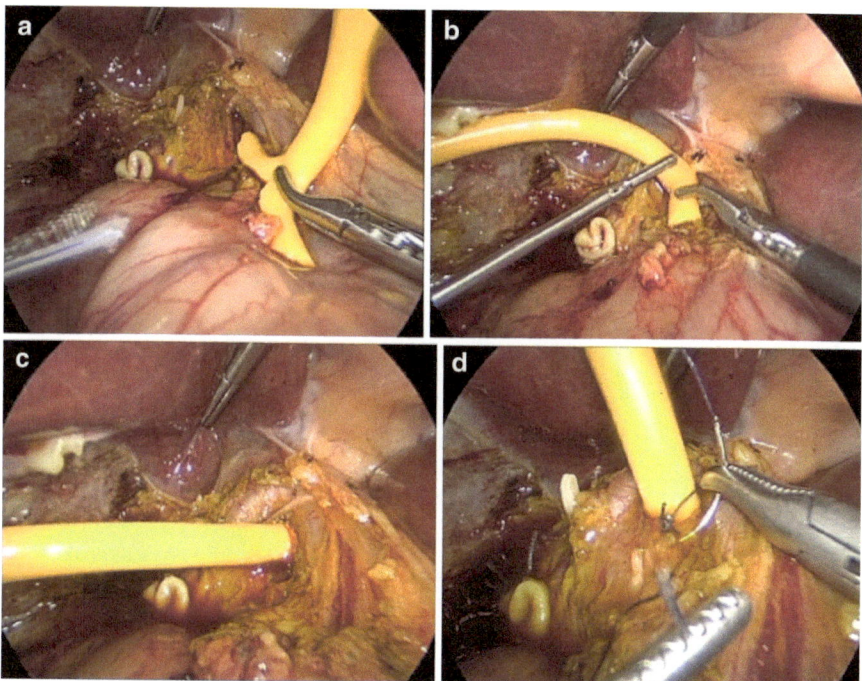

Fig. 16.9 T-tube drainage. The arms of the T-tube are shortened and shaped (**a**), and the T-tube is inserted through the opening in the duct (**b**) and placed cranial side (**c**). The remaining opening below the catheter is closed with absorbable interrupted suture (**d**)

16.4 Tips and Tricks

16.4.1 Port Arrangement and Needle Forceps

Our port arrangement is a co-axial setting in order to exert sufficient motion of the needle grasper. Needlescopic forceps are sharp-pointed, and care should be taken to avoid intraoperative complications such as perforation of liver parenchyma, gallbladder wall, and other viscera. For sufficient retraction of the organs in obese patients, the retraction assistant such as a Silicone disk (Hakko, Tokyo, Japan) is helpful to avoid injury (Fig. 16.10). When a patient has dense adhesion or a thickened gallbladder wall, changing 2-mm forceps to 3-mm would be preferable.

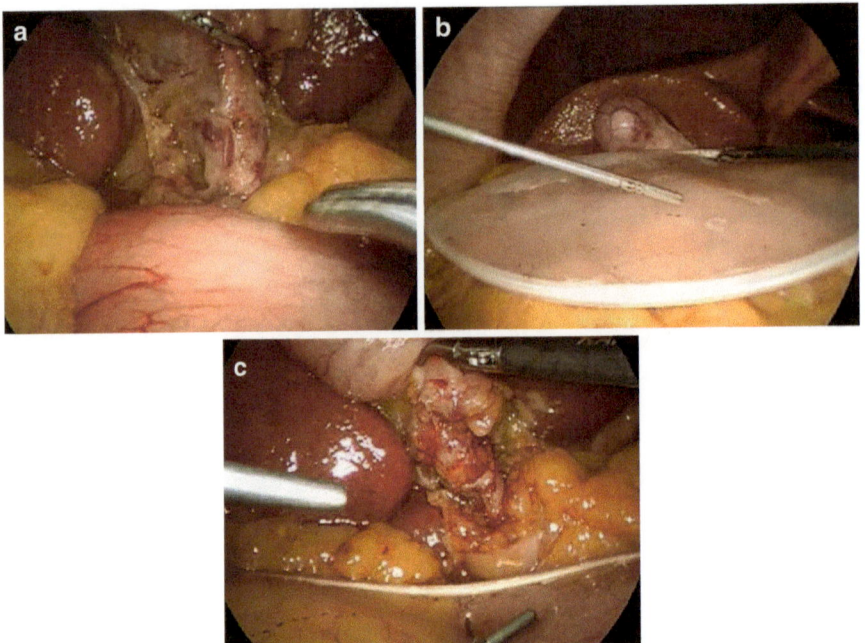

Fig. 16.10 Creating a sufficient operative field. (**a**) Operative field obscured with duodenum. (**b**) and (**c**) Using displacing equipment (Silicone disk) provides enough operative field

16.4.2   LTCE

LTCE uses the cystic duct for exploration. Difficult cannulation may result in tearing of the cystic duct in cases with cicatrice change around the duct, a dense spiral structure, or an extremely thin cystic duct. To avoid this failure, the cystic duct should be skeletonized as long as possible to straighten the duct, and the balloon dilator used routinely. Routine IOC will help to familiarize how to cannulate the cystic duct skillfully. However, when the cannulation to the cystic duct is failing, it is better to switch to LCHE quickly.

Generally, it is not possible to observe the CHD in most of the cases with LTCE. In this case, the completing cholangiography is essential to avoid residual stones. When stones are found in the CHD, move the cholangioscope to the end of the cystic duct. With a reverse Trendelenburg position, fill saline into the bile duct gradually, and wait until the stones have moved to the CBD.

Although there is another method of exploration for LTCE by inserting a basket catheter directly into the CBD through cystic duct under fluoroscopy, it is preferable to use a cholangioscope to avoid perforation of the cystic duct, injury to the CBD, crushing the stone, or unnecessary irradiation of the physician.

We always perform a bile duct exploration (both LTCE and LCBDE) before a cholecystectomy because holding the gallbladder with needle instruments can provide a good operative field.

16.4.3 LCHE

Exposure of the CBD should not be more than half its circumference to avoid ischemia of the CBD, which later causes bile duct stenosis. The length of the opening depends on the size of the stones but should not be too wide because a longer opening may also cause stenotic change. When bleeding occurs during the incision, firm compression for hemostasis is the primary maneuver to prevent thermal damage with electrocautery or LCS.

Stones should be stowed each time in a plastic bag when they flow out from the opening spontaneously during exploration.

For LCHE, a 4.9-mm (or more) cholangioscope is preferable because of a wider view. It requires a 5-mm port in SX. A slimmer, 2.8- to 3.3-mm cholangioscope might not detect the stones during LCHE.

When closing the opening, we routinely use a fine absorbable running suture, 4-0 or 5-0, because it is time-saving. On the other hand, since an interrupted suture is more adjustable and accurate, it is preferable for a longer opening or a thin bile duct wall.

A T-tube is old-fashioned but still needed in certain cases. For instance, it is applied to avoid bile duct stenosis or when there is suspicion of residual stones. Marked dilatation of CBD, persistent sludge, or stacked stones will suggest the possibility of residual stones. The T-tube will need to be removed 3–4 weeks after operation after a cholangiography with confirmation of no remnant stones. Should remnant stones be revealed, they will be removed under the cholangioscopy through the fistula which is formed along the T-tube.

16.5   Recommendations from the Author

Using needle forceps can provide a good cosmetic result, especially with the 2-mm port. In needlescopic LCHE, a thin needle driver is sufficiently functional. In addition, because our co-axial port arrangement facilitates the reordering port site to the umbilicus, it may contribute to a smooth transition to a single site LCBDE (TANKO-LCBDE) as the surgeon's skill improves.

Endoscopic exploration sometimes requires several sessions to clear the CBD, and then might have residual stone or recurrent stone while awaiting LC. Needlescopic LCBDE is obviously preferable for a patient when it is completed successfully in one operation.

Although there are limitations to the indication for needlescopic LTCE, it is feasible and should be the first line of treatment for CBDS because it is not invasive to

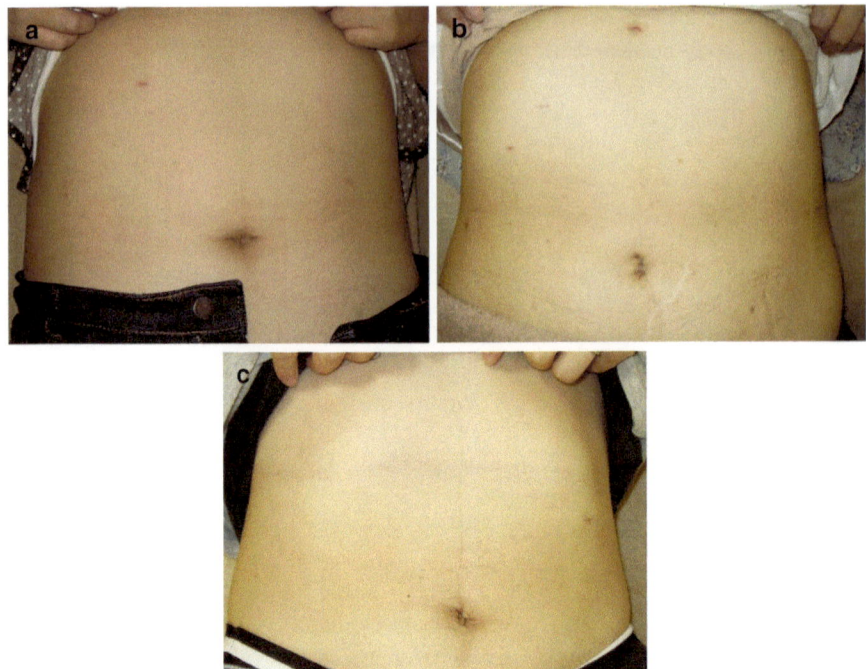

Fig. 16.11 Cosmetic results. (**a**) Operative scars one month after trans-cystic duct exploration. (**b**) Same after choledochal exploration. (**c**) Scars after needlescopic cholecystectomy. Both **a** and **b** are comparable to **c**

the sphincter and does not injure the CBD wall. LTCE can lead to a shorter hospital stay and smaller medical cost compared to EST+LC [2]. Using 2- to 3-mm ports can offer good cosmetic results (Fig. 16.11). With LCHE as a redeeming approach, LCBDE with needle forceps may be the way to pursue in the treatment for CBDs.

References

1. Gagner M, Garcia-Ruiz A (1998) Technical aspects of minimally invasive abdominal surgery performed with needlescopic instruments. Surg Laparosc Endosc 8:171–179
2. Schroppel TS, Schroeppel TJ, Lambert PJ et al (2007) An economic analysis of hospital charges for choledocholithiasis by different treatment strategies. Am Surg 73:472–477

Chapter 17
Distal Gastrectomy

Takeshi Omori and Toshirou Nishida

Abstract Laparoscopic gastrectomy has recently gained acceptance as a less invasive treatment for early stages of gastric cancers. The applications for laparoscopic gastrectomy for malignancy have gradually expanded, with improvements in both surgical techniques and instruments. Although laparoscopic gastrectomy for early gastric cancer is performed in many institutions in Japan now, laparoscopic operations for advanced gastric cancer is currently performed mainly in institutions that deal with many such cases on a regular basis.

More recently, reduced port laparoscopic gastrectomy has been introduced as an advanced technique, in which fewer access trocar points and/or small caliber forceps may prove less invasive than traditional laparoscopic approaches. One of the ultimate goals of this type of surgery is single-incision laparoscopic (SLS) gastrectomy, in which gastrectomy with reconstruction is performed through a single transumbilical incision. Although this approach provides an excellent cosmetic result, the procedure is technically demanding due to the difficulty in creating the proper operative field with the appropriate counter-traction. To overcome these issues, the position of the forceps must be systematized in each surgical field to gain a better view and to prevent the interference of forceps. In this chapter, SLS distal gastrectomy will be described in detail.

Keywords Gastric cancer • Reduced port laparoscopic surgery • Single-incision laparoscopic gastrectomy

T. Omori (✉) • T. Nishida
Department of Surgery, Osaka Police Hospital,
10-31 Kitayama-cho, Tennoji-ku, Osaka 543-0035, Japan
e-mail: ohmori@oph.gr.jp

T. Mori and G. Dapri (eds.), *Reduced Port Laparoscopic Surgery*,
DOI 10.1007/978-4-431-54601-6_17, © Springer Japan 2014

17.1 Introduction

Ever since laparoscopy-assisted gastrectomy was first reported in 1994 by Kitano [1], the laparoscopic approach has gained acceptance as a less invasive treatment for the early stages of gastric cancers [2]. The procedure is accompanied by less pain, faster recovery, shorter hospital stay, decreased blood loss, and better cosmesis compared to open approaches, and has shown similar oncological outcomes [2–4]. The applications for laparoscopic gastrectomy for malignancy have gradually expanded, with advances in both surgical techniques and instruments [5, 6]. Although the merit is yet to be scientifically proven, laparoscopic surgery is also performed for advanced gastric cancer in high volume centers where laparoscopic gastrectomy is regularly done for early cases. In conventional laparoscopy-assisted gastrectomy, a 5-cm mini-laparotomy in the upper abdomen is required for extra-corporeal anastomosis and extraction of resected specimens, after gastric mobilization with lymphadenectomy in laparoscopic approaches. Totally laparoscopic distal gastrectomy, which includes intracorporeal anastomosis and specimen extraction through the umbilical incision, has recently been used as an alternative procedure to conventional laparoscopy-assisted gastrectomy [7, 8].

More recently, reduced port laparoscopic gastrectomy (RPLG) was introduced as a new, minimally invasive technique requiring fewer access trocar points and/or small caliber forceps [9, 10]. Single-incision laparoscopic (SLS) surgery, which is performed through only a small transumbilical incision, can be one of the ultimate goals of RPLG. It offers excellent cosmetic results because the wound appears to be hidden in the umbilicus and may be invisible after scarring. However, ever since transumbilical SLS gastrectomy was first reported by Omori et al. [11], few reports have been available, probably because the procedure is technically difficult. Because laparoscopic gastrectomy for gastric cancer necessitates multiple surgical views where laparoscopic instruments should reach organs throughout the upper abdomen, it is extremely difficult to maintain triangulation, the proper operative field, and retraction of the organs. Therefore, it is necessary to consider ways to overcome these difficulties. In our institute, the positioning of the instruments is formulized in each surgical step to prevent interference of the forceps. The procedure of single-incision laparoscopic distal gastrectomy (SLSDG) will be described in detail.

17.2 Indications and Contraindications

Early gastric cancer seems to be a good indication for RPLG, e.g., cT1N0 gastric cancer in cases endoscopic mucosal resection or endoscopic submucosal dissection is not indicated. Indication can also include advanced gastric cancer, if performed with proper oncologic principle.

Patients with complete obstruction caused by the cancer, cancer invasion to the adjacent organs, and bulky cancer larger than 8-cm in size should be excluded.

17.3 Technique

17.3.1 Patient Positioning and Operating Room Setup

The patient was placed in the supine position with their legs apart. The surgeon was positioned between the patient's legs. The first assistant was on the left side of the patient, and the second assistant (who held the camera) was on the right side. The scrub-nurse stood near the patient's left knee (Fig. 17.1). The team remained in the same position throughout the entire procedure. The laparoscopic unit with the monitor was located above the patient's head.

17.3.2 Port Setting

An umbilical laparotomy through a 2.5- to 3-cm vertical skin incision into the umbilicus was made by the open method. A wound protector (Lap retractor (Hakko Co., Nagano, Japan)) was applied to this wound. A plastic cover (E-Z access (Hakko Co., Nagano, Japan)) with 4 trocars inserted in a diamond-shaped position (Fig. 17.1) is then placed, and pneumoperitoneum was established. The bottom 12-mm trocar was used for introducing the laparoscope. The main surgeon performed the procedures with a co-axial setting using a conventional straight instrument and an energy device through bilateral trocars. An assistant provided counter-traction to maintain the surgical view using forceps through a top trocar in the umbilical access port.

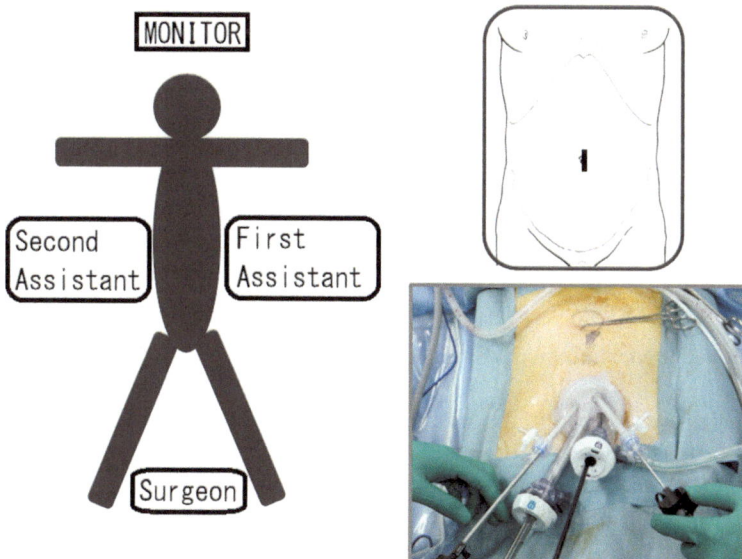

Fig. 17.1 Positions of the equipment and the surgical team and placement of trocars through transumbilical port for the SLS gastrectomy for gastric cancer

17.3.3   Procedure

After establishment of the CO_2 pneumoperitoneum, a careful exploration of the entire peritoneal cavity was done to examine the metastasis of other organs, such as liver metastasis and peritoneal dissemination.

17.3.3.1   Liver Retraction

Proper liver retraction was a key to the success of the laparoscopic gastrectomy. Our preference is the "V-shape retraction technique" as follows: a straight needle with 2-0 nylon was used to puncture first the upper abdomen and then at the right crus and through the abdominal wall again. It was simple and inexpensive without leaving a scar at the punctured site.

17.3.3.2   Suprapancreatic Lymph Nodes Dissection

Suprapancreatic lymphadenectomy is one of the most important and technically difficult aspects of laparoscopic gastrectomy. Various approaches, such as right-to-left, left-to-right (left-sided approach), and medial-to-lateral (medial approach), have been reported in conventional laparoscopic gastric surgery, which can be applied to the single port approach. In these approaches, dissection is initially performed at the cranial edge of the pancreas and then proceeds in a dorsal-to-cranial direction. The medial approach is quite effective for complete dissection of the lymph nodes, with dissection of the layer between the adipose tissue (including lymphatic tissue and the autonomic nerve sheath of major arteries) and medial transection of the left gastric artery [12]. We commonly use the cranial-to-caudal approach (cranial approach), in which the mobilization of the stomach and pancreas and the dissection of the cranial side of the station no. 9 lymph nodes are performed prior to the medial approach. We believe that prior dissection of cranial connections between the lymph nodes and the plexus celiacus will make it easier to perform cephalad dissection of the suprapancreatic lymph nodes in the conventional approach.

17.3.3.3   The Cranial Approach

The patient was placed in the reverse Trendelenburg position. The assistant introduced the intestinal grasping forceps with gauze from the top trocar to retract the stomach caudad. The main surgeon retracted the liver cephalad for retraction of the hepatogastric ligament. The assistant's forceps were placed between the surgeon's bilateral forceps. The procedure was performed smoothly without interference of

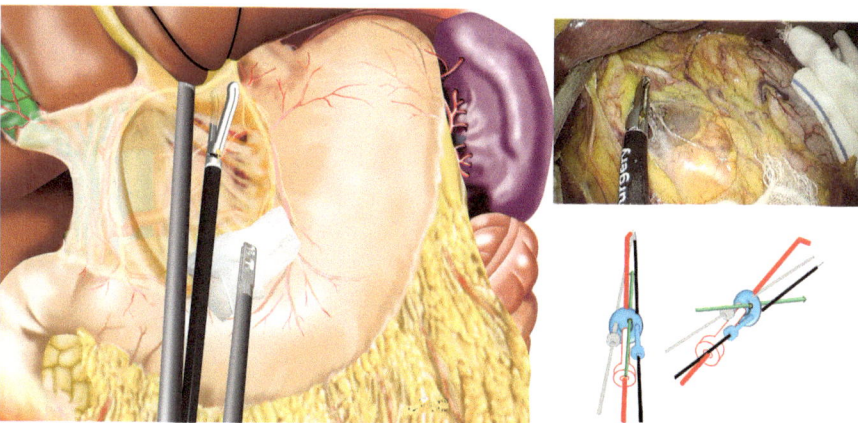

Fig. 17.2 The hepatogastric ligament is dissected with the aid of caudal counter-traction by the assistant's forceps with gauze, preserving the hepatic branches of the vagus nerve

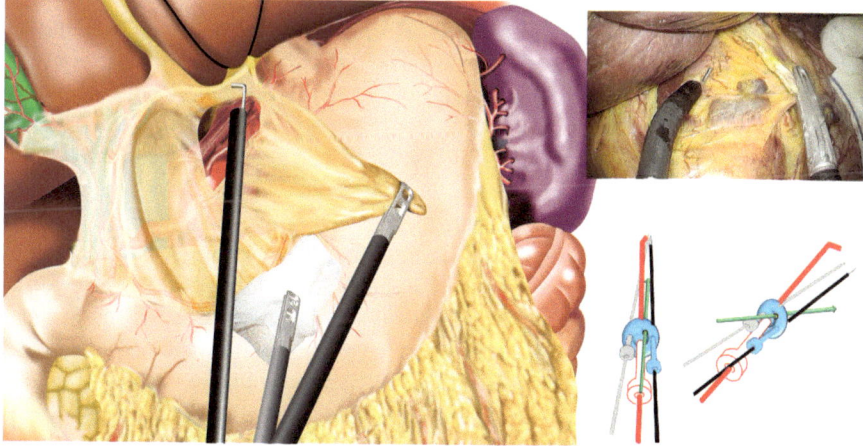

Fig. 17.3 In the cranial approach, the mesogastrium is tented ventro-laterally, and the peritoneum is incised along the right crus of the diaphragm. The plane is dissected between Gerota's fascia and Toldt's fusion fascia to mobilize the stomach and pancreas from the retroperioneum

each instrument in this formation, which is a basic positioning for this surgery (Fig. 17.2). The hapatogastric ligament was then dissected towards the esophagus with preservation of the hepatic branches of the vagus nerve (Fig. 17.2). The mesogastrium was retracted anteriorly using a grasper introduced through the right trocar. The peritoneum was incised at the level of the right crus of the diaphragm (Fig. 17.3). This incision continued downward along the right crus up to the celiac artery. The mesogastrium was retracted anteriorly to expose the posterior space.

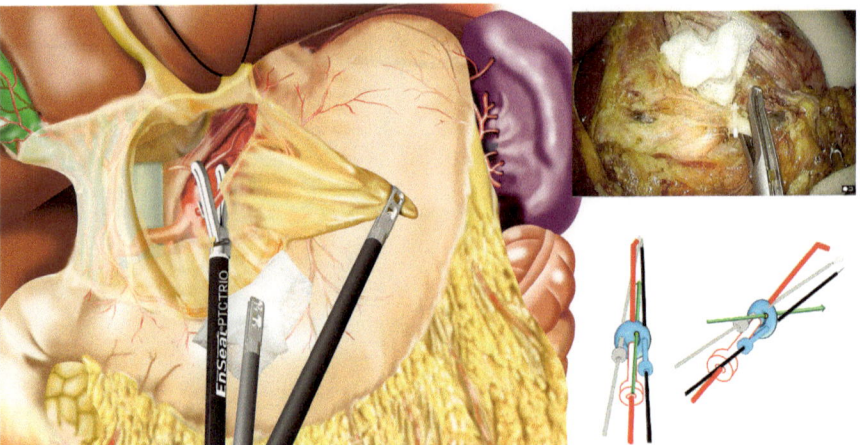

Fig. 17.4 The left gastric artery is clipped and divided at its origin

The plane between Gerota's fascia and Toldt's fusion fascia could then be identified. This plane is avascular and easily divided. The dissection continued posterior to the Toldt's fusion fascia going laterally and caudad. By this dissection, both the pancreatic body and stomach were mobilized.

The left gastric artery was carefully grasped and retracted in a ventro-lateral direction. The adipose tissue including the station no. 9 lymph nodes was separated from the outer layer of plexus celiacus, and we identified the three branches of the celiac artery—the left gastric artery, the common hepatic artery, and the splenic artery. If possible, the left gastric artery should be skeletonized distally, clipped, and divided at its origin using a vessel-sealing device or laparoscopic coagulation shears (Fig. 17.4). This adequate separation of the lymph nodes from the nerve increased the movability of the lymph nodes and facilitated the following caudal-to-cranial dissection of the suprapancreatic lymphadenectomy (Fig. 17.5).

17.3.3.4 Dissection of No. 5 Lymph Nodes and Division of Right Gastric Artery

The assistant introduced the intestinal grasping forceps with gauze from the top trocar to retract the duodenum caudad and stretch the hepatoduodenal ligament. The main surgeon retracted the right gastric artery in a ventro-lateral direction. The ventral peritoneum was initially incised along the duodenum, and the opening window was spread. Under continuous traction, the peritoneum was incised cephalad along the right edge of the proper hepatic artery up to its bifurcation. Using a combination of gentle force and sharp dissection, the right gastric artery with lymph nodes was swept ventrally and the hepatic plexus swept dorsally. Then the right gastric artery was divided using a vessel-sealing device or laparoscopic coagulating shears (Fig. 17.6).

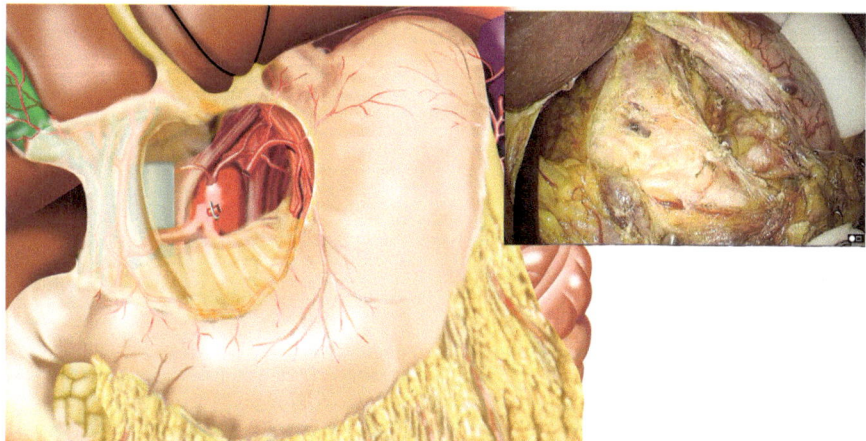

Fig. 17.5 The cranial approach is completed by exposing the celiac plexus. The cranial side of no. 9 lymph node is separated from the nerve ganglion

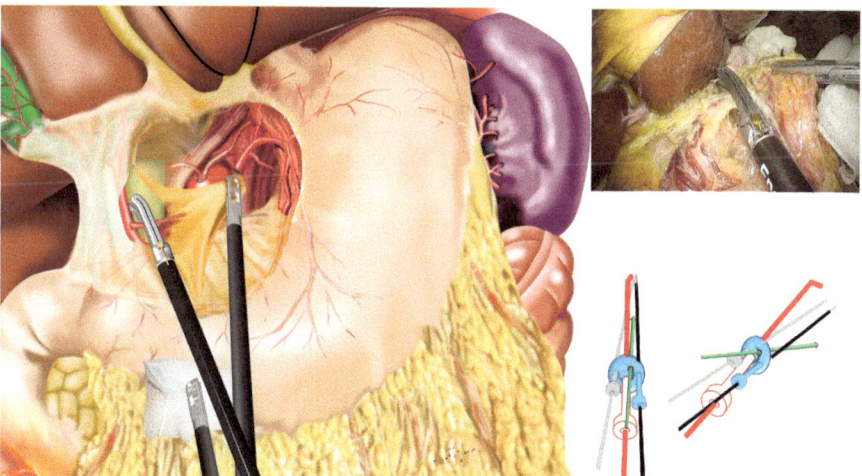

Fig. 17.6 The right gastric artery is retracted ventro-laterally and divided using a vessel-sealing device

17.3.4 Dissection of the Suprapancreatic Lymph Nodes

The assistant introduced the intestinal grasping forceps with gauze from the top trocar to retract and rotated the pancreas in a dorsocaudal direction. After the supra-pyloric lymph nodes were separated from the right gastric artery, the main surgeon provided traction by using the right hand grasper to pick up the cut edge of the peritoneum. The peritoneum was incised toward the left side along the cranial edge of the pancreas, while the adipose tissue with lymph nodes was separated cephalad and laterally from the hepatic plexus and splenic plexus. If the proper plane is

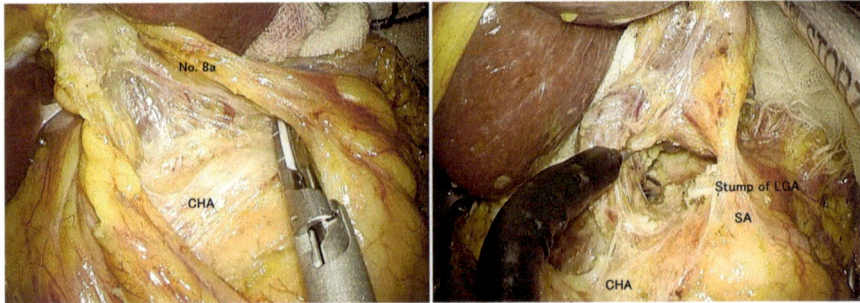

Fig. 17.7 In dissection of the suprapancreatic lymph nodes, the layer between the adipose tissue including lymph nodes and the nerve surrounding the artery, i.e. the outmost layer of the nerve, is dissected. Proceeding along the layer connects to the space created in the cranial approach. CHA: common hepatic artery, SA: splenic artery, LGA: left gastric artery

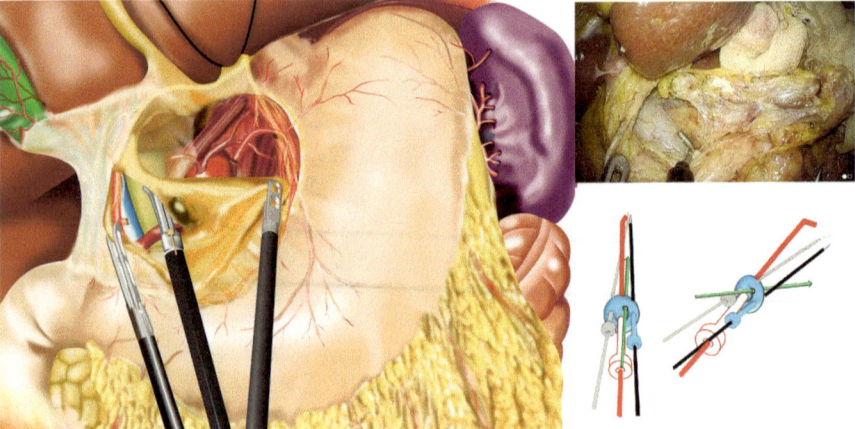

Fig. 17.8 In the station no. 12a dissection, the proper hepatic artery is skeletonized to the line on which the left edge of the portal vein can be seen

entered posteriorly, no bleeding will occur, and the connective tissue in this plane can be divided easily. This plane directly connects the previous dissection plane from the cranial approach, providing a wide space for lymphadenectomy (Fig. 17.7). Dissection continued in a medial-to-lateral direction by applying ventrolateral traction with a grasper along the bilateral celiac ganglion.

The adipose tissues including the station no. 8a, 9, 12a lymph nodes were retracted ventrolaterally. In the station no. 8a dissection, the common hepatic artery and the bifurcation of the proper hepatic artery and the gastroduodenal artery were exposed along the plane of the periarterial plexus. In the station no. 12a dissection, the proper hepatic artery was skeletonized to the line on which the left edge of the portal vein could be seen (Fig. 17.8). Surgeons should make sure not to cut the posterior peritoneum of the hepatoduodenal ligament because retraction of the

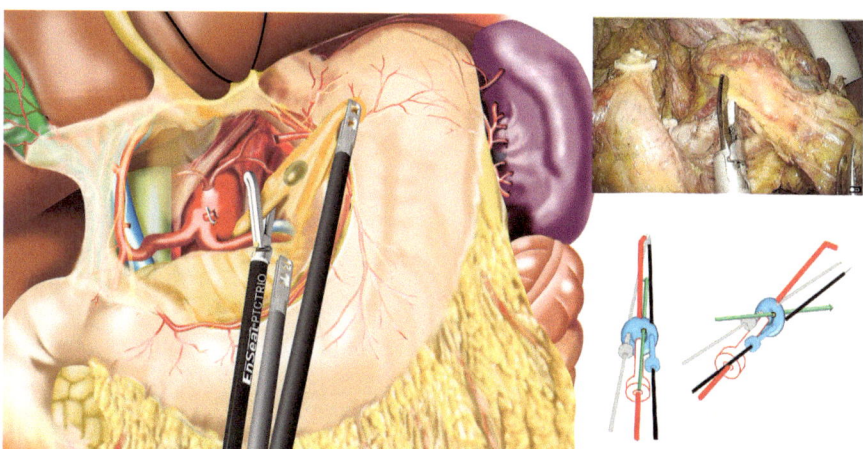

Fig. 17.9 In the station no. 11p dissection, after identifying the splenic artery by incising the gastropancreatic fold, the lymph nodes are dissected on the plane of the splenic plexus by retracting the tissue ventro-laterally

peritoneum allows for proper dissection of the no. 12a lymph nodes. The bifurcation of the proper hepatic artery from the common hepatic artery was the view point to observe the portal vein. Careful dissection with a dissector was used to create a window just lateral to the bifurcation of the proper hepatic artery from the common hepatic artery.

The posterior peritoneum of the hepatoduodenal ligament was incised and the stations no. 7 and 9 lymph nodes were then dissected from the periarterial plexus using a vessel-sealing device and laparoscopic coagulating shears, alternatively. When identifying the left gastric vein during the step of lymphadenectomy, the vessel was transected using a vessel-sealing device or laparoscopic coagulating shears.

In station no. 11p dissection, the splenic artery was identified by incising the gastropancreatic fold. The lymph nodes were dissected on the plane of the splenic plexus. Lymph nodes were dissected to the dorsal plane on which the splenic vein or pancreas could be identified (Fig. 17.9).

17.3.4.1   Dissection of No. 4d, 4sb Lymph Nodes

The assistant introduced the intestinal grasping forceps from the top trocar to hold the gastric body at the greater curvature side and retracted the stomach ventrally toward the right side of the abdomen. The greater omentum was dissected about 4-cm away from the gastroepiploic artery for T1, T2 gastric cancer. The greater omentum was completely resected along the transverse colon for T3, T4 gastric cancer. The omentum was dissected toward the left side. The left gastroepiploic artery was transected using a vessel-sealing device or laparoscopic coagulating shears for dissection of the station no. 4sb lymph nodes.

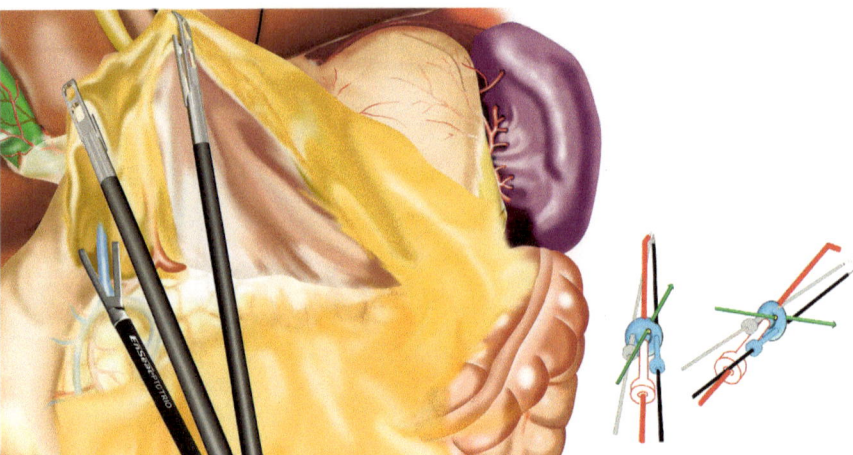

Fig. 17.10 Using triangulating tension, the gastroepiploic vessels are divided after adequate lymphadenectomy

Next, the assistant lifted the stomach to retract the gastroepiploic vessels. Dissection of the greater omentum continued toward the right side. In the station no. 6 dissection, lymph nodes bounded by the inferior edge of the pancreatic head and the anterior plane of the superior mesenteric vein were dissected after exposure of the gastrocolic trunk. The right gastroepiploic vein was divided just distal to the bifurcation of the superior anterior pancreaticoduodenal vein. The right gastroepiploic artery and infraduodenal artery were clipped and divided at these origins (Fig. 17.10).

The duodenum was transected just distal to the pyloric ring using an endoscopic linear stapling device. The stomach was transected with an adequate surgical margin from the malignant lesion using two or three cartridges of the stapling device. The resected specimen was inserted in a retrieval sac and extracted through the umbilical incision.

17.3.4.2 Anastomosis

In SLS gastrectomy, intracorporeal anastomotic techniques are required for reconstruction. Billroth I gastroduodenostomy has long been used for distal gastrectomy because the procedure is technically simple. This reconstruction preserves normal gastrointestinal integrity and provides a better postoperative physiologic result. The Roux-en-Y method should be selected for patients with either small gastric remnants or esophageal hiatus hernia.

Billroth-I Reconstruction Using Intracorporeal Triangular Anastomotic Technique

In conventional laparoscopic gastrectomy, the delta-shaped Billroth-I anastomosis is one of the most common procedures in Japan and Korea [7]. Although this reconstruction method is safe and feasible, a simpler technique is required in the single port approach because of the limited number of access trocars and restricted movement of each instrument. We developed a modified technique named intracorporeal triangular anastomotic technique (INTACT) [13]. Firstly, small holes were made on the greater curvature of the gastric remnant and duodenal stump. A linear stapler was introduced into both the gastric and duodenal stumps through the holes to make posterior anastomosis (Fig. 17.11a). After continuous suturing was used to close the common hole temporarily, the sutured tissues were staple-transected by a linear

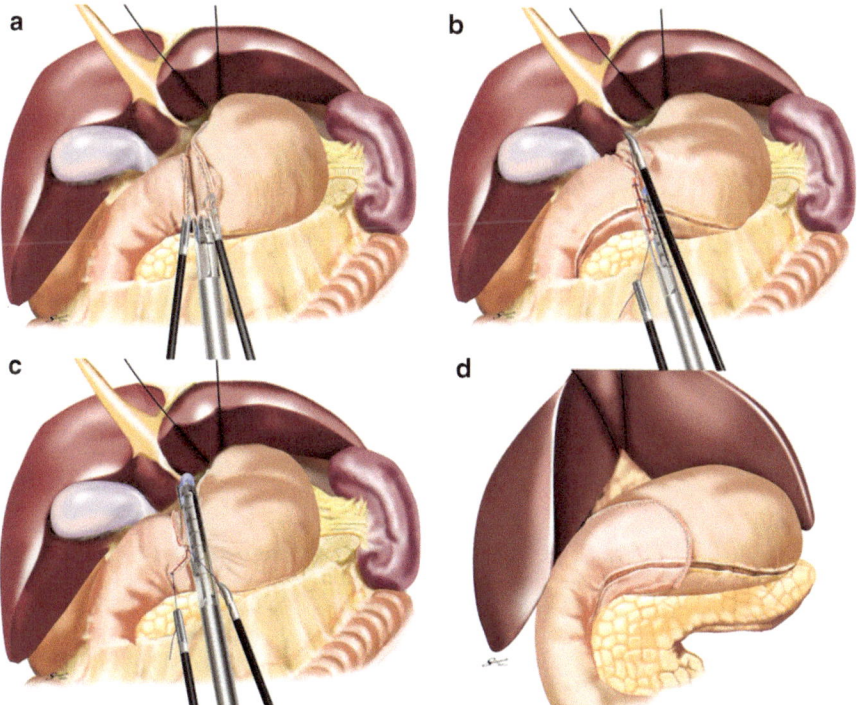

Fig. 17.11 Billroth-I reconstruction is performed using the intracorporeal triangular anastomotic technique (INTACT): (**a**) Firstly, a linear stapler is introduced into both the gastric and duodenal stumps through the small holes to make posterior anastomosis. (**b**) Secondly, after placement of continuous suturing to close the common hole temporarily, the sutured tissues are staple-transected by a linear stapler as a part of anterior anastomosis. (**c**) Finally, both the gastric and duodenal stumps are entirely excised with ventral staple of the first stapling using a linear stapler to complete triangular anastomosis. (**d**) This technique provides end-to-end anastomosis of a triangle orifice

stapler as a part of anterior anastomosis (Fig. 17.11b). Finally, both the gastric and duodenal stumps were entirely excised with a ventral staple of the first stapling using a linear stapler to complete anterior anastomosis (Fig. 17.11c). This technique provided end-to-end anastomosis of a triangular orifice (Fig. 17.11d).

Roux-en-Y Reconstruction

The jejunum was extracted through the umbilical incision and transected 20-cm distal to the Treitz ligament. The jejuno-jejunostomy was performed using hand-sewn sutures or stapling devices under direct vision through the umbilical incision. The gastrojejunstomy was intracorporeally performed by functional end-to-end anastomosis using endoscopic linear stapling devices; small holes were made on the greater curvature of the gastric remnant and antimesenteric side of the jejunum. The anvil fork of the stapler was inserted into the jejunum, and the cartridge side of the stapler was inserted into the gastric remnant through the holes. The common entry hole was closed using the endoscopic linear stapling device to complete anastomosis.

17.4   Recommendations from the Author

SLSDG is a recent surgical procedure that still has many unresolved problems. However, new advances in surgical techniques and equipment have helped solve the issues related to this procedure. By using the above method, we believe that expert laparoscopic surgeons may confidently achieve a safe operation and that this type of surgery will become an attractive alternative to conventional laparoscopic operations.

References

1. Kitano S, Iso Y, Moriyama M, Sugimachi K (1994) Laparoscopy-assisted Billroth I gastrectomy. Surg Laparosc Endosc Percutan Tech 4:146–148
2. Nakamura K, Katai H, Mizusawa J, Yoshikawa T, Ando M, Terashima M, Ito S, Takagi M, Takagane A, Ninomiya M, Fukushima N, Sasako M (2013) A phase III study of laparoscopy-assisted versus open distal gastrectomy with nodal dissection for clinical stage IA/IB gastric Cancer (JCOG0912). Jpn J Clin Oncol 43:324–327
3. Viñuela EF, Gonen M, Brennan MF, Coit DG, Strong VE (2012) Laparoscopic versus open distal gastrectomy for gastric cancer: a meta-analysis of randomized controlled trials and high-quality nonrandomized studies. Ann Surg 255:446–456
4. Kim YW, Baik YH, Yun YH, Nam BH, Kim DH, Choi IJ, Bae JM (2008) Improved quality of life outcomes after laparoscopyassisted distal gastrectomy for early gastric cancer: results of a prospective randomized clinical trial. Ann Surg 248:721–727
5. Pugliese R, Maggioni D, Sansonna F, Costanzi A, Ferrari GC, Di Lernia S, Magistro C, De Martini P, Pugliese F (2010) Subtotal gastrectomy with D2 dissection by minimally invasive

surgery for distal adenocarcinoma of the stomach: results and 5-year survival. Surg Endosc 24:2594–2602

6. Hamabe A, Omori T, Tanaka K, Nishida T (2012) Comparison of long-term results between laparoscopy-assisted gastrectomy and open gastrectomy with D2 lymph node dissection for advanced gastric cancer. Surg Endosc 26:1702–1709

7. Kanaya S, Gomi T, Momoi H, Tamaki N, Isobe H, Katayama T, Wada Y, Ohtoshi M (2002) Delta-shaped anastomosis in totally laparoscopic Billroth I gastrectomy: new technique of intraabdominal gastroduodenostomy. J Am Coll Surg 195:284–287

8. Kinoshita T, Shibasaki H, Oshiro T, Ooshiro M, Okazumi S, Katoh R (2011) Comparison of laparoscopy-assisted and total laparoscopic Billroth-I gastrectomy for gastric cancer: a report of shortterm outcomes. Surg Endosc 25:1395–1401

9. Kawamura H, Tanioka T, Funakoshi T, Takahashi M (2011) Dual-ports laparoscopy-assisted distal gastrectomy compared with conventional laparoscopy-assisted distal gastrectomy. Surg Laparosc Endosc Percutan Tech 21:429–433

10. Kunisaki C, Ono HA, Oshima T, Makino H, Akiyama H, Endo I (2012) Relevance of reduced-port laparoscopic distal gastrectomy for gastric cancer: a pilot study. Dig Surg 29:261–268

11. Omori T, Oyama T, Akamatsu H, Tori M, Ueshima S, Nishida T (2011) Transumbilical single-incision laparoscopic distal gastrectomy for early gastric cancer. Surg Endosc 25:2400–2404

12. Kanaya S, Haruta S, Kawamura Y, Yoshimura F, Inaba K, Hiramatsu Y (2011) Video: laparoscopy distinctive technique for suprapancreatic lymph node dissection: medial approach for laparoscopic gastric cancer surgery. Surg Endosc 25:3928–3929

13. Omori T, Masuzawa T, Akamatsu H, Nishida T (2013) A simple and safe method for Billroth I reconstruction in single-incision laparoscopic gastrectomy using a novel intracorporeal triangular anastomotic technique. J Gastrointest Surg, DOI: 10.1007/s11605-013-2419-7. Dec 3, 2013. [Epub ahead of print]

Chapter 18
Total Gastrectomy

Noriyuki Inaki

Abstract Laparoscopic gastrectomy using five or six 5- or 10-mm ports is widely accepted as surgical treatment for early gastric cancer. The indications for laparoscopic gastrectomy have been expanded to include advanced cancer. Reduced port laparoscopic surgery (RPLS), such as single-port or needlescopic surgery is less invasive than conventional laparoscopic surgery and is considered quite beneficial in the field of endoscopic surgery. The concept of RPLS has been introduced to the surgical treatment of gastric cancer. An approximate 3.5-cm incision at the umbilicus is generally needed for specimen extraction. Therefore, the maximum scar in reduced port laparoscopic gastrectomy (RPLG) is the scar that results from this incision. RPLG, then, is actually performed as single-port laparoscopic gastrectomy (SPLG). The author uses inexpensive silicone access device as an umbilical platform to perform SPLG, maintaining the same quality lymphadenectomy and reconstruction that achieved with the multiport technique. SPLG ensures minimal injury to the abdominal wall and a good cosmetic outcome. In this chapter, our single-port laparoscopic total gastrectomy performed for gastric cancer is described in detail and illustrated with laparoscopic photos and a picture of the single platform viewed externally. The needle-assisted technique is also falls under the RPLS concept.

Keywords Laparoscopic total gastrectomy • Needlescopic surgery • Reduced port laparoscopic surgery • Single-port surgery

N. Inaki (✉)
Department of Gastroenterological Surgery, Ishikawa Prefectural Central Hospital,
Kanazawa, Japan
e-mail: n.inaki@viola.ocn.ne.jp

T. Mori and G. Dapri (eds.), *Reduced Port Laparoscopic Surgery*,
DOI 10.1007/978-4-431-54601-6_18, © Springer Japan 2014

18.1 Introduction

Since the first laparoscopic gastrectomy for gastric cancer was performed in 1994 by Kitano et al. [1], the laparoscopic technique has become common. The procedure has seen refinement with developments in the technique and technology. More detailed images displayed by high definition endoscope have apparently renewed our knowledge of surgical anatomy, resulting in more precise procedure. Multiport laparoscopic subtotal gastrectomy for early gastric cancer is widely accepted for both tumor resection with lymphadenectomy and reconstruction. The indications for laparoscopic surgery in case of gastric cancer have expanded to include advanced cancer. Reduced port laparoscopic surgery (RPLS), which includes both single-port surgery and needlescopic surgery, has been developed and is well-known in the field of endoscopic surgery. The concept has also been introduced to laparoscopic surgery for gastric cancer [2–4]. Generally, an incision of approximately 3.5 cm is needed at the umbilicus through which the resected specimen is extracted. Therefore, the maximum scar for single-port laparoscopic gastrectomy (SPLG) or reduced port laparoscopic gastrectomy (RPLG) is the 3.5-cm umbilical incision. The author uses an inexpensive, silicone-access device as an umbilical platform. With SPLG or RPLG, lymphadenectomy and reconstruction are of the same quality as obtained by the multiport technique. SPLG ensures minimal injury to the abdominal wall and a good cosmetic outcome.

In this chapter, our single-port laparoscopic total gastrectomy (SPLTG) procedure performed for gastric cancer is described in detail and illustrated with laparoscopic photos and a picture of the single platform viewed externally. The needle-assisted technique is also falls under the RPLS concept.

18.2 Indications

As is widely recognized, technical difficulty in RPLS is closely related to the distance from the access site to the surgical field. We would recommend performing RPLG, at least in the first few cases, in patients with a distance from the umbilicus to the xiphoid process 15 cm or less and with BMI 30 kg/m² or less. Indication can then be expanded as surgeon's skill and the surgical team's experience increase.

18.3 Technique

18.3.1 Positioning

The set-up for RPLG is identical to that for conventional laparoscopic distal gastrectomy (CLDG). The patient is placed supine in the dorsosacral position (Fig. 18.1). The surgeon stands between the patient's legs, the camera assistant

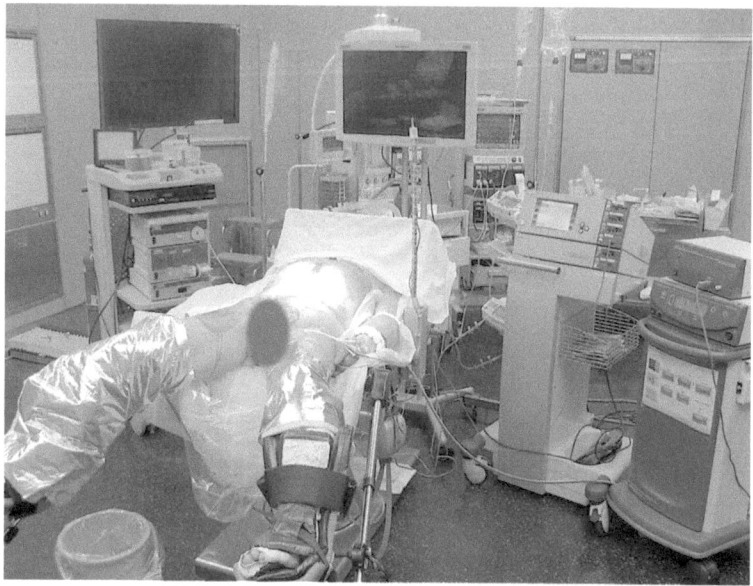

Fig. 18.1 Patient positioning

stands at the patient's right side, and the first assistant stands at the patient's left side. A monitor is placed above the patient's head, and the laparoscopic system is positioned behind the patient's right shoulder. A 5- or 10-mm endoscope with a 3-CCD high-definition camera (Karl Storz-Endoskope, Tuttlingen, Germany) is preferred (Fig. 18.2).

18.3.2   Access Device

A 3.5-cm incision is made at the umbilicus. We prefer use of the Lap-protector FF1010™ and the EZ access™ for the protector (Hakko Co. Ltd., Nagano, Japan) (Fig. 18.3), which can be assembled as an umbilical access device (Fig. 18.4). A 12-mm trocar and three 5-mm trocars are inserted through the EZ access™ device. A 5-mm, 30-degree endoscope, both of the surgeon's forceps, and the assistant's forceps are inserted through the respective trocars (Fig. 18.5). The energy device, stapler, and gauze are inserted and removed through the 12-mm trocar.

18.3.3   Liver Retraction

The liver retraction procedure is important for gastrectomy. We retract the left lobe of the liver in two steps without the use of a trocar or retractor (Fig. 18.6). The round ligament of the liver is lifted with 2-0 nylon thread attached to a straight needle that

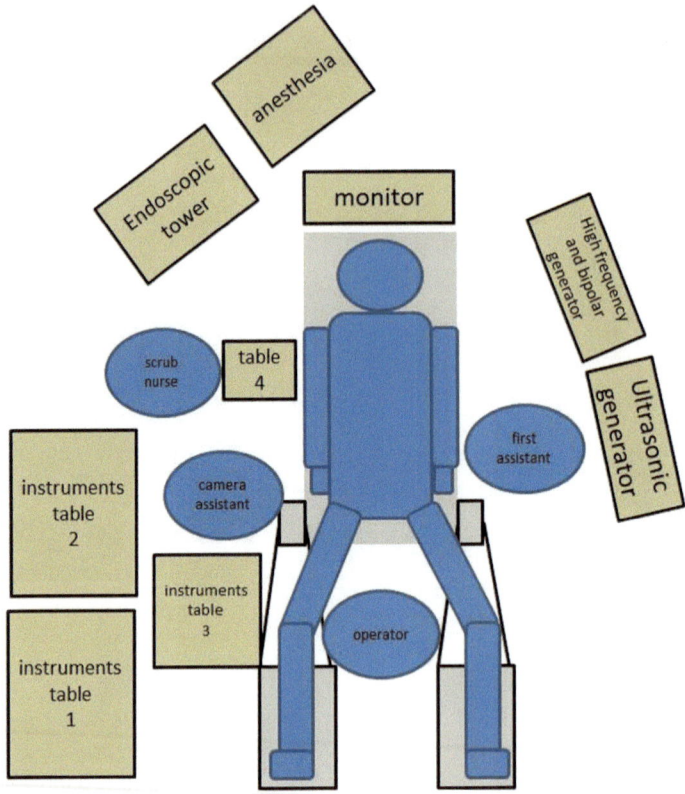

Fig. 18.2 Operation room set-up

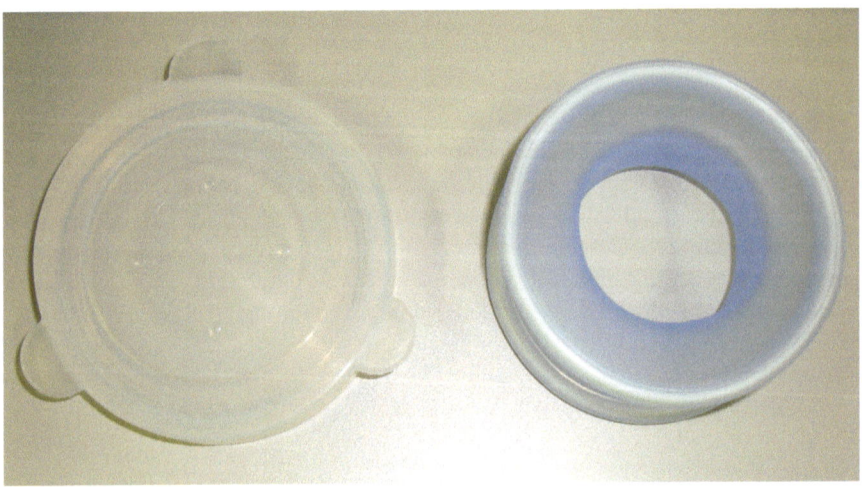

Fig. 18.3 The Lap protector FF1010™ (Hakko) and EZ access™ (Hakko) for FF1010 are assembled

Fig. 18.4 Desktop
simulation

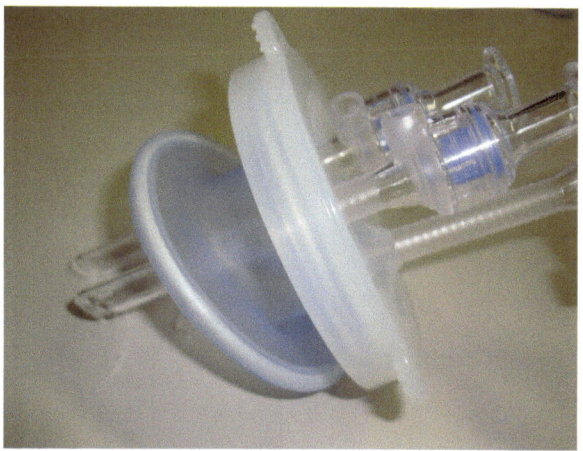

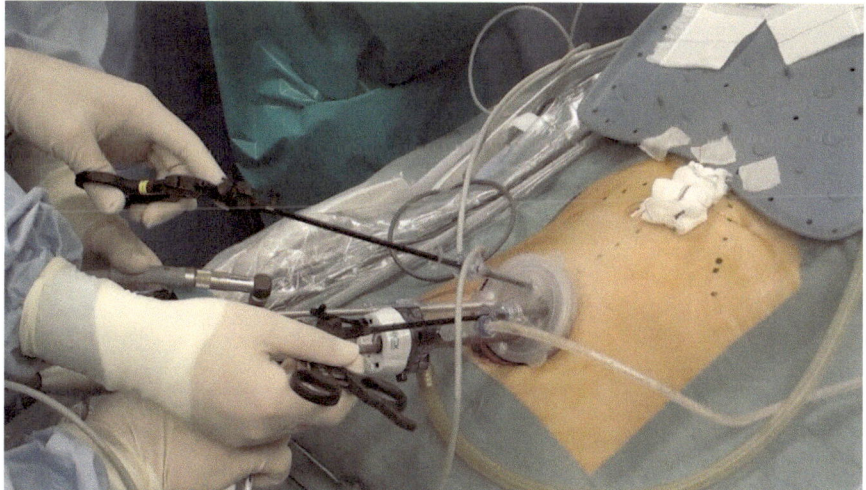

Fig. 18.5 External view of the single-port at the umbilicus

has been inserted percutaneously into the abdominal cavity. The needle is passed over the round ligament and then out through the skin. A medium size silicon-disc (Hakko Co.) is introduced into the abdominal cavity and placed under the left lobe of the liver. The straight needle with the 2-0 nylon thread is introduced by percutaneous puncture, directed through the front side of the disc, the central tendon of the diaphragm at the dorsal side of the disc, and again through the disc on the patient's right, withdrawn percutaneously, and tied extracorporeally. With experience, this series of step is performed within 5 min. We believe this method of liver retraction without scaring is effective and that it prevents postoperative transaminase elevation.

Fig. 18.6 A silicon disc is placed for liver retraction

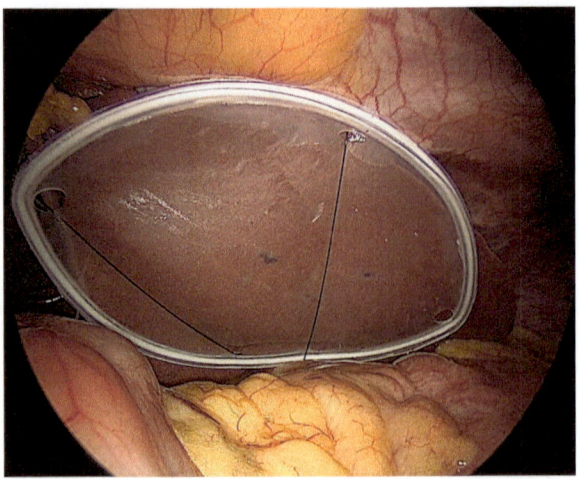

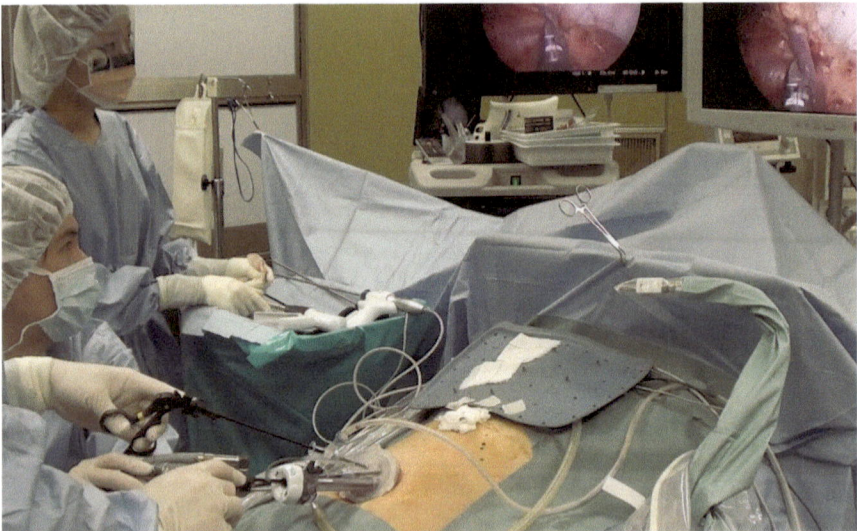

Fig. 18.7 Dorsosacral and head-up tilt position

18.3.4 Procedure

Dissection of the left side of the greater omentum: the lymph nodes are dissected in the same manner as in CLDG. The difference between SPLG and CLDG is how the tissue is manipulated. In SPLG, two forceps are used instead of three. To begin laparoscopic insufflation, the operation table is tilted into the head-up position (Fig. 18.7).

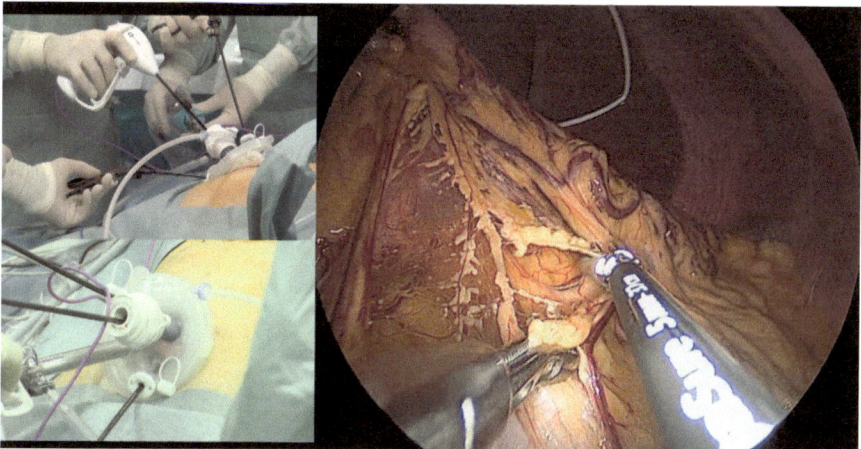

Fig. 18.8 The middle portion of the greater omentum is opened

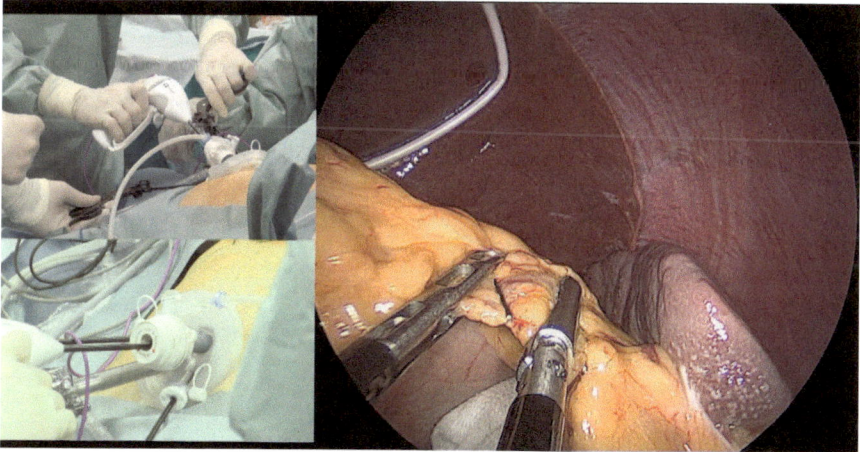

Fig. 18.9 The origins of left gastroepiploic artery and vein are clipped and cut with a bipolar sealing device

The first surgical step is opening the greater omentum. The greater curvature of the middle stomach is grasped by the assistant and lifted upward, and the middle portion of the greater omentum is cut with a bipolar sealing device toward the origin of the left gastroepiploic artery and vein (Fig. 18.8), which are then clipped and cut (Fig. 18.9). The short gastric arteries and veins are then coagulated and cut with the use of a bipolar sealing device and no clips (Fig. 18.10). The gastro-splenic mesentery should be carefully treated during dissection, otherwise bleeding can occur.

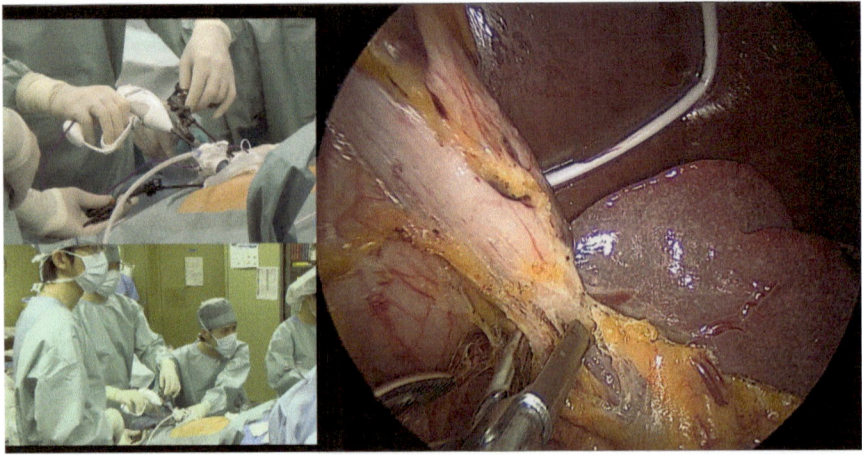

Fig. 18.10 Short gastric arteries and veins are coagulated and cut with a use of a bipolar sealing device and no clips

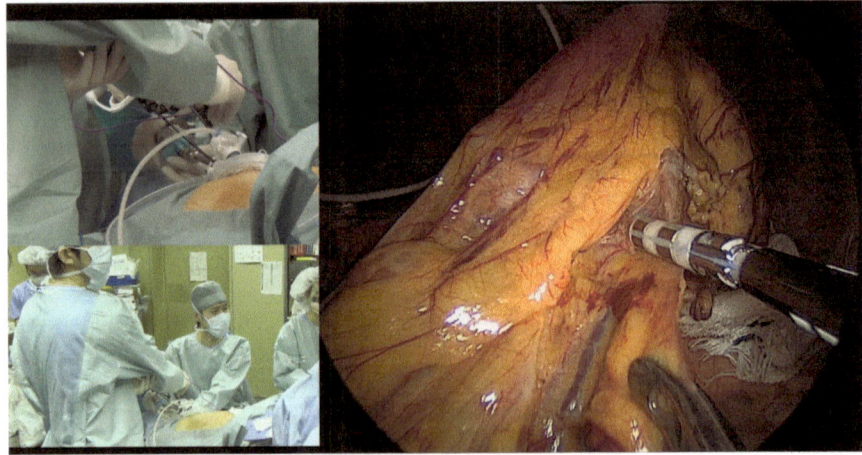

Fig. 18.11 The right side of the greater omentum is opened

Dissection of the right side of the greater omentum: the central portion of the greater omentum is cut with a bipolar sealing device toward the right side of the omentum (Fig. 18.11). This means the greater omentum is taken off the transverse mesocolon. The goal of the right-side dissection is the wall of the descending duodenum. In dissection around the root of right gastroepiploic artery and vein in the pyloric area, the assistant grasps the peripheral part of the gastroepiploic vessels, and the surgeon creates traction by applying gauze and pushing downward on the mesocolon. The artery and vein are clipped and cut, and the remaining tissue,

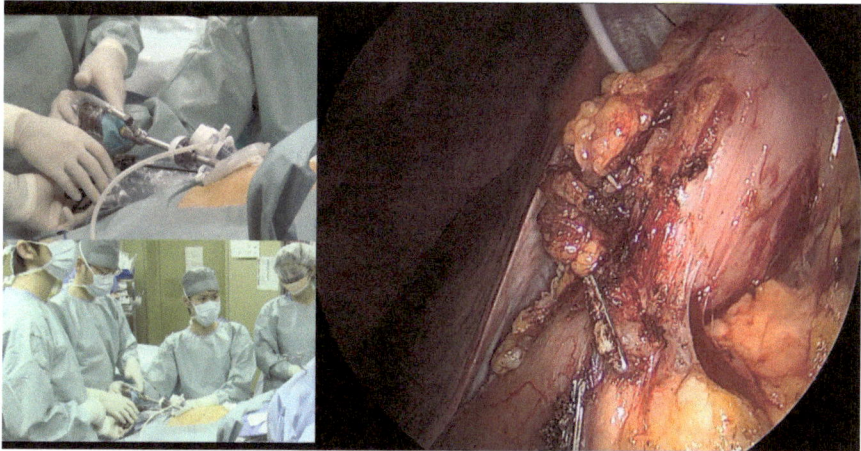

Fig. 18.12   No. 6 lymph node is completely dissected

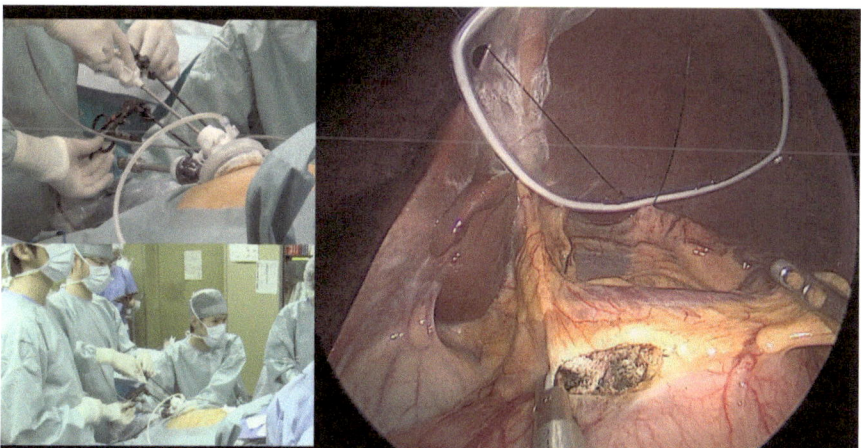

Fig. 18.13   The lesser omentum is opened around the pyloric area

including No. 6 lymph node, is completely dissected (Fig. 18.12). An ultrasonically activated device (USAD) is generally used for precise dissection. In using a USAD, the surgeon must take care to avoid cavitation, which can occur at the tip of the active USAD blade. To avoid cavitation, it is important to incline the pedicle of the gastroepiploic artery and vein to both sides in a flag-like motion, freeing the tip of the active blade from other vessels and pancreatic tissue. A titanium clip is used in the same manner.

Dividing the duodenum: before dividing duodenum, we open the lesser omentum around the pyloric area (Fig. 18.13). The stapler is inserted through the 12-mm

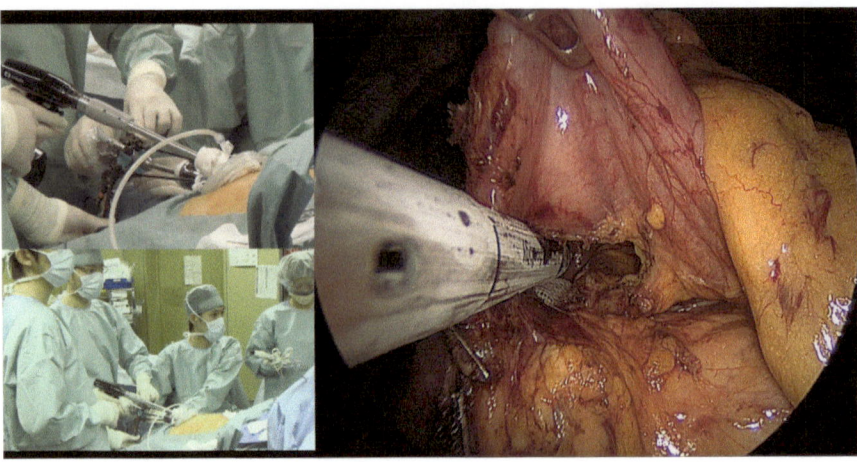

Fig. 18.14 Duodenal dividing with a liner stapler

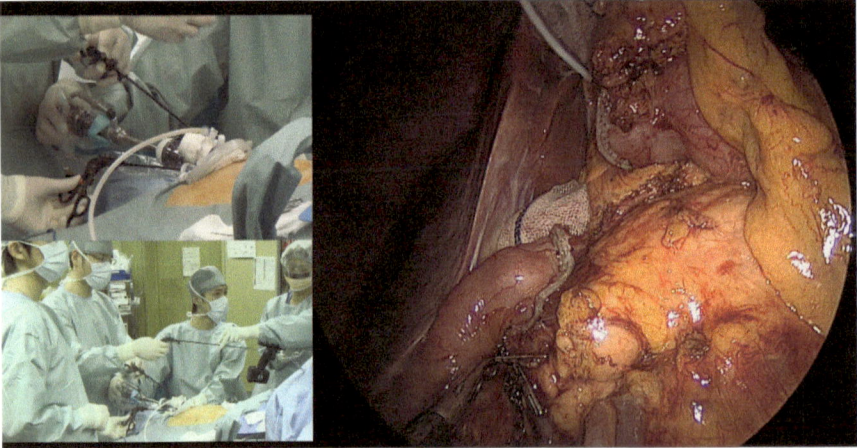

Fig. 18.15 Appropriate duodenal dividing

trocar (Fig. 18.14), the cartridge should be appropriately articulated for identification of the staple line, and the duodenal bulb is divided (Fig. 18.15).

Dissection around the hepato-duodenal ligament: after division of the duodenum, the field around the hepato-duodenal ligament, including the root of the right gastric artery and vein, can be clearly seen. Dissecting along the surface of the gastro-duodenal artery, we first cut the serosa along the proper hepatic artery and open the lesser curvature up to the crura of the diaphragm (Fig. 18.16). In case of early gastric cancer, we preserve the hepatic branch of the vagus nerve.

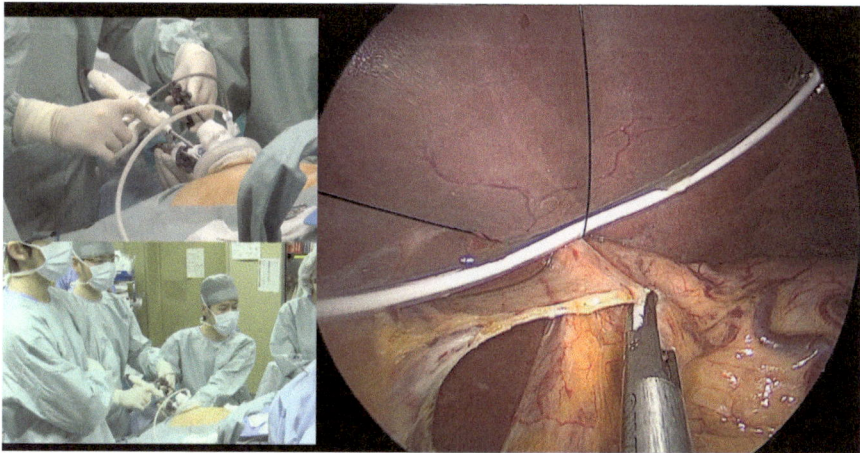

Fig. 18.16 The lesser curvature is opened to the crura of the diaphragm

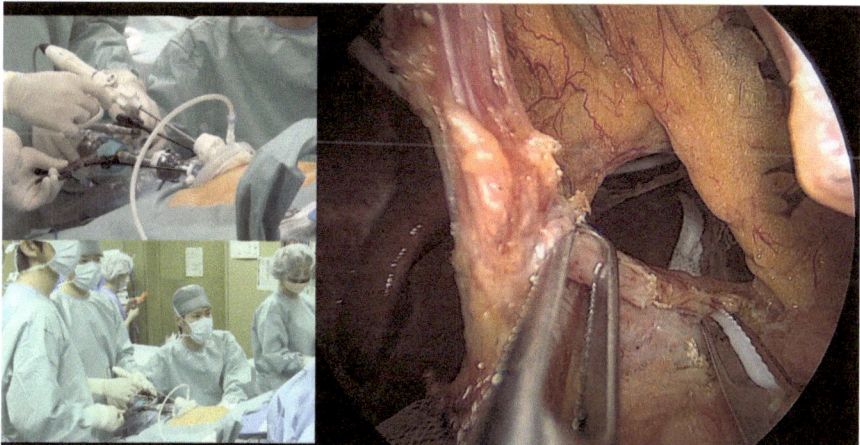

Fig. 18.17 Finding the surface of the neural layer around the common hepatic artery

We then look for the surface of the neural layer around the common hepatic artery (Fig. 18.17), which is referred to as the "outer-most layer" [5], or "dissectable layer." The outer-most layer should be preserved during the next step, dissection around the suprapancreatic area. The root of the right gastric artery and vein is encircled, clipped, and divided (Fig. 18.18). The lymph node at the left of the portal vein is appropriately dissected or preserved, according to the level of nodal dissection planned.

Dissection of the suprapancreatic area: the Assistant grasps the middle part of gastro-splenic fold, and the surgeon creates traction by pushing gauze downward

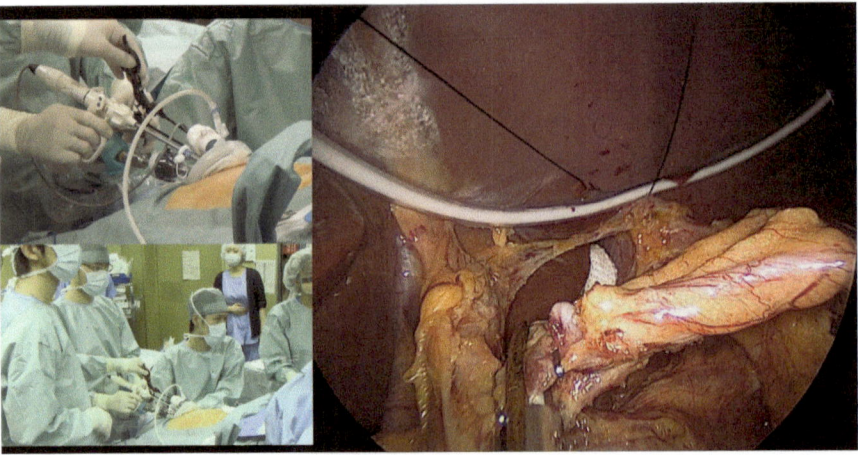

Fig. 18.18 The root of the right gastric artery and vein is encircled, clipped, and divided

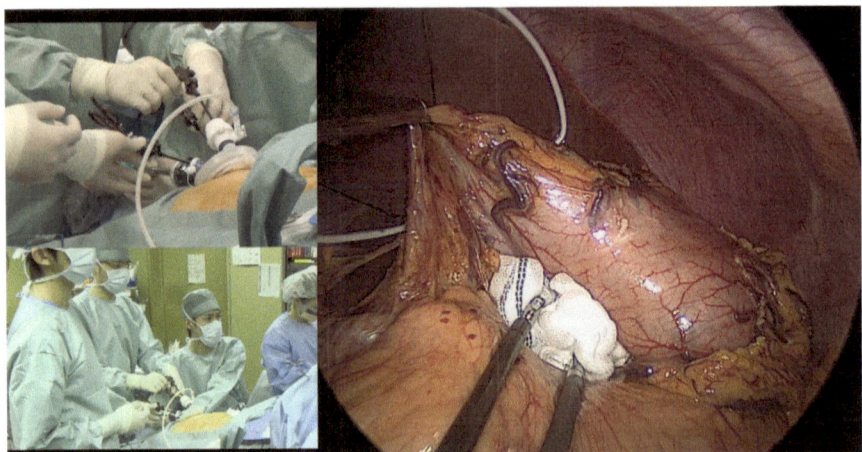

Fig. 18.19 Gauze is inserted to create working space and absorb blood

on the spleen. In using the forceps in the area, the surgeon's approach angle is the aspect of the procedure that differs most from CLDG. Lymph node dissection around the common hepatic artery or splenic artery can be difficult because of the horizontal angle. One of the solutions to the difficult manipulation is to use gravity; this leads to a falling away of the pancreas, making dissection around the arteries easy. Gauze packing behind the gastro-splenic fold and on the pancreatic tail is also useful for creating working space and absorbing blood (Fig. 18.19). We respect the medial approach [6] for dissection of the suprapancreatic lymph nodes.

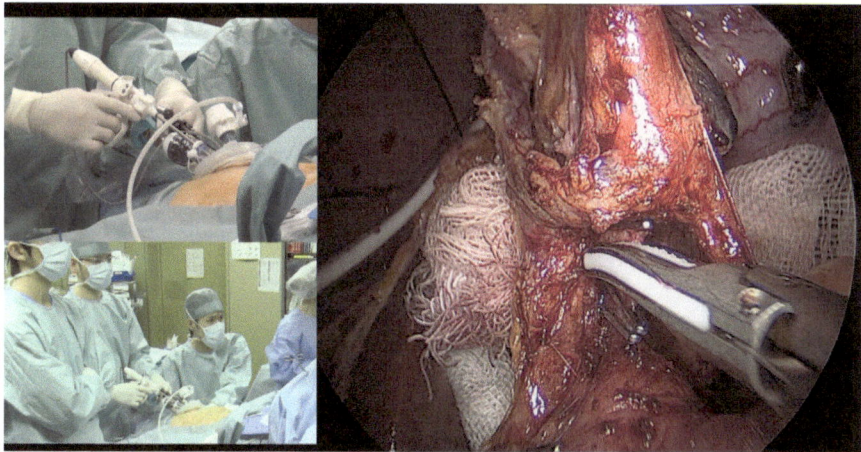

Fig. 18.20 The root of the left gastric artery is cut

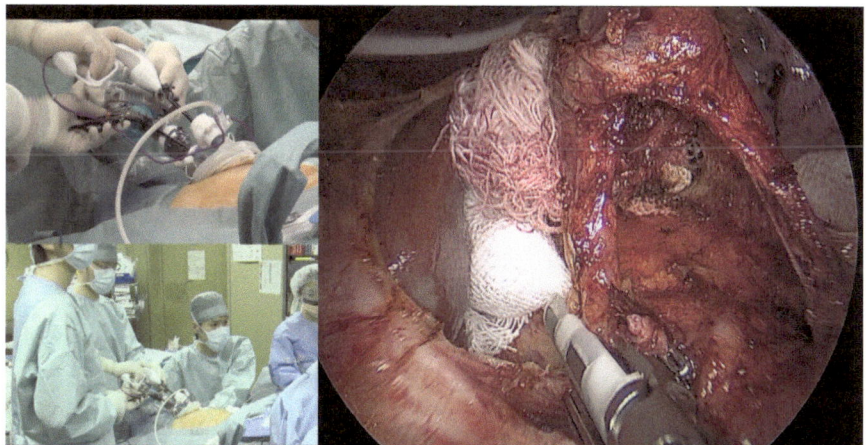

Fig. 18.21 The left side of the celiac artery is dissected

Dissecting the lateral sides of the left gastric artery, we cut the root of the left gastric artery (Fig. 18.20). We then dissect the right side of the gastro-splenic fold including No. 9 and No. 8a lymph node stations (Fig. 18.21), and the left side of the celiac artery including, No. 9 and No. 11p lymph node stations are dissected upward in the same way (Fig. 18.22). The remaining suprapancreatic tissue is dissected completely (Fig. 18.23).

Trimming around the abdominal esophagus: the tissue around the abdominal esophagus is dissected. Both vagus nerves are cut up (Fig. 18.24), and the 60-mm-cartridge stapler is applied to the esophago-gastric junction (Fig. 18.25).

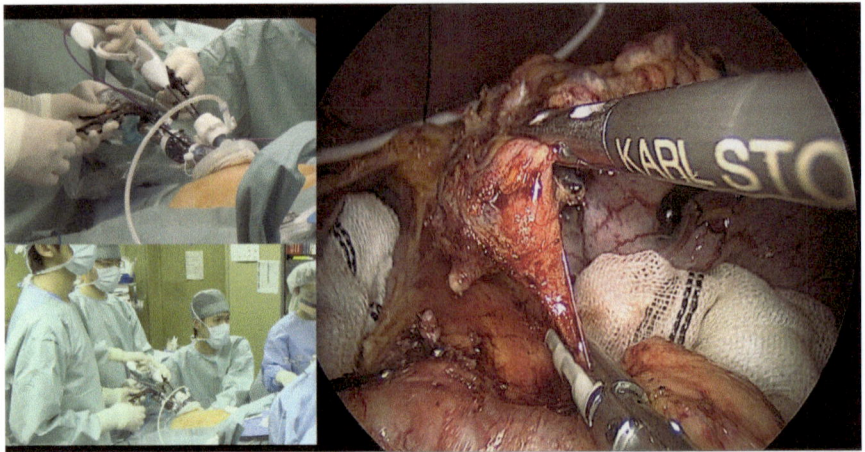

Fig. 18.22 The right side of the celiac artery is dissected

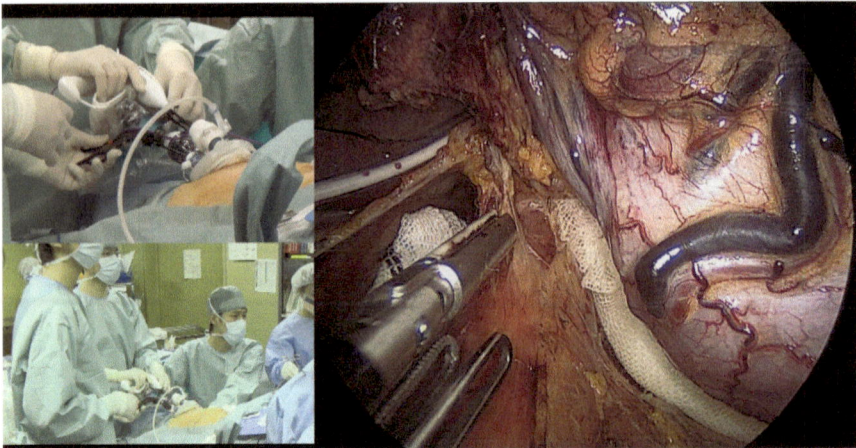

Fig. 18.23 The remaining suprapancreatic tissue is dissected

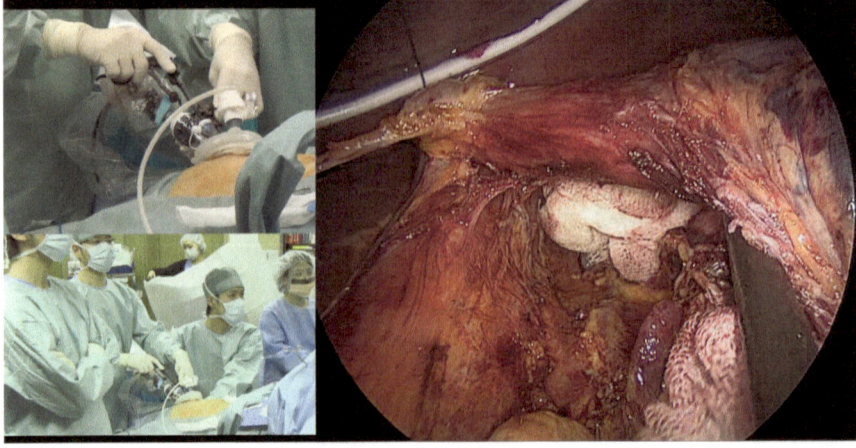

Fig. 18.24 Paraesophageal tissue is dissected

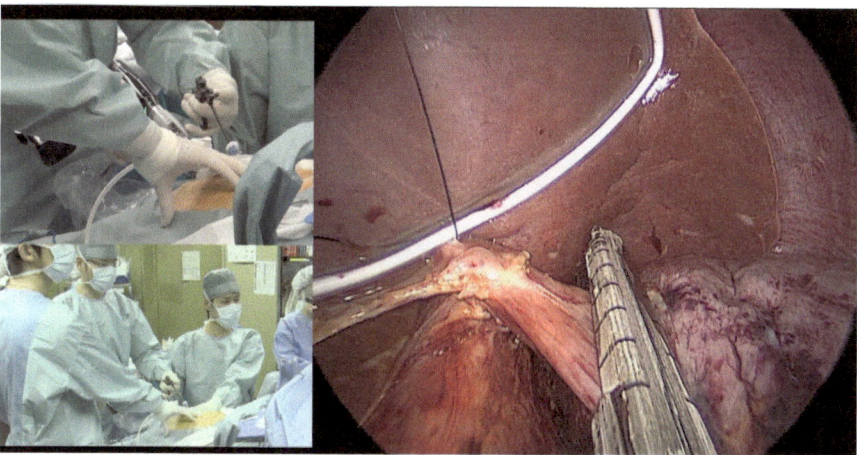

Fig. 18.25 A 60-mm cartridge stapler is applied to the esophagogastric junction

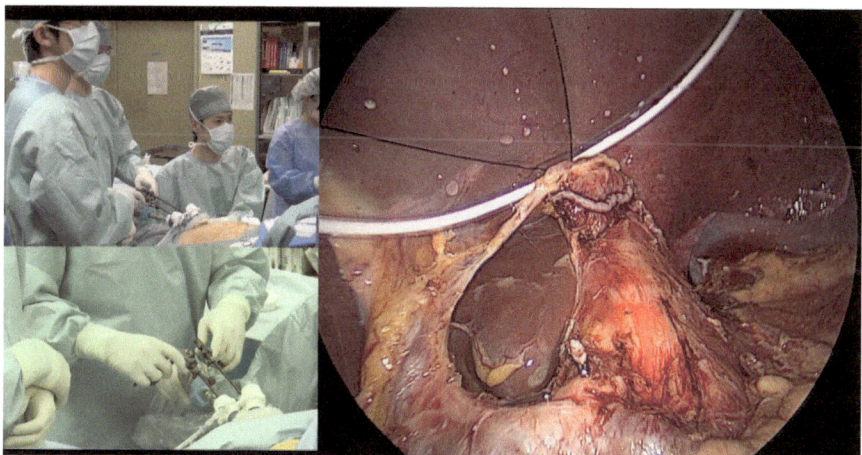

Fig. 18.26 A certain esophageal margin

Dividing the esophagus and specimen extraction: the abdominal esophagus is divided with a certain margin (Fig. 18.26). The resected specimen is placed in a plastic bag (Fig. 18.27), and extracted through the umbilical port (Fig. 18.28). Laparoscopic insufflation is restarted, and the dissected field is appropriately washed with saline. The lymphadenectomy field is inspected endoscopically for any missed suspicious nodes (Figs. 18.29, 18.30, and 18.31).

Reconstruction: we perform Roux-en-Y reconstruction after total gastrectomy with the use of a linear stapler. We first measure 25 cm from the Treiz ligament and

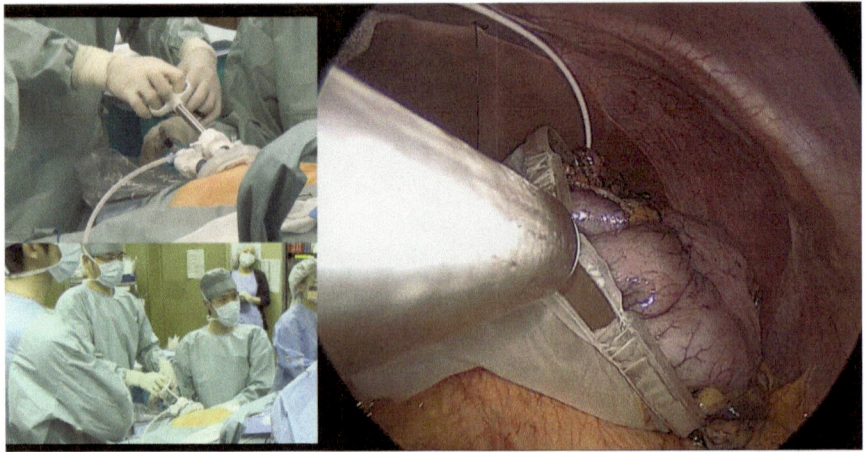

Fig. 18.27 The resected specimen is place intracorporeally into a plastic bag

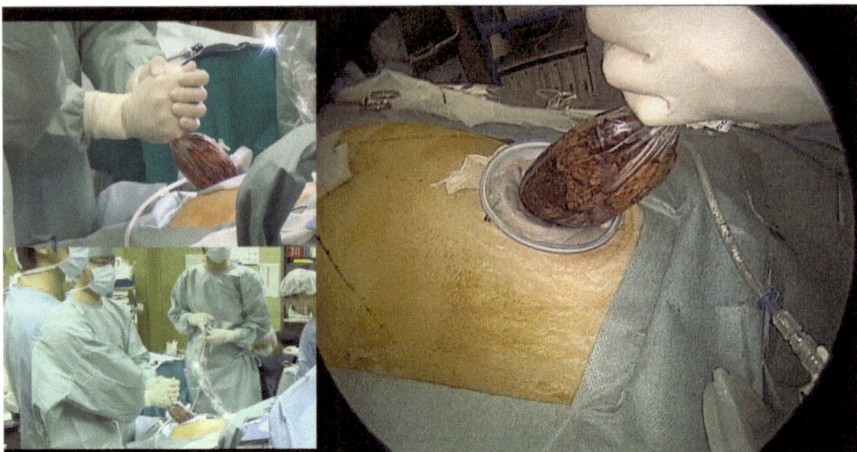

Fig. 18.28 The resected specimen is extracted through the umbilical port

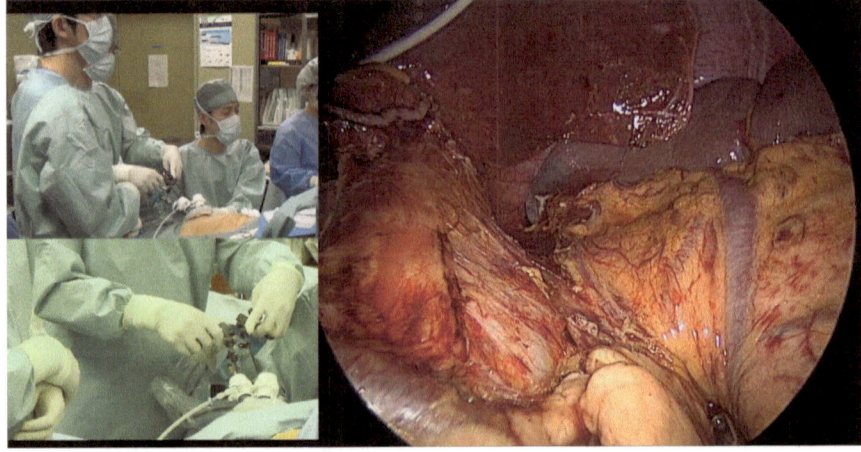

Fig. 18.29 Final inspection of the lymphadenectomy: left side of the celiac artery

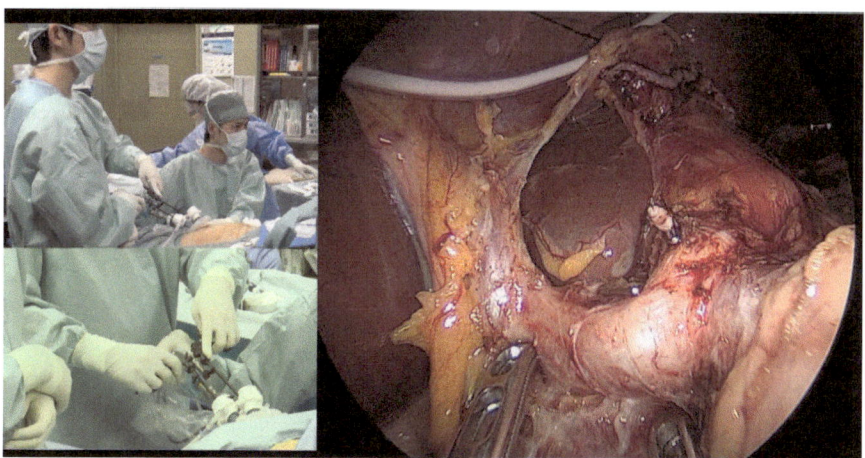

Fig. 18.30 Final inspection of the lymphadenectomy: right side of the celiac artery

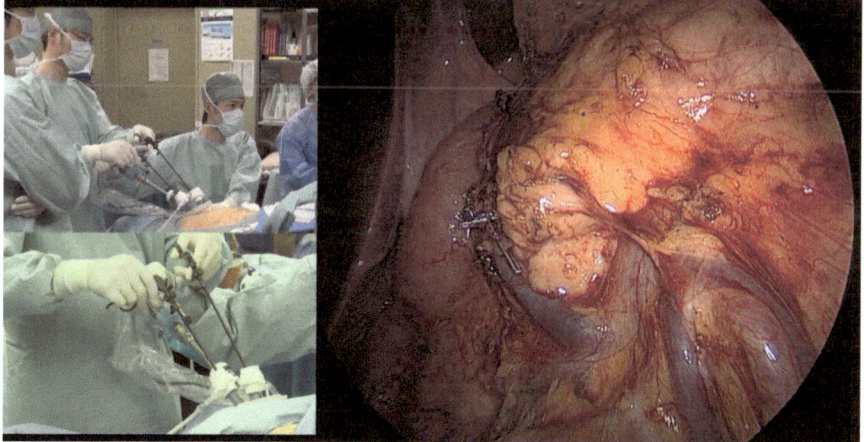

Fig. 18.31 Final inspection of the lymphadenectomy: around the pancreatic head

lift the jejunum (Fig. 18.32). A small hole is made near the jejunum. Under laparoscopic observation, the jejunum is divided with a linear stapler (Fig. 18.33). About 20 cm of the Roux limb is sacrificed for safe reconstruction (Fig. 18.34). Esophago-jejunosotomy is simulated, and the Y limb is measured and inked at a point 40 cm away from the point of simulated esophagojejunosotomy. The Y limb is then created extracorporeally by means of a side-to-side anastomosis achieved

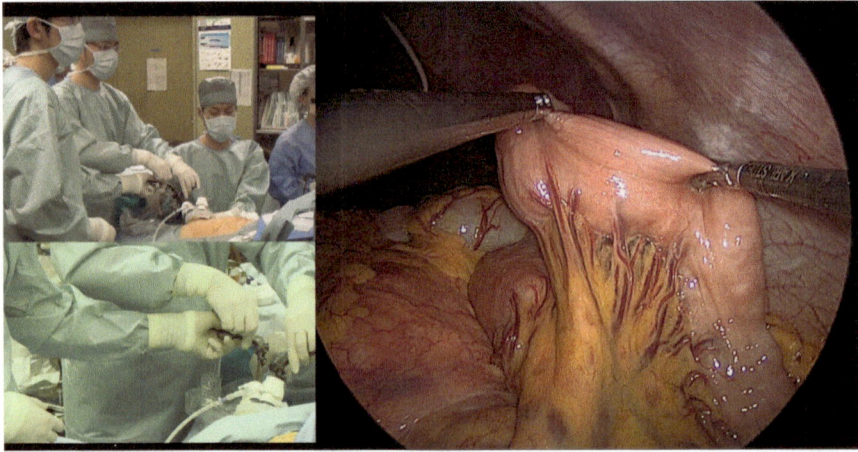

Fig. 18.32 The jejunum is lifted at a point 25 cm from the ligament of Treitz

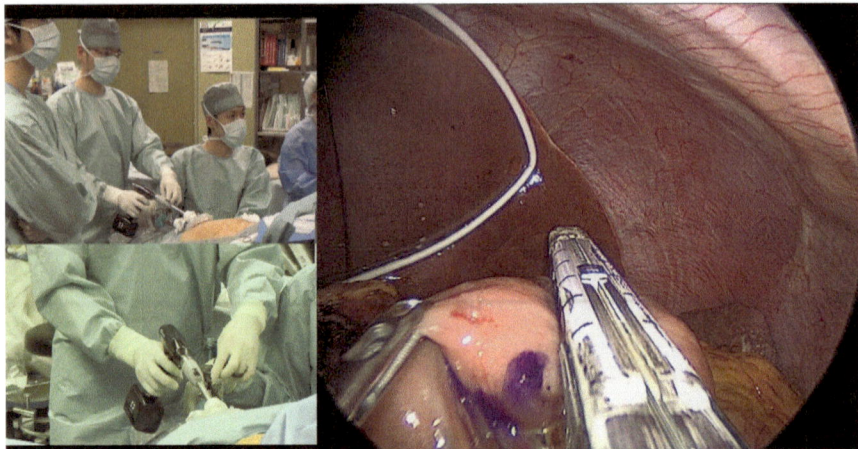

Fig. 18.33 The jejunum is divided with a use of a linear stapler

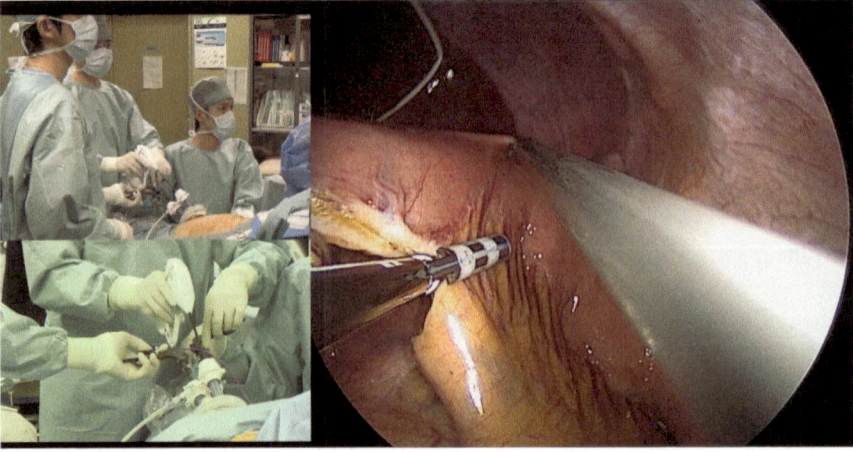

Fig. 18.34 Sacrificing the jejunum

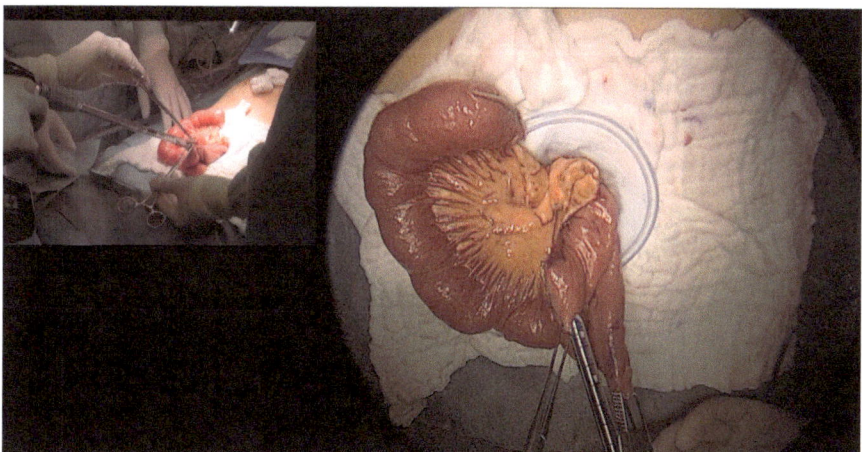

Fig. 18.35 Extracorporeal side-to-side anastomosis created with a 60-mm linear stapler

Fig. 18.36 Closing the stapler entry hole by hand suturing

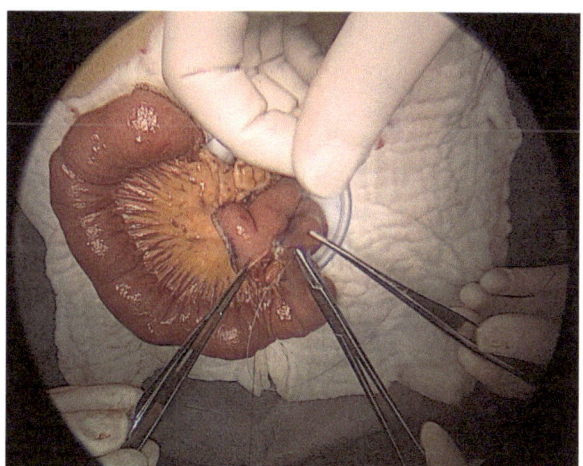

with a 60-mm linear stapler (Fig. 18.35). The stapler entry hole is hand sutured with 4-0 controlled-release braided absorbable thread (Fig. 18.36). A continuous one-layer suture is adequate for the closure. We can choose either intracorporeal or extracorporeal suturing for the Y limb. This is because it is usually easy to lift the Y limb outside from the umbilical port in patients meeting the criteria for SPLTG. Esophagojejunostomy is performed intracorporeally. We always choose side-to-side anastomosis using a 45-cm linear stapler, the so-called overlap technique (Fig. 18.37). The stapler entry hole is sutured intracorporeally (Fig. 18.38).

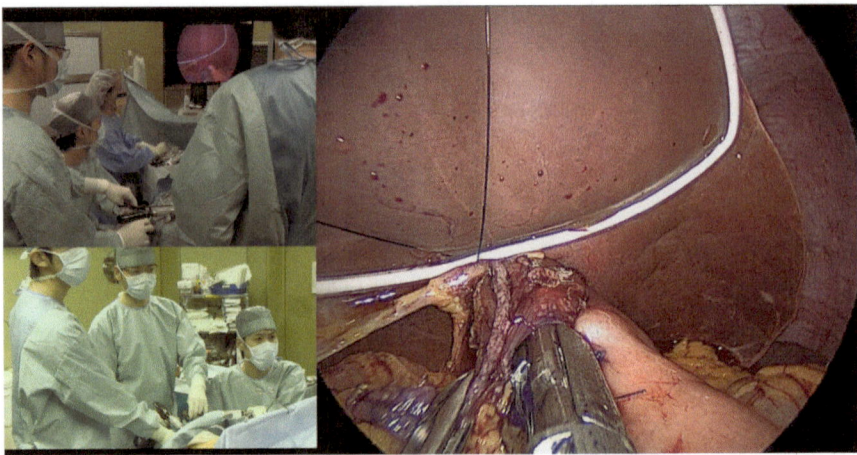

Fig. 18.37 Esophagojejunostomy achieved by the overlap technique

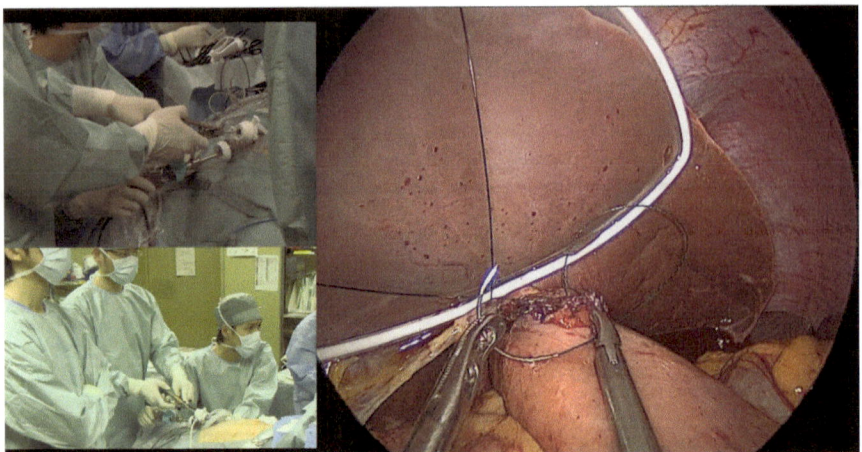

Fig. 18.38 Intracorporeal suturing with barbed suture material

Barbed suture material, 15 cm 3-0 V-Loc™ 180 (Covidien, New Haven, CT, USA), is used for the suturing. This material prevents line slack during the suturing and does not require knotting. After the closure, we check for leakage by pumping air through the naso-gastric tube. Finally, both the Petersen's defect and mesenterial space of the Y limb are closed with a continuous barbed suture, as described previously (Figs. 18.39 and 18.40).

We do not place any drain tubes. After rewashing and checking the abdominal cavity, we apply a Seprafilm adhesion barrier (Kaken Pharmaceutical Co. Ltd.,

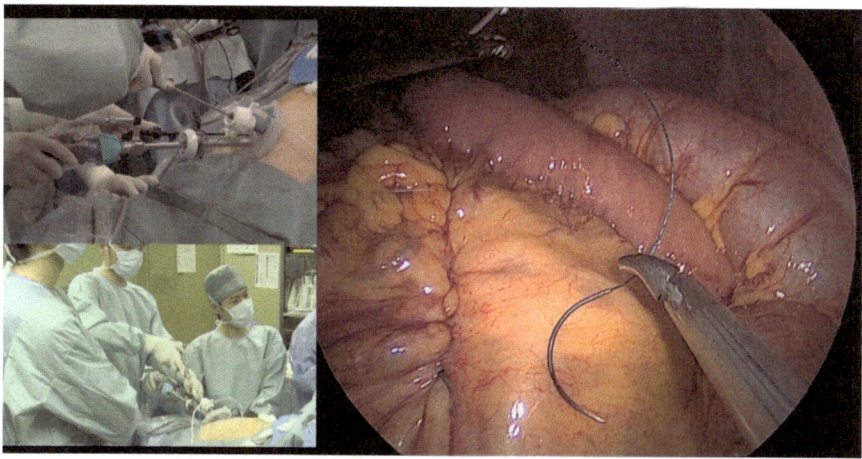

Fig. 18.39 Closing Petersen's defect

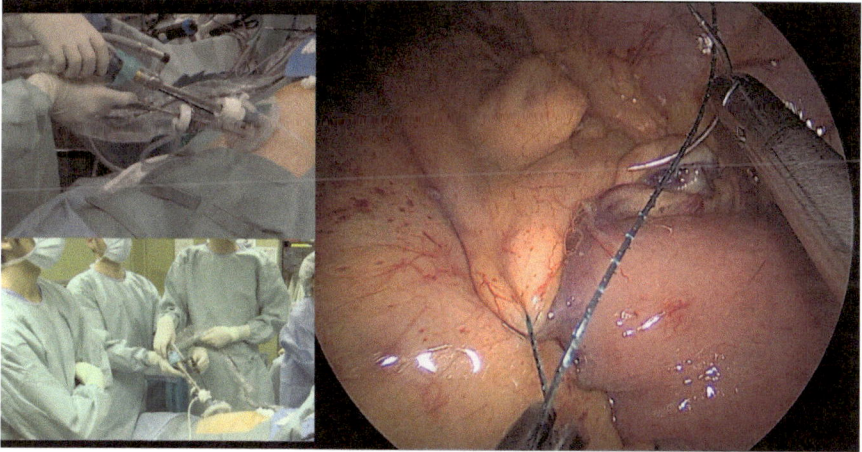

Fig. 18.40 Closing the mesenterial space of the Y limb

Tokyo, Japan) just below the umbilical scar. Finally the single umbilical opening is cosmetically closed with an appropriate buried suture, and the scar is generally invisible after 3 months (Fig. 18.41).

18.4 Tips, Tricks and Recommandations from the Author

1. One of the most difficult technical demands is the resolution of instrument conflicts outside the port. To resolve the problem, we use EZ trocar™ (Hakko Co., Ltd.) (Fig. 18.42), which is 5-mm in diameter. The housing is also small, although

Fig. 18.41 The scar at the umbilicus is nearly invisible after 3 months

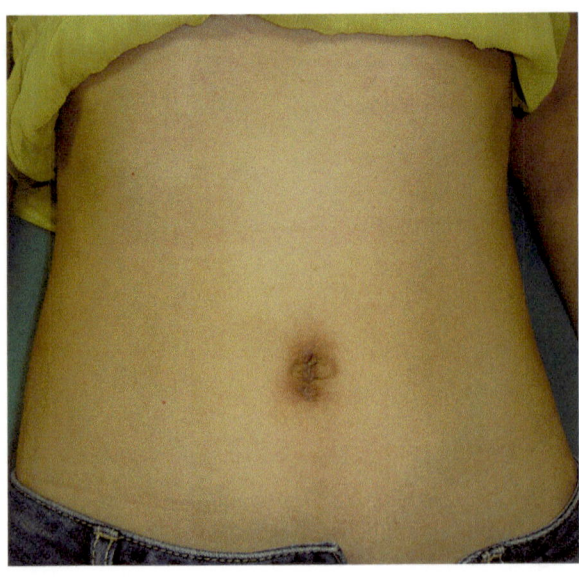

Fig. 18.42 The EZ trocar™ housing is small (Hakko)

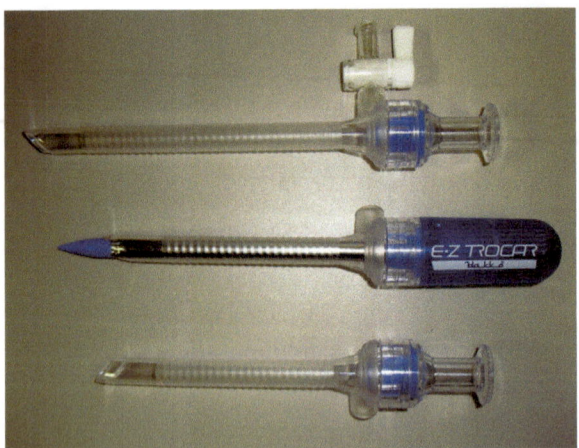

a trocar of at least 10- to 12-mm is needed for inserting the stapler, the gauze, and the suture needle. Actually, a trocar of different size can be selected, if necessary. In that case, the trocar housing will not cause interference (Fig. 18.43).

2. When we perform SPLTG, we introduce gauze into the abdominal cavity at various sites. This helps create space and organ traction without the need for traction assistance, as in CLTG. The gauze also absorbs blood and lymphatic fluid (Fig. 18.19).

Fig. 18.43 The small housing prevents instrument conflicts

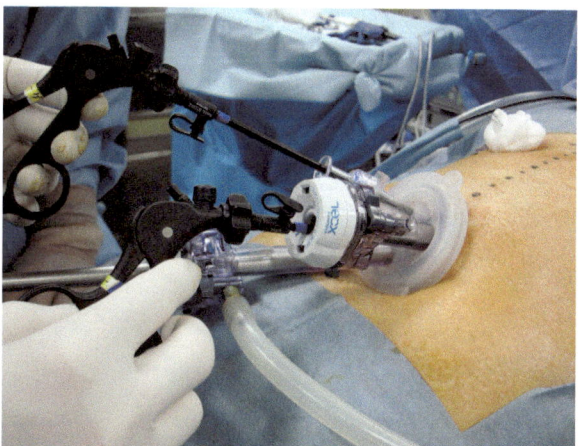

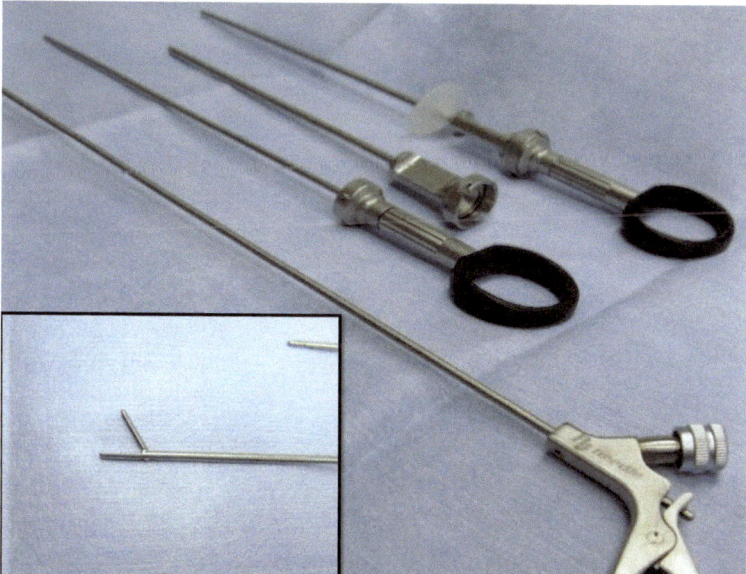

Fig. 18.44 BJ needle™ (Niti-On)

3. We use straight instruments, which are also use in conventional laparoscopic surgery. Sometimes we encounter instrument conflicts at the single-port and cannot maintain an adequate working angle. In such situations, it is sometimes necessary to abandon the single-port. If necessary, additional ports should be inserted but in a minimally invasive manner. We prefer to use the 2.1-diameter BJ needle™ (Nition Co., Ltd., Chiba, Japan) forceps, not through an additional port but via puncture (Fig. 18.44). A trocar made especially for BJ needle can be easily

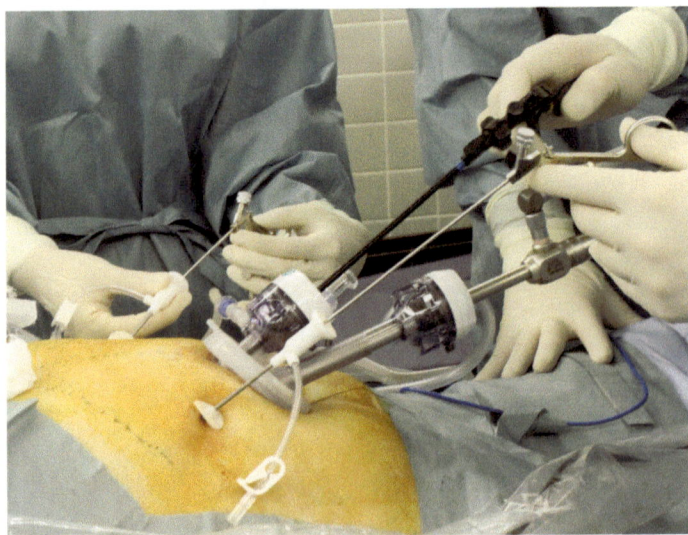

Fig. 18.45 Use of needle instruments creates a good working angle

inserted without causing postoperative pain or an unsatisfactory cosmetic outcome. Even one additional BJ needle in the surgeon's left hand is helpful for
obtaining the proper manipulation angle in the laparoscopic view. According to
our experience, three additional BJ needles at most, one in the surgeon's left hand
and one each in the assistant's right and left hands will create almost the same
tissue traction as in conventional laparoscopic surgery (Fig. 18.45). We believe
the needle instruments to be helpful not only in single-port surgery, but also to
facilitate RPLS performed under the concept of minimally invasive surgery.

References

1. Kitano S, Iso Y, Moriyama M et al (1994) Laparoscopy-assisted Billroth I gastrectomy. Surg
   Laparosc Endosc 4:146–148
2. Omori T, Oyama T, Akamatsu H et al (2011) Transumbilical single-incision laparoscopic distal
   gastrectomy for early gastric cancer. Surg Endosc 25:2400–2404
3. Kawamura H, Tanioka T, Kuji M et al (2013) The initial experience of dual port laparoscopy-
   assisted total gastrectomy as a reduced port surgery for total gastrectomy. Gastric Cancer
   16(4):602–608
4. Kunisaki C, Ono HA, Oshima T et al (2012) Relevance of reduced-port laparoscopic distal
   gastrectomy for gastric cancer: a pilot study. Dig Surg 29:261–268
5. Uyama I, Suda K, Satoh S (2013) Laparoscopic surgery for advanced gastric cancer: current
   status and future perspectives. J Gastric Cancer 13:19–25
6. Kanaya S, Haruta S, Kawamura Y et al (2011) Video: laparoscopy distinctive technique for
   suprapancreatic lymph node dissection: medial approach for laparoscopic gastric cancer surgery. Surg Endosc 25:3928–3929

Chapter 19
Wedge Gastric and Endo-Gastric Resection

Eiji Kanehira, Aya Kamei, and Takashi Tanida

Abstract Two different operative techniques for resection of gastric submucosal tumors through a single incision and one needle-puncture are described. One involves an extragastric approach, which is indicated for tumors at a location distant from the esophagogastric junction. The other involves an endoluminal approach, which is indicated for tumors located at the esophagogastric junction. We use the x-Gate® multichannel port (Sumitomo Bakelite, Tokyo, Japan), through which two or three instruments are inserted. In addition we use BJ needle® (Niti On Co., Chiba, Japan), a 2-mm grasper, through a puncture site. With the extragastric approach, tumors are excised in full-thickness by an ultrasonically activated device, and this is followed by manual suturing. With the endoluminal approach a temporary gastrostomy is constructed at the navel, through which the x-Gate® (Sumitomo Bakelite) is fixed in the gastric cavity. Under percutaneous gastroscopic view, tumors at the esophagogastric junction are resected in full thickness, and this is followed by manual suturing. The techniques described here can be safely performed, and the cosmetic result of both techniques is satisfactory.

Keywords Gastric submucosal tumor • Gastrointestinal stromal tumor • Intragastric surgery • Single-incision laparoscopic surgery (SLS) • Wedge resection

19.1 Introduction

Single-incision laparoscopic surgery (SLS) might be as applicable to local gastrectomy for submucosal tumor as it is to cholecystectomy because such a complicated procedure such as meticulous lymphadenectomy or anastomosis is not required [1, 2].

E. Kanehira (✉) • A. Kamei • T. Tanida
Department of Surgery, Medical Topia Soka,
1-11-18 Yatsuka, Soka City, Saitama 340 0028, Japan
e-mail: kanehiraxy@yahoo.co.jp

T. Mori and G. Dapri (eds.), *Reduced Port Laparoscopic Surgery*,
DOI 10.1007/978-4-431-54601-6_19, © Springer Japan 2014

Fig. 19.1 Cosmetic result of a representative Technique II case

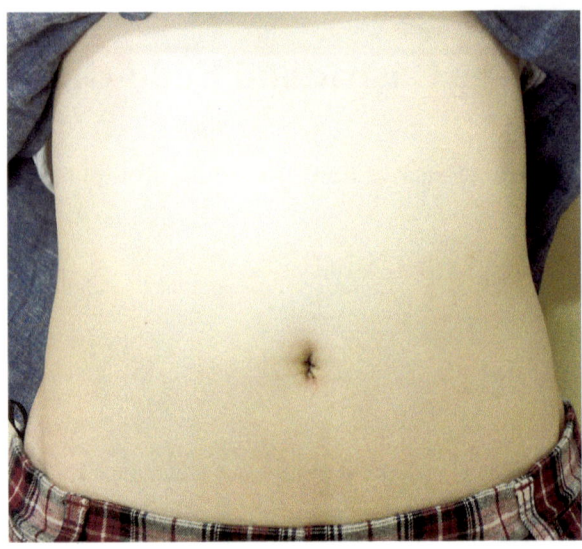

However, unlike laparoscopic cholecystectomy, the operative technique cannot be described as a single method because the resection strategy must be tailored according to the location, size, and growth type of the tumor itself [3, 4]. Between January 2009 and April 2013, we performed laparoscopic local gastrectomy in 121 patients, 63 of whom underwent a single-incision procedure. Reviewing our experience herein, we introduce the two basic methods of single-incision laparoscopic local gastrectomy. One comprises an extragastric approach with manual resection (Technique I), and the other comprises a percutaneous endoluminal approach to the stomach [2, 5] (Technique II). The cosmetic result of Technique II is shown in Fig. 19.1.

19.2   Technique I: Extragastric Approach

19.2.1   Setup

The patient is placed in a supine position with legs spread apart. The surgeon stands between the patient's legs, and the assistant surgeon stands on the right side of the patient to hold the laparoscope. The scrub nurse stands on the left side (Fig. 19.2).

19.2.2   Establishment of the Main Access Route

A 2.5-cm longitudinal incision is made at the navel. The ligament beneath the navel is incised. The fascia is opened with a 2.5-cm longitudinal incision so that the peritoneum is incised for entry into the abdominal cavity. The inner ring of a multichannel

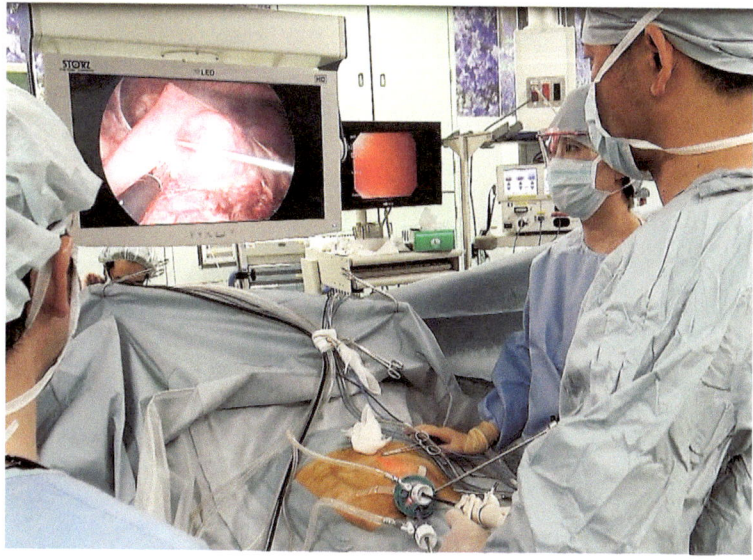

Fig. 19.2 The main surgeon stands between the patient's legs. The multichannel port called x-Gate® (Sumitomo Bakelite) is placed under the navel via a 2.5-cm incision

Fig. 19.3 The main body of x-Gate® (Sumitomo Bakelite) consists of a hard outer ring and a flexible inner ring. The converter has four flexible channels, one of which one allows 12-mm instruments

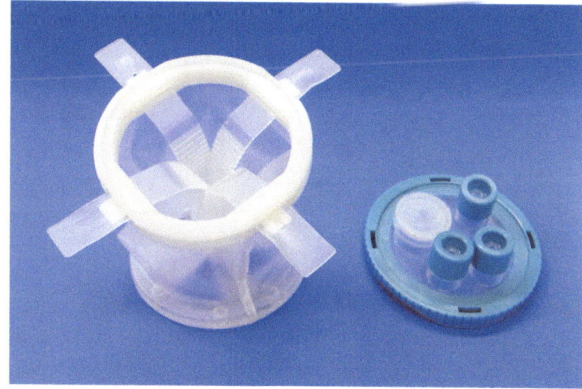

port, x-Gate® (Sumitomo Bakelite, Tokyo, Japan) (Fig. 19.3) [6], is inserted into the abdominal cavity. The inner ring of the port is brought close to the outer ring by pulling up the four belts attached to the inner ring. This manipulation also enlarges the opening in the abdominal wall as the belts force the parietal incision to expand from the inside. The converter is then attached to the outer ring of the main unit by rotating it clockwise. A long 5-mm cannula and a short 5-mm cannula are inserted through the channels on the cephalic side of the converter. To complete establishment of the access port, the gas supply tube is connected to one cannula, and the smoke evacuation tube is connected to the other. We use a 5-mm long-shafted laparoscope with a forward viewing angle of 30° and to which a high definition charge-coupled device camera is attached (Karl Storz-Endoskope, Tuttlingen, Germany).

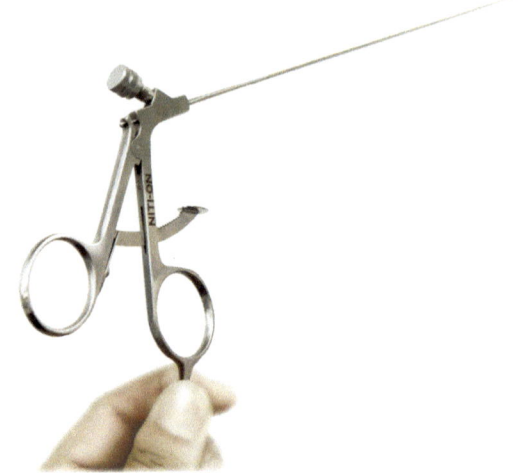

Fig. 19.4 A 2-mm grasper (BJ needle® (Niti On Co.)), which adds remarkable assistance in reduced port surgery, helps preserve the cosmetic appearance of the port-site wound

19.2.3 Insertion of 2-mm Forceps

BJ Needle® (Niti On Co., Chiba, Japan) (Fig. 19.4) is a very thin-caliber grasping forceps with a shaft diameter of 2 mm. The access port specially manufactured for BJ Needle® (BJ Port® (Niti On Co.)) is inserted into the abdominal cavity. The puncture site depends on the tumor location and the surgeon's preference. Generally, the left upper quadrant is chosen. BJ Needle® (Niti On Co.) is rigid enough to manipulate the stomach and surrounding tissue with adequate traction and expose the target.

19.2.4 Resection

We limit use of a stapling device to tumors that protrude well outside the stomach. This is because resection of a tumor with a stapling device can remove too much of the healthy gastric wall, which results in severe stomach deformity. Moreover, when the tumor is located at the lesser curvature, resection with a stapling device can damage the vagal nerve and thus cause gastric dysmotility [7, 8].

When the tumor is identified, traction is exerted on the gastric wall with the BJ needle® (Niti On Co.), and another forceps is inserted through one of the x-Gate® channels (Sumitomo Bakelite) (Fig. 19.5a). For this, we usually use a 5-mm bendable grasper (Diamond Flex®, Snowden Spencer, USA). With the two graspers, appropriate tension is applied to the target point on the gastric wall, which is incised with SonoSurg® (Olympus, Tokyo, Japan), a reusable ultrasonically activated device. When the margin of the tumor is not clearly identifiable on the serosal aspect, intraoperative peroral gastroscopy is performed to identify the safety margin from inside. Full-thickness resection of the stomach wall containing the tumor is performed. The procedure involves only minimal resection of healthy tissue around the tumor (Fig. 19.5b). The specimen is enclosed in a retrieval bag (Fig. 19.5c).

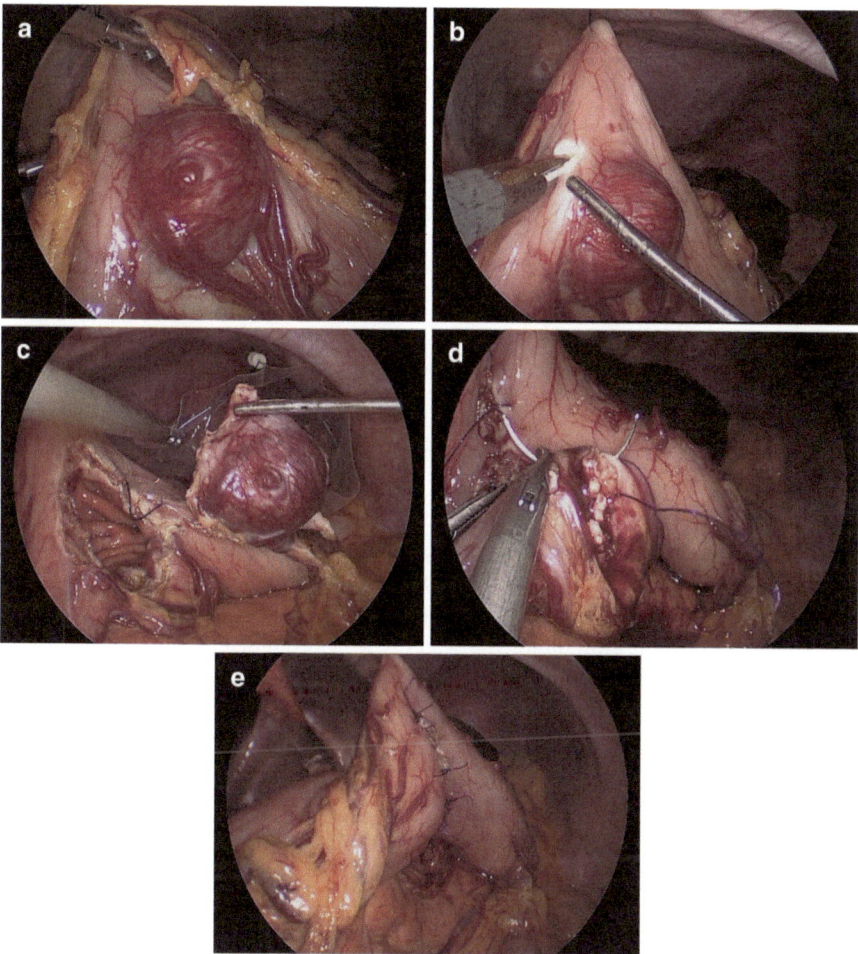

Fig. 19.5 (**a**) To expose the submucosal tumor, effective traction is applied to the stomach with a bendable grasper and a needle grasper. (**b**) The tumor, with an adequate safety margin, is removed by full-thickness gastric resection with an ultrasonically activated device. (**c**) The resected specimen is captured in an extraction bag. (**d**) The defect is closed by suturing. The full-thickness is approximated by a continuous running suture with absorbable 3-0 monofilament material. (**e**) The seromuscular layer is closed with interrupted sutures

19.2.5   Closure of the Defect

The full-thickness defect on the gastric wall is closed by manual suturing. We use a "parrot jaw" needle grasper (Karl Storz-Endoskope), which is inserted through the x-Gate® (Sumitomo Bakelite) and driven by the left hand, and a BJ needle® (Niti On Co.) as an assistant forceps held in the right hand. Absorbable monofilament 3-0 suture with a 26-mm half-circle needle is used. The x-Gate® channels (Sumitomo Bakelite) are flexible enough to facilitate swift insertion and withdrawal of the 26-mm needle.

Fig. 19.6 When the tumor is
located on the posterior
gastric wall, the greater
curvature is lifted to turn
stomach over by
percutaneous suture with a
straight needle

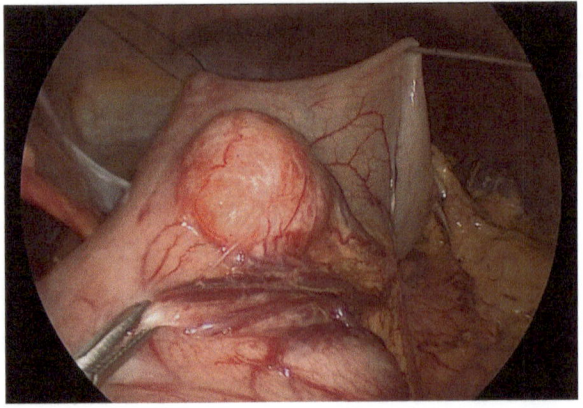

The suture line is completed transversely, crossing the longitudinal axis of the
stomach at a right angle. The idea is to avoid stenosis. The full thickness of the gastric
wall is first closed by continuous running suture (Fig. 19.5d), and the seromuscular
layer is then approximated by interrupted suture (Fig. 19.5e). After closure, peroral
gastroscopy is performed to confirm hemostasis, smooth passage, and peristalsis.

The retrieval bag containing the specimen is brought out through the navel.
We usually do not leave any drainage tube. The wounds are closed in a cosmetic
manner.

19.2.6   Tips and Tricks

19.2.6.1   Turning the Stomach Over

When the tumor is located in the posterior wall of the stomach, the stomach must be
turned over. To achieve this, the greater omentum is divided caudal to the gastroepiploic vessels, and the greater curvature is stitched at an appropriate point with a 3-0
thread and a straight needle. The needle is pushed through the abdominal wall into
the abdomen. It penetrates the stomach wall, finally returning to the abdominal wall.
Both ends of the thread are pulled up or loosened extracorporeally to control the
degree of traction (Fig. 19.6). There are several alternative devices, such as
EndoGrab® (Virtual Ports Ltd., Caesaera, Israel), [9]), an internal retractor that can
be used to turn the stomach.

19.2.6.2   Layout of the Channels

To avoid instrument conflicts, we recommend the following layout of the x-Gate®
channels (Sumitomo Bakelite). The channel positions are described as clock positions,
for example, 0 o'clock, which indicates the cephalic direction, and 9 o'clock, which

refers to the patient's right. The 5-mm laparoscope is inserted through the 9 o'clock channel, the energy device is inserted through the 2 o'clock channel, and the bendable forceps is inserted through the 5 o'clock channel. The bendable forceps is brought under the laparoscope toward the patient's right side and is curved back toward the target. This is the basic layout, which we use frequently. However, it is often necessary to adjust the layout whenever a significant conflict is anticipated or encountered.

19.3 Technique II: Endoluminal Approach

19.3.1 Indication

When the tumor is located at the esophagogastric junction and the dominant portion of the tumor is not outside the stomach, the endoluminal approach [2, 5] is indicated.

19.3.2 Setup

The setup described for Technique I is applied to Technique II.

19.3.3 Construction of a Temporary Gastrostomy

The navel is incised 2.5 cm longitudinally, and the abdominal cavity is entered as described for Technique I. When the approach site is cephalad to the navel, we prefer transverse skin incision. Through the parietal wound, the greater curve of the gastric angle is caught and pulled to the outside. The full-thickness gastric wall is incised approximately 2 cm in length. The edge of this opening is sutured to the skin around the wound at eight points so that a temporary gastrostomy is constructed (Fig. 19.7). Through this gastrostomy, the inner ring of the x-Gate® (Sumitomo Bakelite) is inserted into the stomach and fixed in the manner as described above. The stomach is insufflated to 8 mmHg with CO_2 gas.

19.3.4 BJ Needle® (Niti On Co.) Insertion

For the endoluminal procedure, we use BJ needle® (Niti On Co.) as an assistant forceps. Thus, BJ port® (Niti On Co.) is inserted by puncture into the gastric cavity. The puncture point is usually at the left upper quadrant.

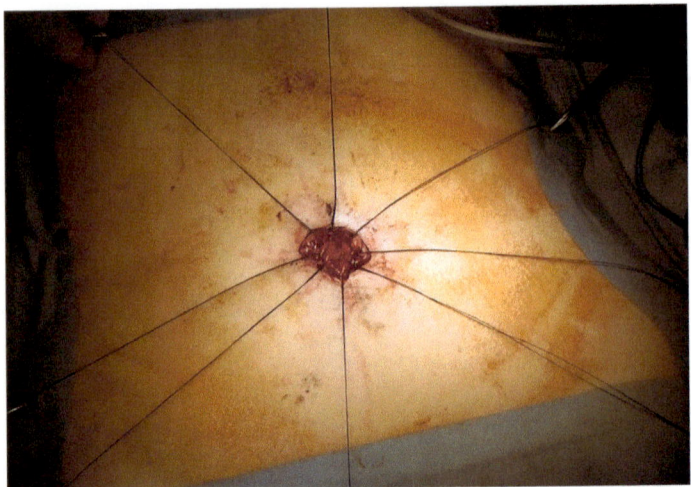

Fig. 19.7 A temporary gastrostomy (2 cm in diameter) is constructed in the lower gastric body for percutaneous entrance into the stomach

19.3.5 Resection

When the esophagogastric junction is seen from the lower gastric body by a rigid laparoscope, the tumor is well visualized (Fig. 19.8a). Through the x-Gate® channels (Sumitomo Bakelite), various instruments are inserted into the gastric cavity to facilitate resection and closure. The planned resection area is first marked by coagulation dots. The submucosa is then injected with normal saline via Pettit Needle® (Hakko Co., Nagano, Japan). This injection expands the space between the mucosa and the tumor surface and allows us to avoid unintended cuts to the tumor surface. The mucosa is cut with a high-frequency hook, tracing the coagulation dots marked around the tumor. BJ needle® (NitiOn Co.) is used to retract the tumor-containing tissue by grasping the overlying mucosa. The magnified endoscopic view makes it possible to distinguish the healthy muscularis propria from the neoplasm. Moreover, meticulous use of a high-frequency hook helps in judging whether the tissue is soft or tough and where to cut.

Usually, during resection, the gastric wall is perforated and the perigastric fat is recognized (Fig. 19.8b). However, in most cases, the insufflation is maintained. When the perforation is significant and the gastric cavity is collapsed, the perforation must be closed by suturing. When vessels are encountered, precoagulation should be performed before they are cut. Our standard method of hemostasis is to pinch the bleeder with a dissecting forceps and then apply a high frequency current for coagulation. The SonoSurg® energy device (Olympus) is our secondary option for this procedure, and it is selected when the tissue bleeds easily.

When the resection is completed, the tumor is enclosed in a retrieval bag and brought out through the x-Gate® (Sumitomo Bakelite).

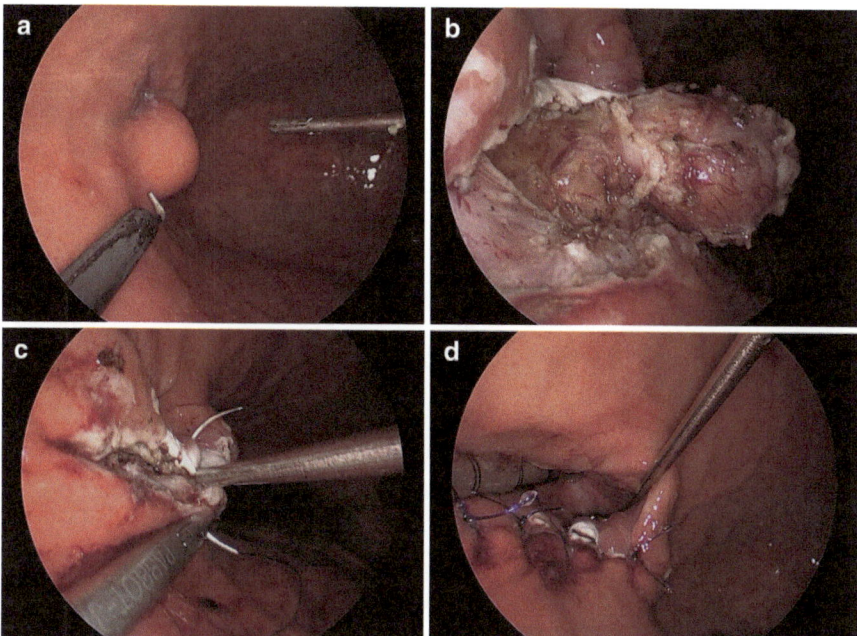

Fig. 19.8 (**a**) A submucosal tumor is located at the esophagogastric junction. A 2-mm grasper (BJ needle (Niti On Co.)) is inserted in the left subcostal margin, and a high-frequency hook and 5-mm laparoscope are inserted through the gastrostomy. (**b**) With the tumor excised almost in full thickness, the perigastric fat is recognized at the bottom of the defect. (**c**) The defect is closed by manual suturing with absorbable 3-0 monofilament material. The muscle layer of the esophagus and the stomach must be approximated to avoid postoperative regurgitation. (**d**) The closure line must be circumferential to avoid stenosis. Passage through the esophagogastric junction is preserved

19.3.6   Closure of the Defect

Closure of the defect when Technique II is applied is mandatory because the defect involves the full thickness of the gastric wall. Reconstruction of the muscularis propria has significant meaning from the standpoint of preventing gastro-esophageal reflux. Also, because the defect usually reaches the esophagus, the direction of the suture line must be considered to avoid possible stenosis. Thus, we always direct the suture line transversely (circumferentially around the esophagus). For this closure, we apply interrupted sutures with absorbable 3-0 monofilament thread using a 26-mm half-circle needle. Knot tying is very well facilitated with the assistance of BJ needle® (Niti On Co.) (Fig. 19.8c, d). When the closure is completed, peroral endoscopy is performed to make sure the junction is not stenotic.

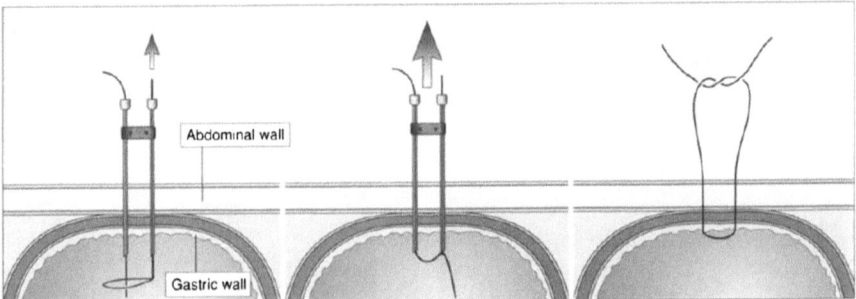

Fig. 19.9 Fixation of the gastric wall to the abdominal wall is facilitated by a Funada gastropexy instrument

19.3.7   Repair of the Gastrostomy

After the intragastric procedure, the x-Gate® (Sumitomo Bakelite) is removed. The gastrostomy sutures are freed from the skin, and the gastrotomy is closed with a continuous running suture of absorbable 3-0 thread. The tiny puncture wound in the upper gastric body made by the BJ port® (Niti On Co.) is left open. Generally, we do not use a drainage tube.

19.3.8   Tips and Tricks

19.3.8.1   Location of the Temporary Gastrostomy

Preoperative gastroscopy is performed to check whether the stomach can be stretched down to the navel. During this examination, the navel is pressed with a finger to see if the compression is recognized at the greater curvature of the lower gastric body. If so, the navel is chosen as the approach site. When the stomach does not reach the navel, the approach site must be amended accordingly in the cephalic direction.

19.3.8.2   Gastropexy

Prior to insertion of the BJ port® (Niti On Co.), we fix the anterior wall of the gastric wall to the abdominal wall by suturing it with the aid of the Funada Gastropexy Instrument® (Create Medic, Yokohama, Japan) (Fig. 19.9) [5]. This assures precise puncture into the gastric cavity and avoids slippage of the needle on the surface of the stomach. Moreover, even in cases in which the port is dislodged, re-puncture at the same point can be performed.

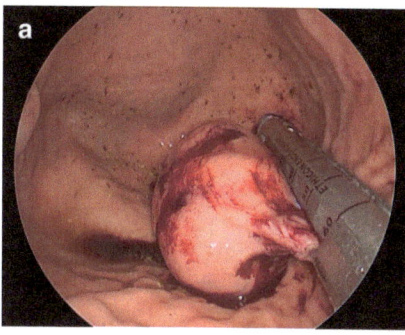 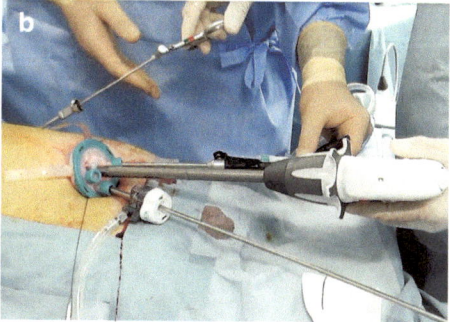

Fig. 19.10 (**a**) A submucosal tumor measuring 3 cm in diameter protruding into the gastric cavity is resected with a stapling device in single-incision endoscopic intragastric surgery. (**b**) One of the flexible x-Gate® channels (Sumitomo Bakelite) allows insertion of a 12-mm stapler

19.3.8.3 Stapler Resection

In limited cases, a stapler may be used to excise a tumor in the gastric cavity. This procedure is indicated when the tumor definitely protrudes into the gastric cavity and when it is located in the upper stomach away from the esophagogastric junction (Fig. 19.10). A tumor located in the upper body along the greater curvature at the fornix is the ideal indication for stapler resection. The x-Gate® channels (Sumitomo Bakelite) are flexible, and one of them can accommodate 12-mm instruments.

References

1. Takahashi T, Takeuchi H, Kawakubo H et al (2012) Single-incision laparoscopic surgery for partial gastrectomy in patients with a gastric submucosal tumor. Am Surg 78:447–450
2. Park JY, Eom BW, Yoon H et al (2012) Transumbilical single-incision laparoscopic wedge resection for gastric submucosal tumors: technical challenges encountered in initial experience. J Gastric Cancer 12:173–178
3. Sexton JA, Pierce RA, Halpin VJ et al (2008) Laparoscopic gastric resection for gastrointestinal stromal tumors. Surg Endosc 22:2583–2587
4. Lee CH, Hyun MH, Kwon YJ et al (2012) Deciding laparoscopic approaches for wedge resection in gastric submucosal tumors: a suggestive flow chart using three major determinants. J Am Coll Surg 215:831–840
5. Kanehira E, Omura K, Wakasa R et al (1998) A technique of percutaneous endoscopic intragastric surgery. Minim Invasive Ther Allied Technol 7:15–20
6. Kanehira E, Siozawa K, Kamei A et al (2012) Development of a novel multichannel port (x-Gate(®)) for reduced port surgery and its initial clinical results. Minim Invasive Ther Allied Technol 21:26–30
7. Shafi MA, Pasricha PJ (2007) Post-surgical and obstructive gastroparesis. Curr Gastroenterol Rep 9:280–285
8. Dong K, Yu XJ, Li B et al (2006) Advances in mechanisms of postsurgical gastroparesis syndrome and its diagnosis and treatment. Chin J Dig Dis 7:76–82
9. Schlager A, Khalaileh A, Shussman N et al (2010) Providing more through less: current methods of retraction in SIMIS and NOTES cholecystectomy. Surg Endosc 24:1542–1546

Chapter 20
Antireflux Procedures

Giovanni Dapri

Abstract In the last decade, a new philosophy to be less invasive in minimally invasive surgery and to perform laparoscopy without visible scars invested surgeons, researchers and companies. The purpose was basically the improved cosmesis, but the postoperative pain, the hospital stay, and the patient's convalescence were also attempted to be reduced.

Natural orifices transluminal endoscopic surgery (NOTES) and single-port/single-incision laparoscopy (SPL/SLS) were the two principal fields of researches and investments. Due to the difficulties to perform the conventional multiport laparoscopic procedures through NOTES and sometimes also through SPL/SLS, a new philosophy to keeping in mind the desire of less invesivity of minimally invasive surgery started to be popular and named reduced port laparoscopic surgery (RPLS). In RPLS, the classic multiport laparoscopic procedures can be performed in a similar method, but through a reduced number of trocars, a reduced size of each trocar and use of needlescopic instruments. Furthermore, some intrabdominal devices can be inserted in the abdomen and used like an assistant's help or to improve the operative field's exposure.

In this chapter two main antireflux procedures, Nissen fundoplication (360°) and Toupet fundoplication (270°), are described step by step using the transumbilical access, and curved reusable instruments. Each step is represented by specific drawings showing the internal triangulation, which characterizes the conventional multiport laparoscopy, and the external surgeon's ergonomy.

Keywords Fundoplication • Reduced port laparoscopy • Single-access • Single-incision • Single-port • Single-site

Giovanni Dapri (✉)
Department of Gastrointestinal Surgery, European School of
Laparoscopic Surgery, Saint-Pierre University Hospital, Brussels, Belgium
e-mail: giovanni@dapri.net

T. Mori and G. Dapri (eds.), *Reduced Port Laparoscopic Surgery*,
DOI 10.1007/978-4-431-54601-6_20, © Springer Japan 2014

20.1   Introduction

Reduced port laparoscopic surgery (RPLS) antireflux procedures are performed through the umbilicus as main access-site, which represents the embryonic natural orifice of the scarless surgery [1]. A patient's selection (body mass index, height, left liver lobe size) is required because the umbilicus sometimes is located too distally from the xyphoid process and hiatus. The left lobe of the liver may eclips the hiatus. An option to increase the exposure of the hiatal region is the insertion of the 1.8-mm trocarless grasping forceps according to DAPRI (Karl Storz-Endoskope, Tuttlingen, Germany), under the left liver lobe and against the diaphragm. Other possibilities described in literature are:

- the insertion of a classic 5-mm liver retractor [2],
- the insertion of a penrose drain in the triangular ligament [3],
- the fixation of a penrose drain to the abdominal wall by endohernia stapler [4] or by sutures [5],
- the placement of an expandable sponge under the left liver lobe [6],
- the use of cyanocrylate between the left liver lobe and the diaphragm [7],
- the anchoring of the bulldog to the falciform ligament [8],
- the use of the magnet forceps manoeuvred by external magnets [9],
- the insertion of the percutaneous transhepatic sutures [10] or superficial hepatic sutures [11, 12],
- the insertion of the percutaneous Cerrahpasa retractor [13],
- the insertion of the boxing glove retractor [14].

In this chapter two techniques of antireflux procedures by transumbilical access are described using a particular technique with a classic 11-mm trocar and DAPRI curved reusable instruments (Karl Storz-Endoskope) inserted in the umbilicus without trocars. This technique respects two basic rules of conventional multiport laparoscopy: the video screen, the operative field and the surgeon's head on the same axis [15], and the optical system in the middle as the bisector of the working triangulation formed by two ancillary effectors [16].

20.2   Technique

20.2.1   Patient and Team Positioning

The patient is placed in a supine position, with the arms along side the body and the legs apart. The surgeon stands between the patient's legs, and the camera assistant to the patient's right. The scrub-nurse stands to the patient's left. The video monitor is placed in front of the surgeon and camera assistant (Fig. 20.1).

Fig. 20.1 Patient and team positioning

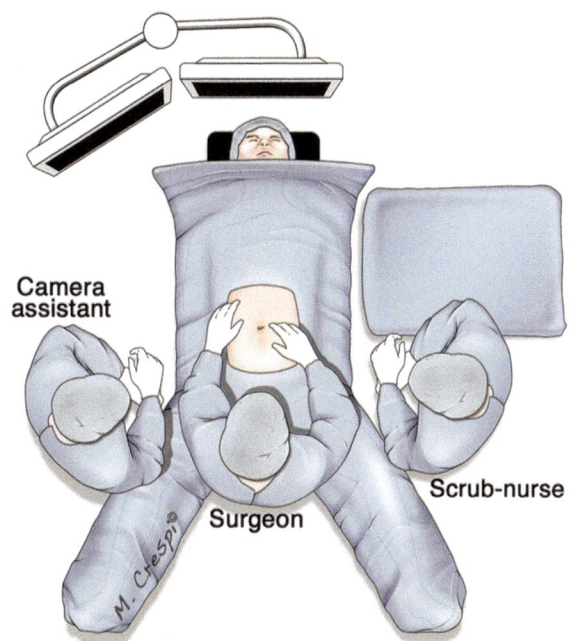

20.2.2   Beginning of RPLS

The umbilicus is incised (Fig. 20.2), and the fascia opened until to reach the peritoneum, which is opened as well. A purse-string suture using PDS 1 is placed in full-thickness method in the umbilical fascia and peritoneum at 2, 4, 6, 8, 10, 12 o'clock positions (Fig. 20.3). An 11-mm reusable metallic trocar is introduced into the peritoneal cavity inside the purse-string suture, and the pneumoperitoneum is created (Fig. 20.4). A 10-mm, 30° rigid and standard length scope (Karl Storz-Endoskope) is advanced through the 11-mm trocar, and curved reusable instruments according to DAPRI (Karl Storz-Endoskope) are inserted into the abdomen through the umbilical scar without trocars. The bicurved grasping forceps III (Fig. 20.5) is inserted through a separate fascia window, created by a sharp obturator of 5-mm trocar, at some of 5 mm outside the purse-string suture at 10 o'clock position in the respect of the patient head (Fig. 20.6). The other instruments like the monocurved coagulating hook (Fig. 20.7a), the monocurved scissors (Fig. 20.7b), the monocurved bipolar grasping forceps and scissors (Fig. 20.7c, d), the bicurved needle holder II (Fig. 20.7e), the monocurved suction and irrigation cannula, the straight 5-mm clip applier, and the straight 5-mm grasping forceps are introduced on the other side of the bicurved grasping forceps III at 3 o'clock position, parallel to the 11-mm trocar and inside the purse-string suture (Fig. 20.8). The suture is adjusted to maintain a tight seal around the 5-mm tools and the 11-mm trocar, and open only for the change of the instruments and evacuation of the smoke created with the dissection. The operative table is positioned in a reversed Trendelenburg position.

Fig. 20.2 Transumbilical access: incision of the original umbilical scar

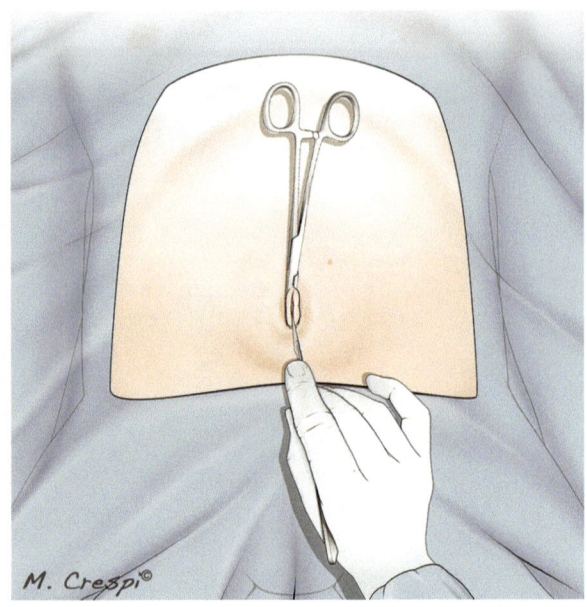

Fig. 20.3 Transumbilical access: placement of the purse-string suture (PDS 1) in the umbilical fascia and peritoneum at 2, 4, 6, 8, 10, 12 o'clock positions

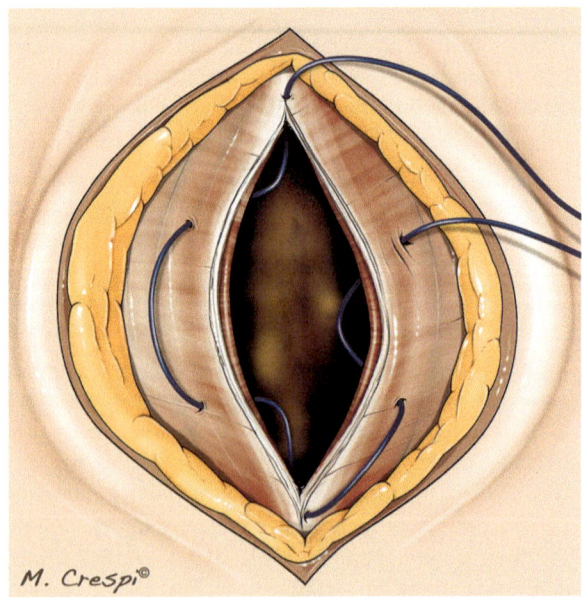

Fig. 20.4 Transumbilical access: insertion of the 11-mm reusable metallic trocar

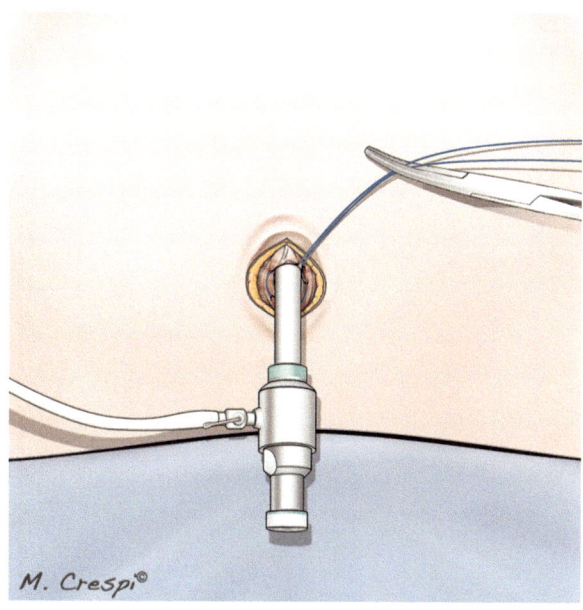

Fig. 20.5 Bicurved reusable grasping forceps III according to DAPRI (Karl Storz-Endoskope)

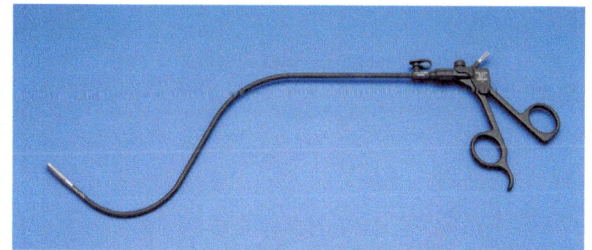

Fig. 20.6 Transumbilical access: insertion of the grasping forceps III through a separate fascia window at some of 5 mm outside the purse-string suture at 10 o'clock position

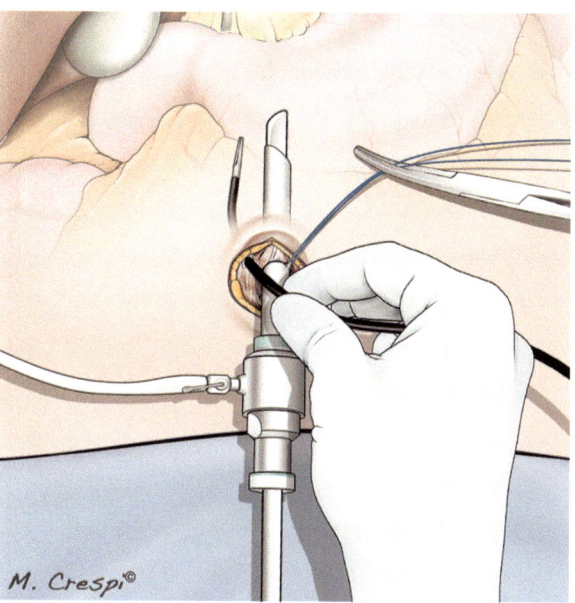

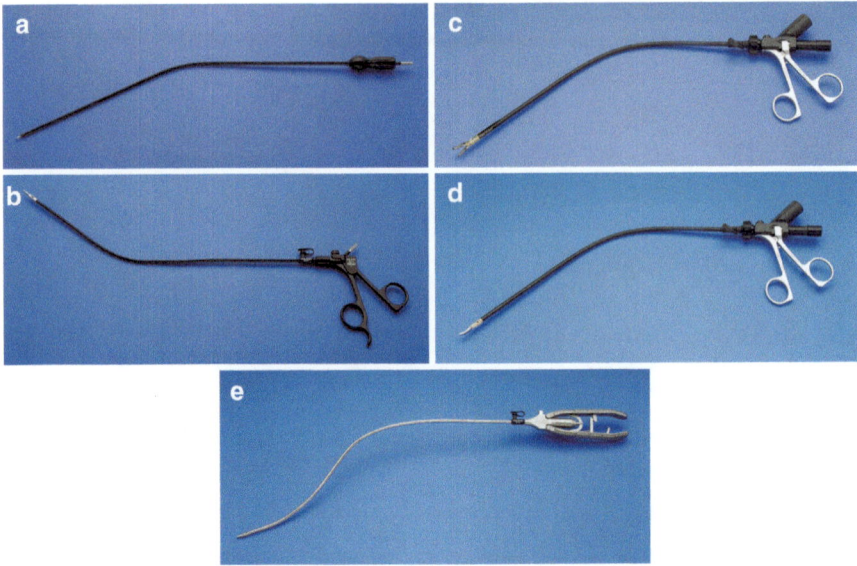

Fig. 20.7 Other curved reusable instruments according to DAPRI (Karl Storz-Endoskope): mono-curved coagulating hook (**a**), monocurved scissors (**b**), monocurved bipolar grasping forceps (**c**), monocurved bipolar scissors (**d**), bicurved needle holder II (**e**)

Fig. 20.8 Transumbilical access: insertion of the other curved instruments at 3 o'clock position, parallel to the 11-mm trocar and inside the purse-string suture

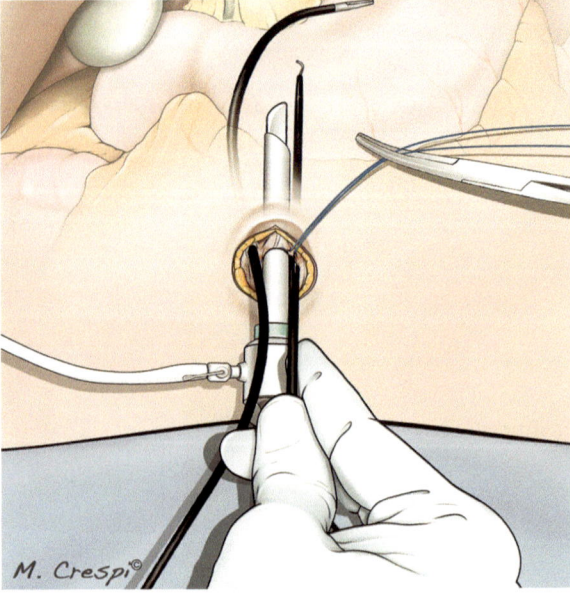

Fig. 20.9 Use of the distal curve of the bicurved grasping forceps III to retract the left liver lobe and to contemporary expose the opening of the hepatogastric ligament (**a**), without any conflict between the surgeons' hands (**b**)

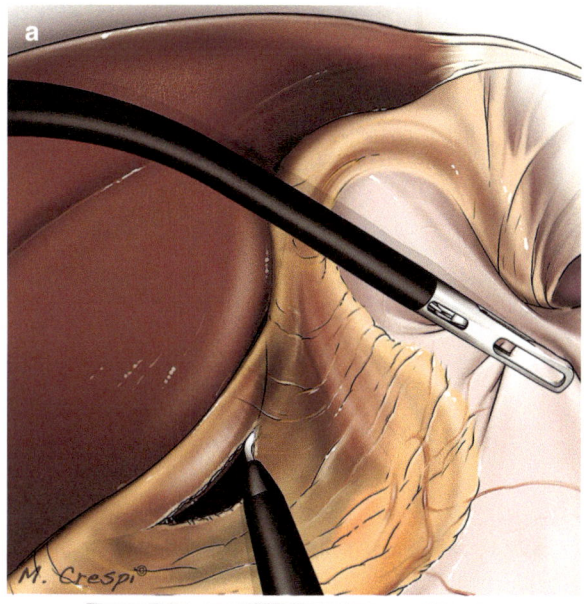

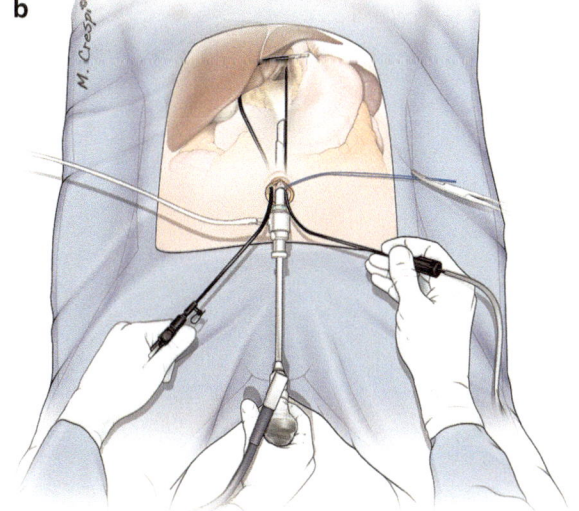

The distal curve of the bicurved grasping forceps III is used to retract the left liver lobe and to contemporary expose the opening of the hepatogastric ligament on the lesser curvature (Fig. 20.9a, b). Thanks to the peculiar shape of the instruments, the scope never appeared in conflict with the instruments' tips, and the conflict between the surgeon's hands and the scope is avoided.

If an insufficient exposure of the hiatal region is evidenced, the DAPRI 1.8-mm trocarless grasping forceps (Fig. 20.10) is inserted percutaneously under the xyphoid

Fig. 20.10 1.8-mm trocarless grasping forceps according to DAPRI (Karl Storz-Endoskope)

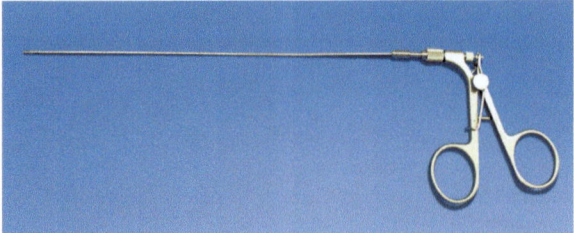

Fig. 20.11 Placement of the DAPRI 1.8-mm trocarless grasping forceps percutaneously under the xyphoid access

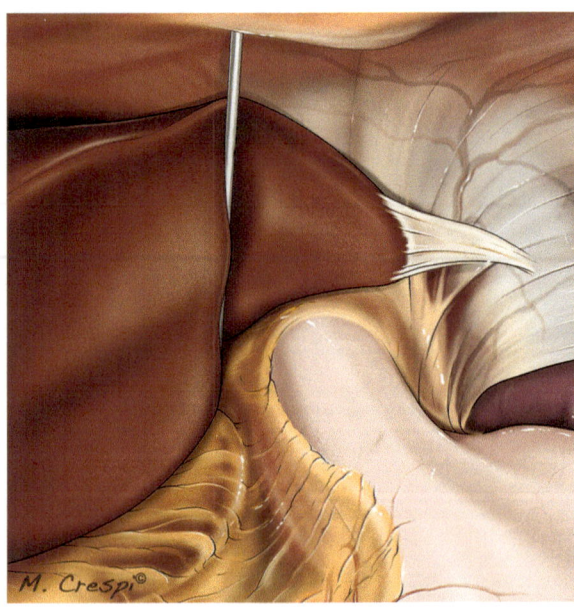

access, through a skin puncture created by a Veress needle (Fig. 20.11). This grasper is placed under the left liver lobe and against the diaphragm.

The hepatogastric ligament is opened close to the liver segment 1, and the right phrenogastric ligament is incised as well (Fig. 20.12), dividing its anterior and posterior sheets. The right crus is freed from bottom to top (Fig. 20.13). The left

Fig. 20.12 Incision of the
right phrenogastric ligament
using the coagulating hook

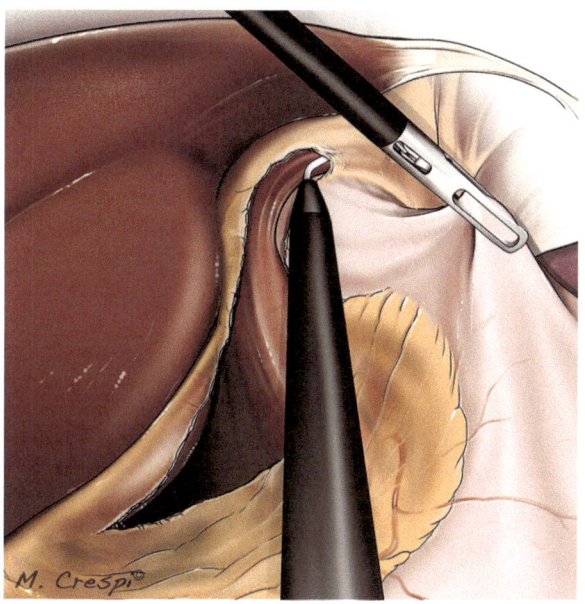

Fig. 20.13 Skeletonization
of the right crus using the
coagulating hook from
bottom to top

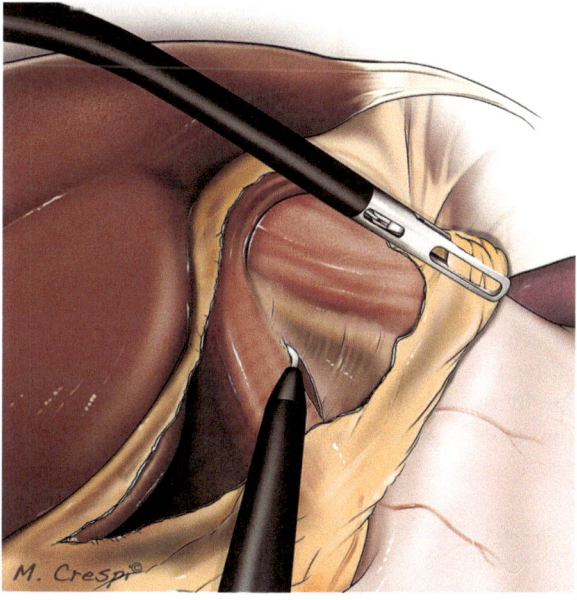

phrenogastric ligament is incised (Fig. 20.14), and the left crus is exposed. The
lower esophagus is freed, encircled and suspended by a piece of cotton tape using
the bicurved grasping forceps III (Fig. 20.15a, b). Thanks to this maneuver, both
crura under the esophagus are better exposed and more easily freed (Fig. 20.16).

Fig. 20.14 Incision of the left phrenogastric ligament using the coagulating hook

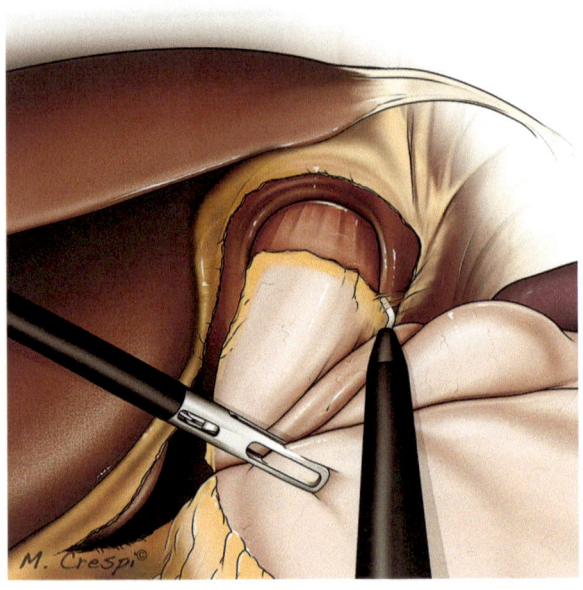

The operative table is maintained in a reversed Trendelenburg position with right-sided tilt, permitting an increased exposure of the splenic region. The gastrosplenic ligament is incised starting from the previous dissection of the left phrenogastric ligament, until to control the first short gastric vessel (Fig. 20.17). Then, the operative table is replaced without any tilt and maintaining the Trendelenburg position, in order to move the upper part of the gastric fundus behind the lower esophagus. The other short gastric vessels are just dissected "à la demand" giving a more slack to the wrap (Fig. 20.18a, b), using the monocurved coagulating hook or the monocurved bipolar grasping forceps and scissors.

Figure of eight sutures using silk 2/0 are used to close the crura (Fig. 20.19), using intracorporeal sutures and knotting technique (Fig. 20.20). This maneuver is performed without the orogastric bougie in place. Only after cruraplasty, the anesthesiologist pushes down a 34 French orogastric bougie.

20.2.2.1 Nissen Fundoplication

The floppy 360° fundoplication is performed by silk 2/0 sutures, using intracorporeal sutures and knotting technique, under ergonomic position, without clashing of the instruments' tips (Fig. 20.21). A gastro-gastric suture, a gastro-eso-gastrique suture (Fig. 20.22), and two gastro-esophageal sutures inferiorly to the first previous and on both sides of the lower esophagus (Fig. 20.23) are performed (Fig. 20.24).

Fig. 20.15 Suspension of the lower esophagus by a piece of cotton tape (**a**) using the bicurved grasping forceps III and the straight 5-mm grasping forceps (**b**)

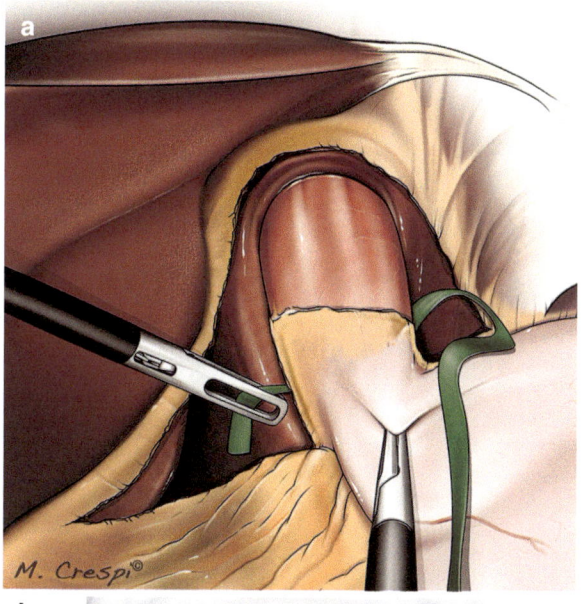

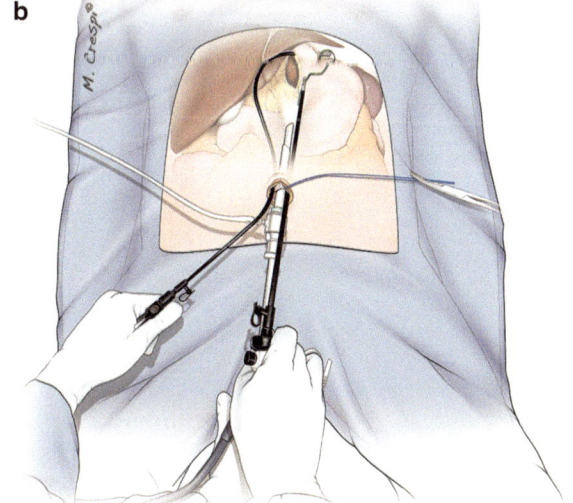

20.2.2.2 Toupet Fundoplication

The 270° fundoplication is performed by silk 2/0 sutures. The right side of the wrap is fixed by four simple sutures to the right crura (Fig. 20.25), starting with the first suture at the apex of the right crura. Then, the right side of the wrap is anchored to

Fig. 20.16 Easier
mobilization of both crura
thanks to the cotton tape's
tension

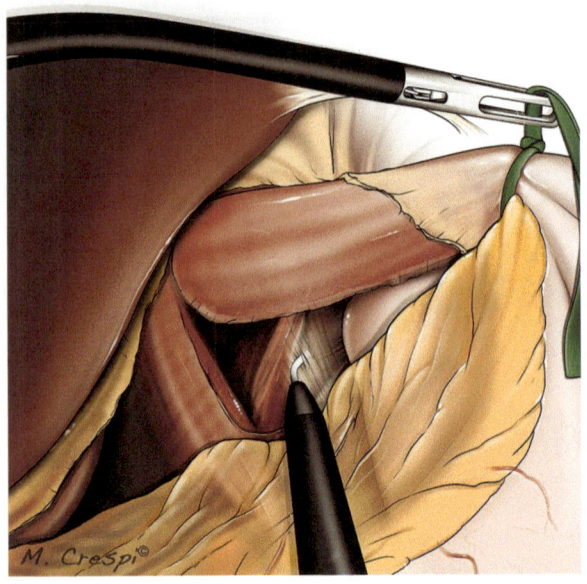

Fig. 20.17 Incision of the
gastrosplenic ligament from
the left phrenogastric
ligament until to the first
short gastric vessel

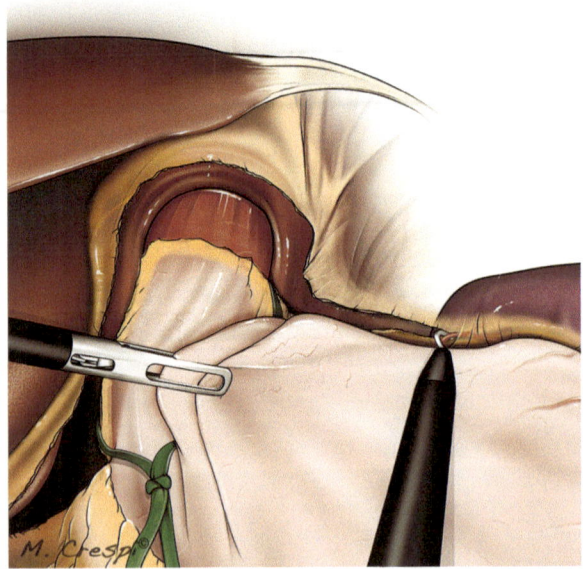

the lower esophagus by three other simple sutures (Fig. 20.26). As well, the left side
of the wrap is fixed to the left crura by two simple sutures (Fig. 20.27), and then the
left side of the wrap is anchored to the lower esophagus by three other simple sutures
(Fig. 20.28).

Fig. 20.18 Dissection of the other short gastric vessels just "à la demand" (**a**) with a medial-to-lateral approach (**b**)

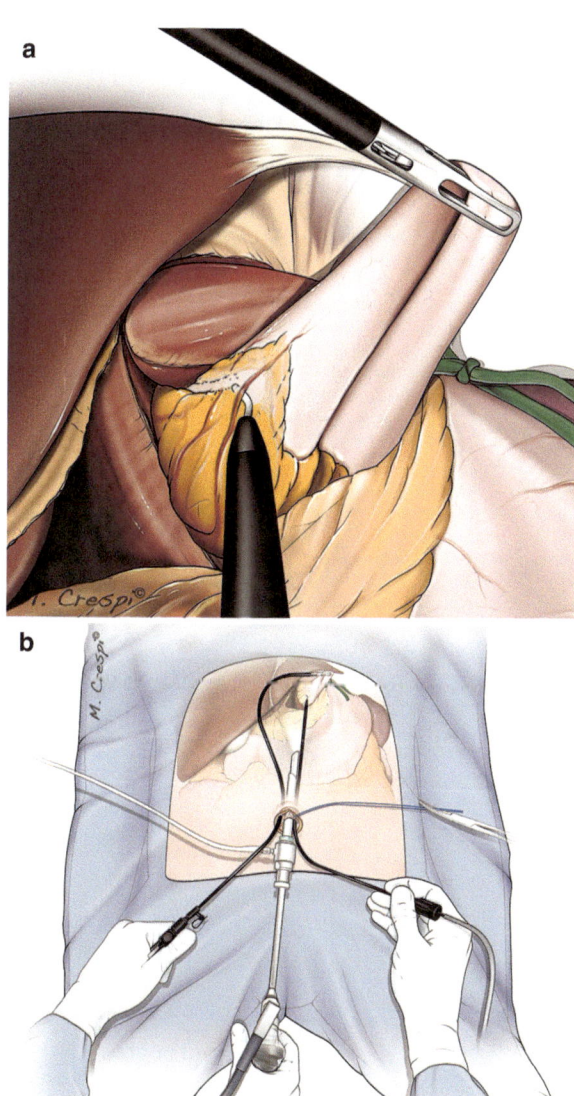

20.2.2.3   End of RPLS

At the end of the procedure, the operative table is replaced like in the beginning of the procedure, without any Trendelenburg position and tilt. The orogastric bougie, the piece of cotton tape, the sutures and all the instruments are removed under view. The curved instruments are retrieved following their curves at 45° in the respect of the abdominal wall.

Fig. 20.19 Closure of the
crura using silk 2/0
intracorporeal sutures and
knotting technique

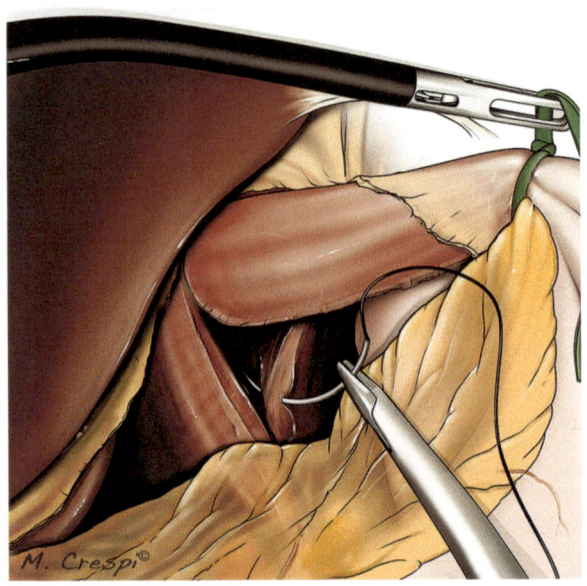

Fig. 20.20 Final aspect of
the closed crura using figure
of eight sutures

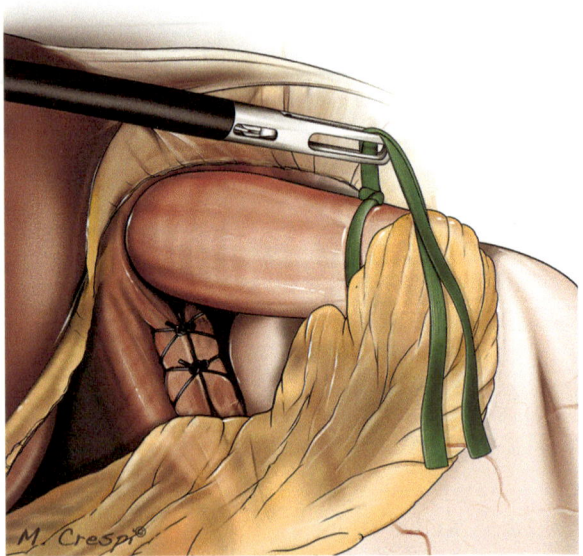

After having removed the 11-mm trocar for the scope, Vicryl 1 sutures are placed
as figure of eight to close the umbilical fascia, including the separate fascia opening
for the bicurved grasper III (Fig. 20.29). The cutaneous scar is closed by intradermal
sutures (Fig. 20.30).

Fig. 20.21 Nissen
fundoplication: intracorporeal
sutures and knotting
technique, under ergonomic
position and without
instruments' tips clashing

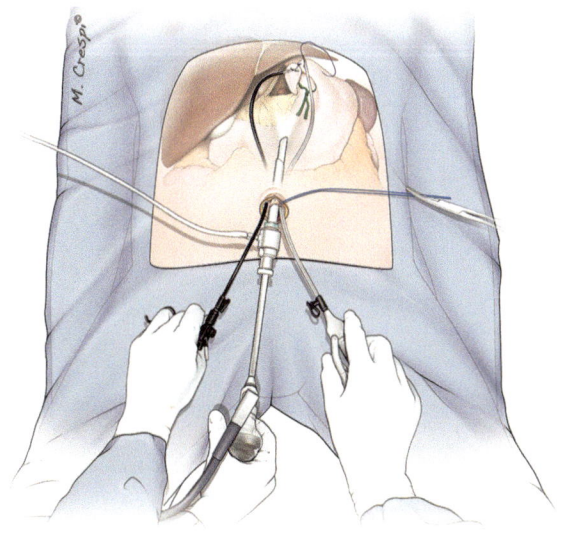

Fig. 20.22 Nissen
fundoplication:
gastro-eso-gastrique
suture using silk 2/0

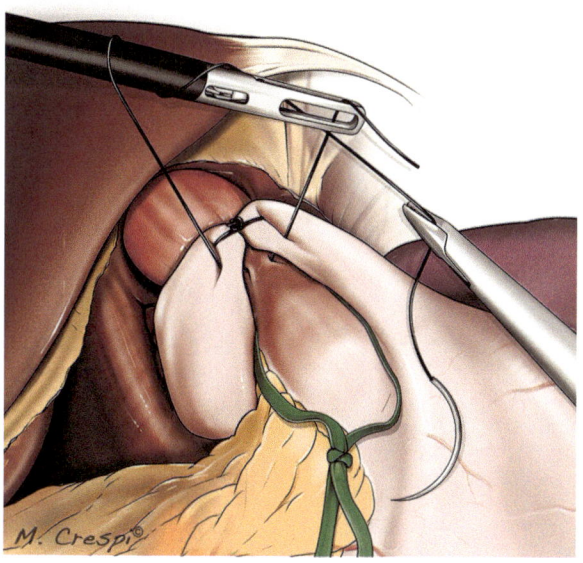

Fig. 20.23 Nissen
fundoplication: gastro-
esophageal suture inferiorly
to the first previous and on
the left side of the lower
esophagus

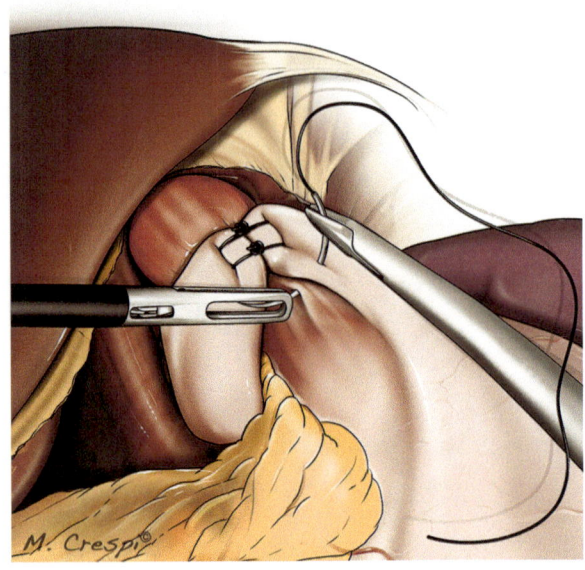

Fig. 20.24 Nissen
fundoplication: gastro-
esophageal suture inferiorly
to the first previous and on
the right side of the lower
esophagus

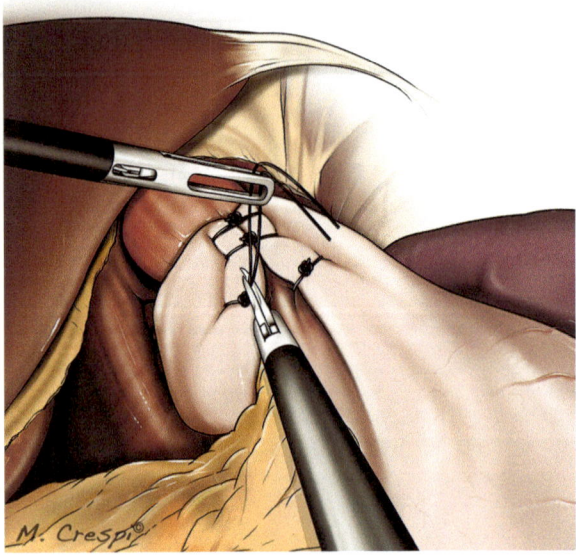

Fig. 20.25 Toupet
fundoplication: the right
side of the wrap is fixed to
the right crura by four simple
silk 2/0 sutures

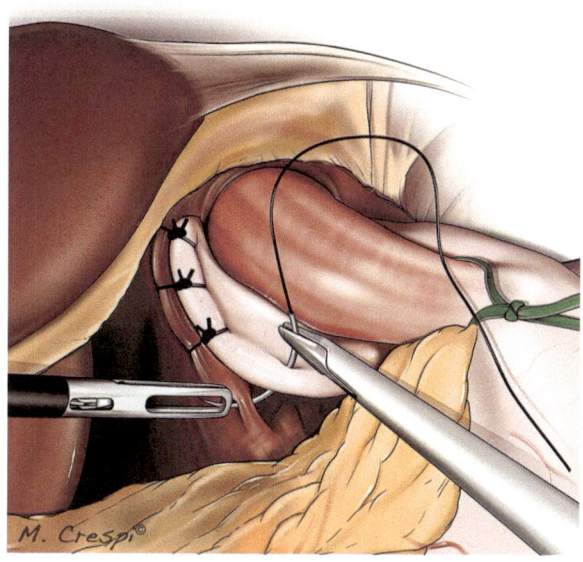

Fig. 20.26 Toupet
fundoplication: the right side
of the wrap is fixed to the
lower esophagus by three
simple silk 2/0 sutures

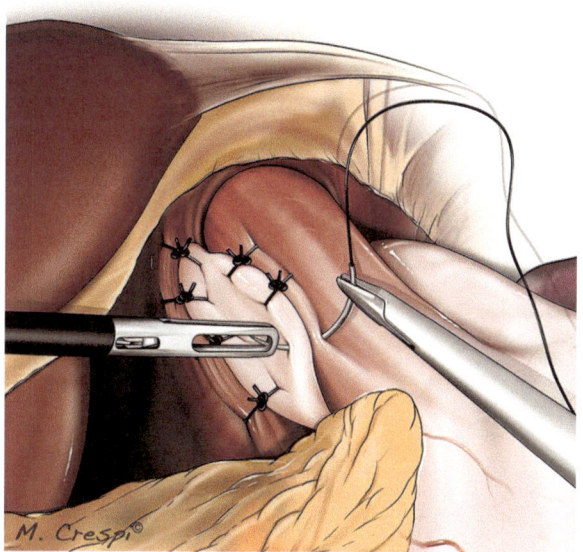

Fig. 20.27 Toupet
fundoplication: the left side
of the wrap is fixed to the left
crura by two simple silk 2/0
sutures

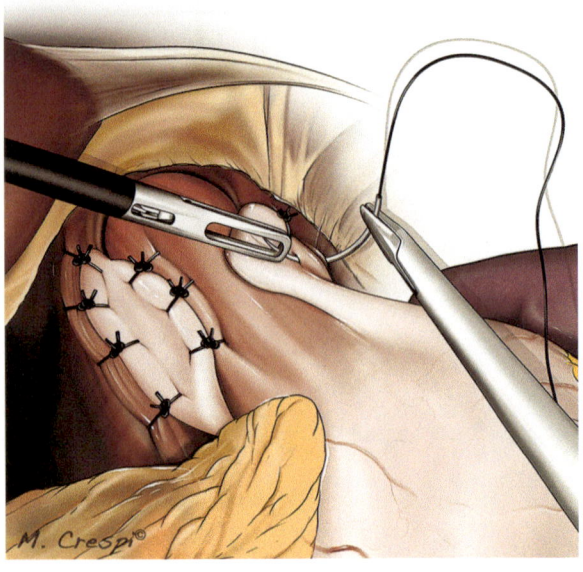

Fig. 20.28 Toupet
fundoplication: the left side
of the wrap is fixed to the
lower esophagus by three
simple silk 2/0 sutures

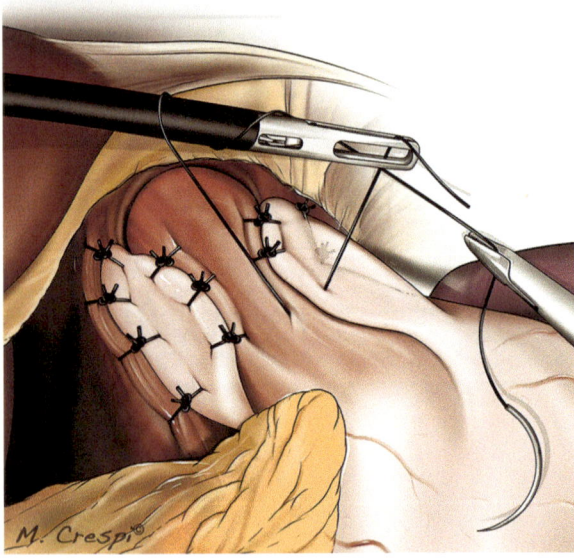

Fig. 20.29 Closure of the
umbilical access including
the separate fascia opening
(used for the bicurved
grasper III) by figure
of eight Vicryl 1 sutures

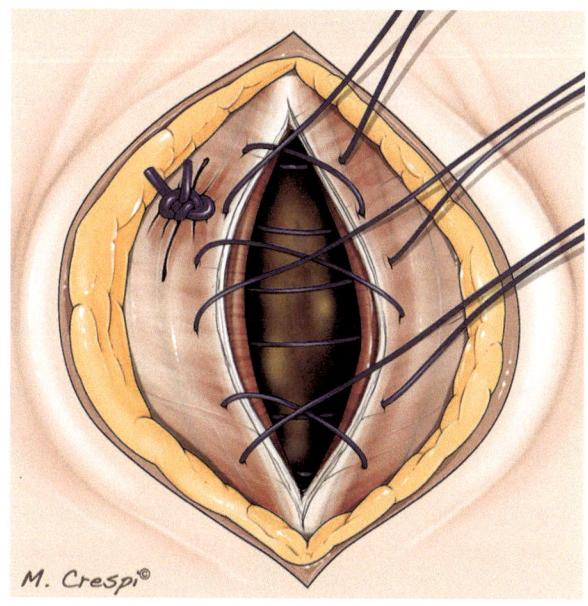

Fig. 20.30 Transumbilical
access: final aspect

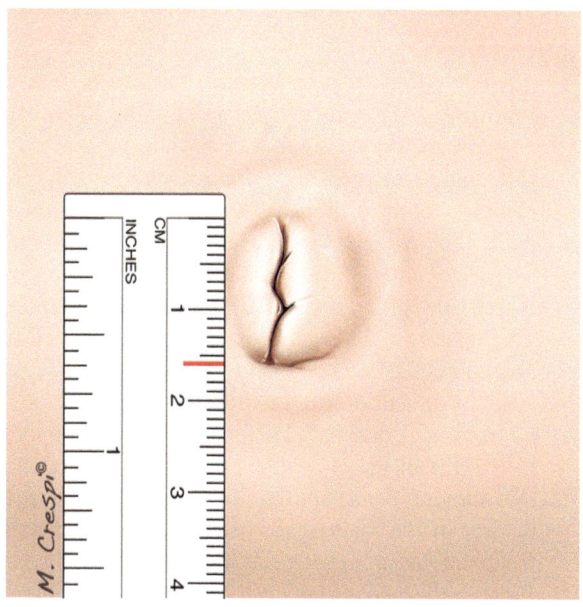

20.2.3 Post-operative Care

One gram paracetamol is given i.v. at the end of the surgical procedure. Postoperative analgesia is given following the WHO visual analog pain scale (VAS). In the recovery room the following scheme is followed: for VAS between 1 and 3, 1 g paracetamol i.v. is pushed; for VAS between 4 and 8, 100 mg tramadol i.v. is used; for VAS > 8, 1 mg piritamide i.v. is incremented.

After the patient left the recovery room, pain is assessed every 6 h, with 1 g paracetamol administered i.v. if VAS is between 1 and 3, 100 mg tramadol administered i.v. if VAS is between 4 and 8, and 1 mg piritamide administered i.v. if VAS > 8.

A gastrograffin swallow check is scheduled on the first postoperative day, and if negative the patient is allowed to drink water, and after 24 h to tolerate a light diet. If there are no complications, the patient is discharged on the second postoperative day.

Upon discharge, 1 g paracetamol perorally or 50 mg tramadol perorally are prescribed only if needed.

Office visits are scheduled at 10 days, 1, 3, 6, 12 months after the procedure. The barium swallow checks are performed at 6 and 12 months.

20.3   Recommendations from the Author

– The curved reusable instruments have to be inserted into the abdominal cavity following a 45° angle in the respect of the abdominal wall. Their removal have to be performed in the same way as well.
– If the hiatal region is not sufficiently exposed by the distal curve of the bicurved grasping forceps III, some other options are available and useful to improve the field.
– The use of a piece of cotton tape to encircle the gastroesophageal junction, helps in exposing the right and left crus and in performing the cruraplasty.
– The operative table has to be used as an assistant's help during the entire procedure.
– After having sectioned the first short gastric vessels, the rest of the fundus has to be freed "à la demand" by a medial-to-lateral approach.
– Use of the bicurved needle holder II helps in minimizing the movement during the intracorporeal sutures. The instrument's tip has a 45° orientation in the respect of the main shaft, hence only a 15° rotation of the surgeon's wrist is needed to insert and remove the needle from the tissue.
– Finally, the choice between the two fundoplications mainly comes from the results of the patient's preoperative work-up.

References

1. Remzi FH, Kirat HT, Kaouk JH, Geisler DP (2008) Single-port laparoscopy in colorectal surgery. Colorectal Dis 10:823–826
2. Ross S, Roddenbery A, Luberice K et al (2013) Laparoendoscopic single site (LESS) vs. conventional laparoscopic fundoplication for GERD: is there a difference? Surg Endosc 27:538–547
3. Hamzaoglu I, Karahasanoglu T, Aytac E, Karatas A, Baca B (2010) Tranumbilical totally laparoscopic single-port Nissen fundoplication: a new method of liver retraction: the Istanbul technique. J Gastrointest Surg 14:1035–1039
4. Huang CK, Lo CH, Asim S, Houng JY, Huang SF (2011) A novel technique for liver retraction in laparoscopic bariatric surgery. Obes Surg 21:676–679
5. Yano F, Omura N, Tsuboi K et al (2012) Single-incision laparoscopic Heller myotomy and Dor fundoplication for achalasia: report of a case. Surg Today 42:299–302
6. Takahashi T, Takeuchi H, Kawakubo H, Saikawa Y, Wada N, Kitagawa Y (2012) Single-incision laparoscopic surgery for partial gastrectomy in patients with a gastric submucosal tumor. Am Surg 78:447–450
7. Fan Y, Wu SD, Kong J, Su Y, Tian Y (2013) Transumbilical single-incision laparoscopic fundoplication: a new technique for liver retracion using cyanoacrylate. J Laparoendosc Adv Surg Tech A 23:1–5
8. Galvani CA, Gallo AS, Gorodner MV (2012) Single-incision and dual-incision laparoscopic adjustable gastric band: evaluation of initial experience. Surg Obes Relat Dis 8:194–200
9. Morales Conde S, Dominguez G, Cañete Gomez J et al (2013) Magnetic-assisted single-port sleeve gastrectomy. Surg Innov 20:NP9–NP11
10. Huang CK (2011) Single-incision laparoscopic bariatric surgery. J Minim Access Surg 7:999–1003
11. Nakajima J, Sasaki A, Obuchi T, Baba S, Umemura A, Wakabayashi G (2011) Single-incision laparoscopic Heller myotomy and Dor fundoplication for achalasia: report of a case. Surg Today 41:1543–1547
12. Yilmaz H, Alptekin H (2012) Single-port laparoscopic Nissen fundoplication: a new method for retraction of the left lobe of the liver. Surg Laparosc Endosc Percutan Tech 22:e265–e266
13. Eyuboglu E, Ipek T, Atasoy D (2012) Single-port laparoscopic floppy Nissen fundoplication: a novel technique with the aid of the Cerrahpasa retractor. J Laparoendosc Adv Surg Tech A 22:173–175
14. Omori T, Oyama T, Akamatsu H, Tori M, Ueshima S, Nishida T (2011) Transumbilical single-incision laparoscopic distal gastrectomy for early gastric cancer. Surg Endosc 25:2400–2404
15. Hanna GB, Shimi SM, Cuschieri A (1998) Task performance in endoscopic surgery is influenced by location of the image display. Ann Surg 227:481–484
16. Hanna G, Drew T, Clinch P, Hunter B, Cuschieri A (1998) Computer-controlled endoscopic performance assessment system. Surg Endosc 12:997–1000

Chapter 21
Hepatectomy

Minoru Tanabe

Abstract Thanks to the recent advances in multiport laparoscopic liver resection and the development of single-port access surgery (SPAS), several groups have reported the feasibility of SPA hepatectomy. Moreover, the SPA hepatectomy instruments and the technique are applicable to conventional laparoscopic hepatectomy, allowing a reduction in the number and size of the ports. In this chapter, we present our SPA and reduced-port laparoscopic hepatectomy methods and discuss the feasibility of the SPA approach as well as its potential benefits and limitations.

Keywords Liver resection • Reduced port surgery • Single-port surgery

21.1 Introduction to Single-Port Access (SPA) Hepatectomy

Single-port access surgery (SPAS) is of growing interest in the effort to minimize abdominal wall trauma. SPAS provides a desirable cosmetic effect because the surgical scar is hidden in the umbilical orifice. Beyond the cosmetic advantage, the other benefits of SPAS remain to be elucidated, but they may include reduced morbidity and postoperative pain, relatively short hospital stay, and speedy recovery. Various abdominal surgeries have already been performed by SPAS, including appendectomy [1], cholecystectomy [2], splenectomy [3], sleeve gastrectomy [4], colectomy [5], and ventral hernia [6].

M. Tanabe (✉)
Department of Hepatobiliary and Pancreatic Surgery, Tokyo Medical and Dental University, 1-5-45 Yushima, Bunkyo-ku, Tokyo 113-8510, Japan
e-mail: tana.msrg@tmd.ac.jp

T. Mori and G. Dapri (eds.), *Reduced Port Laparoscopic Surgery*, DOI 10.1007/978-4-431-54601-6_21, © Springer Japan 2014

Since the first report of laparoscopic partial hepatectomy in 1992 [7], laparoscopic liver resection has become an accepted procedure for treatment of liver tumors. The current international position on laparoscopic liver surgery as expressed in the Louisville Statement (8), is that the procedure is "a safe and effective approach for the management of surgical liver disease in the hands of trained surgeons with experience in hepatobiliary and laparoscopic surgery." Thanks to the recent advances in multiport laparoscopic liver resection and the development of SPAS, several groups have reported the feasibility of SPAS hepatectomy [9–24]. Moreover, the instruments and techniques are applicable to conventional laparoscopic hepatectomy, allowing the number and size of the port. In this chapter, we present our hepatectomy techniques based on SPAS and reduced port surgery (RPS) and discuss the feasibility of this approach as well as its potential benefits and limitations, particularly in comparison to conventional multiport laparoscopic hepatectomy.

21.2 Indications and Contraindications for SPA Hepatectomy

The superior and dorsal parts of the right hepatic lobe are beyond the reach of the umbilical port instruments, suggesting that resection of these parts is contraindicated. Tumors located in the anterolateral segment of the liver (Fig. 21.1). Hepatectomy of the entire left lateral segment r a part of this segment is particularly suited to the SPA approach because this part of the liver is not thick and the transection line can be adjusted easily in line with the axis of the umbilical trocar by mobilizing the liver. In addition, the resected specimen should not exceed 6–7 cm in size. A larger specimen may require extension of the umbilical incision for extraction. The lateral segment represents the upper limit in terms of the size, of a specimen that can be extracted from a small umbilical incision without marked deformity of the navel.

21.3 Procedural Techniques

21.3.1 Position of the Patient and Layout of the Instruments

The patient, under general anesthesia, is placed supine with the legs apart. The operator stands between the patient's legs. If the tumor is located on the patient's left side, the assistant holding the scope stands at the patient's right side, and vice versa (Fig. 21.2).

Fig. 21.1 Indications for SPAS hepatectomy. A good indication for SPAS hepatectomy is a tumor located in the anterolateral segment of the liver. In addition, the resected specimen should not exceed 6-7 cm in size

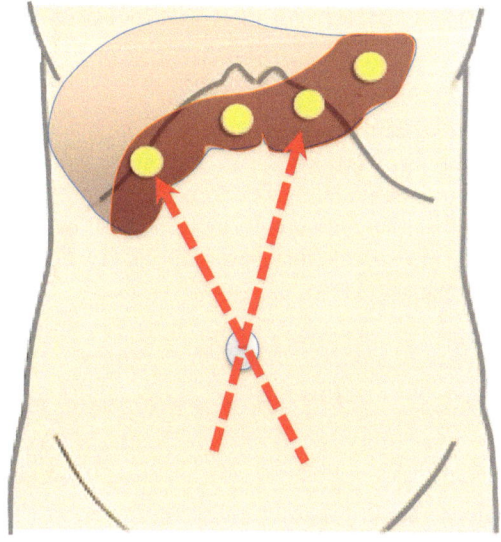

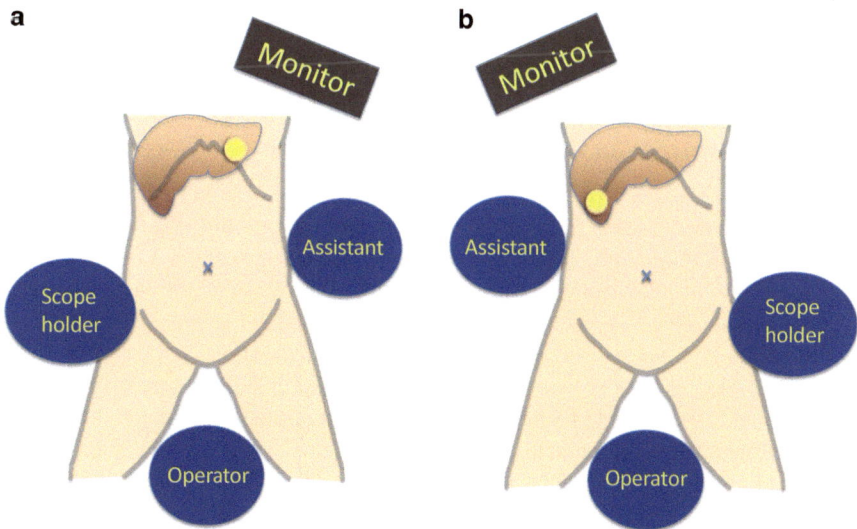

Fig. 21.2 Position of the patient and layout of the instruments for SPA hepatectomy

21.3.2   Insertion of a Multi-Access Port and Establishment of Pneumoperitoneum

A multi-access port is inserted through a 25-mm longitudinal incision made at the umbilicus. The port is fixed so that the working channels form an inverted triangle. Pneumoperitoneum is established at 8 mmHg. Upon transection of the liver parenchyma, the pressure is increased to 13 mmHg to suppress venous bleeding. A 5-mm deflectable laparoscope and two instruments are inserted through the port channels.

21.3.3   Mobilization of the Liver

Under cross-placement of the devices, an ultrasonic scalpel (SonoSurg™, Olympus Corporation, Tokyo, Japan or Harmonic ACE™, Ethicon Endosurgery, Cincinnati, OH, USA) is used to mobilize the liver (Fig. 21.3a). It is usually possible to cut the falciform ligament, left coronary ligament, and bilateral triangular ligament by means of dissecting devices inserted through the umbilical port. Extended mobilization of the right lobe is not possible in SPAS hepatectomy because the instruments inserted through the umbilical port cannot reach the superior and dorsal parts of the right lobe.

21.3.4   Transection of the Liver Parenchyma

Intra-operative ultrasonography must be performed to determine the tumor location and the transection line. If the tumor is located at the edge of the liver, pre-coagulation will allow for bloodless transection with scissors and without energy devices. Generally, the pre-coagulation is performed along the intended line of transection with articulating microwave ablation instruments (Fig. 21.4).

hen a bulky part of the liver is transected, a more subtle technique is used. As in conventional laparoscopic hepatectomy, transection of the liver parenchyma in SPA hepatectomy can be done with an ultrasonic scalpel [17, 22] and the Cavitron Ultrasonic Surgical Aspirator (CUSA EXcel, ValleyLab, Inc., Boulder, CO, USA) [20] (Fig. 21.5). The superficial part of the liver can be cut with an ultrasonic scalpel (Fig. 21.3b), as there are no large vessels in this part. In contrast, in the deeper part of the liver, isolation of the vessels with the CUSA and meticulous hemostasis achieved with energy devices is necessary (Fig. 21.3c, d). We usually use a biclamp for hemostasis with a saline drip from an additional needle device inserted directly from the upper abdominal quadrant.

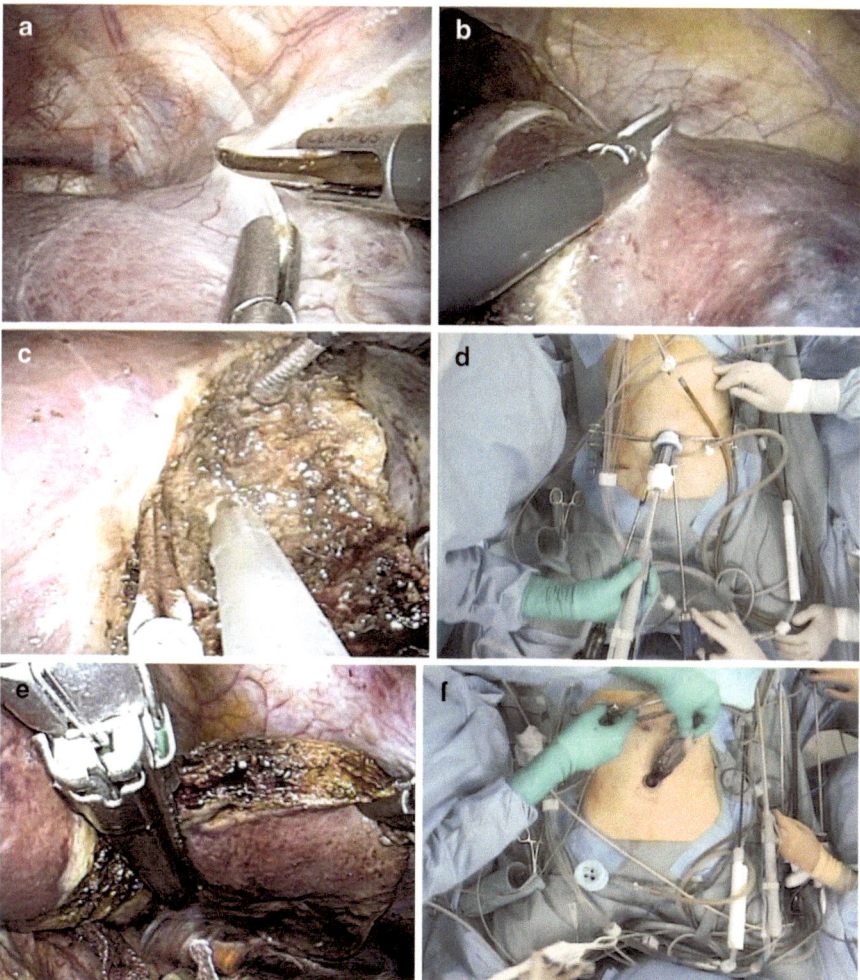

Fig. 21.3 SPAS lateral segmentectomy. (**a**) The falciform ligament is cut with an ultrasonic scalpel to mobilize the liver. (**b**) The superficial part of the liver can be cut with an ultrasonic scalpel. (**c**, **d**) We usually use CUSA Excel and BiClamp for transection of the deep part of the liver. (**e**) Large vascular pedicles are divided with a laparoscopic stapler. (**f**) The specimen is extracted transumbilically

21.3.5 Hemostasis

Hemostasis is technically difficult in laparoscopic liver resection, making uncontrollable bleeding the main reason for conversion to laparotomy. In SPAS hepatectomy in particular, special attention must be paid to parenchymal transection. Thanks to recent innovations in the energy devices, laparoscopic transection of the liver parenchyma is now relatively safe. Low-voltage coagulation devices are useful for

Fig. 21.4 Pre-coagulation performed with articulating microwave ablation instruments

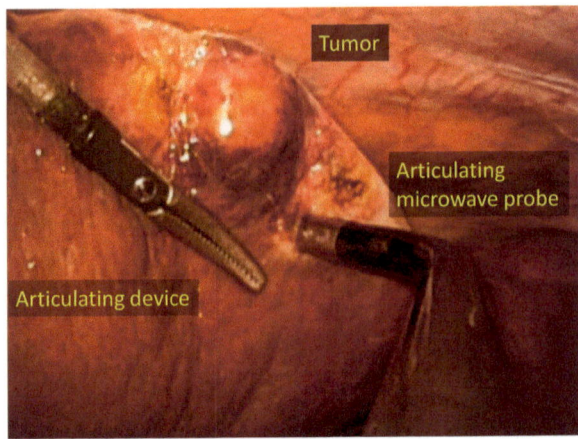

Fig. 21.5 Cavitron Ultrasonic Surgical Aspirator (CUSA Excel Plus, Integra Lifesciences). A handpiece for both laparoscopic and open laparotomy procedures is available

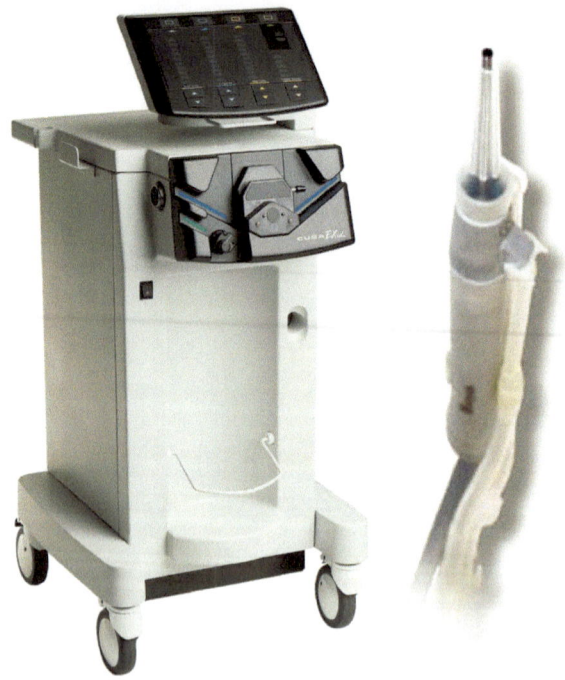

controlling bleeding during parenchymal transection [21]. The VIO electrosurgical unit (Erbe Elektromedizin GmbH, Tubingen, Germany) (Fig. 21.6a) can be operated in low-voltage "Soft Coag" mode, which allows rapid in-depth coagulation without carbonization and little sticking of the electrode. The VIO electrosurgical unit can be connected to the CUSA EXcel. The concurrent use of ultrasonic aspiration and low-voltage coagulation dramatically decreases bleeding upon parenchymal transection. The dripping of saline at the coagulation site enhances the hemostatic effect. We use a supplemental needle device inserted from the subcostal or intercostal region for the saline drip.

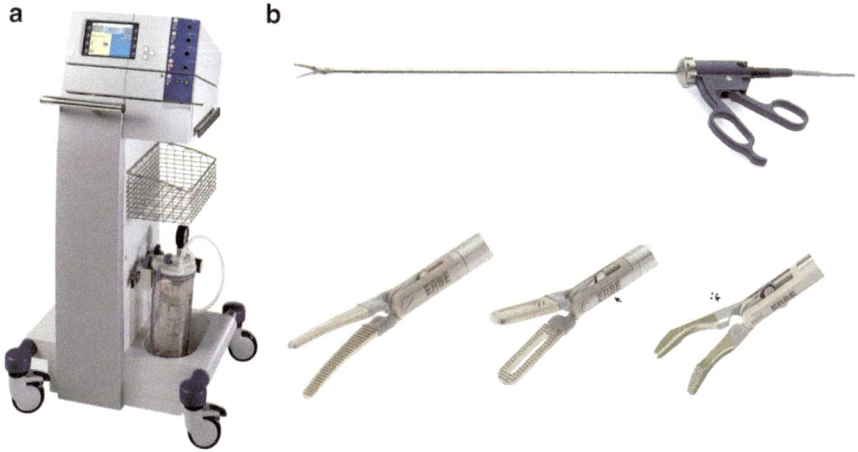

Fig. 21.6 The Electrosurgical system VIO300D generator (Erbe Elektromedizin GmbH, Tubingen, Germany) (**a**) and BiClamp LAP forceps, Maryland, deep-ribbed (Erbe Elektromedizin GmbH, Tubingen, Germany) (**b**)

The development of bipolar vessel-sealing devices has also contributed to safe parenchymal transection. The BiClamp forceps (Erbe Elektromedizin GmbH, Tubingen, Germany) (Fig. 21.6b) are bipolar and allow for firm grasping and reliable coagulation of vessels less than 3 mm in size. BiClamp is quite useful for stopping active bleeding and sealing the small vessels. LigaSure (Covidien, New Haven, CT, USA) (Fig. 21.7a) and EnSeal (Ethicon Endosurgery) (Fig. 21.7b) can seal and cut small vessels less than 3 mm in a sequential action, and no clipping is required. The number of instruments that can be used simultaneously in SPAS is limited, compelling the surgeon to change the instruments frequently. Thus, it is quite advantageous that the vessels can be sealed and cut in one action without clipping.

Vessels larger than 3 mm are clipped and transected. When the transection line is in the left lateral segment, the vascular pedicles are divided with the use of a laparoscopic stapler (Fig. 21.3e). An articulating laparoscopic stapler (Fig. 21.8a, b) is useful to achieve the ideal staple deployment angle.

21.3.6 Completion of the Procedure

A plastic bag is introduced into the abdomen through the 12-mm trocar, and the specimen is extracted transumbilically (Fig. 21.3f). Because of the meticulous hemostasis, no suction drain is left in place. The umbilical fascia is closed with absorbable sutures.

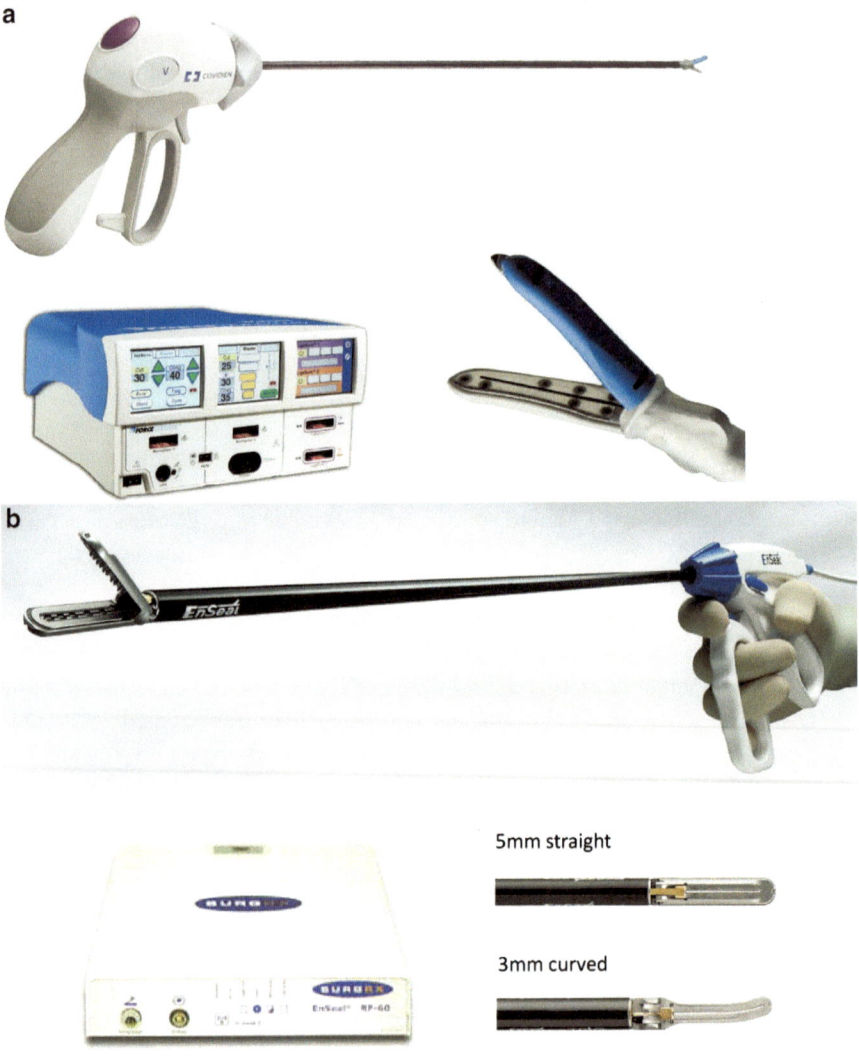

Fig. 21.7 (**a**) LigaSure (Covidien, New Haven, CT, US). (**b**) EnSeal (Ethicon Endosurgery, Cincinnati, OH, USA)

21.4 Tips and Tricks

21.4.1 *Crossed and Parallel Device Configuration*

For the basic intra-abdominal procedure, a crossed device configuration (Fig. 21.9a) is useful because articulating devices allow non-parallel access to the surgical field and offer free movement of the manipulating devices. SPAS remains a demanding procedure; however, the cross-configuration makes it possible to triangulate even

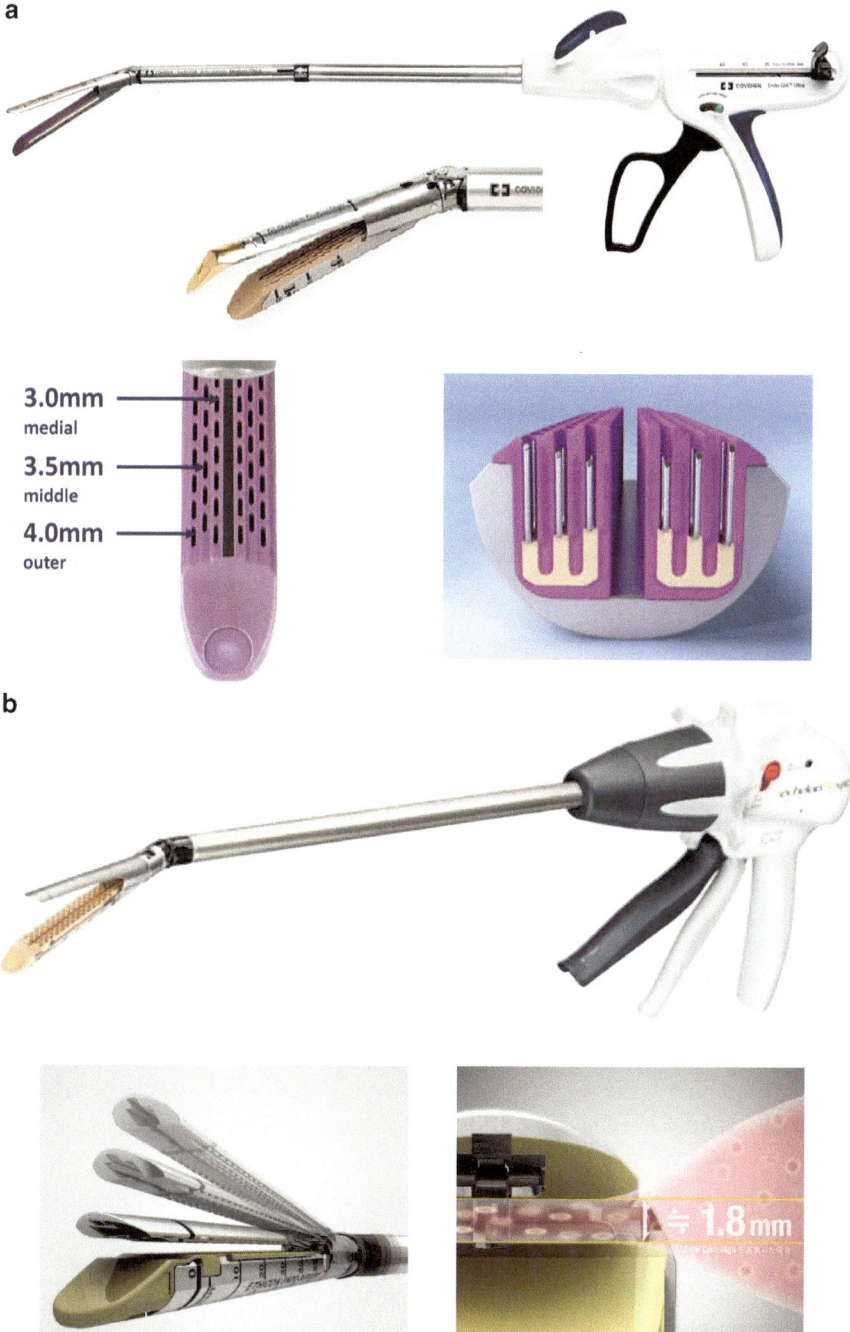

Fig. 21.8 (**a**) Endo GIA™ Ultra Universal staplers with Tri-Staple™ technology (Covidien, New Haven, CT, USA). (**b**) ECHELON FLEX (Ethicon Endosurgery, Cincinnati, OH, USA)

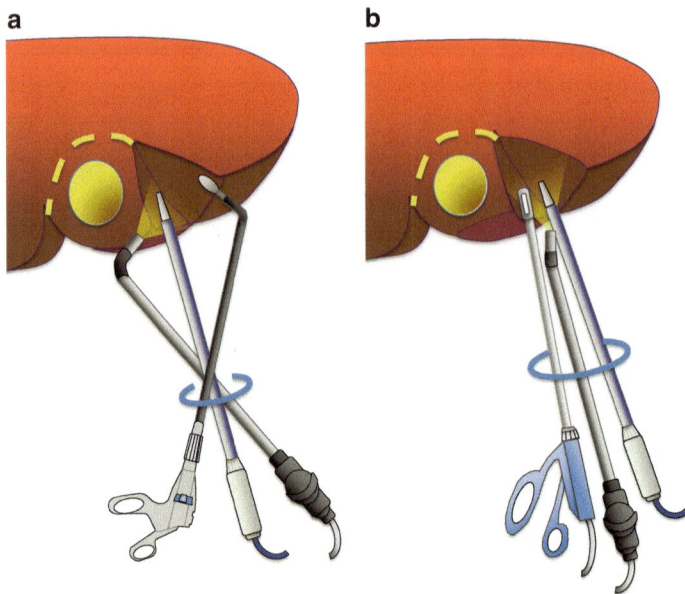

Fig. 21.9 (**a**) Crossed and (**b**) parallel device configurations

with 10-mm instruments such as the aspirator, stapling devices, and ultrasound probes. For the articulating device, we commonly use the SILS™ Clinch (Covidien, New Haven, CT, USA) (Fig. 21.10) or Autonomy™ Laparo-Angle™ grasper (Cambridge Endo, Framingham, MA, USA). These articulating graspers play an important role in exposing the operative field.

In transecting the liver parenchyma, simultaneous use of the CUSA EXcel (10-mm shaft) and BiClamp/bipolar forceps (5-mm shaft) is very effective. Both devices have a straight shaft; thus, parallel device configuration is necessitated (Fig. 21.9b). With this configuration, the channel distance must be more than 3 cm to avoid device conflicts.

21.4.2 RPS

The feasibility of SPAS has been well demonstrated, but standardization and safety need additional assessment. In this context, RPS could represent an interim target without concerns related to procedural safety and additional skills. A significant contribution of SPAS has been the development of innovative devices such as multi-access ports, curved instruments, and needle-type devices. Application of the SPAS instruments may reduce the number and size of the ports needed for conventional laparoscopic hepatectomy, normally requiring three to five ports (Fig. 21.11). Thus, SPAS contributes to the RPS technique. Even one additional standard trocar at the subcostal region allows the surgeon to maintain the ideal triangulation, avoiding

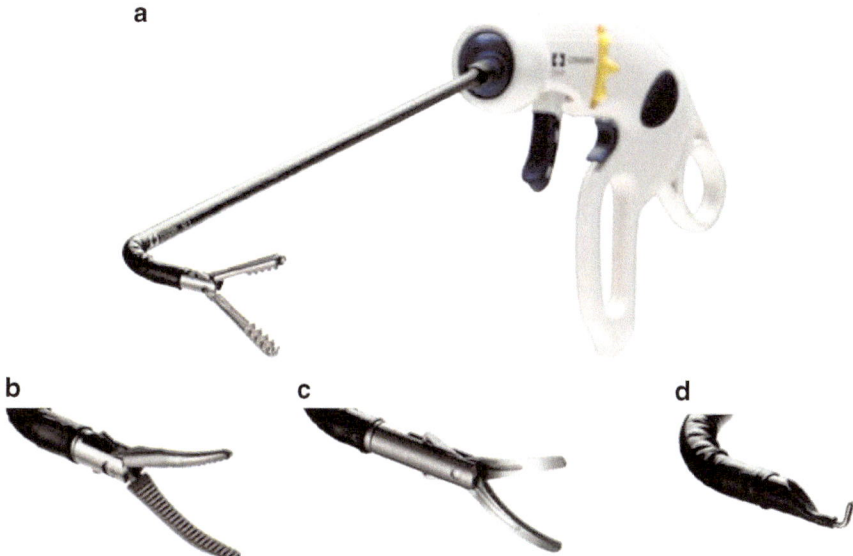

Fig. 21.10 The SILS™ hand instruments (Covidien). SILS™ hand instruments are the (**a**) SILS™ Clinch, (**b**) SILS™ Dissector, (**c**) LS™ Shears, (**d**) SILS™ Hook. Each device allows infinite dynamic articulation and locking of the instrument shaft and angle by means of an articulation lock lever

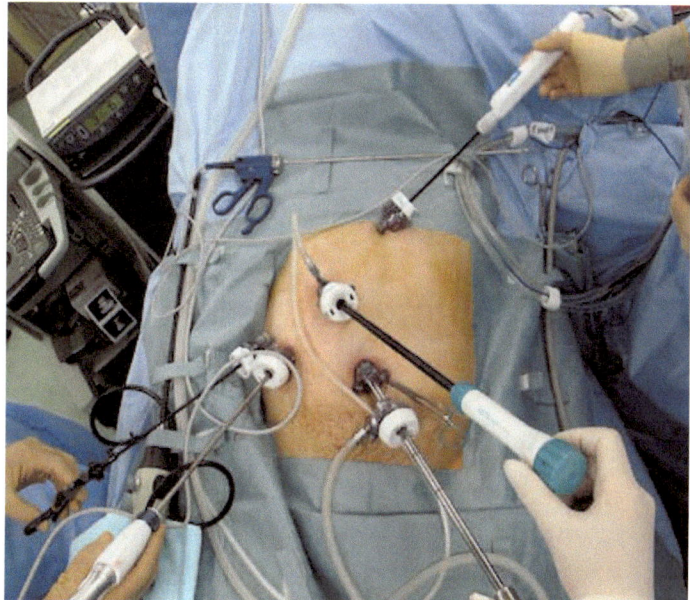

Fig. 21.11 Conventional laparoscopic hepatectomy

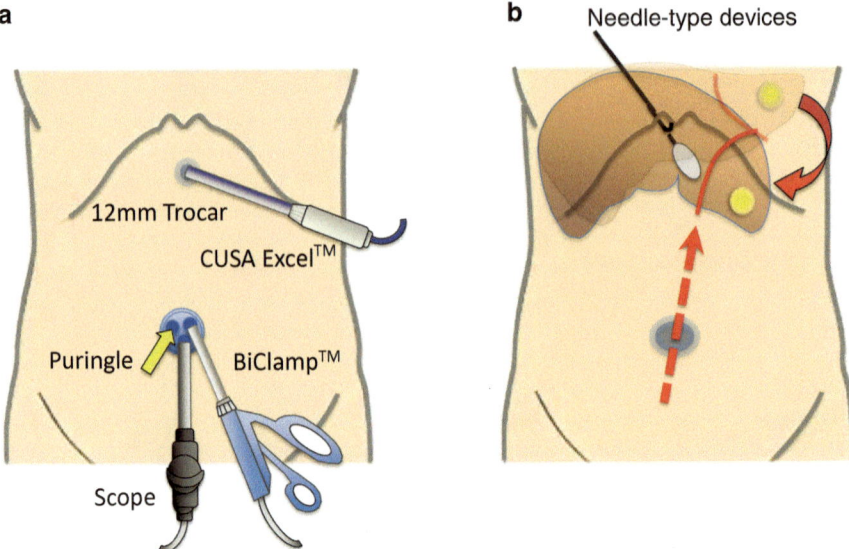

Fig. 21.12 Reduced-port surgery (RPS). (**a**) An additional standard trocar at the subcostal region allows the surgeon to maintain the ideal triangulation, avoiding clashing of instruments. (**b**) Using an additional needle-type instrument, the assistant retracts the liver to properly align the transection line

conflict between the instruments (Fig. 21.12a). This is very effective in resolving problems associated with SPAS, such as poor tissue manipulation, compromised visualization, and the limited reach of instruments from the umbilical port.

Additional puncture can be applied by inserting needle-type instruments. Instruments less than 3 mm in diameter do not leave a visible scar, in keeping with the goal of SPAS. Various needle-type instruments have been developed. The limited number of instruments that can be used during SPAS means that the surgeon must perform solo surgery. The use of needle-type instruments, however, enables the assistants to help with the procedure and ensures a scarless operation. The line of the intended liver parenchymal transection is not always in the same axis as the umbilical port sites. In this case, needle-type or standard devices inserted from the upper abdominal quadrant can be used to retract the liver and thus properly align the transection line (Fig. 21.12b).

21.5   Recommendations from the Author

21.5.1   Laparoscope

To avoid the clashing of instruments, an oblique-view, small-diameter laparoscope is essential. Neither a rigid laparoscope with a straight view nor a 10-mm laparoscope should be used (Fig. 21.13a). We use a 5-mm deflectable laparoscope (EndoEye Flex

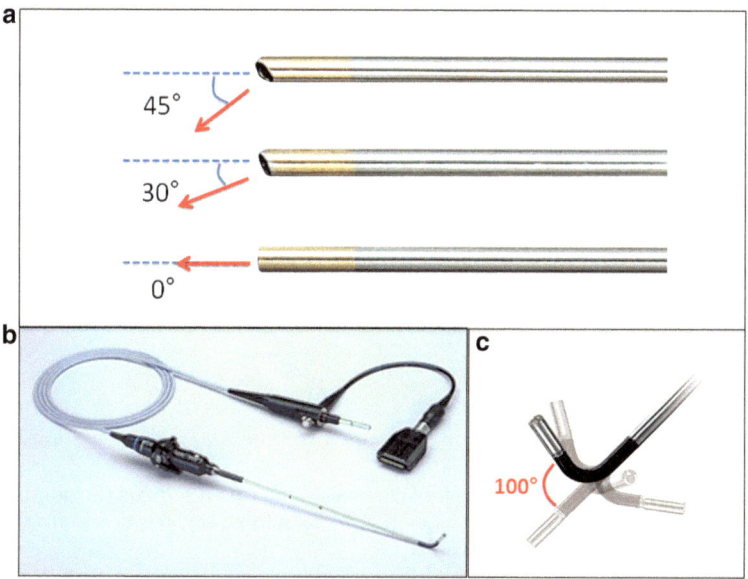

Fig. 21.13 Rigid (**a**) and flexible (**b**) laparoscope. (**c**) EndoEye Flex 5 (Olympus Corporation, Tokyo, Japan)

5, Olympus Corporation, Tokyo, Japan) (Fig. 21.13b) It allows 100-degree angulation and an 85-degree field of view for exceptional visualization and surgical dexterity.

21.5.2   Multi-Access Port

The multi-access port was developed for SPAS, and various makes and models are commercially available. A multi-access port allows multiple instruments to pass simultaneously through a single umbilical incision. One of the most commonly used products is the SILS™ Port (Covidien, Norwalk, Connecticut, USA) (Fig. 21.14a), which is a flexible soft-form port with three access channels arranged 15 mm apart. It comes with three 5-mm and one 12-mm cannula, which can be mounted inside the access channels.

When straight instruments are used together, a greater port distance is advantageous to avoid clashing of the instruments. X-gate (Johnson & Johnson K.K. Medical Company, Tokyo, Japan) (Fig. 21.14b) has four separate access channels with a maximum channel distance of 35 mm, which allows freedom in the handling of straight devices. We prefer to use X-gate, especially when the CUSA EXcel and hemostatic bipolar forceps are used simultaneously for transection of the liver parenchyma. GelPoint (Applied Medical, Rancho Santa Margarita, CA, USA) (Fig. 21.14c) is another candidate multi-access port for SPA hepatectomy. An accompanying wound retractor maximizes the working diameter of the umbilical wound, and exclusively designed trocars with small housings offer maximum freedom of movement.

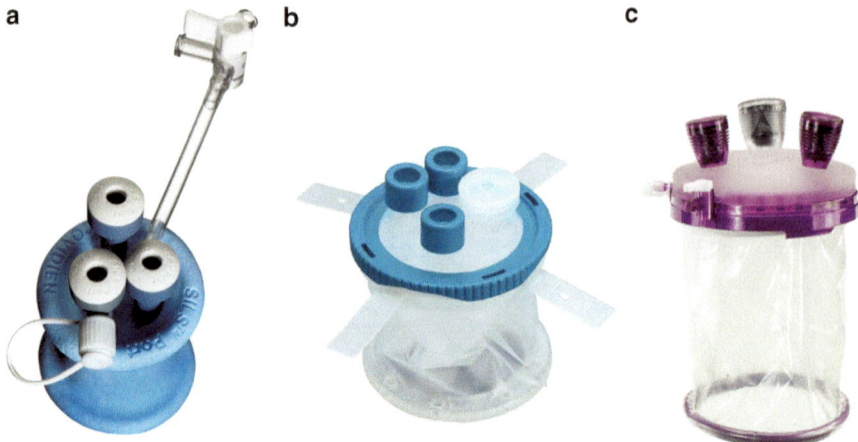

Fig. 21.14 Various multi-access ports for SPA hepatectomy. (**a**) SILS™ Port (Covidien, Norwalk, CT, USA). (**b**): X-gate (Johnson & Johnson K.K. Medical Company, Tokyo, Japan). (**c**) GelPoint (Applied Medical, Rancho Santa Margarita, CA, USA)

References

1. Nguyen NT, Reavis KM, Hinojosa MW, Smith BR, Stamos MJ (2009) A single-port technique for laparoscopic extended stapled appendectomy. Surg Innov 16:78–81
2. Nguyen NT, Reavis KM, Hinojosa MW, Smith BR, Wilson SE (2009) Laparoscopic transumbilical cholecystectomy without visible abdominal scars. J Gastrointest Surg 13:1125–1128
3. Barbaros U, Dinccag A (2009) Single-incision laparoscopic splenectomy: the first two cases. J Gastrointest Surg 13:1520–1523
4. Nguyen NT, Reavis KM, Hinojosa MW, Smith BR, Wilson SE (2009) Laparoscopic transumbilical sleeve gastrectomy without visible abdominal scars. Surg Obes Relat Dis 5:275–277
5. Bucher P, Pugin F, Morel P (2008) Single-port-access laparoscopic right hemicolectomy. Int J Colorectal Dis 23:1013–1016
6. Ahmed I and Paraskeva P. A clinical review of single-incision laparoscopic surgery. Surgeon, 9:341–351, 2011.
7. Gagner, Rheault M, Dubuc J. Laparoscopic partial hepatectomy for liver tumor. Surg Endosc 6:99, 1992.
8. Buell JF, Cherqui D, Geller DA, O'Rourke N, Iannitti D, Dagher I, et al. The international position on laparoscopic liver surgery: the Louisville Statement, 2008. Ann Surg 250:825–830, 2009.
9. Kobayashi S, Nagano H, Marubashi S, et al. A single incision laparoscopic hepatectomy for hepatocellular carcinoma: initial experience in a Japanese patient. Minim Invasive Ther Allied Technol 19:367–371, 2010.
10. Patel AG, Belgaumkar AP, James J, Singh UP, Carswell KA, Murgatroyd B. Video. Single-incision laparoscopic left lateral segmentectomy of colorectal liver metastasis. Surgical Endosc 25:649–650, 2011.
11. Aldrighetti L, Guzzetti E, Ferla G. Laparoscopic hepatic left lateral sectionectomy using the LaparoEndoscopic Single Site approach: evolution of minimally invasive liver surgery. J Hepatobiliary Pancreat Sci 18:103–105, 2011.
12. Chang SKY, Mayasari M, Ganpathi IS, Wen VLT, Madhavan K. Single port laparoscopic liver resection for hepatocellular carcinoma: a preliminary report. Int J Hepatol 2011: doi: 10.4061/2011/579203.

13. Belli G, Fantini C, D'Agostino A, et al. Laparoendoscopic single site liver resection for recurrent hepatocellular carcinoma in cirrhosis: first technical note. Surg Laparosc Endosc Percutan Tech 21:166–168, 2011.
14. Hu MG, Zhao GD, Xu DB, Liu R. Transumbilical single-incision laparoscopic hepatectomy: an initial report. Chin Med J 124:787–789, 2011.
15. Barbaros U, Demirel T, Gozkun O, et al. A new era in minimally invasive liver resection (MILR) single-incision laparoscopic liver resection (SIL-LR): the first two cases. Surg Technol Int 21:81–84, 2012.
16. Røsok BI and B. Edwin B. Single-incision laparoscopic liver resection for colorectal metastasis through stoma site at the time of reversal of diversion ileostomy: a case report. Minim Invasive Surg 2011: http://www.hindawi.com/journals/mis/2011/502176/ Accessed 20 Feb 2014
17. Gaujoux S, Kingham TP, Jarnagin WR, D'Angelica MI, Allen RJ, Fong Y, Single-incision laparoscopic liver resection. Surg Endosc 25:1489–1494, 2011.
18. Zhao G, Hu M, Liu R, et al. Laparoendoscopic single-site liver resection: a preliminary report of 12 cases. Surg Endosc 25:3286–3293, 2011.
19. Cipriani F, Catena M, Ratti F, Paganelli M, F. Ferla F, L. Aldrighetti L. LESS technique for liver resection: the progress of the mini-invasive approach: a single-centre experience. Minim Invasive Ther Allied Technol 21:55–58, 2012.
20. Shetty GS, You YK,. Choi HJ, Na GH, Hong TH, Kim DG. Extending the limitations of liver surgery: outcomes of initial human experience in a high-volume center performing single-port laparoscopic liver resection for hepatocellular carcinoma. Surg Endosc 26:1602–1608, 2012.
21. Aikawa M, Miyazawa M, Okamoto K, Toshimitsu Y, Okada K, Ueno Y. Single-port laparoscopic hepatectomy: technique, safety, and feasibility in a clinical case series. Surg Endosc 26:1696–1701, 2012.
22. Tan EK, Lee VT, Chang SK, Ganpathi IS, Madhavan K, Lomanto D. Laparoendoscopic single-site minor hepatectomy for liver tumors. Surg Endosc 26:2086–2091, 2012.
23. Cai W, Xu J, Zheng M, Qin M, Zhao H. Combined laparoendoscopic single-site surgery: initial experience of a single center. Hepatogastroenterology 59:986–989, 2012.
24. Dapri G, DiMarco L, Cadiere GB, Donckier V. Initial experience in single-incision transumbilical laparoscopic liver resection: indications, potential benefits, and limitations. HPB Surg 2012:1–9, 2012

Chapter 22
Splenectomy

Eduardo M. Targarona, Carlos Rodriguez Luppi, Julio Lopez Monclova, Carmen Balague, and Manuel Trias

Abstract Multiport laparoscopic splenectomy is the current standard technique for spleen removal. However, the concept of minimally invasive surgery has progressed to natural orifices translumenal endoscopic surgery and single-port access (SPA). A concept of reduced port laparoscopic surgery has emerged trying to overcome the difficulties of SPA. The best indication for single-port or reduced port laparoscopic splenectomy is slim patients with normal or slightly enlarged spleen. Splenomegaly or liver cirrhosis are not an absolute contraindication but may increase the technical difficulty. Massive splenomegaly is a formal contraindication. These two options offer optimal aesthetic outcomes with the counterpart of increased technical difficulty. Optimal technological resources, proper patient selection with adequate preoperative information and technical skill training are of paramount importance to assure the best clinical outcome. However, clearly-defined clinical advantages of these approaches are not well established and we should wait for the outcome of proper, statistically-powered clinical studies before drawing any definitive conclusions.

Keywords Reduced port laparoscopic surgery • Single-port laparoscopic surgery • Splenectomy

E.M. Targarona (✉) • C.R. Luppi • J.L. Monclova
C. Balague • M. Trias
Service of Surgery, Hospital de la Santa Creu i Sant Pau., Universitat Autònoma de Barcelona (UAB), Mas Casanovas 90, 4th floor, 08041 Barcelona, Spain
e-mail: etargarona@santpau.cat

T. Mori and G. Dapri (eds.), *Reduced Port Laparoscopic Surgery*,
DOI 10.1007/978-4-431-54601-6_22, © Springer Japan 2014

22.1 Introduction

Multiport laparoscopic splenectomy is considered the "gold standard" for the management of surgical diseases in normal or slightly enlarged spleens [1]. Its effectiveness and low-complication rate, together with patient comfort, decreased hospital stay and enhanced recovery make it the procedure of choice for most surgeons.

The concept of minimally-invasive surgical techniques has progressed since the early 1990s, from standard multiport laparoscopy to natural orifice translumenal endoscopic surgery (NOTES) and, more recently, to single-port access (SPA). Experience with SPA has been reported sporadically since minimally invasive procedures (appendectomy, cholecystectomy) first appeared, but the number of papers on the subject has increased consistently since 2007, perhaps because surgeons view this technique as a bridge to the even less invasive NOTES [2]. Simultaneously, a concept of reduced port laparoscopic surgery has emerged trying to overcome the difficulties of SPA. The reduction of the number and size of incisions as well the use of natural orifices or scars, permits the preservation of the integrity of the abdominal wall, reduces the number and size of wounds, and improves the aesthetic outcome [3].

22.2 Indications and Contraindications

The best indication for single-port laparoscopic splenectomy (SPLS) or reduced port laparoscopic splenectomy (RPLS) is the case of a slim patient with normal or slightly enlarged spleen [4]. Previous surgery is not a definitive contraindication, but, undoubtedly, increases the difficulty when adhesions should be taken down. There are two anatomic features that also may increase the difficulty or preclude the performance of SPLS or RPLS. They are the belly shape and an extremely tall patient. In the case of a prominent belly, the distance from the belly bottom to the splenic fossa increases, and in some cases it is not possible to reach the top of the posterior adhesions of the upper pole of the spleen. Also, in extremely tall patients, the distance from the umbilicus to the diaphragm is too long for the use of conventional endoscopic instruments. A solution for these situations may be the placement of the device just in a subcostal midclavicular point, thereby reducing significantly the working distance. Another technical alternative is to introduce an additional 2- or 5-mm trocar in the left hypochondrium, since the use of this new instrument may allow the surgeon to overcome dissection difficulties. This port site may be used as a drainage exit in case it proves necessary.

Splenomegaly or liver cirrhosis are not an absolute contraindication but increase the dissection and removal maneuvers. Massive splenomegaly is a formal contraindication.

22.3 Surgical Technique

22.3.1 SPLS

The patient is placed in the standard right decubitus position for LS, with the table flexed at the flank (Fig 22.1). A transumbilical approach can be chosen for thin patients and in cases of splenic cyst. In cases in which the patient is tall, obese, or has a non-compliant abdomen, a left 2-cm subcostal incision is placed at a point between the subcostal margin and the umbilicus in the midclavicular line.

SPLS can be performed through two approaches. (Fig. 22.2)

1. SPLS using multiple trocars: a 15-mm skin incision is made inside the umbilicus and a 12-mm bladeless trocar (Excel Endopath (Ethicon, Cincinnati, OH, USA)) is bluntly introduced into the abdomen under optic control with a flexible tip 10-mm HD scope (Olympus, Tokyo, Japan). After exploring the abdominal cavity, a 5-mm trocar with a flexible threaded cannula (Karl Storz-Endoskope, Tuttlingen, Germany) is inserted to the left of the 12-mm trocar and another 5-mm trocar with a small valve is placed to the right.

Single Incision Laparoscopic Splenectomy

Hospital de la Santa Creu i Sant Pau

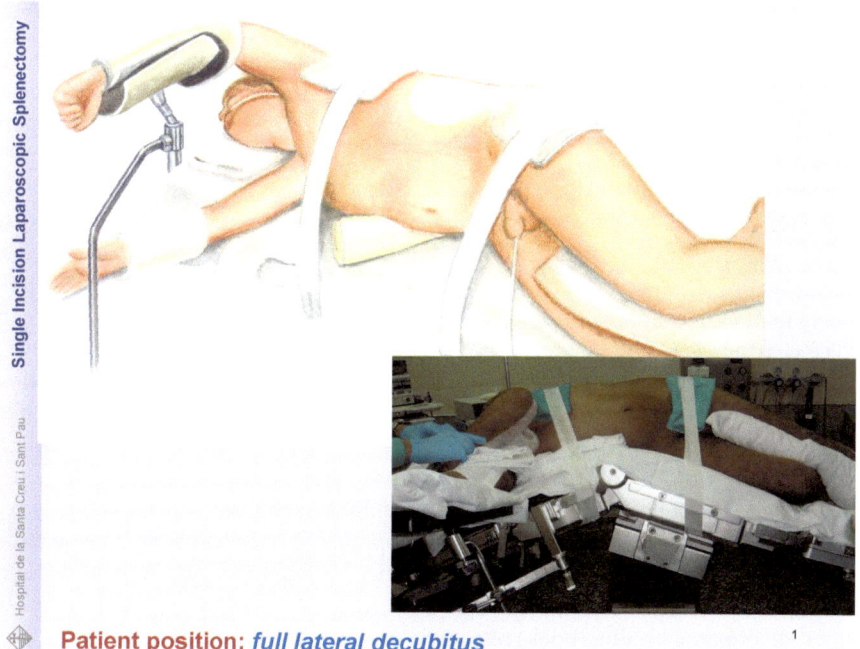

Patient position: *full lateral decubitus*

Fig. 22.1 Surgical position. The patient is placed in a full lateral position, with a flexion to open the costo-pelvic space

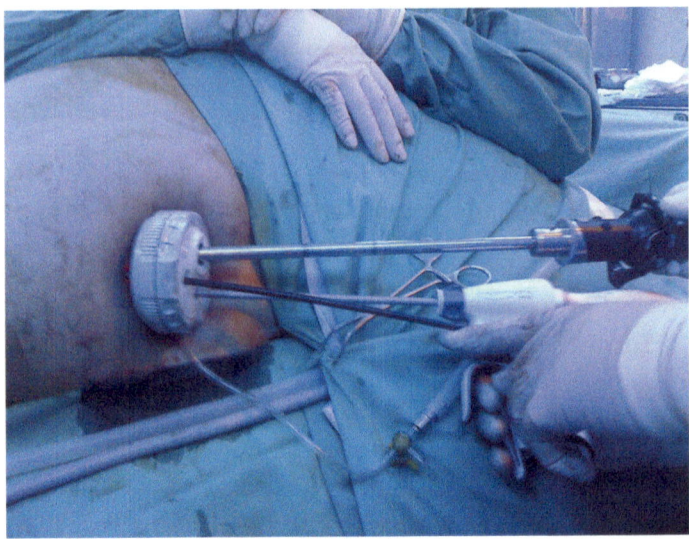

Fig. 22.2 External intraoperative view of instruments handling during a SPLS

2. SPLS using a multiport device. After the insertion of the Veress needle, a 20-mm
   incision is made and a multiple-port device (Triport, Quadriport, (Olympus),
   Uno (Ethicon)) is inserted (Fig. 22.2).

The technique used for splenic dissection is similar to that used in standard LS.
After an explorative laparoscopy, the possible existence of accessory spleens is
ruled out. A 5-mm curved grasper used for transanal endoscopic microsurgery
(TEM) (Richard Wolf, Vernon Hills, IL, USA) is placed through the left port. The
slightly curved end of this instrument fits into the flexible trocar or through a port of
the mutichannel device, and it is sufficiently curved to work intrabdominally without causing instruments to clash. A 5-mm harmonic scalpel (Harmonic Ace
(Ethicon)) is then introduced through the right port. Using this approach, it is possible to mobilize the splenic colon flexure and to reach the lower pole of the spleen.
The next step is to gain access to the retrogastric pouch and to severe the short vessels at the upper pole of the spleen (Fig. 22.3). With this view, and due to the flexible
tip of the scope, it is possible, if desired, to ligate or clip the splenic artery. The
instruments are then moved to the posterior aspect of the spleen and the table is
tilted to the right to take advantage of gravity and obtain exposure of the retrosplenic area. The posterior spleno-renal attachments are freed.

Sometimes, especially if the umbilical approach is used and there are some difficulties with the more posterior and upper part of the upper splenic pole, a 3-mm
instrument can be introduced through the left flank. This mini-instrument can be
used to retract or section (hook) retroperitoneal adhesion.

Once the spleen is completely mobile, the flexible scope is withdrawn and the
intraabdominal visual control is changed to a 5-mm scope. If the multichannel has
several large bore ports (Quadriport (Olympus)), the 10-mm scope can be

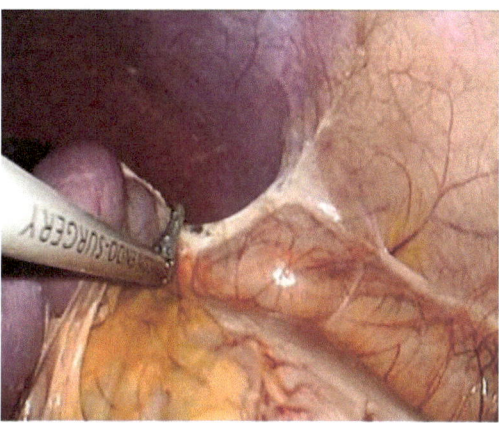

Fig. 22.3 Intraoperative steps: spleen mobilization

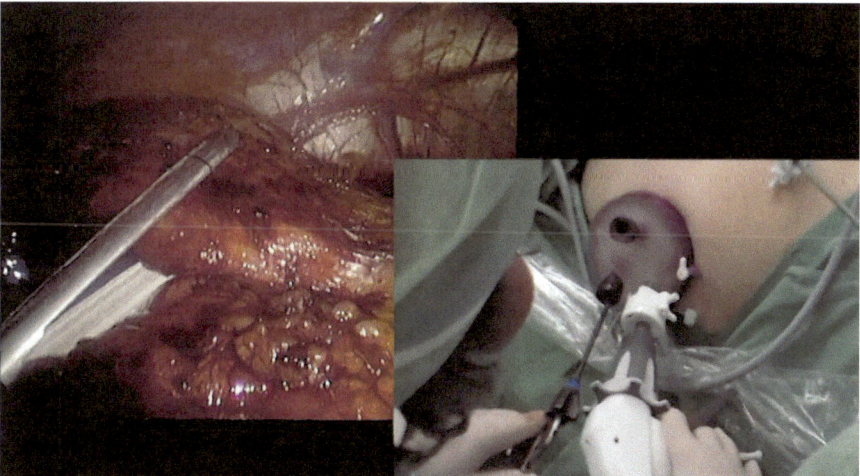

Fig. 22.4 Transection of the splenic hilum with an endostapler

maintained. A probe inserted through the left 5-mm trocar lifts up the splenic hilum, providing sufficient space for the placement of the endostapler. An endoscopic linear stapler with a 6-cm white cartridge (Echelon (Ethicon)) is inserted through a 12-mm trocar/port and advanced to the splenic fossa. After adjusting the jaws, the endostapler is fired several times until the splenic hilum is completely severed (Fig. 22.4).

Once the spleen is completely free, a 15-mm endobag (Endocatch II (Covidien, New Haven, CT, USA)) is inserted. The spleen is grasped with a 5-mm instrument and hung in the splenic fossa. The bag is deployed below the organ and the spleen is introduced. The bag is pulled to the umbilical incision and the spleen is retrieved intact or morcellated (Fig. 22.5). Lastly, the operating field is revised and complete hemostasis is achieved.

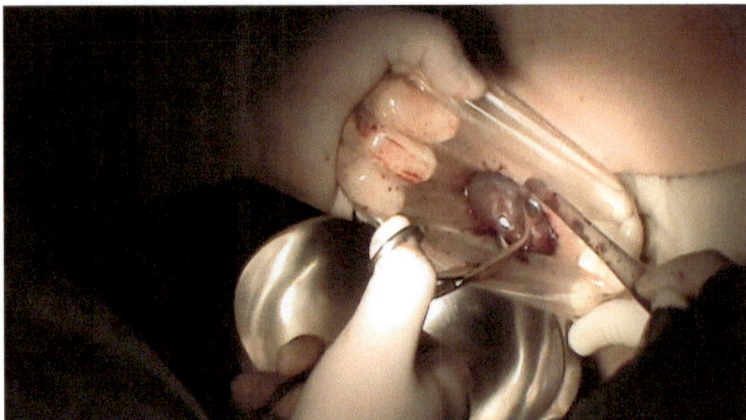

Fig. 22.5 Spleen morcellation and extraction inside a bag

Fig. 22.6 Postoperative
wound appearance

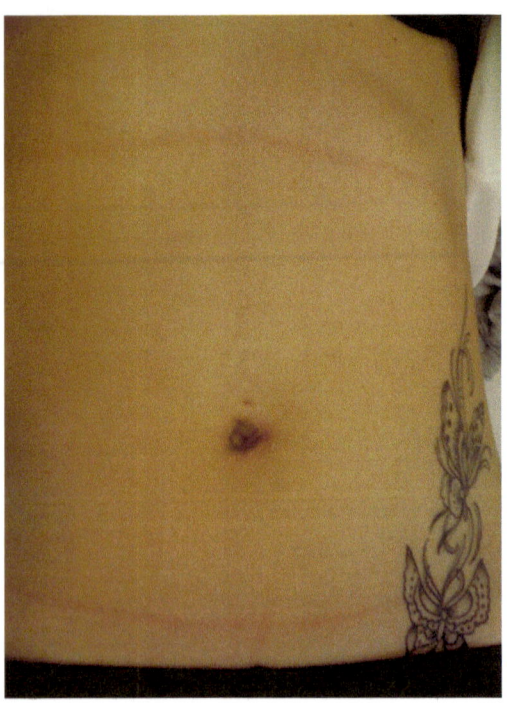

In the case of fenestration of a splenic cyst, the first step is to puncture and evacu-
ate the cyst contents. Then, with the aid of the harmonic scalpel, we excise as much
cystic wall as possible, until the splenic parenchyma is reached. Once hemostasis is
completed, cyst wall fragments are extracted in an endobag.

The umbilicus is closed and carefully reconstructed, obtaining an optimal aesthetic result (Fig. 22.6).

Fig. 22.7 Trocars placement

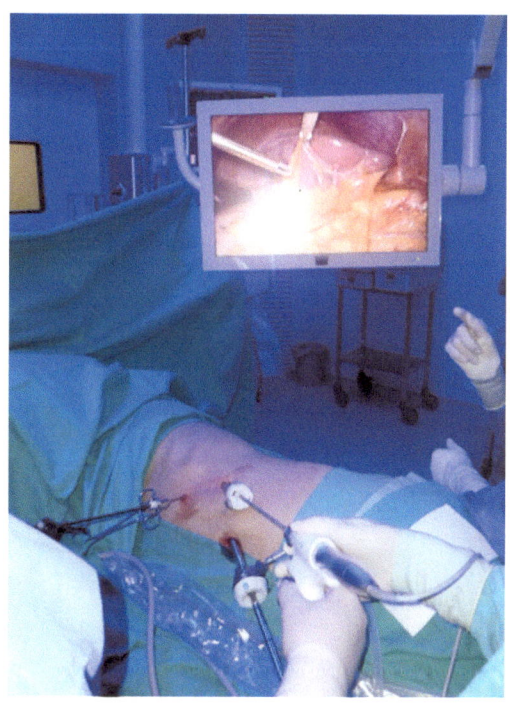

22.3.2 RPLS

The patient is placed in lateral decubitus, and the access to the abdominal cavity is gained using a 12-mm optic bladeless trocar (Excel Endopath (Ethicon)) introduced through the umbilicus. A 10-mm flexible tip HD scope (Endoeye (Olympus)) is routinely used. A subcostal 5-mm trocar is placed under direct vision at the level of the anterior axillary line and a 3-mm port is inserted at the midepigastric region (Fig. 22.7).

The sequential steps are the same as with SPLS. Using a 5-mm harmonic scalpel (Harmonic Ace (Ethicon)) and 3-mm instruments (Karl Storz-Endoskope), access is gained to the lesser sac by dividing the gastrosplenic ligament and short vessels until the upper pole of the spleen is reached (Fig. 22.8). Every attempt is made to ligate the splenic artery at the superior border of the pancreas to allow some shrinkage of the spleen.

The splenic flexure of the colon is mobilized to get the lower pole of the spleen freed. The table is then tilted to the right to obtain a good exposure of the retrosplenic area, taking advantage of gravity. The posterior splenorenal ligament is then severed.

Once the spleen is completely dissected free from all of its attachments, the optic is changed for a 5-mm, 30-degree scope introduced through the left hypocondrium trocar, and an endostapler with a 60-mm white cartridge (Echelon (Ethicon)) is

Fig. 22.8 Section of the
short vessels

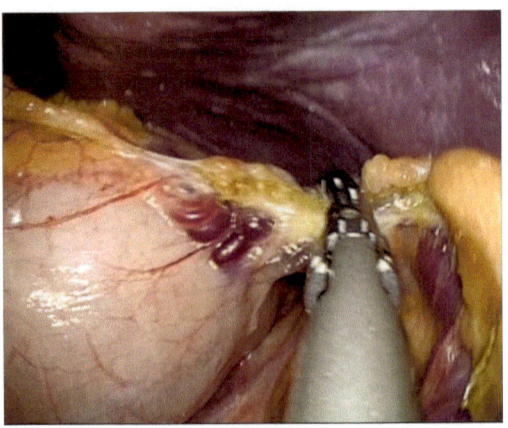

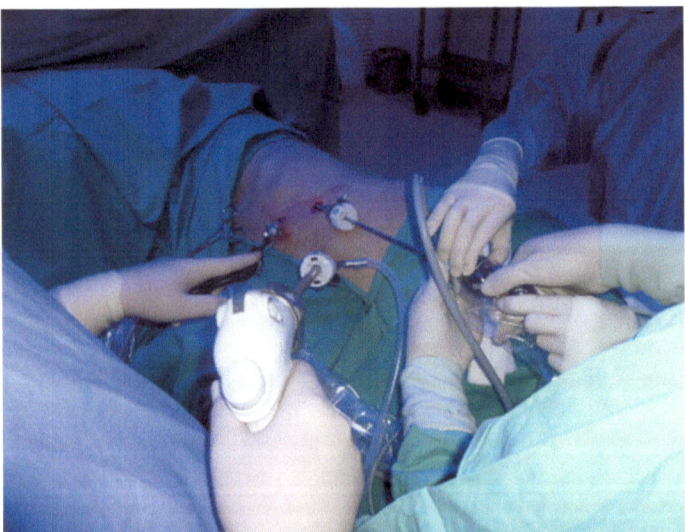

Fig. 22.9 Splenic hilum is severed with a 12-mm endostapler introduced trough the umbilicus

inserted through the umbilical port, advanced to the splenic fossa, and fired to divide
the splenic artery and vein at the level of the hilum (Fig. 22.9). A 15-mm endobag
(Endocatch II (Covidien)) is used to retrieve the spleen after being morcellated trough
the umbilical incision (Fig. 22.10). A drain, exteriorized through the lateral 5-mm
trocar, is used selectively. Hemostasis of the operating field is obtained and a subcuticular suture permits obtaining small scars with a satisfactory aesthetic outcome
(Fig. 22.11).

Fig. 22.10 Spleen extraction inside a large size bag introduced through the umbilicus

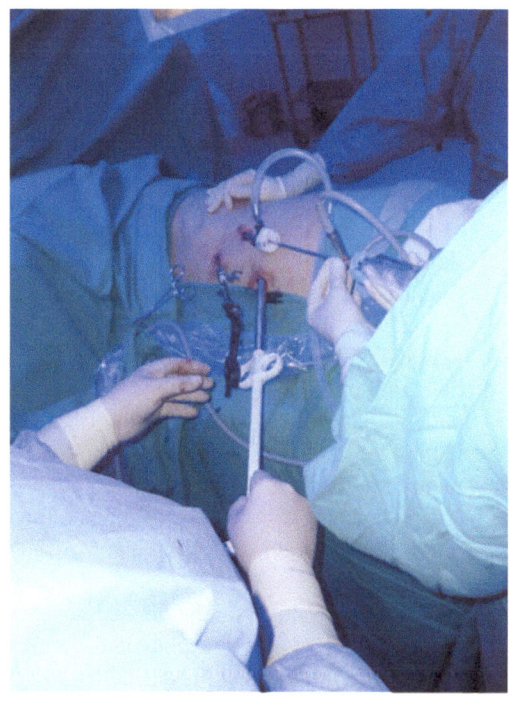

Fig. 22.11 Postoperative aesthetic outcome

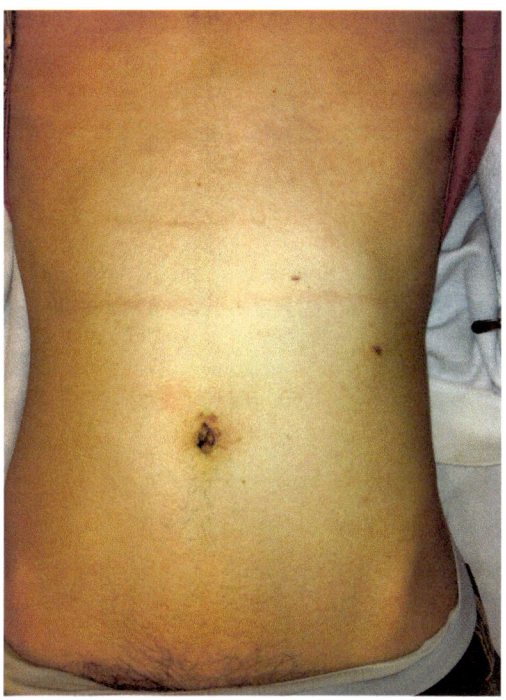

22.4   Tips and Tricks

1. Evaluate the distance from the umbilicus to the splenic fossa. In very tall patients the instruments or the endostapler may not reach the splenic fossa.
2. In case of a large belly, also the spleen is located too high and difficulties may exist in reaching the posterior attachments of the upper pole. This situation can be overcome by inserting a small diameter instrument trough the left flank.
3. The use of a flexible scope through the umbilicus is advised because, due to the angled view obtained, it allows the vision of anatomic areas that are very difficult to reach with 0° or 30° scopes.
4. Selection of the patients is of paramount importance. Enlarged spleens or obese patients may increase the difficulty of the procedure.
5. If the placement of a drain is planned, the insertion site can be used for placement of an additional small instrument.
6. A 5-mm scope is necessary to replace the 10-mm scope when the endostapler is inserted through the umbilicus or when the bag is inserted for the spleen retrieval.
7. Additional trocars of small diameter shorten the operative time and prevent complications if anatomic or technical difficulties develop during the surgical procedure, without impairing the aesthetic outcome.
8. Closure of the umbilical wound should be carefully attained in order to avoid late umbilical complications.

22.4.1   Recommendations from the Author

SPLS and RPLS are the latest conceptual advances in the trend to reduce the invasiveness of minimally invasive surgery of the spleen. These two options allow the achievement of optimal aesthetic outcomes at the expense of increased technical difficulty. Optimal technological resources, proper patient selection with adequate preoperative information and technical skill training are of paramount importance to assure the best clinical outcome. However, definitive clinical advantages of these approaches are not well established and we should hold on for the outcome of properly, statistically powered clinical studies before drawing any definitive conclusions.

References

1. Gamme G, Birch DW, Karmali S (2013) Minimally invasive splenectomy: an update and review. Can J Surg 56:280–285
2. Curcillo PG 2nd, Podolsky ER, King SA (2011) The road to reduced port surgery: from single big incisions to single small incisions, and beyond. World J Surg 35:1526–1531
3. Ahmed I, Ciancio F, Ferrara V et al (2012) Current status of single-incision laparoscopic surgery: European experts' views. Surg Laparosc Endosc Percutan Tech 22:194–199
4. Targarona E, Lima M, Balague C, Trias M (2011) Single-port splenectomy: current update and controversies. J Minim Access Surg 7:61–64

Chapter 23
Distal Pancreatectomy

Takeyuki Misawa

Abstract Recent interest in improved cosmetic outcomes has led to application of single-incision laparoscopic surgery (SLS) to a variety of organs. However, this innovative technique has been applied only rarely to pancreatic surgery, and, it is regarded as quite challenging. In this chapter, we describe techniques we use to perform single-incision laparoscopic distal pancreatectomy (DP) with or without splenic preservation. A 2.5-cm intra-umbilical mini-laparotomy is made for placement of a SILS™ Port (Covidien, New Haven, CT, USA) as a single access site. The overall procedure is similar to that of standard laparoscopic DP with multiple trocars. To obtain adequate exposure of the operative field, we applied suture suspension of the greater curvature of the stomach, the tug-exposure technique, a balloon retractor, and the use of gravity by changing the patient's position. The pancreas is transected with a linear stapler, and the specimen is extracted through the umbilical wound. The resulting umbilical scar is nearly invisible by 1 month after surgery. We conclude that SLS can be safely applied to DP if specific technical refinements are implemented. Although the cosmetic benefit of single-incision laparoscopic DP is clear, several issues, including the extent of invasiveness, the costs, the indications, and the learning curve, remain to be investigated.

Keywords Laparoscopic distal pancreatectomy • Single-incision laparoscopic surgery (SLS) • Single-port laparoscopic surgery • Splenic preservation

T. Misawa (✉)
Department of Surgery, The Jikei University School of Medicine, Kashiwa, Chiba, Japan

Hepato-Biliary-Pancreatic Surgery, Jikei University Kashiwa Hospital,
163-1 Kashiwashita, Kashiwa, Chiba, Japan
e-mail: take-misawa@jikei.ac.jp

T. Mori and G. Dapri (eds.), *Reduced Port Laparoscopic Surgery*,
DOI 10.1007/978-4-431-54601-6_23, © Springer Japan 2014

23.1 Introduction

Since the initial reports of distal pancreatectomy (DP) performed by laparoscopic approach [1, 2], laparoscopic DP (LDP) with multiple trocars rapidly gained popularity, and a number of case series and multi-institutional studies have documented the safety and efficacy of LDP [3]. Recent interest in improved cosmetic outcomes has led to performance of single-incision laparoscopic surgery (SLS) for a variety of target organs, which itself has drawn a great deal of attention [4–10]. However, the application of SLS to DP is highly challenging, and published reports on SLS-DP have been limited to case series [11–14]. Therefore, we consider SLS-DP as an emerging procedure with much room for technical improvement to ensure its safe performance. Herein, we describe the technical refinements we have developed for performance of SLS-DP, both with and without splenic preservation.

23.2 Indications and Contraindications

Currently, we perform SLS-DP for benign or borderline malignant pancreatic lesions. Examples include intraductal papillary mucinous neoplasm, mucinous cystic neoplasm, and neuroendocrine tumor, for which systematic lymph node dissection is unnecessary. Whether pancreatic cancer is indicated for SLS-DP remains to be clarified; the oncologic outcomes of even conventional LDP with multiple trocars are not yet clearly understood [15]. Therefore, application of SLS-DP to pancreatic cancer is not recommended because the oncologic picture is unclear and the procedure is technically difficult. SLS-DP is also not recommended when chronic pancreatitis is present. Dense adhesions around the pancreas may be encountered. In such cases, placement of additional trocars, or conversion to hand-assisted laparoscopic surgery [16] or open surgery should be performed without hesitation. Preservation of the spleen together with the splenic artery and vein should be chosen when the lesion is rather small and located in the pancreatic tail. However, when the lesion is rather large, and it compresses and adheres tightly to the splenic vessels, or when the tumor is located in the pancreatic body rather close to the portal vein, splenectomy should be considered because dissection of the pancreatic parenchyma from the splenic vessels becomes problematic.

23.3 Techniques

The operating room setup for SLS-DP is the same as for conventional laparoscopic DP. The patient is placed in the semilateral position on the right side with the left arm fixed over the head. The surgeon stands on the patient's right, and an assistant stands on the patient's left (Fig. 23.1). With cosmesis in mind, the umbilicus is

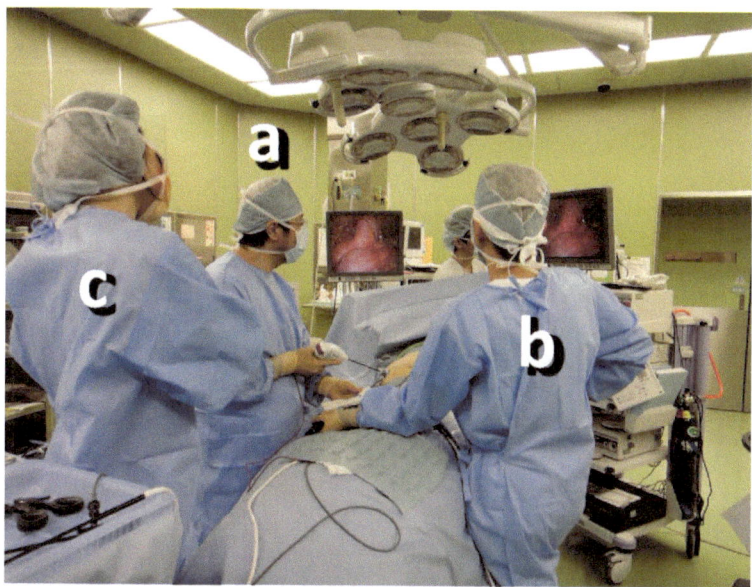

Fig. 23.1 Operating room set-up. (**a**) Operator, (**b**) assistant, (**c**) nurse

chosen as the access site. In tall or obese patients, the access site is sometimes placed closer to the splenic hilum to compensate for the limited length of the instruments used. With the patient under general anesthesia, an intra-umbilical skin incision is made for an approximate 2.5-cm mini-laparotomy. A SILS™ Port (Covidien, New Haven, CT, USA) with three 5-mm trocars is then placed in this wound and used for access. Pneumoperitoneum is created at a maximum 10 mmHg CO_2, and the operating table is tilted into a reverse Trendelenburg position. A flexible 5-mm laparoscope (Olympus LTF Type VH; Olympus Surgical, Tokyo, Japan) and an articulating grasper (Roticulator™ EndoGRASP™; Covidien) are used in addition to conventional laparoscopic equipment (Fig. 23.2). Once the laparoscope, grasper, and dissector are introduced, the overall procedure is similar to that of conventional LDP performed with multiple trocars [17]. The technical refinements that we apply to SLS-DP, with or without splenic preservation, are described below.

23.4 S-DP Without Splenic Preservation

The first step is dissection of the ligamentous attachments around the spleen for its mobilization. A 5-mm LigaSure V (Valleylab; Covidien) is used for the dissection of all ligaments as well as small vessels such as the short gastric vessels. By dissecting the gastrocolic and gastrosplenic ligaments, the omental bursa is opened toward the superior pole of the spleen, and the splenic hilum is well exposed. The inferior pole of the spleen is then freed by dissecting the splenocolic

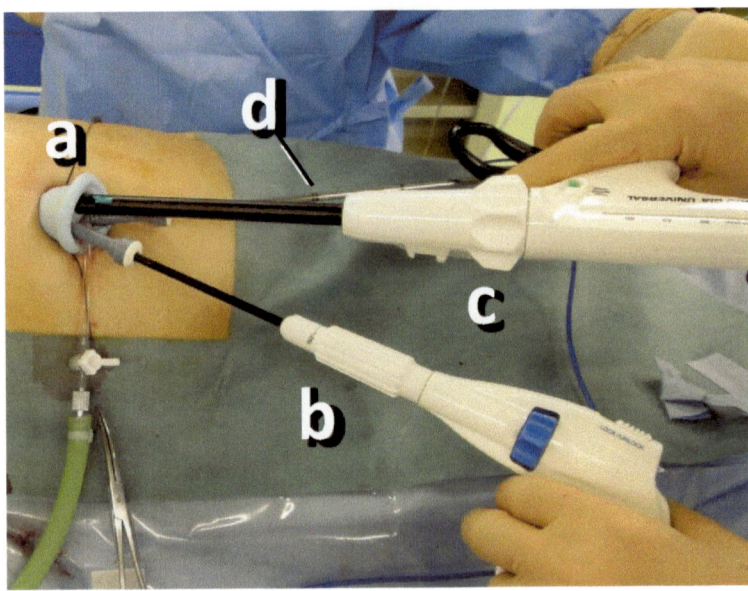

Fig. 23.2 Access through the umbilicus. (**a**) SILS Port™ (Covidien), (**b**) articulating grasper, (**c**) linear stapler, (**d**) 5-mm flexible scope (behind the scope)

ligament. The phrenosplenic ligament is also dissected. After dissection of both the superior and inferior poles of the spleen, the retroperitoneum lateral to the spleen (the splenorenal ligament) is dissected toward the superior pole of the spleen. After rough completion of splenic hilar dissection, one of the three 5-mm trocars is temporarily replaced by a 12-mm trocar, through which a 3- to 5-mm width cloth tape is introduced intraperitoneally to encircle and tug the splenic hilum. Both ends of the tape are grasped and exteriorized with the use of a laparoscopic suture passer or mini-loop retractor (Mini Loop Retractor II; Hakkou-shoji, Tokyo, Japan) through a needle hole that is approximately 2 mm in diameter and placed on the left midaxillary line 1 cm inferior to the costal margin (Fig. 23.3a, b). By pulling the tape with the use of an extracorporeal clamp or laparoscopic graspers in appropriate directions, excellent exposure of the splenic hilum and the pancreatic tail is obtained. This method is known as the tug-exposure technique [10]. This technique is also helpful for dissecting the remnant ligaments around the spleen and for detaching the pancreas, tail to body, from the retroperitoneum. Another 5-mm trocar is replaced by a 12-mm trocar that allows introduction of an endostapler (60 mm in length, 4.8-mm staples; Covidien). Although we have reported use of a six-row stapler to prevent postoperative pancreatic fistula, the six-row stapler does not have an articulating function for closing the pancreatic stump in LDP [18]. The articulating function of the linear stapler is indispensable; it ensures an optimal angle in transecting the pancreatic parenchyma. The pancreas,

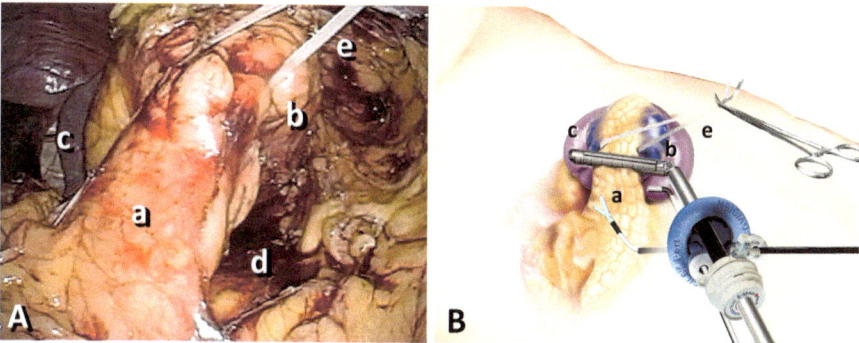

Fig. 23.3 Photograph of an actual SLS-DP (**a**) and an illustration of SLS-DP (**b**) in which the tug-exposure technique is used for a large cystic tumor in the pancreatic tail. The pancreas is mobilized, tail to body, and lifted from the retroperitoneum with a cloth tape. (*a*) pancreas, (*b*) cystic tumor, (*c*) spleen, (*d*) retroperitoneal space, (*e*) cloth tape

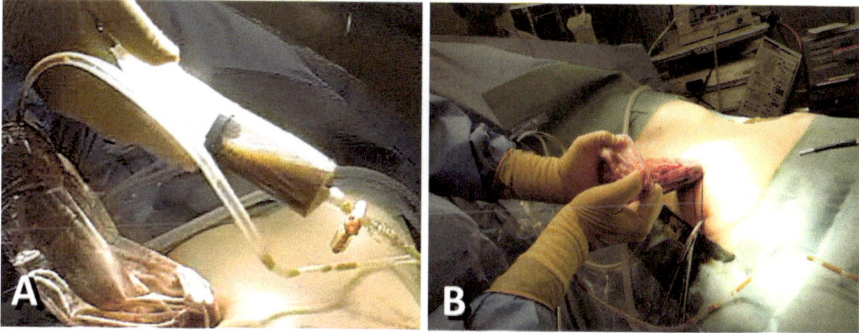

Fig. 23.4 The cystic contents are aspirated within the retrieval bag (**a**). Extraction of the pancreatic tail, the cyst, and the spleen from the umbilical wound (**b**)

together with the splenic vessels, is divided with the stapler. If minor bleeding from the arterial stump occurs, application of a metal clip is effective. If there is any oozing from the parenchymal stump, argon beam coagulation is useful. The12-mm trocar is then temporarily removed, and an EndoCatch II retrieval bag (Covidien) is introduced directly through a channel of the SILS™ Port. In the case of a cystic tumor, the fluid content is aspirated within the retrieval bag by direct puncture with an 18G needle through the umbilical wound; careful attention must be paid to avoid spillage. Then, through the umbilical wound, the spleen is pierced with Péan forceps to suction an aliquot of blood into the bag. These techniques facilitate extraction of the specimen through the umbilical wound without any need to extend the skin incision (Fig. 23.4a, b). A small silicone drain is placed in the splenic fossa, and the drain tube is extracted from the bottom of the umbilicus. Finally the umbilical wound is closed, with 0-Vicryl used for the fascia and 5-0 PDS used for subcutaneous suture.

23.5   SLS-DP with Splenic Preservation

The greater curvature of the stomach is suspended with two sutures of 2-0 Ethibond Excel (Ethicon, Cincinnati, OH, USA), which provides excellent exposure of the pancreas from body to tail and of the tumor behind the stomach after the omentum is opened (Fig. 23.5). This technique is applicable to any SLS-pancreatectomy including the SLS-DP described above. The tail of the pancreas is then carefully detached from the retroperitoneum and the splenic vessels. Careful attention should be paid to the treatment of the branches of the splenic vein and artery. A 5-mm LigaSure™V with a dolphin tip is useful for sealing and cutting the small branches. A balloon-type retractor (Cat Hand; Hakko Co., Nagano, Japan) provides excellent exposure by gentle retraction of the pancreas during the dissection. When the splenic artery and vein, and sometimes the inferior mesenteric vein, are well freed and exposed (Fig. 23.6), the pancreatic parenchyma is divided with use of the end-ostapler (60 mm in length, 4.8-mm staples; (Covidien) as performed in S-DP

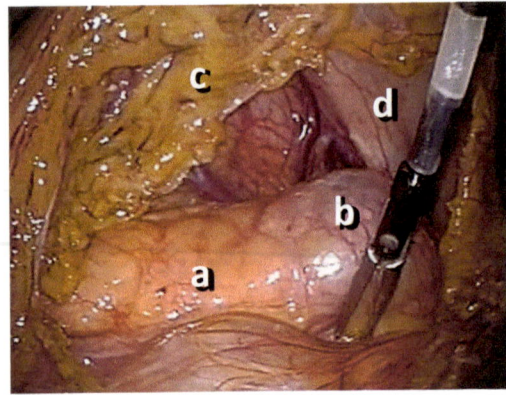

Fig. 23.5 The pancreas and the tumor behind the stomach are well visualized after the omentum is opened. The greater curvature of the stomach is suspended by two sutures. (**a**) Pancreas, (**b**) tumor, (**c**) omentum, (**d**) stomach

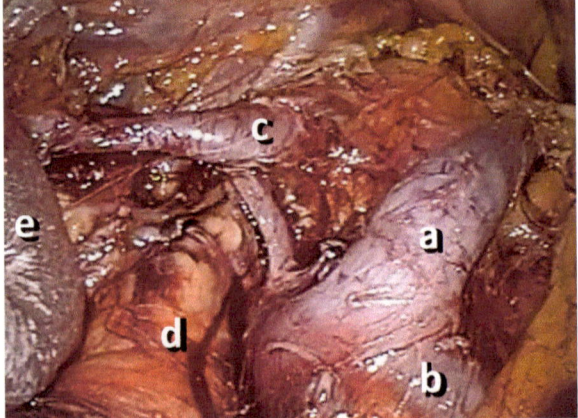

Fig. 23.6 The splenic vein (**a**), inferior mesenteric vein (**b**), and splenic artery (**c**) are well visualized behind the pancreas (**d**), which is retracted toward the right side with a balloon retractor (**e**)

Fig. 23.7 The umbilical
wound is almost invisible
1 month after surgery

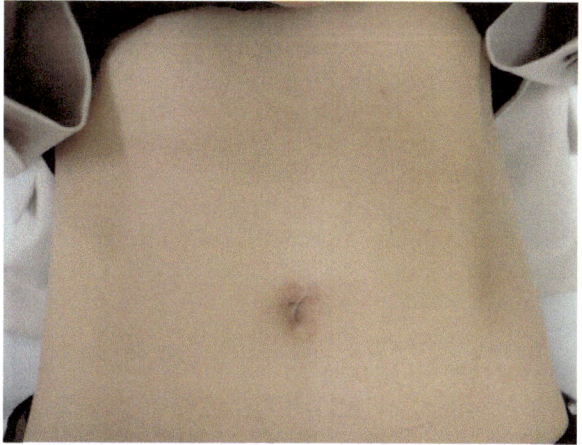

without splenic preservation. The resected specimen is extracted through the umbilical
site in a retrieval bag. A small silicone drain is placed in the splenic fossa through
the umbilical wound, which is closed in the same manner as described above. The
umbilical wound is nearly invisible 1 month after surgery (Fig. 23.7).

23.6   Tips and Tricks

In performing SLS-DP, one of the critical points is optimum exposure of the pancreas, which lies behind the stomach. This is achieved by sufficient organ retraction.
Because SLS tends to be a "solo surgery," additional instruments are not used by the
assistant to retract the surrounding organs and thus increase the working space. The
solution to this inconvenience is twofold: (1) making use of gravity by inclining or
tilting the operating table, (2) applying the tug-exposure technique [10] or the suspension technique by using stay sutures [14]. These two methods are effective for removing the obstructing organs from the operative field. When the reverse Tredelenburg
position is used together with a 60–90-degree tilt (right-side down), gravity pulls the
stomach down, putting the gastrosplenic and the splenocolic ligaments under strain,
and finally, placing the splenic pedicle under tension [19]. Furthermore, gravity pulls
the pancreas and the spleen downward, close to the umbilicus and thus assists in the
maintenance of good exposure throughout the operation.

23.7   Recommendations from the Author

SLS-DP is clearly an advanced and challenging procedure that should be performed
by a surgeon with plenty of experience in both LDP and a basic single-incision
procedure such as SLS cholecystectomy. Although some researchers have reported

decreased pain with SLS [20, 21], superiority of SLS over conventional laparoscopic surgery remains controversial [22]. The superiority might be limited to the cosmetic advantage. Therefore, a decision to perform SLS-DP must be made carefully by weighing the advantages and disadvantages in each case. Whether to introduce SLS-DP for malignant lesions such as invasive ductal cell carcinoma of the pancreas requires thorough investigation. Nevertheless, even the very notion of SLS-DP should alert surgeons to the possibility of reducing the number of the ports in any one case. Although surgeons usually use more than four trocars in conventional LDP [23, 24], they will be able to perform LDP comfortably using a SILS port™ with one or two additional access sites, minimizing abdominal wall disruption and superficial scarring. For safe and comfortable performance of SLS-DP, the energy devices, i.e., the coagulation shears and vessel sealing system, should be made flexible, like the articulating graspers and dissectors. We look to the future for further improvement in the instruments, which we consider crucial for safe SLS-DP. Finally, whenever technical difficulties and risk are encountered during SLS-DP despite application of the technical refinements described above, placement of additional trocars or conversion to open surgery should be done without delay. Several issues, such as the extent of invasiveness, the costs, and the SLS-DP learning curve relative to those of conventional multitrocar LDP, remain to be investigated, but the cosmetic benefit of SLS-DP is clear. Thus, we conclude that SLS-DP can be safely performed by experienced surgeons by applying appropriate technical refinements in selected cases.

References

1. Cuschieri A (1994) Laparoscopic surgery of the pancreas. J R Coll Surg Edinb 39:178–184
2. Gagner M, Pomp A, Herrera MF (1996) Early experience with laparoscopic resections of islet cell tumors. Surgery 120:1051–1054
3. Borja-Cacho D, Al-Refaie WB, Vickers SM et al (2009) Laparoscopic distal pancreatectomy. J Am Coll Surg 209:758–765
4. Hama T, Takifuji K, Uchiyama K et al (2008) Laparoscopic splenectomy is a safe and effective procedure for patients with splenomegaly due to portal hypertension. J Hepatobiliary Pancreat Surg 15:304–309
5. Esposito C (1998) One-trocar appendectomy in pediatric surgery. Surg Endosc 12:177–178
6. Piskun G, Rajpal S (1999) Transumbilical laparoscopic cholecystectomy utilizes no incisions outside the umbilicus. J Laparoendosc Adv Surg Tech A 9:361–364
7. Remzi FH, Kirat HT, Kaouk JH et al (2008) Single-port laparoscopy in colorectal surgery. Colorectal Dis 10:823–826
8. Reavis KM, Hinojosa MW, Smith BR et al (2008) Single-laparoscopic incision transabdominal surgery sleeve gastrectomy. Obes Surg 18:1492–1494
9. Ponsky LE, Cherullo EE, Sawyer M et al (2008) Single access site laparoscopic radical nephrectomy: initial clinical experience. J Endourol 22:663–666
10. Misawa T, Sakamoto T, Ito R et al (2011) Single-incision laparoscopic splenectomy using the "tug-exposure technique" in adults: results of ten initial cases. Surg Endosc 25:3222–3227
11. Barbaros U, Sümer A, Demirel T et al (2010) Single incision laparoscopic pancreas resection for pancreatic metastasis of renal cell carcinoma. JSLS 14:566–570

12. Kuroki T, Adachi T, Okamoto T et al (2011) Single-incision laparoscopic distal pancreatectomy. Hepatogastroenterology 58:1022–1024
13. Chang SK, Lomanto D, Mayasari M (2012) Single-port laparoscopic spleen preserving distal pancreatectomy. Minim Invasive Surg 2012:197429
14. Misawa T, Ito R, Futagawa Y, Fujiwara Y et al (2012) Single-incision laparoscopic distal pancreatectomy with or without splenic preservation: how we do it. Asian J Endosc Surg 5:195–199
15. Marangos IP, Buanes T, Røsok B et al (2012) Laparoscopic resection of exocrine carcinoma in central and distal pancreas results in a high rate of radical resections and long postoperative survival. Surgery 151:717–723
16. Misawa T, Shiba H, Usuba T et al (2007) Systemic inflammatory response syndrome after hand-assisted laparoscopic distal pancreatectomy. Surg Endosc 21:1446–1449
17. Takaori K, Tanigawa N (2007) Laparoscopic pancreatic resection: the past, present, and future. Surg Today 37:535–545
18. Misawa T, Shiba H, Usuba T et al (2008) Safe and quick distal pancreatectomy using a staggered six-row stapler. Am J Surg 195:115–118
19. Katkhouda N (1998) Advanced laparoscopic surgery: techniques and tips. Saunders, Philadelphia
20. Asakuma M, Hayashi M, Komeda K et al (2011) Impact of single-port cholecystectomy on postoperative pain. Br J Surg 98:991–995
21. Tsimoyiannis EC, Tsimogiannis KE, Pappas-Gogos G et al (2010) Different pain scores in single transumbilical incision laparoscopic cholecystectomy versus classic laparoscopic cholecystectomy: a randomized controlled trial. Surg Endosc 24:1842–1848
22. Luna RA, Nogueira DB, Varela PS et al (2013) A prospective, randomized comparison of pain, inflammatory response, and short-term outcomes between single port and laparoscopic cholecystectomy. Surg Endosc 27:1254–1259
23. Kneuertz PJ, Patel SH, Chu CK et al (2012) Laparoscopic distal pancreatectomy: trends and lessons learned through an 11-year experience. J Am Coll Surg 215:167–176
24. Cuschieri A, Jakimowicz JJ, van Spreeuwel J (1996) Laparoscopic distal 70 % pancreatectomy and splenectomy for chronic pancreatitis. Ann Surg 223:280–285

Chapter 24
Pancreatico-Jejunostomy

Chinnusamy Palanivelu and Palanisamy Senthilnathan

Abstract Reduced port laparoscopic surgery (RPLS) is now being performed for various procedures usually done by the conventional laparoscopic approach. Advanced procedures are now possible with RPLS, and pancreatic surgery is no exception. Chronic calcifying pancreatitis with dilated duct and intraductal calculus is one such condition wherein for properly selected patients lateral pancreaticojejunostomy (LPJ) can be safely performed by this approach. Though many access devices are available, the single incision multipuncture technique allows performing this procedure without compromising the patient's safety while at the same time facilitating intracorporeal suturing. We use three trocars through a 2.5-cm umbilical incision that are spaced 1 cm from each other. A long scope with an axial light cable connection and varying length of routine instruments make this procedure ergonomically sound. Varying retraction techniques are used, including hooking the stomach to the anterior abdominal wall. Key steps of this procedure include complete exposure of pancreas, removal of the entire stone from the pancreatic duct, and Roux-en-Y reconstruction. The wound is closed with facial sutures. Our preliminary experience shows that single incision laparoscopic LPJ is feasible and safe when performed by an experienced laparoscopic surgeon. It has a cosmetic advantage over laparoscopic LPJ.

Keywords Chronic calcific pancreatitis • Lateral pancreaticojejunostomy • Reduced port laparoscopic surgery

C. Palanivelu (✉) • P. Senthilnathan
GEM Hospital and Research Centre, 45 Pankaj Mill Road,
Ramanathapuram, Coimbatore, Tamil Nadu, India
e-mail: info@geminstitute.in; Senthilnathan94@yahoo.com

T. Mori and G. Dapri (eds.), *Reduced Port Laparoscopic Surgery*,
DOI 10.1007/978-4-431-54601-6_24, © Springer Japan 2014

293

24.1 Introduction

Reduced port laparoscopic surgery (RPLS) is now being performed for various procedures usually done by the conventional laparoscopic approach. It has gained tremendous attention in the past few years, and pancreatic surgery is no exception. Though the literature on reduced port pancreatic surgery is sparse, we believe this surgery has the potential to improve cosmesis, decrease parietal trauma, and hence, result in better patient satisfaction compared to standard multiport laparoscopy [1, 2]. Many see it as a natural progression to minimize the number of incisions. The acceptance among patients is high when they are told that one incision will be used instead of four or five.

Lateral pancreaticojejunostomy (LPJ) is one such procedure that can be performed in a select set of patients with chronic obstructive calcifying pancreatitis with dilated duct and intraductal calculus. We published a series of NOTES: transvaginal endoscopic cholecystectomy in eight patients using an endoscope and conventional endoscopic instruments, and we took a new step in minimal invasive surgery towards making it scarless [3]. Soon after, we published the first report on laparoendoscopic single site lateral pancreaticojejunostomy (LESS LPJ) for chronic calcifying pancreatitis with dilated pancreatic duct, using conventional laparoscopic instruments [4].

24.2 Indications for LPJ

Chronic calcifying pancreatitis is a disease found in tropical countries, with high prevalence in regions like southern India [5]. The pattern of disease presentation differs from that of the west, as it shows more duct dilatation and intraductal calculus than mass formation, a sign that is more typical of alcoholic pancreatitis. Even though chronic pancreatitis is mainly managed with drugs, surgery is required in select groups of patients. In symptomatic patients with dilated duct and intraductal calculus, which acts as a surrogate for increased intraductal pressure, decompression surgeries are indicated. Chronic pain and intractable steatorrhoea form the majority of indications. In 1958, Puestow and Gillesby proposed longitudinal decompression of the duct into the Roux limb of the jejunum [6], a process that was later modified by Partington and Rochelle by describing longitudinal side-to-side anastomosis [7]. It relieves the ductal hypertension that is considered one of the main etiology of pain in chronic pancreatitis and, at the same time, preserves endocrine and exocrine function [8]. Moreover, LPJ improves the survival of patients with chronic calcifying pancreatitis [9].

Palanivelu et al. [10] have already reported that the same result can be achieved by the laparoscopic approach.

24.3   Specific Considerations for RPLS LPJ

Lateral pancreaticojejunostomy (LPJ) is a relatively complex procedure to be performed by RPLS. However, using the reduced port approach requires even more expertise, stricter case selection, and other conditions. Though these criteria are not standardized and vary from center to center, the following items are to be considered before opting for RPLS LPJ:

1. BMI less than 30 kg/m^2
2. No previous upper abdominal surgeries
3. Pancreatic duct diameter more than 10 mm
4. No obvious inflammatory mass in the pancreatic parenchyma
5. No evidence of portal hypertension

24.4   Setup

The patient is placed in the supine position with legs split (Fig. 24.1). The table is tilted in different directions to gain gravity-aided exposure when required. The need for an additional port for retraction can be avoided by liberal use of gravity and

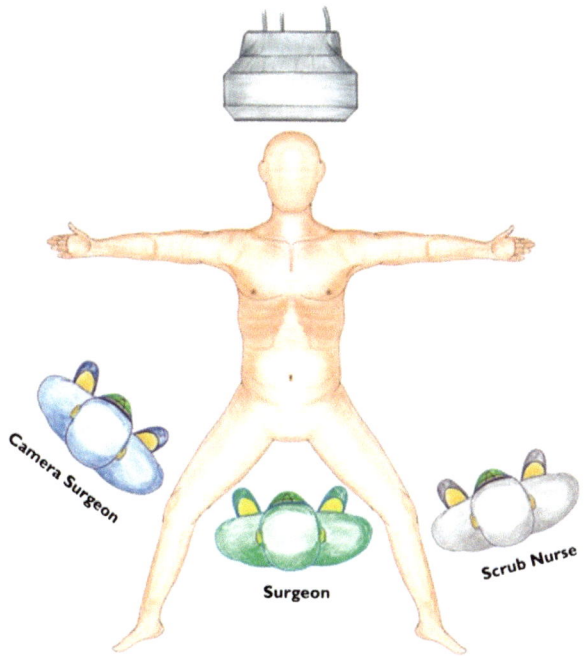

Fig. 24.1 The patient is placed in the supine position with legs split

some of the novel retraction techniques described below. The surgeon stands between the legs of the patient during the initial exposure of the pancreas and later moves to either side for duct opening and anastomosis. The camera surgeon stands on the right side initially and changes place depending on the surgeon's position. Usually one monitor at the head end of the patient is sufficient for this procedure, with slight change in direction of the screen.

24.5 Access Devices and Instrumentation

RPLS can be performed in many ways using different access devices and specially designed instruments. These devices are generally expensive and cumbersome to use, increasing the cost and prolonging the operative time. However, these short-comings can be overcome with the single-incision multi-puncture technique. A curvilinear 2.5-cm incision is made around the umbilicus and deepened up to the fascia. The area surrounding the fascia is cleaned by blunt and sharp dissection. A Veress needle is inserted through the fascia into the peritoneal cavity, and a pneumoperitoneum of 12 mmHg is created using carbon dioxide gas. One 10-mm and two 5-mm ports are inserted through the fascia, making multiple punctures via the same incision and maintaining 1 cm distance between these ports. If needed, a 0.5-cm slit on either side of the curvilinear incision can be made to achieve this 1-cm distance between the trocars. This arrangement provides a narrow triangulation for the working instruments, facilitating intracorporeal suturing, a vital prerequisite for this procedure (Fig. 24.2). The 10-mm port is placed first in the center of the incision, and one 5-mm port is placed on each side at 2 o'clock and 10 o'clock. Furthermore, to reduce the clashing of instruments, two modifications are incorporated. First, instruments of different lengths are used for both hands which makes them to work at different distances from the abdomen. Second, a long telescope with a co-axial light

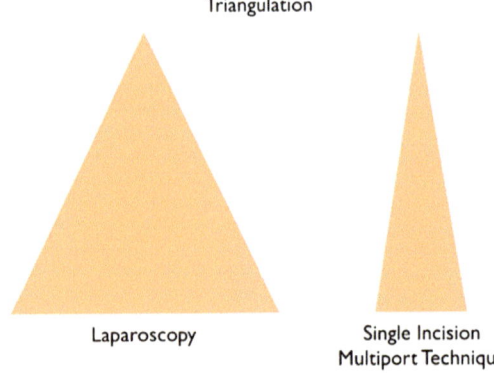

Fig. 24.2 Achieving narrow triangulation in single-incision multiport technique

Fig. 24.3 Instruments of different lengths with a long telescope with a co-axial light cable is used to further reduce the crowding and clashing

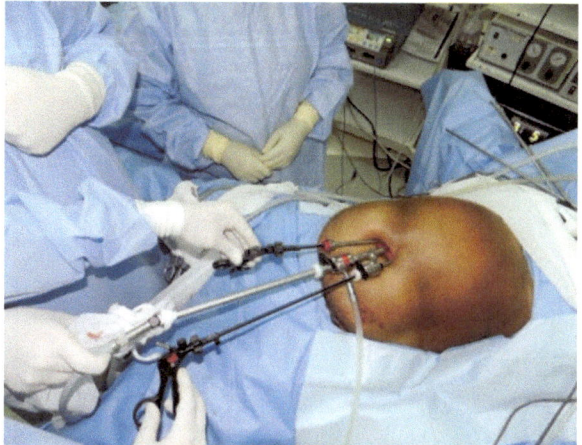

cable is used to further reduce the crowding and clashing (Fig. 24.3). Using an endostapler, the 10-mm port is changed to a 12-mm, and a 5-mm scope is used briefly. No extra ports (or needlescopic ports) are needed for this procedure.

24.6 Retraction of Tissues

The retraction of tissues is a contentious issue in RPLS. Apart from the liberal use of gravity, there are many methods for retracting the stomach and liver. Liver retraction is usually not required during LPJ, but in the case of a large left lateral segment, sometimes it is necessary to retract the liver. We fix a piece of corrugated drain to sutures at both ends to lift up the liver. Retraction of the stomach, on the other hand, is critical to expose the entire length of pancreas. This is done using retracting sutures placed in the posterior wall of the stomach close to the greater curvature. The suture ends are then brought out through a suture passer. This arrangement hooks the stomach to the anterior abdominal wall (Fig. 24.4).

24.7 Operative Technique

The lesser sac is entered by dividing the gastrocolic omentum using ultrasonic shears, and the stomach is separated from the pancreas. The stomach is retracted as previously described. The pancreas is exposed completely after dividing the right gastroepiploic vessels. The duct is then opened from head to tail using ultrasonic shears. The location of the pancreatic duct is confirmed using needle aspiration or, in difficult situations, an intra-operative ultrasound probe. Intraductal stones are

Fig. 24.4 Stomach hooked to anterior abdominal wall

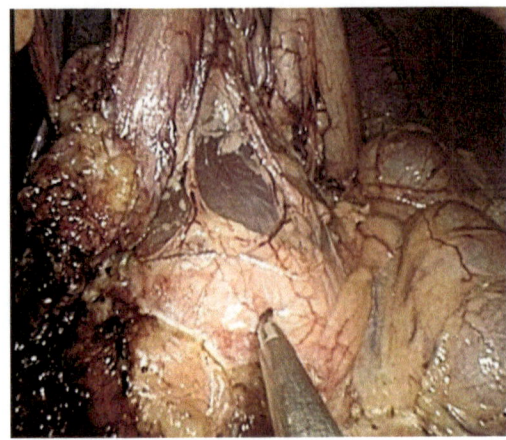

Fig. 24.5 Intraductal stones are cleared completely along its entire length

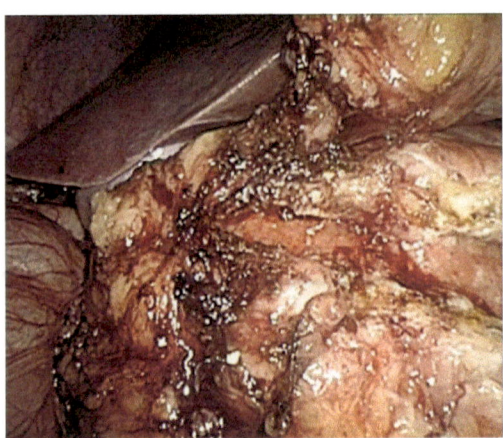

cleared completely along the entire length of the duct (Fig. 24.5). Care must be taken to open the duct in the head region, a process that requires safe parenchymal division to avoid bleeding. From our experience in laparoscopic surgery, we have learnt that the most common complication during the procedure is bleeding from the edge of duct opening. If branches from the gastroduodenal arcade are damaged, they can be suture ligated, as using cautery alone may be insufficient. Ultrasonic shears are best to open the duct. The entire procedure is similar to already prevalent techniques for LPJ, except for the type of access and stomach elevation. The single-incision technique requires no compromise, and the entire dissection is performed under clear display of the surgical field.

The jejunum is divided 30 cm from the ligament of Treitz using an endostapler. The distal limb is taken to the lesser sac by creating a window in transverse

Fig. 24.6 Duct to mucosa anastomosis

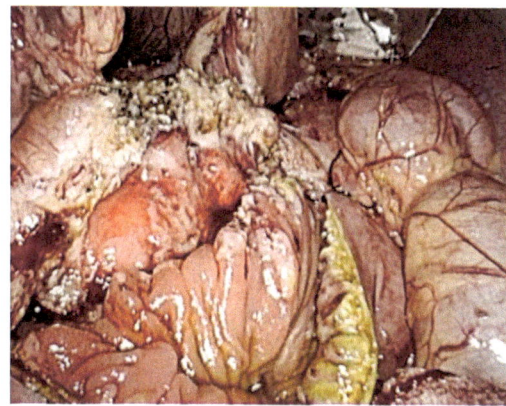

Fig. 24.7 Skin closed at the end of the surgery

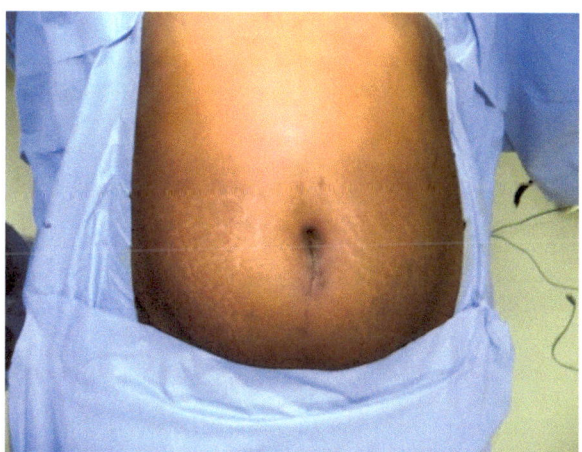

mesocolon. Enterotomy is made on jejunum according to the size of the open pancreatic duct. Side-to-side LPJ is created using a continuous 2-0 PDS suture, taking care to approximate the pancreatic duct to the jejunal mucosa (Fig. 24.6). Because of the narrow triangulation between the instruments, to-and-fro movement instead of left-and-right movement facilitates intracorporeal suturing. The first posterior layer is sutured from the left to the right side, and then the anterior layer is closed. The stapled jejuno-jejunostomy is made distally.

All the defects in the fascia are repaired using polypropylene 1 suture. The skin is closed using polyglactin 3-0 subcutaneous suture (Fig. 24.7). Local anesthetic bupivacaine 0.25 % is injected locally at the end of surgery.

24.8 Post-operative Care

Post-operative pain is managed by using diclofenac suppository. An oral diet is usually started on the first post-operative day. Generally the patient is discharged from the hospital on the third or fourth day, as in the conventional laparoscopic approach. After 1 month, the wound is hardly noticeable.

24.9 Conclusion

As with any new surgical technique, there is a learning curve. Some golden rules of laparoscopy need to be broken in order to perform RPLS. For example, all the working instruments and the camera must be inserted into one incision, therefore losing the basic principle of triangulation to an extent. For an inexperienced laparoscopic surgeon, this may lead to increased risk of intraoperative complications. Visualization also may not be optimal at all times during the procedure. Thus, surgeons must take caution. Our preliminary experience shows that RPLS LPJ is feasible and safe when performed by an experienced laparoscopic surgeon. It has a cosmetic advantage over laparoscopic LPJ. However, it remains to be seen if this technique offers additional advantages of decreased analgesia, decreased hospital stay, or cost effectiveness.

References

1. Rieger NA, Lam FF (2010) Single-incision laparo-scopically assisted colectomy using standard laparoscopic instrumentation. Surg Endosc 24:888–890
2. Ostrowitz MB, Eschete D, Zemon H, DeNoto G (2009) Robotic-assisted single-incision right col-ectomy: early experience. Int J Med Robot 5:465–470
3. Palanivelu C, Rajan PS, Rangarajan M et al (2009) NOTES: transvaginal endoscopic cholecystectomy in humans – preliminary report of a case series. Am J Gastroenterol 104:843–847
4. Palanivelu C (2011) Laparoendoscopic single-site lateral pancreaticojejunostomy. Gastrointestinal and Laparoscopic Surgery, GEM Hospital, Coimbatore, India. Pancreatology 11(5):500–505
5. Geevarghese PJ (1985) Calcified pancreatitis. Varghese Publishing House, Bombay
6. Puestow CB, Gillesby WJ (1958) Retrograde surgical drainage of pancreas for chronic relapsing pancreatitis. AMA Arch Surg 76:898
7. Partington PF, Rochelle RE (1960) Modified Puestow procedure for retrograde drainage of the pancreatic duct. Ann Surg 152:1037
8. Isaji S (2009) Has the Partington procedure for chronic pancreatitis become a thing of the past? A review of the evidence. J Hepatobiliary Pancreat Sci 17:763–769
9. Sakorafas GH, Zobolas B (2001) Lateral pancreatojejunostomy in the surgical management of chronic pancreatitis: current concepts and future perspectives. Department of Surgery, Greece. Dig Liver Dis 33(2):187–191
10. Palanivelu C, Rajan PS, Kumar KS, Parthasarathi R (2001) Role of laparoscopy in pancreatic surgery. Bombay Hosp J 43:119–123

Chapter 25
Adrenalectomy

Riccardo Autorino, Marco De Sio, and Abhay Rane

Abstract Multiple series have demonstrated the benefits of laparoscopic adrenalectomy techniques when compared to open surgery. Laparoendoscopic single-site surgery (LESS) for adrenal gland has been effectively performed for a number of indications and a wide variety of approaches have been described. That said, there are still obvious technical difficulties associated with LESS and, in particular, LESS adrenalectomy is regarded as a highly challenging procedure. "Reduced port laparoscopic surgery" has been implemented as a way of moving forward towards the path of *scarless* surgery by overcoming the constraints of LESS. Herein we describe the techniques for reduced port laparoscopic adrenalectomy (RPLA), in both supine and prone position. As far as the approach is concerned, both transperitoneal and retroperitoneal techniques have demonstrated similar outcomes with appropriate patient selection criteria. The anterior transperitoneal route is used with the patient is supine position. This technique can present few advantages, including easy positioning of the patient on the operative table, clear evidence of anatomical landmarks, wider exposure of the adrenal gland, early ligature of the main adrenal vein before gland manipulation, the possibility to perform a bilateral procedure, easy immediate conversion to open in the case of major bleeding. Adrenalectomy with the patient in the prone position can also be used. Overall, RPLA represents a viable option in the surgical management of adrenal diseases. Its main feature is represented by the possibility of restoring the triangulation needed to optimize working angles while minimizing the scar associated with the procedure.

R. Autorino
Glickman Urological and Kidney Institute, Cleveland Clinic, Cleveland, OH, USA

Second University of Naples, Naples, Italy

M. De Sio
Second University of Naples, Naples, Italy

A. Rane (✉)
Department of Urology, East Surrey Hospital, Redhill, Surrey, UK
e-mail: a.rane@btinternet.com

T. Mori and G. Dapri (eds.), *Reduced Port Laparoscopic Surgery*,
DOI 10.1007/978-4-431-54601-6_25, © Springer Japan 2014

Keywords Adrenalectomy • Prone position • Reduced port laparoscopy • Supine position

25.1 Introduction

Since 1992 [1], laparoscopic adrenalectomy (LA) has been performed using different approaches, including the anterior [2] and lateral [3] transperitoneal approach, as well as via the lateral [4] and posterior [5] retroperitoneal approach. Multiple series have demonstrated the benefits of LA techniques, specifically the decreased requirements for analgesics, improved patient satisfaction, and shorter hospital stay and recovery time when compared to open surgery [6].

Over the last 5 years, a step towards *scarless* surgery has been made with the introduction and development of single-site or single-port laparoscopic techniques [7], comprehensively defined as laparoendoscopic single site surgery (LESS) [8, 9].

LESS adrenal surgery has been effectively performed for a number of indications and a wide variety of approaches (transperitoneal versus retroperitoneal, multichannel trocar versus multiple ports, trans- or extraumbilical) have been described [10]. That said, there are still obvious technical difficulties associated with LESS surgery and, in particular, LESS adrenalectomy is regarded as a highly challenging procedure [11].

In general, laparoscopic surgery is done with one hand performing dissection and the other hand providing traction, thus making it necessary to coordinate bimanual motions. The difficulties encountered in LESS surgery mainly arise from the "sword fighting" of the instruments. Bent instruments can be used to minimize this "fighting", but the angle of the bent instruments needs to be adjusted, and these maneuvers require quite a bit of time. Moreover, because the distance from the port to the tissue in the transumbilical approach is longer than in the conventional laparoscopic approach, the approach becomes more tangential in direction in LESS.

Thus, the concept of "reduced port laparoscopic surgery (RPLS)" has been implemented [12], and seen as a way of moving forward towards the path of *scarless* surgery by overcoming the constraints of LESS (Fig. 25.1). Several series have been reported in the field of general surgery [13, 14], whereas limited evidence is available in urology [15, 16].

Herein we describe the techniques for reduced port laparoscopic adrenalectomy (RPLA), in both supine and prone position.

25.2 Surgical Indications

As a general principle, all eligible laparoscopic surgery patients may be considered for LESS depending on surgeons' own experience. The same criterion can be used for RPLS (Table 25.1). When starting out with a new technique, patient selection

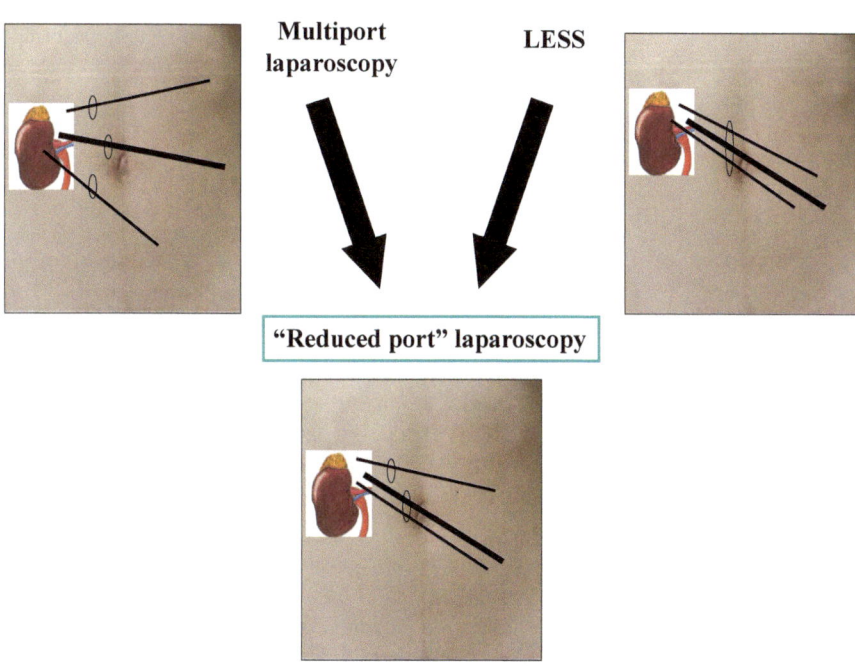

Multiport laparoscopy

LESS

"Reduced port" laparoscopy

Fig. 25.1 Overcoming the challenges of LESS: the concept of RPLS

Table 25.1 Indications to RPLS (adapted from [10])

Factor	Feature	Initial indication	Advanced indication
Adrenal mass	Size	<4 cm	Up to 10 cm
	Type	Nonfuncitoning and functioning adenoma	Adrenal metastasis; pheochromocytoma; adrenocortical carcinoma
	Number	Single	Multiple (including bilateral)
	Stage[a]	Localized	Localized
Patient	BMI	Non-obese	Obese
	Previous surgery	No	Yes

[a]For malignant masses

criteria are expected to be stringent. Disease as well as patient features should considered. With growing experience, indications can be expanded to include more challenging cases, which is likely to be facilitated by a RPLS versus a pure LESS approach. In general, there should be a low threshold for conversion to standard laparoscopy, or even open surgery if necessary.

As far as the approach is concerned, both transperitoneal and retroperitoneal techniques have demonstrated similar outcomes with appropriate patient selection criteria. Overall, patients with smaller tumors and previous abdominal operation seem to be more suitable for the retroperitoneal approaches for the prone approach.

On the other hand it can become more challenging to proceed with a retroperitoneal approach in patients with a high body mass index and thick posterior back soft tissue planes.

25.3 Technique

25.3.1 RPLA: Transperitoneal Approach in Supine Position

The anterior transperitoneal route is used with the patient is supine position [17]. This technique can present few advantages, including easy positioning of the patient on the operative table, clear evidence of anatomical landmarks, wider exposure of the adrenal gland, early ligature of the main adrenal vein before gland manipulation, the possibility to perform a bilateral procedure, easy immediate conversion to open in the case of major bleeding.

A 2.5-cm vertical incision is made within the umbilical ring, through which a SILS™ port (Covidien, New Haven, CT, USA). In alternative, other commercially available multi-channel ports can be used, such as the Triport™ (Olympus, Tokyo, Japan) or standard trocars placed within the same skin incision but through different fascial incisions (in this case a 5-mm nonbladed trocar can be placed side-by-side with the camera trocar). Besides the umbilical site, a 3-mm or a 5-mm nonbladed trocar is then placed along the anterior axillary line. This access site is used for the left or the right hand depending on the site of the surgery. A variety of instruments can be used depending on surgeon's preference, including vessel-sealing devices such as Ligasure™ (Covidien) or Harmonic™ scalpel (Ethicon, Cincinnati, OH, USA).

The surgical strategy follows a conventional transperitoneal adrenalectomy. Once the white line of Toldt's fascia is incised, the junction of the colonic mesentery and Gerota's fascia is identified. This plane is then dissected to the renal vein. The adrenal veins are identified, clipped with 5-mm Hem-O-Lok clips (Teleflex Medical, Research Triangle Park, NC, USA), and divided. A vessel-sealing device can be used to complete the adrenal dissection. The specimen is extracted by removing the 10-mm bag through the enlarged paraumbilical trocar site.

25.3.2 RPLA: Retroperitoneal Approach in Prone Position

Adrenalectomy with the patient in the prone position (and with moderately bent hip joints) has been detailed for both standard retroperitoneoscopy [18] and single-site retroperitoneoscopy [19]. The same principles are used for the RPLS technique. Regardless the technique, besides the number of access points, the procedure remains the same.

Initially, a 1.5 cm transverse incision just below the tip of the 12th rib is performed. After having prepared the subcutaneous and muscle layer by sharp and blunt dissection, the retroperitoneal space was easily accessible by digital perforation of the dorsolumbar fascia. A small cavity is prepared digitally for balloon dilatation with a special distension balloon trocar, which is insufflated under endoscopic control for a few minutes. After removing the distension trocar, a 5-mm standard trocar is introduced with internal finger guidance 4–5 cm laterally (medioaxillary line) to the initial incision site. Thus safe trocar placement is possible without visual control. Finally, a blunt trocar with an inflatable balloon and an adjustable sleeve is introduced into the initial incision site and blocked. Pneumoretroperitoneum is created by high (20 mmHg) CO_2 pressure. Retroperitoneoscopy is performed by a 10-mm 30° endo-scope which is introduced into the port. The endoscope itself can eventually allow a step-by-step creation of the retroperitoneal space by disruption of the Gerota's fascia and by pushing the retroperitoneal fatty tissue bluntly downwards. Thereby, the area of the adrenal gland and the upper renal pole are exposed.

As the next step, a 5-mm bipolar scissor (LigaSure® (Covidien)) can be introduced through the lateral port so that following steps of dissection are completely performed in a single hand technique with the non-dominant hand holding the camera.

First of all, the upper pole of the kidney is mobilized. Dissection of the adrenal gland begins from lateral to medial on the backside of the peritoneum identifying the lower pole of the adrenal gland. On the right side, the adrenal arteries cross the vena cava medially posteriorly. These vessels are separated with a bipolar scissor. By lift-ing up the adrenal gland, the inferior vena cava is visualized posteriorly in its retro-peritoneal cranial segment. The short suprarenal vein thus becomes clearly visible running postero-laterally. This vessel is followed for a length of 0.5–1 cm and divided by bipolar scissor. Eventually, clips can be used for the main adrenal vein. Preparation of the right adrenal gland is completed by lateral and cranial dissection. For the left-sided adrenalectomy, an extended mobilization of the upper pole of the kidney is essential as the lower pole of the adrenal gland lies in front of the kidney. Thereafter, the inferior part of the gland can be visualized and dissected. The typical main left adrenal vein joins the diaphragmatic vein between the upper pole of the kidney and the spine. After dissection of the adrenal vein with the bipolar scissor the gland is mobilized. In case of partial adrenalectomy, extent of dissection depends on the localization of the neoplasia. The parenchyma is divided with the bipolar scissor.

To prevent injury of the adrenal capsule an en-bloc resection of the gland with the surrounding fatty tissue must always be pursued. The completely mobilized tis-sue is placed in a retrieval bag, which is inserted directly through the skin incision and pulled through the initial sub-costal incision after removal of camera and its port. After specimen removal, the surgical field is checked for hemostasis.

An alternative option in the disposition of the ports is to remove the initially placed 10-mm port and place in the same site a 5-mm port and a 3.5-mm port inserted through the same incision. Then, a 3.3-mm 30° endoscope is used and the 5-mm port, which lies on the same axis of the camera mini-port, can be used for suction or counter-traction.

25.4 Conclusions

RPLA represents a viable option in the surgical management of adrenal diseases. Its main feature is represented by the possibility of restoring the triangulation needed to optimize working angles while minimizing the scar associated with the procedure. The technique can be regarded as a safe way to move towards the more challenging LESS, whose intrinsic limitations can translate into a steep learning curve. Further clinical research is warranted to define the role of both RPLS and LESS in the advancing field of minimally invasive adrenal surgery.

References

1. Gagner M, Lacroix A, Bolté E (1992) Laparoscopic adrenalectomy in Cushing's syndrome and pheochromocytoma. N Engl J Med 327(14):1033
2. Rassweiler JJ, Henkel TO, Potempa DM, Coptcoat M, Alken P (1993) The technique of trans-peritoneal laparoscopic nephrectomy, adrenalectomy and nephroureterectomy. Eur Urol 23(4):425–430
3. Gagner M, Pomp A, Heniford BT, Pharand D, Lacroix A (1997) Laparoscopic adrenalectomy: lessons learned from 100 consecutive procedures. Ann Surg 226(3):238–246
4. Gasman D, Droupy S, Koutani A et al (1998) Laparoscopic adrenalectomy: the retroperitoneal approach. J Urol 159(6):1816–1820
5. Baba S, Miyajima A, Uchida A, Asanuma H, Miyakawa A, Murai M (1997) A posterior lumbar approach for retroperitoneoscopic adrenalectomy: assessment of surgical efficacy. Urology 50(1):19–24
6. Gumbs AA, Gagner M (2006) Laparoscopic adrenalectomy. Best Pract Res Clin Endocrinol Metab 20(3):483–499
7. Rané A, Rao P, Rao P (2008) Single-port-access nephrectomy and other laparoscopic urologic procedures using a novel laparoscopic port (R-port). Urology 72(2):260–263
8. Gill IS, Advincula AP, Aron M et al (2010) Consensus statement of the consortium for laparo-endoscopic single-site surgery. Surg Endosc 24(4):762–768
9. Autorino R, Cadeddu JA, Desai MM et al (2011) Laparoendoscopic single-site and natural orifice transluminal endoscopic surgery in urology: a critical analysis of the literature. Eur Urol 59(1):26–45
10. Rane A, Cindolo L, Schips L, De Sio M, Autorino R (2012) Laparoendoscopic single site (LESS) adrenalectomy: technique and outcomes. World J Urol 30(5):597–604
11. Ishida M, Miyajima A, Takeda T, Hasegawa M, Kikuchi E, Oya M (2013) Technical difficulties of transumbilical laparoendoscopic single-site adrenalectomy: comparison with conventional laparoscopic adrenalectomy. World J Urol 31(1):199–203
12. Curcillo PG 2nd, Podolsky ER, King SA (2011) The road to reduced port surgery: from single big incisions to single small incisions, and beyond. World J Surg 35(7):1526–1531
13. Costedio MM, Aytac E, Gorgun E, Kiran RP, Remzi FH (2012) Reduced port versus conventional laparoscopic total proctocolectomy and ileal J pouch-anal anastomosis. Surg Endosc 26(12):3495–3499
14. Monclova JL, Targarona EM, Vidal P et al (2013) Single incision versus reduced port splenectomy—searching for the best alternative to conventional laparoscopic splenectomy. Surg Endosc 27(3):895–902
15. Cho HJ, Choi YS, Bae WJ et al (2012) Two-port laparoscopic donor nephrectomy with simple retraction technique. Urology 80(6):1379–1382

16. Sumino Y, Nakano D, Mori K, Nomura T, Sato F, Mimata H (2011) Left transperitoneal adrenalectomy with a laparoendoscopic single-site surgery combined technique: initial case reports. Case Rep Med 2011:651380
17. Lezoche E, Guerrieri M, Crosta F, Paganini A, D'Ambrosio G, Lezoche G, Campagnacci R (2008) Perioperative results of 214 laparoscopic adrenalectomies by anterior transperitoneal approach. Surg Endosc 22(2):522–526
18. Walz MK, Alesina PF, Wenger FA et al (2006) Posterior retroperitoneoscopic adrenalectomy–results of 560 procedures in 520 patients. Surgery 140(6):943–948
19. Walz MK, Alesina PF (2009) Single access retroperitoneoscopic adrenalectomy (SARA)–one step beyond in endocrine surgery. Langenbecks Arch Surg 394(3):447–450

Chapter 26
Right Colectomy

Giovanni Dapri

Abstract With the advent of natural orifices translumena endoscopic surgery (NOTES) and single-port/single-incision laparoscopy (SPL/SLS), minimally invasive surgery recently underwent to an impressive evolution, mainly improving the cosmesis and reducing the abdominal wall trauma. A new concept to be less invasive in minimally invasive surgery started to be popular and named reduced port laparoscopic surgery (RPLS). A reduced number of trocars associated to a reduced size of each trocar and instrument chracterizes this new technique.

During conventional multiport laparoscopic colorectal surgery, the specimen has to be retrieved, hence an enlargement of the trocar or a new opening of the abdominal wall is necessary. With NOTES, surgeons started to consider the natural orifices to remove the specimen from the abdomen (vagina/rectum), and with SPL/SLS to minimize the abdominal trauma and to improve the cosmesis.

In this chapter a right colectomy is described using the suprapubic scar as the main access to perform RPLS and also to remove the specimen from the abdomen at the end. This access remains under the bikini line, hence cosmetically acceptable. The procedure is performed using three reusable trocars inserted close each others in the same suprapubic incision, and curved reusable instruments. Each step is represented by specific drawings showing the internal triangulation, which characterizes the conventional multiport laparoscopy, and the external surgeon's ergonomy.

Keywords Right colectomy • Reduced port laparoscopy • Single-access • Single-incision • Single-port • Single-site

Giovanni Dapri (✉)
Department of Gastrointestinal Surgery, European School
of Laparoscopic Surgery, Saint-Pierre University Hospital, Brussels, Belgium
e-mail: giovanni@dapri.net

T. Mori and G. Dapri (eds.), *Reduced Port Laparoscopic Surgery*,
DOI 10.1007/978-4-431-54601-6_26, © Springer Japan 2014

26.1   Introduction

During reduced port laparoscopic surgery (RPLS), the main access-site used is usually the umbilicus, because it represents the embryonic natural orifice, which avoids a new incision in the abdomen [1]. The umbilicus can also be used during solid organs RPLS, because the specimen is morcellated at the access-site, maintaining a satisfactory cosmetic outcome.

In colorectal surgery, the access-site has to be open enough to remove the specimen, which oncologically varies in dimensions. As well, the mesocolon with all the lymphnodes has to be maintained intact. For these reasons during colorectal RPLS a different umbilical access-site has to be considered.

During conventional multiport laparoscopic colorectal surgery, an abdominal opening is necessary to remove the specimen, and frequently the suprapubic area is chosen [2]. Hence, the suprapubic scar can be used as the main access-site for the entire procedure of RPLS, which is finally also cosmetically acceptable because it remains under the bikini line. Furthermore, the suprapubic access, traditionally used for cesarean section, is known to be less painful [3]. Then, the risk of incisional hernia associated with the transumbilical surgery [4], is most likely avoided, because of easier opening of the fascial edges, predominance of muscle-splitting incisions and final closure of the fascia multiple layers [5, 6].

In this chapter the technique of right colectomy is described using the suprapubic scar as the main access-site of the entire procedure and as the abdominal window to remove the specimen. Three reusable trocars are inserted close each other in the same suprapubic incision, to accomodate curved reusable instruments. A 10-mm standard optical system is used and inserted in the central trocar, permitting to respect the two basic rules of conventional multiport laparoscopy: the video screen, the operative field and the surgeon's head located on the same axis [7], and the optical system in the middle as the bisector of the working triangulation formed by two ancillary effectors [8]. During the step of the intracorporeal anastomosis, a 5-mm long scope is adopted to permit the insertion of the linear stapler through the central trocar. Obviously, an intracorporeal anastomosis is required, which moreover avoids the potential traction of the mesentery and of the transverse mesocolon. Finally the positioning of the operative table is considered as the main assistant help and in case of perioperative difficulties or complications, an additional 1.8-mm trocarless grasping forceps according to DAPRI (Karl Storz-Endoskope, Tuttlingen, Germany) is inserted in the left hypocondrium under the rib.

26.2   Technique

26.2.1   Patient and Team Positioning

The patient is placed in a supine position, with the arms along side the body and the legs apart; a urinary catheter is inserted. The surgeon stands between the patient's legs, and the camera assistant to the patient's left. The scrub-nurse stands to the

Fig. 26.1 Patient and team
positioning

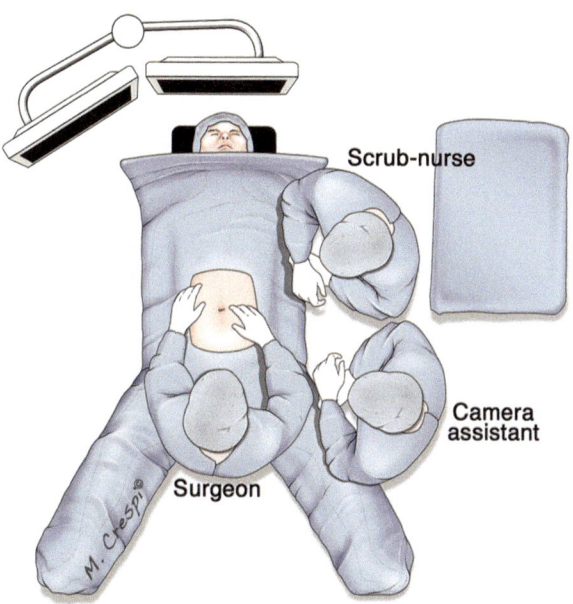

Scrub-nurse

Camera
assistant

Surgeon

M. Crespi

camera assistant's right. The video monitor is placed in front of the surgeon and
camera assistant (Fig. 26.1).

26.2.2   RPLS

A 3.5 cm transverse skin incision is made in the midline, 1 cm above the pubic
symphysis (Fig. 26.2). The underlying fascia is divided in a transverse fashion for
1.5 cm, which expose the rectus abdominis muscle. Anterior and posterior flaps are
developed in the avascular plane separating the fascia from the underlying muscle.
A purse-string suture using PDS 1 is placed in the fascia. The peritoneum is entered
through the midline with a 1 cm incision, and a new purse-string suture using Vicryl
1 is placed. An 11-mm reusable metallic (or a 12-mm disposable) trocar is inserted
into both purse-string sutures in order to accomodate a 10-mm, 30° rigid and standard length scope (Karl Storz-Endoskope), and the pneumoperitoneum is created.
Two 6-mm reusable flexible trocars (Karl Storz-Endoskope) are inserted at 3 and 9
o'clock position in the respect of the patient head, outside the purse-string sutures
(Fig. 26.3). Curved reusable instruments according to DAPRI (Karl Storz-
Endoskope) are inserted through the 6-mm flexible trocars (Fig. 26.4a–h). The flexible trocar located at 9 o'clock position accomodates only one instrument, which is
the bicurved grasping forceps I (Fig. 26.4a), and the flexible trocar located at 3
o'clock position accomodates the other tools like the monocurved grasping forceps
IV (Fig. 26.4b), the monocurved coagulating hook (Fig. 26.4c), the monocurved
bipolar grasping forceps and scissors (Fig. 26.4d, e), the monocurved dissecting
forceps (Fig. 26.4f), the monocurved scissors (Fig. 26.4g), the monocurved needle

Fig. 26.2 Suprapubic access: a 3.5 cm transverse skin incision is made in the midline, 1 cm above the pubic symphysis

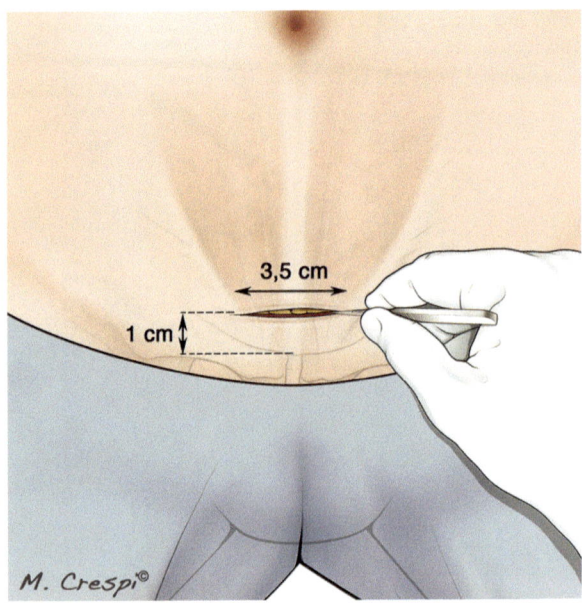

Fig. 26.3 Suprapubic access: insertion of an 11-mm reusable metallic and two 6-mm reusable flexible trocars (Karl Storz-Endoskope)

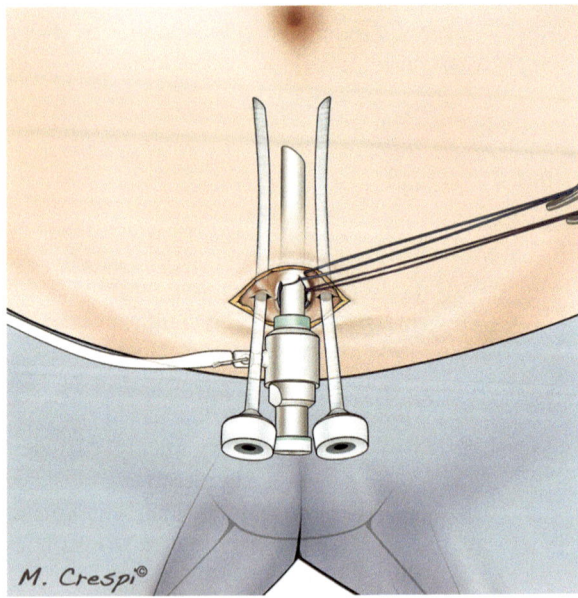

holder I (Fig. 26.4h), the monocurved suction and irrigation cannula, and the straight 5-mm clip applier (Weck Hem-o-lok, Teleflex Medical, Brussels, Belgium).

During this procedure if an assistant grasper is necessary, a needlescopic grasper, or the DAPRI 1.8-mm trocarless grasping forceps (Karl Storz-Endoskope)

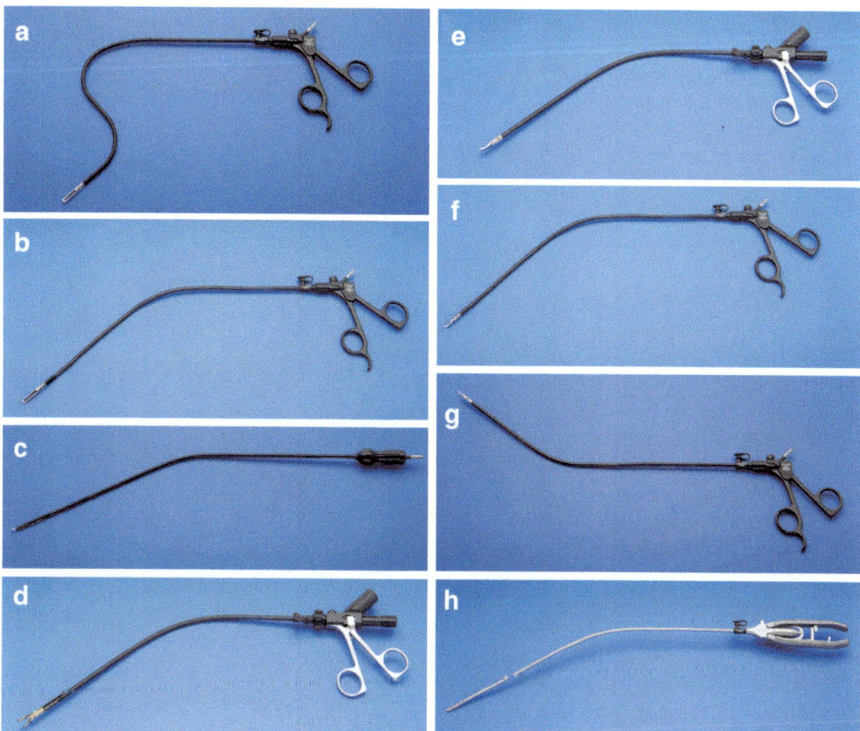

Fig. 26.4 Curved reusable instruments according to DAPRI (Karl Storz-Endoskope): bicurved grasping forceps I (**a**), monocurved grasping forceps IV (**b**), monocurved coagulating hook (**c**), monocurved bipolar grasping forceps (**d**), monocurved bipolar scissors (**e**), monocurved dissecting forceps (**f**), monocurved scissors (**g**), monocurved needle holder I (**h**)

Fig. 26.5 1.8-mm trocarless grasping forceps according to DAPRI (Karl Storz-Endoskope)

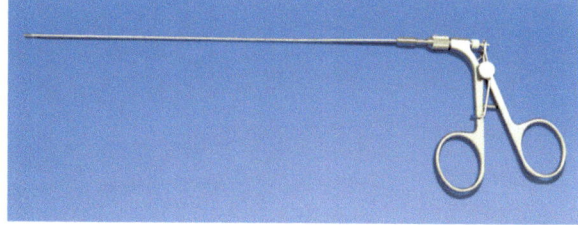

(Fig. 26.5), or a classic 5-mm instrument, is inserted in the left hypocondrium under the rib.

The abdominal cavity is explorated to rule out the presence of peritoneal metastases, superficial hepatic lesions and free peritoneal fluid.

The operative table is initially placed in a moderate Trendelenburg position with left-sided tilt. The transverse colon is exposed by reflecting the greater

Fig. 26.6 Lateral-to-medial
approach: incision of the
mesentery of the last bowel
loop and separation from the
parietal peritoneal sheet using
the monocurved coagulating
hook (**a**), under ergonomic
surgeon's conditions (**b**)

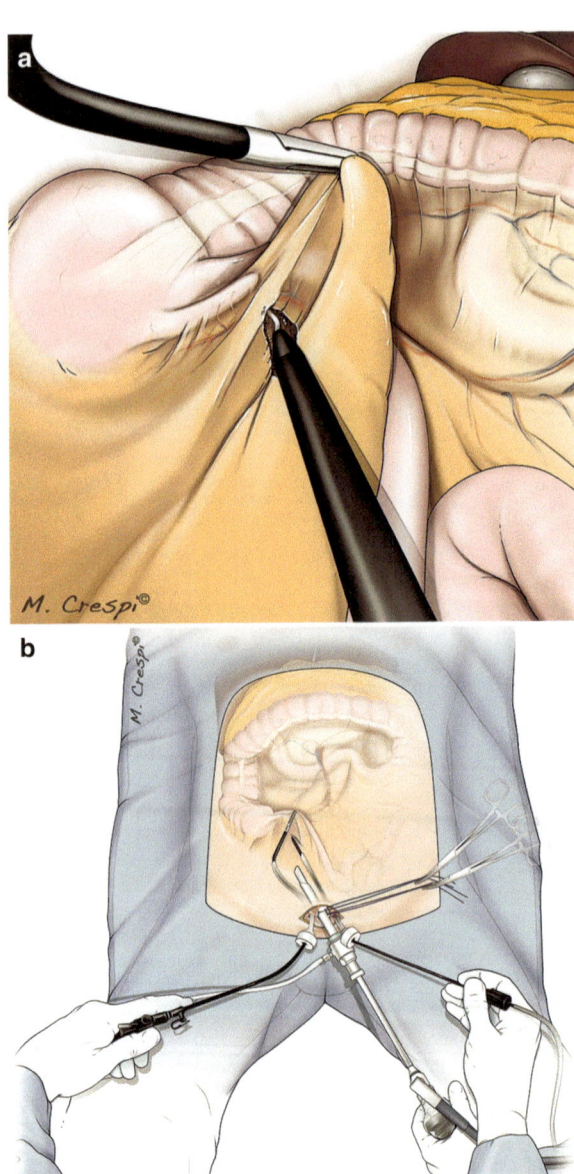

omentum, and the small bowel is gently swept out of the right quadrants of the
abdomen, until the last bowel loop is identified. This loop is grasped by the
bicurved grasping forceps I, and the mesentery is separated from the peritoneal
sheet using the monocurved coagulating hook (Fig. 26.6a, b). The terminal ileum,
cecum and the ascending colon are freed from the subperitoneal fascia. The right
mesocolon is also mobilized and the right mesocolon is dissected using a

Fig. 26.7 Lateral-to-medial
approach: mobilization of the
ileo-caecal valve and of the
right mesocolon from the
parietal peritoneal sheet (**a**),
under ergonomic surgeon's
conditions (**b**)

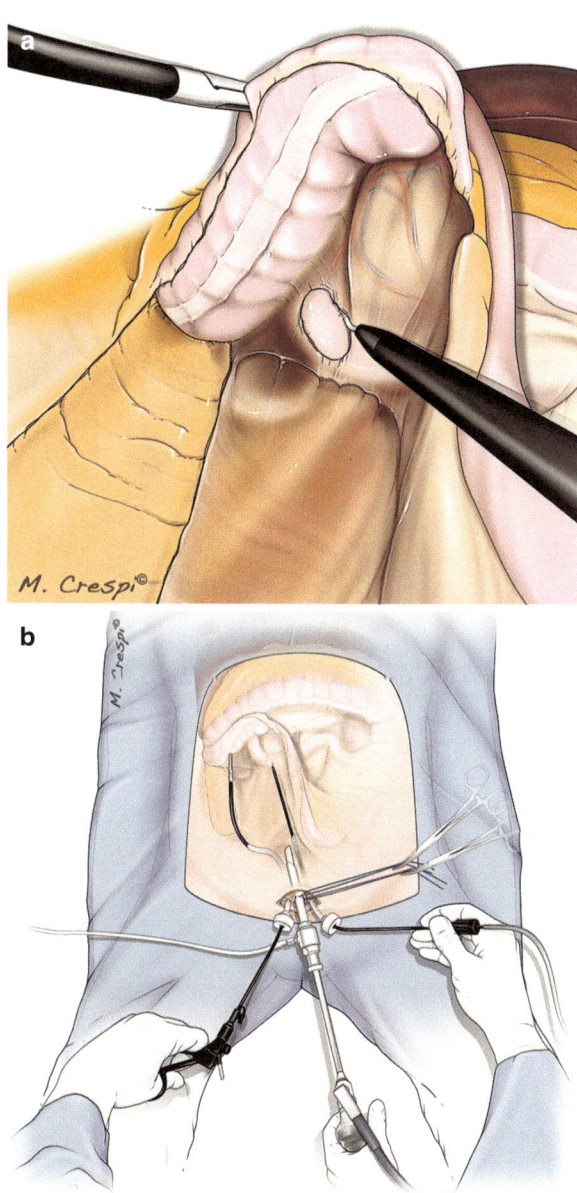

lateral-to-medial approach. This dissection is carried superiorly, respecting
Gerota's fascia, until the second and the third portion of the duodenum are idienti-
fied (Fig. 26.7a, b). An internal working triangulation as well as an external surgeon's ergonomy like in multiport laparoscopy is established thanks to the curves
of the instruments.

Fig. 26.8 Mesocolic dissection (**a**) without clashing of the instruments' tips or crossing of the surgeons' hands (**b**)

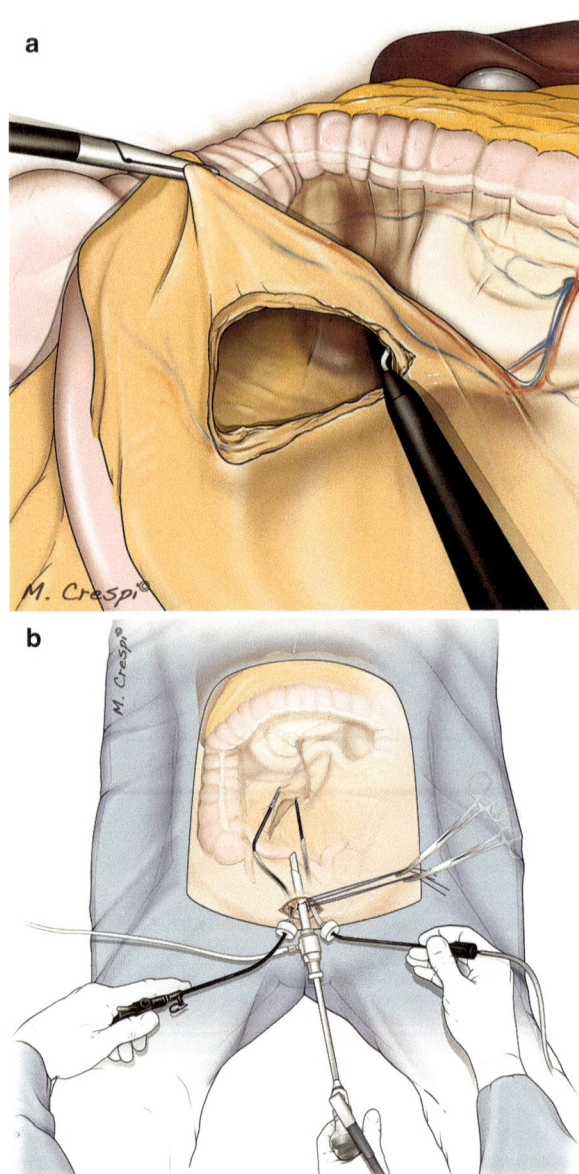

For the mesocolon mobilization, the operative table is positioned without any Trendelenburg and tilt. By grasping the mesentery and the right mesocolon with the bicurved grasping forceps I, sufficient tension is applied for section, using the monocurved coagulating hook or the monocurved bipolar scissors and forceps, respecting the medial limit of the superior mesenteric vein (Fig. 26.8a). The surgeon is able to work without crossing hands or clashing instruments' tips and with an optimal

Fig. 26.9 Internal (**a**) and external (**b**) view of 5-mm clips placement at the root of the ileo-cecal vessels

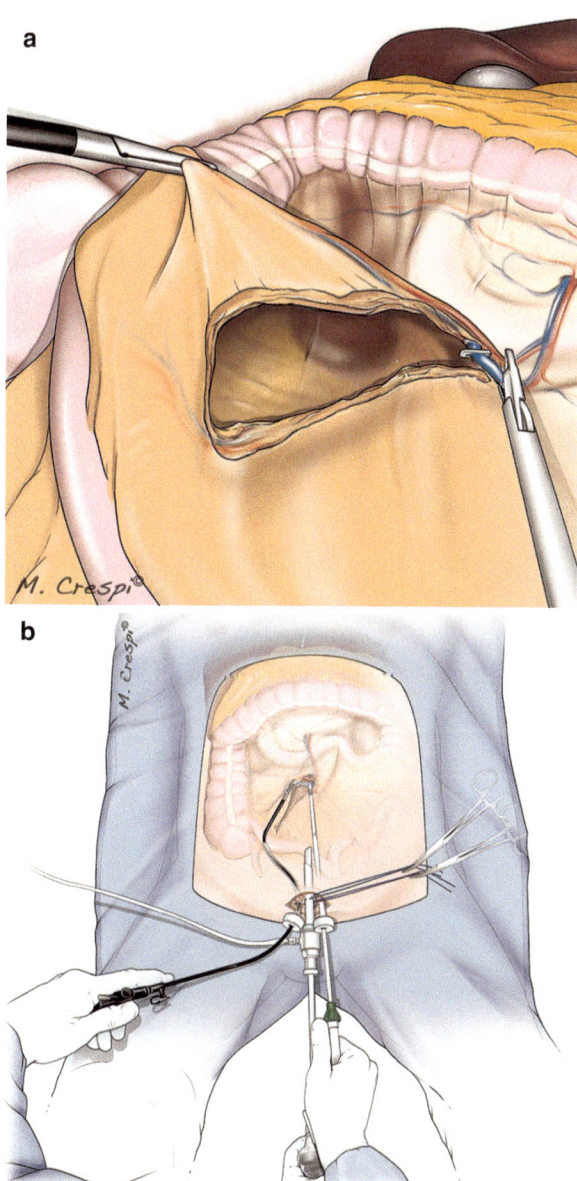

triangulation (Fig. 26.8b). The ileo-cecal vessels, the right colic vessels, and the right branch of the middle colic vessels are exposed at their root and dissected using the monocurved dissecting forceps. These vessels are individually clipped at their root using a 5-mm straight clip applier (Fig. 26.9a, b), and divided with the mono-curved scissors (Fig. 26.10a, b).

Fig. 26.10 Internal (**a**) and external (**b**) view of the ileo-cecal vessels section, with both curved instruments

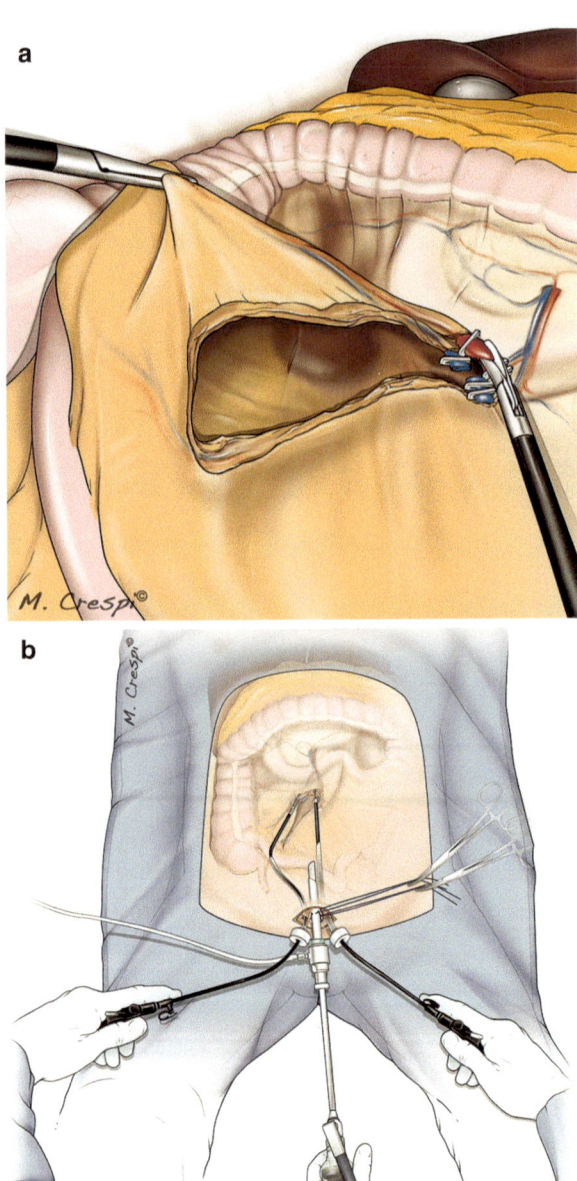

For the mobilization of the hepatic flexure, the operative table is placed in a reversed Trendelenburg position with left-sided tilt. The hepatic flexure attachments are dissected using a lateral-to-medial approach (Fig. 26.11a, b). The portion of the omentum attached to the proximal transverse colon is also dissected.

For the anastomosis, the operative table is placed in a moderate Trendelenburg position with right-sided tilt. The 11-mm trocar is replaced by a 13-mm reusable

Fig. 26.11 Lateral-to-medial approach: mobilization of the hepatic colic flexure (**a**), under ergonomic surgeon's conditions (**b**)

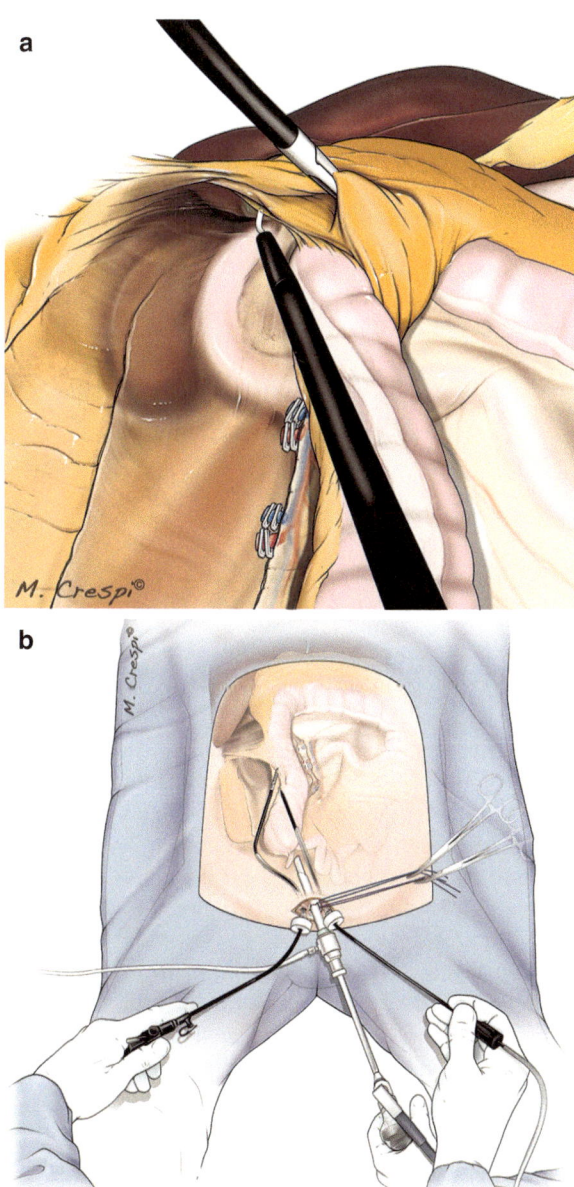

metallic trocar (Karl Storz-Endoskope) (if the 12-mm disposable trocar is used, this replacement is not needed), to accomodate a 45 flexible linear stapler. The 10-mm scope is switched into a 5-mm, 30° long scope (Karl Storz-Endoskope), which is inserted through the 6-mm flexible trocar at 3 o'clock position. The small bowel is divided by a firing of linear stapler white load (Fig. 26.12), and the proximal transverse colon by two firings blue load (Fig. 26.13a, b).

Fig. 26.12 Anastomotic step: replacement of the 11-mm trocar by a 13-mm reusable metallic trocar (Karl Storz-Endoskope) to accomodate a 45 flexible linear stapler. A 5-mm, 30° long scope (Karl Storz-Endoskope) is inserted through the 6-mm flexible trocar at 3 o'clock position, and the last small bowel is sectioned

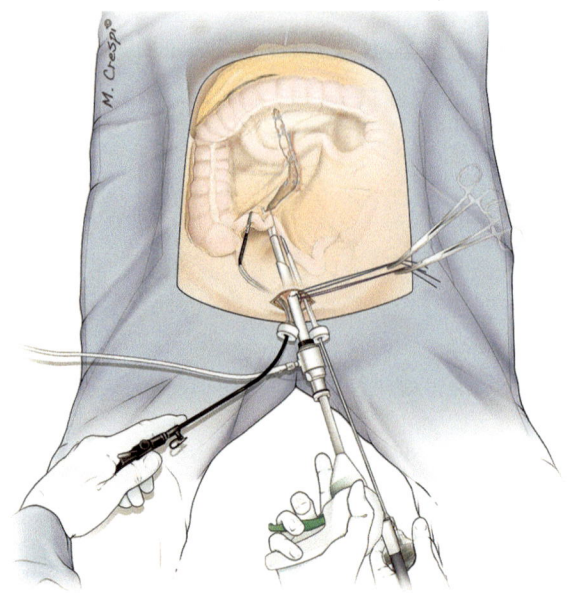

An intracorporeal linear mechanical side-to-side ileo-colic anastomosis is performed. The remnant transverse colon and small bowel are placed next each other, and 1 cm opening is made in each lumen using the monocurved coagulating hook. A linear stapler blue load is inserted in both viscera and fired (Fig. 26.14). The 13-mm trocar is replaced by the 11-mm trocar, together with the changement of the scope into 10-mm. The enterocolotomy is closed by two converting PDS 2/0 running sutures using the bicurved grasping forceps I and the monocurved needle holder I (Fig. 26.15a). Surgeon performs intracorporeal sutures and knotting technique in the same ergonomy as in multiport laparoscopy (Fig. 26.15b). The mesenteric window (between the right mesocolon and the small bowel mesentery) is closed by a PDS 2/0 running suture (Fig. 26.16).

The operative table is positioned without any Trendelenburg and tilt, and no drain is left in the abdominal cavity. Both purse-string sutures are retrieved together with the three trocars. The three trocars fascia openings on the rectus abdominis muscle are joined together (Fig. 26.17), and a plastic protection (Vi-Drape, Medical Concepts Development, MN, USA) is inserted into the peritoneal cavity to protect the suprapubic access. The specimen is removed through the suprapubic incision (Fig. 26.18). The peritoneum and the rectus abdominis muscle fascia are meticulously closed by Vicryl 1 and 2 sutures respectively (Fig. 26.19), and the cutaneous scar by intradermal sutures. The urinary catheter is removed. The final scar length depends from the specimen's size.

Fig. 26.13 Under the control of the 5-mm scope (**a**), the proximal transverse colon is sectioned (**b**)

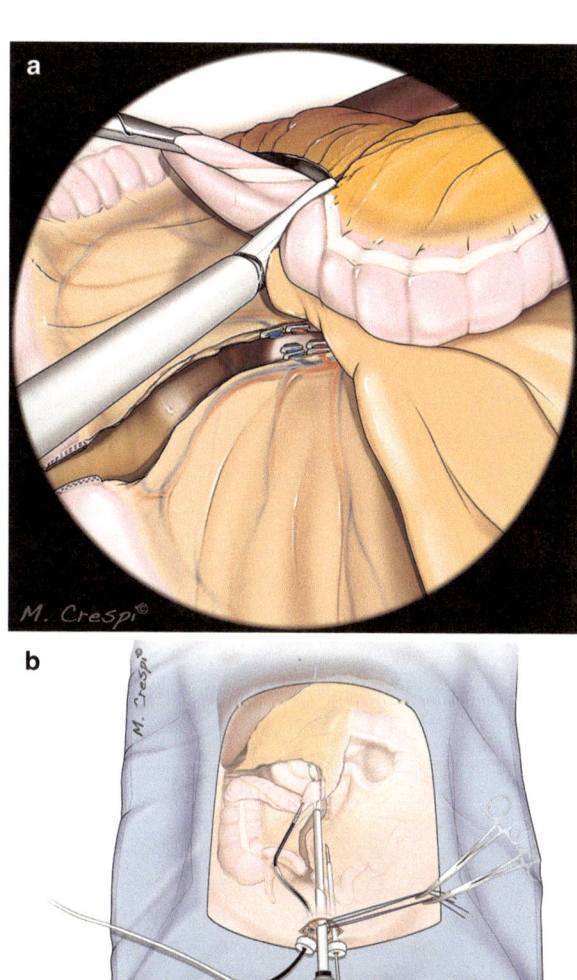

Fig. 26.14 Intracorporeal
linear mechanical side-to-side
ileo-colic anastomosis

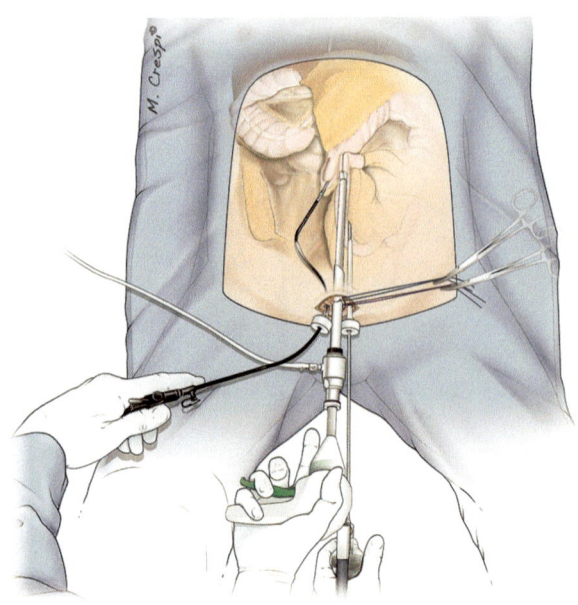

26.2.3 Post-operative Care

One gram paracetamol is given i.v. at the end of the surgical procedure, and
intraoperatively 2 g of cefazoline and 500 mg of metronidazole are administered.
Postoperative analgesia is given following the WHO visual analog pain scale
(VAS). In the recovery room the following scheme is followed: for VAS between 1
and 3, 1 g paracetamol i.v. is pushed; for VAS between 4 and 8, 100 mg tramadol
i.v. is used; if VAS > 8, 1 mg piritamide i.v. is incremented.

After the patient leaves the recovery room, pain is assessed every 6 h, with 1 g
paracetamol administered i.v. if VAS is between 1 and 3, 100 mg tramadol administered i.v. if VAS is between 4 and 8, and 1 mg piritamide administered i.v. if
VAS > 8.

The patient is allowed to drink water after 24 h from the procedure, and to tolerate a light diet after 48 h. If there are no complications, the patient is discharged on
the fourth postoperative day.

Upon discharge, 1 g paracetamol perorally or 50 mg tramadol perorally are prescribed only if needed.

Office visits are scheduled at 10 days, 1 and 3, 6, 12 months after the procedure.

Fig. 26.15 Closure of the
enterocolotomy by two
converting PDS 2/0 running
sutures using the bicurved
grasping forceps I and the
monocurved needle holder I
(**a**), under the same surgeon's
ergonomy as in multiport
laparoscopy (**b**)

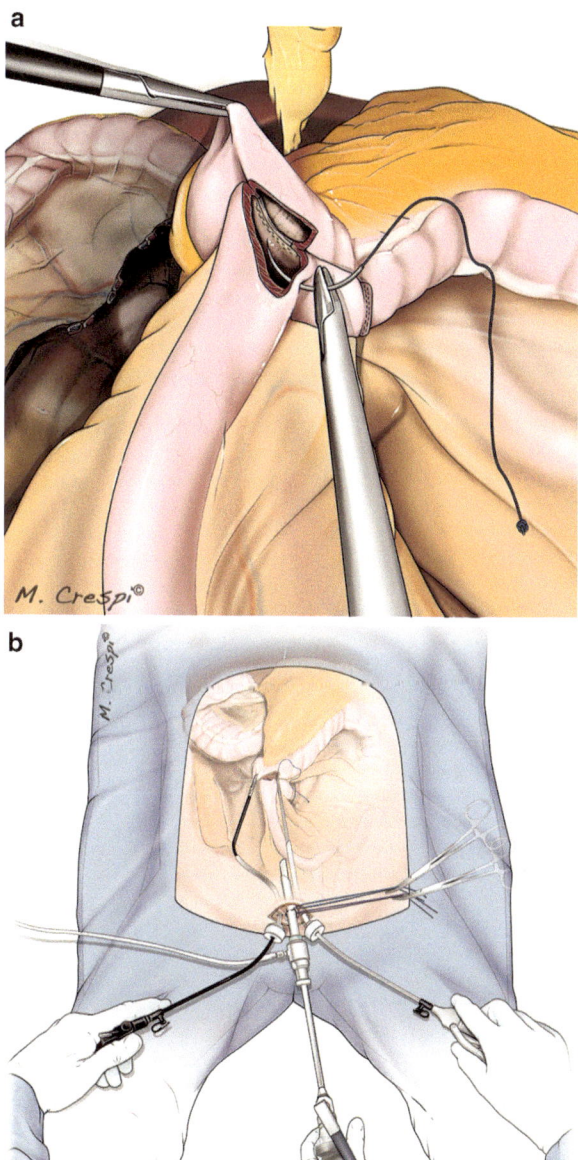

Fig. 26.16 Closure of the
mesenteric window, between
the right mesocolon and the
small bowel mesentery, using
PDS 2/0 running suture

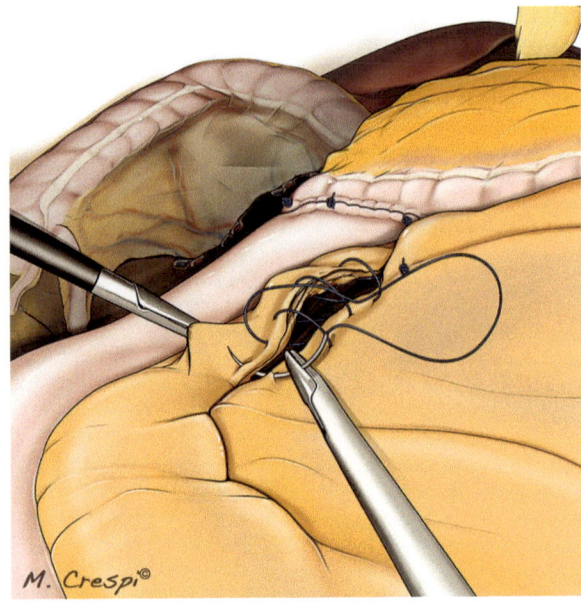

Fig. 26.17 Suprapubic
access: opening of the rectus
abdominis muscle fascia,
joining together each single
trocar's hole

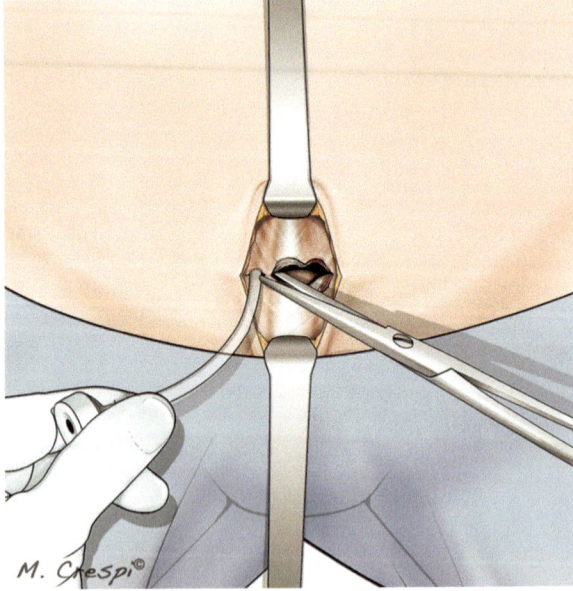

Fig. 26.18 Suprapubic
access: removal of the
specimen, after insertion of
the plastic protection into the
peritoneal cavity

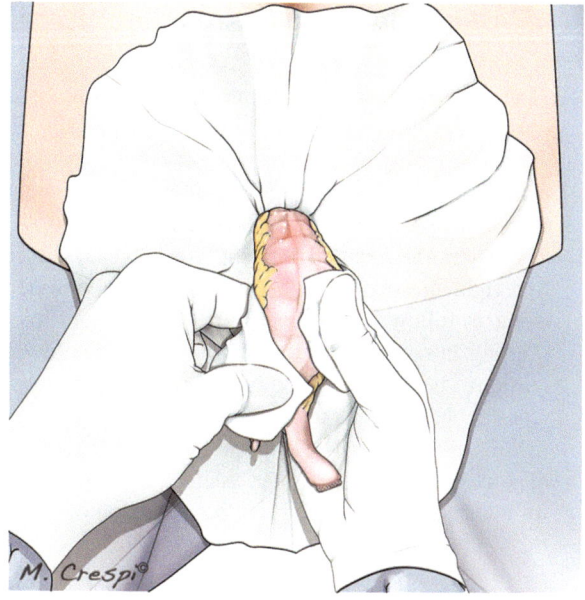

Fig. 26.19 Meticulousely
closure of the peritoneal sheet
and of the rectus abdominis
muscle fascia

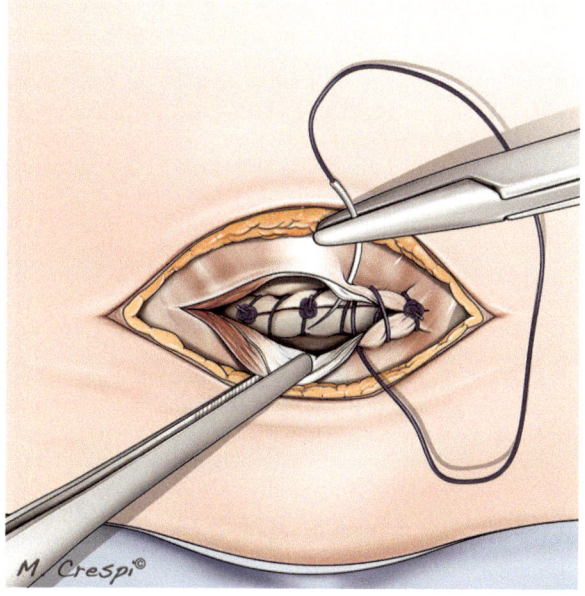

26.3   Recommendations from the Author

- The curved reusable instruments have to be inserted into the abdomen and removed, following a 45° angle with the respect of the abdominal wall.
- The positioning of the operative table has to be considered as the main assistant. The different table positionings allow the permanent good exposure of the operative field, due to the use of the gravity force.
- The lateral-to-medial approach offers an easy dissection of the mesentery and of the right mesocolon because the pneumoperitoneum help to individualize the route to follow for the dissection.
- During intracorporeal anastomosis, a 45 flexible linear stapler is used because easier to be inserted in both visceral lumen through the suprapubic access. The enterocolotomy has to be closed by two converting running sutures because it avoids any potential stricture obtained with a firing of linear stapler.
- The closure of the mesenteric defect, at the end of the procedure, avoids the risk of internal hernia and subsequent intestinal occlusion.

References

1. Remzi FH, Kirat HT, Kaouk JH, Geisler DP (2008) Single-port laparoscopy in colorectal surgery. Colorectal Dis 10:823–826
2. Laurent C, Leblanc F, Bretagnol F, Capdepont M, Rullier E (2008) Long-term wound advantages of the laparoscopic approach in rectal cancer. Br J Surg 95:903–908
3. Malvasi A, Tinelli A, Serio G, Tinelli R, Casciaro S, Cavallotti C (2007) Comparison between the use of the Joel-Cohen incision and its modification during Stark's cesarean section. J Matern Fetal Neonatal Med 20:757–761
4. Advani V, Ahad S, Hassan I (2011) Single incision laparoscopic right hemicolectomy for colon cancer: less is more? Surg Innov 18:NP4–NP6
5. Duepree HJ, Senagore AJ, Delaney CP, Fazio VW (2003) Does menas of access affect the incidence of small bowel obstruction and ventral hernia after bowel resection? Laparoscopy versus laparotomy. J Am Coll Surg 197:177–181
6. Singh R, Omiccioli A, Hegge S, McKinley C (2008) Does the extraction-site location in laparoscopic colorectal surgery have an impact on incisional hernia sites? Surg Endosc 22:2596–2600
7. Hanna GB, Shimi SM, Cuschieri A (1998) Task performance in endoscopic surgery is influenced by location of the image display. Ann Surg 227:481–484
8. Hanna G, Drew T, Clinch P, Hunter B, Cuschieri A (1998) Computer-controlled endoscopic performance assessment system. Surg Endosc 12:997–1000

Chapter 27
Left Colectomy

Ichiro Takemasa, Mamoru Uemura, Junichi Nishimura,
Tsunekazu Mizushima, Hirofumi Yamamoto,
Yuichiro Doki, and Masaki Mori

Abstract Current efforts in minimally invasive laparoscopic surgery have led to reduced port laparoscopic surgery (RPLS). The aim is to decrease trauma by reducing the number of ports and/or size of the trocars. Single-site laparoscopic colectomy (SLC) performed entirely through one incision is considered the ultimate RPLS for colectomy because it is thought to improve cosmesis, reduce postoperative pain, and reduce abdominal wall morbidity. Several reports have described the feasibility and benefits of SLC, but there are technical limitations. In addition, oncologic clearance in SLC has not been fully investigated.

Laparoscopic left colectomy for a tumor located near the left colic flexure is difficult because the procedure includes extensive dissection in the area of the left colic mesentery with splenic flexure mobilization and appropriate lymphadenectomy corresponding to the individual patient's vessel network. The technical difficulties have delayed standardization of the procedure. Reduced port laparoscopic left colectomy (RPLLC) is an even more difficult procedure.

We routinely create a virtual three-dimensional multi-imaging to understand the precise anatomy of the target organs and neighboring structures. Herein, we describe our techniques for RPLLC with D3 lymphadenectomy in detail, including some tips and tricks. Our procedure makes standardization of safe and certain RPLLC possible.

Keywords Colon cancer • Left side colectomy • Reduced port laparoscopic surgery • Single-port laparoscopic surgery

I. Takemasa (✉) • M. Uemura • J. Nishimura • T. Mizushima
H. Yamamoto • Y. Doki • M. Mori
Department of Gastroenterological Surgery, Graduate School of Medicine, Osaka University,
2-2 Yamadaoka, Suita, Osaka 565-0871, Japan
e-mail: itakemasa@gesurg.med.osaka-u.ac.jp

T. Mori and G. Dapri (eds.), *Reduced Port Laparoscopic Surgery*,
DOI 10.1007/978-4-431-54601-6_27, © Springer Japan 2014

27.1 Introduction

Current efforts in minimally invasive treatment have shifted toward decreasing trauma by reducing the number of ports and/or the size of the trocars [1]. Conventional multiport laparoscopic colectomy (MLC) requires several ports and abdominal incisions [2]. The concept of reduced port laparoscopic surgery (RPLS) has been introduced to laparoscopic colectomy. Single-site laparoscopic colectomy (SLC) performed entirely through one extraction site is considered the ultimate RPLS colectomy procedure for improving cosmesis and theoretically reducing postoperative pain and the risk of abdominal wall morbidities including bleeding and hernia. Several groups have reported the feasibility and benefits of SLC including improved cosmesis, reduced postoperative pain, and shortened recovery time, but there are some limitations such as instrument crowding, in-line viewing, insufficient counter-traction, somewhat narrow patient applicability, and increased costs [3–11]. In addition, concerns over oncologic clearance in SLC remain unsettled. The less invasive procedure may bring patient satisfaction, but oncologic clearance and technical safety are of utmost importance in the surgical treatment of colon cancer.

Intraoperative palpation around the target organs and an overview of the operative field are difficult to achieve in laparoscopic surgery. Understanding the three-dimensional anatomy of the target organs and the neighboring structures along with a precise preoperative diagnosis is essential in individual cases for completion of an appropriate laparoscopic procedure. Laparoscopic left colectomy for transverse or descending colon cancer located near the left colic flexure is difficult [12] in comparison to laparoscopic left hemicolectomy or sigmoidectomy because the procedure includes extensive dissection of the left colic mesentery with splenic flexure mobilization and appropriate lymphadenectomy corresponding to patients' individual vessel patterns. In addition, the anatomical relations between the left colon and neighboring structures including the pancreas, spleen, and greater omentum are complex. The technical difficulties, especially with respect to D3 lymphadenectomy or complete mesocolic excision (CME), may delay standardization of the procedure. Aside from the fact that reduced port laparoscopic left colectomy (RPLLC) is a particularly difficult procedure; there are only a few reports of the procedure [13, 14].

We routinely create a virtual three-dimensional multi-imaging integrating FDG-PET/CT scan for localization of the tumor and any lymph node metastases, CT colonography for a complete picture of the entire colon, and CT angiography for depiction of the arteries and veins and their variations. This is used for preoperative simulation and intraoperative navigation (Fig. 27.1). The dissection area with complete lymphadenectomy depends on the location of the tumor (Fig. 27.2). In left colectomy for a transverse or descending colon cancer, preoperative virtual imaging for tumor localization and the corresponding arterial network is essential because the major arteries feeding the tumor are supplied by the middle colic artery (MCA), the left colic artery (LCA), or both.

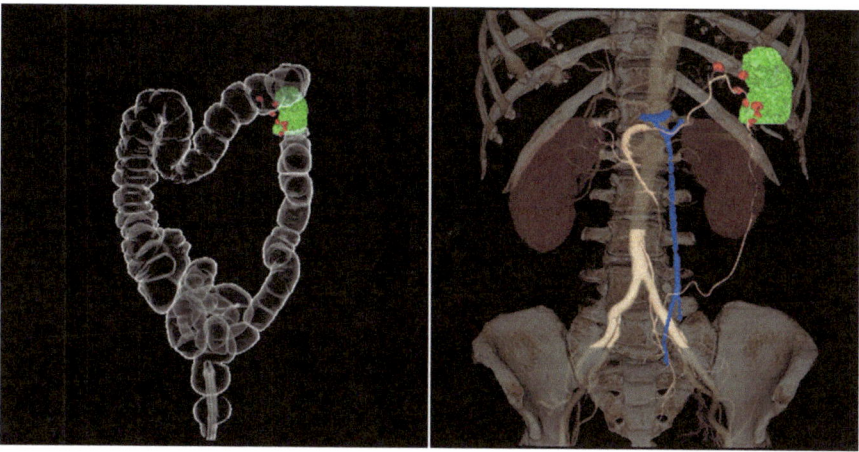

Fig. 27.1 A three-dimensional virtual multi-imaging derived from FDG-PET/CT scan, CT colonography, and CT angiography (*right*). The tumor is indicated in green, and the metastatic lymph nodes are indicated in red by FDG-PET/CT scan, and the entire colon is visualized by CT colonography (*left*). The arteries and veins related to the tumor are also visualized by CT angiography

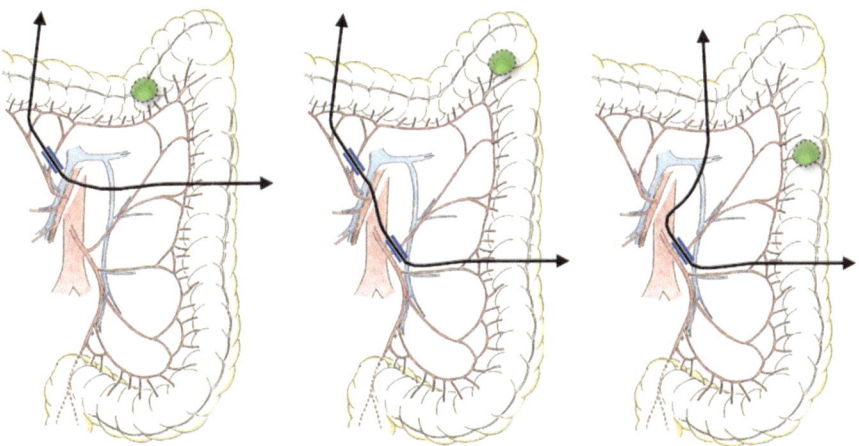

Fig. 27.2 Dissection area with complete lymphadenectomy, depending on the tumor location

Here, we introduce our techniques for RPLLC with D3 lymphadenectomy. Our medial-to-lateral approach makes it possible to standardize the procedure for mobilization of the mesentery, ligation of the vessels at their origin, and complete lymphadenectomy in a safe and a certain manner.

27.2   Indications and Contraindications

Indications for RPLLC, like those for MLC, are Tis-T3 tumor, tumor diameter <4 cm, body mass index (BMI) <35 kg/m^2, and American Society of Anesthesiologists (ASA) class <2. Advanced T4 tumor, a huge or bulky tumor ≥4 cm, severe obesity, perforated tumor, stenosis with bowel distention, prior abdominal polysurgery, and any severe comorbidity are contraindications. Complete informed consent is imperative.

27.3   Technique

27.3.1   Patient Positioning and Operative Set-up

The patient, under general anesthesia, is positioned on the operating table between sides supports mounted on the table. The patient's feet are placed in boot-type leg holders with the legs spread apart and knees only slightly flexed. The arms are tucked along the patient's sides. The operator, the camera assistant, and the scrub nurse stand on the right of the patient, and the first assistant and the laparoscopic monitor are on the left.

27.3.2   Access to the Abdominal Cavity

A 2–3-cm vertical skin incision and mini-laparotomy incision are made in the umbilicus. A multichannel access device such as EZ Access (Hakko Co., Nagano, Japan) with a previously installed 12-mm trocar for the laparoscope and two 5-mm trocars is fitted into the incision. We prefer to use ultrasonic laparoscopic coagulation shears (LCS) as the dissection device and atraumatic graspers or fine dissectors as forceps. An additional incision or trocar port is made without hesitation if necessary to complete the procedure, and conversion to open laparotomy is kept as an option. The indication and timing of trocar insertion or conversion to open surgery depend on the surgeon's judgment.

27.3.3   Operative Exposure

CO_2 pneumoperitoneum is established and maintained at 10 mmHg. After complete exploration of the abdomen to identify any metastatic nodules or superficial hepatic metastases with a 30-degree 10-mm rigid laparoscope, the patient is tilted into a deep Trendelenburg position and inclined to the right. The small intestine is moved into the right upper quadrant, exposing the root of the left colonic mesentery. The greater omentum is then flipped to expose the transverse colon and the splenic flexure.

Fig. 27.3 Medial-to-lateral
approach for dissection of the
left colonic mesentery and
the mesorectum, preserving
the right hypogastric nerve

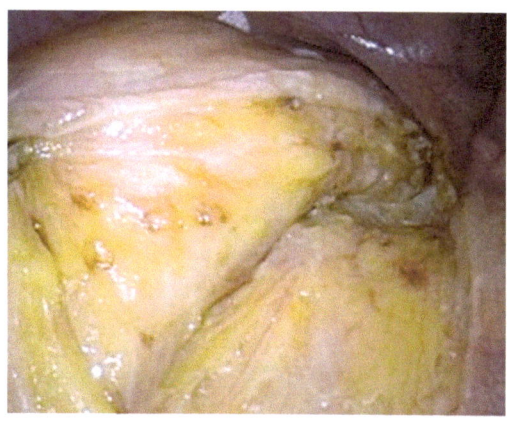

27.3.4   Dissection of the Left Colonic Mesentery and the Mesorectum

By tenting the left colonic mesentery with an atraumatic grasper held in the surgeon's left hand, the root of the left colonic mesentery is incised with LCS, starting at the sacral promontory, in a medial to lateral approach. The appropriate plane is dissected, preserving the right hypogastric nerve (Fig. 27.3). Continuous dissection below the inferior mesenteric artery (IMA) is performed by sweeping down the retroperitoneal fascia to preserve the left ureter and the gonadal vessels in the posterior plane (Fig. 27.4a). The mesorectum is dissected posteriorly in the plane of total mesorectal excision, in front of the hypogastric plexus nerves. The peritoneum is then incised cephalad beside the duodenum beyond the origin of the IMA (Fig. 27.4b). The medial dissection is continued until the inferior border of the pancreas on Gerota's fascia is reached.

27.3.5   Ligation of the Inferior Mesenteric Vessels

The inferior mesenteric vessels are ligated, depending on the tumor location. When there is a need to ligate the IMA at its origin, the IMA is dissected between clips 0.5-cm away from its aortic origin so as not to injure the lumbar splanchnic nerves. When possible, to preserve blood flow to the superior rectal artery (SRA), the left colic artery (LCA) is dissected between clips at its origin with or without D3 lymphadenectomy around the origin of the IMA (Fig. 27.5a, b). The inferior mesenteric vein is exposed and dissected below the duodenojejunal junction between two clips (Fig. 27.6a, b).

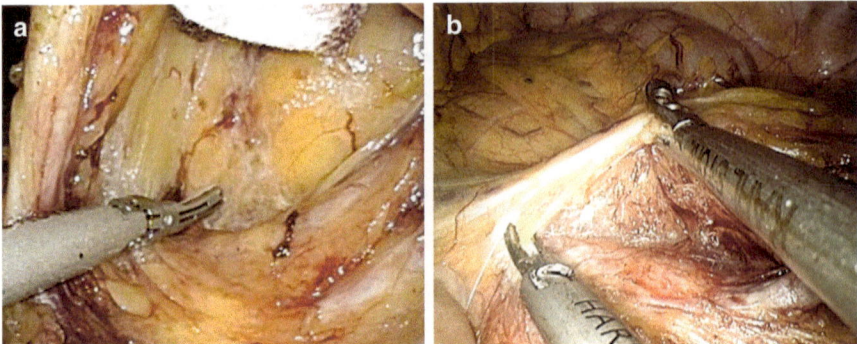

Fig. 27.4 (**a**) Dissection below the inferior mesenteric artery (IMA) by sweeping down the retroperitoneal fascia to preserve the left ureter and gonadal vessels. (**b**) Cephalad incision of the peritoneum beside the duodenum beyond the origin of the IMA

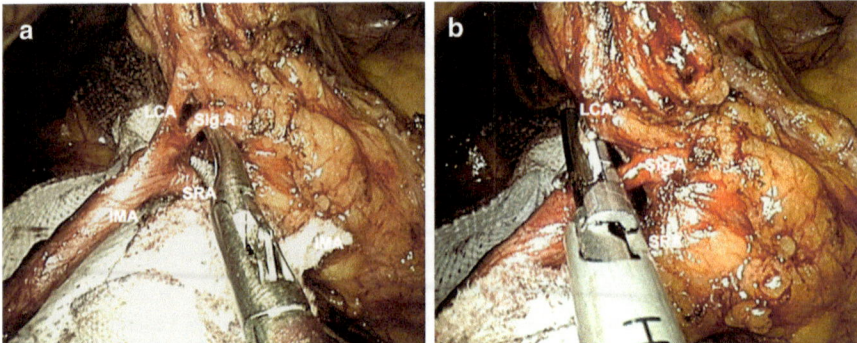

Fig. 27.5 (**a**) To preserve the superior rectal artery (SRA), skeletonization of the IMA and its branches with D3 lymphadenectomy around the origin of the IMA is performed. (**b**) Ligation of the left colic artery (LCA) by clips at its origin, preserving the SRA

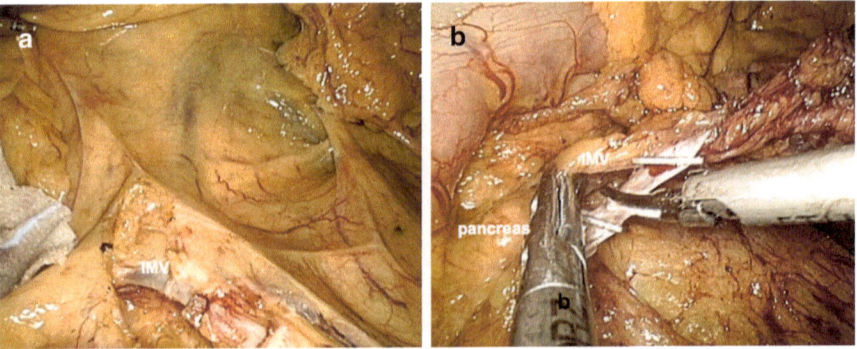

Fig. 27.6 (**a**) Exposure of the inferior mesenteric vein (IMV) below the duodenojejunal junction. (**b**) Ligation of the IMV between two clips

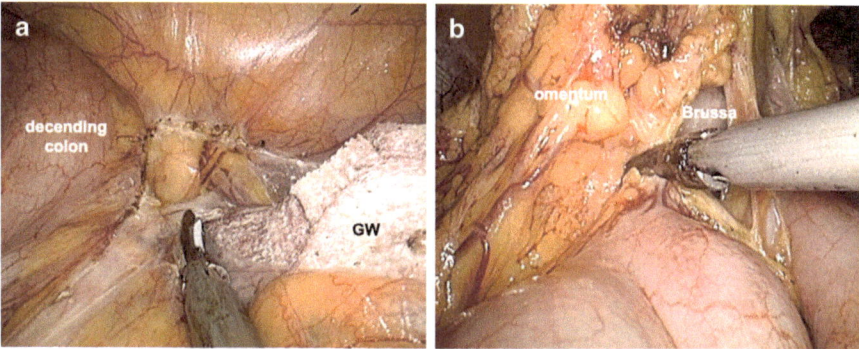

Fig. 27.7 (**a**) Dissection of the lateral attachment of the left colon up to the splenic flexure. (**b**) Separation of the greater omentum from the middle of the transverse colon to the splenic flexure by opening the bursa omentalis

27.3.6   Mobilization of the Splenic Flexure

The lateral attachment of the left colon and rectum is dissected from bottom to top and is freed up to the splenic flexure (Fig. 27.7a). The operating table is then moved to a head-up position (reverse Trendelenburg position) in preparation for mobilization of the splenic flexure. The greater omentum is lifted cephalad with a retracting device such as the EndoGrab Retractor (Virtual Ports Ltd., Caesaera, Israel), and the transverse colon is pulled caudad with an atraumatic grasper held in the surgeon's left hand. Thus, the greater omentum is separated by sharp dissection from the middle of the transverse colon to the splenic flexure by opening the bursa omentalis (Fig. 27.7b). The root of the transverse colonic mesentery is dissected laterally and freed from the inferior border of the pancreas (Fig. 27.8a, b). The splenic flexure is mobilized completely with sharp division of the splenocolic ligaments joining previous dissection of the left Toldt fascia (Fig. 27.9a, b).

27.3.7   Transection of the Rectum

When the IMA is ligated at its origin, the fat surrounding the rectum at the transection line, and usually near the promontory below Sudeck's point, is removed, and the superior rectal vessels are dissected. In preparation for transection of the rectum, a 5-mm trocar in the access device is changed to a 12-mm trocar for the introduction of a linear stapler. The rectum is clamped and transected by one firing of an

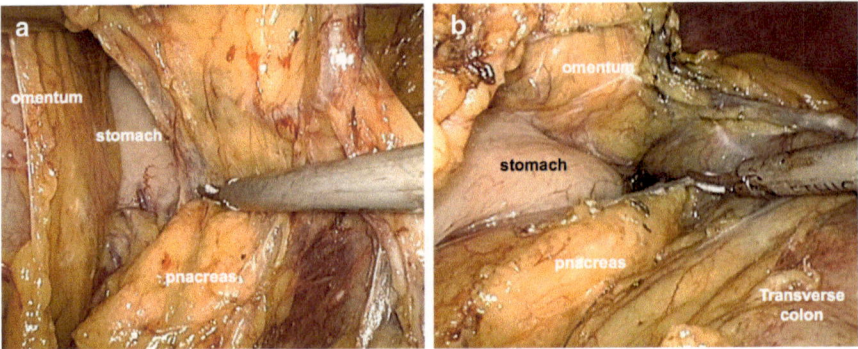

Fig. 27.8 (**a**) Dissection of the root of the transverse colonic mesentery laterally from the inferior border of the pancreas. (**b**) Complete separation of the transverse colonic mesentery from the surface of the pancreas

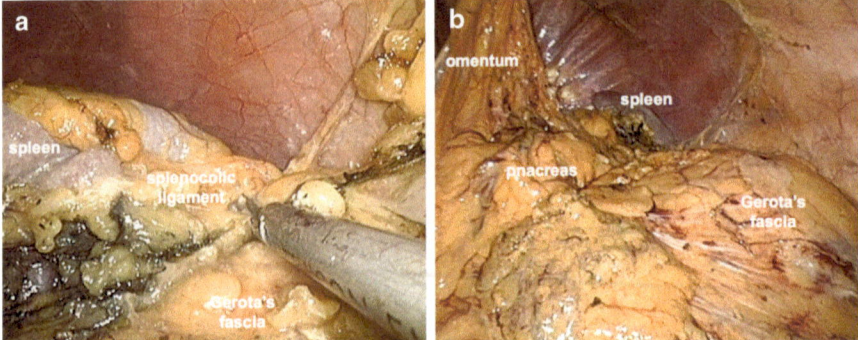

Fig. 27.9 (**a**) Mobilization of the splenic flexure with sharp division of the splenocolic ligaments. (**b**) Complete mobilization of the splenic flexure joining the previous dissection of the left Toldt fascia

articulated linear stapler with a 60-mm cartridge. The rectum is drawn cephalad so that the staple line is perpendicular to the axis of the rectum. When the SRA is preserved, the mesentery is dissected cuneately at least 10-cm both distal and proximal to the lesion from the ligated stump of the LCA.

27.3.8 Extraction of the Specimen

After removal of the access device with the wound protector remaining in place, the left colon and rectum are extracted through the mini-laparotomy incision in the umbilicus. The descending colon or the transverse colon and its mesentery are divided 10-cm proximal to the lesion after ligation of the mesentery vessels and the adjacent vascular arcade.

27.3.9   Anastomosis

When the IMA is ligated, the anvil of the circular stapling device is introduced into the stump of the proximal colon for anastomosis. The colon, with the anvil, is replaced in the abdomen, and the access device is re-applied for re-establishment of the pneumoperitoneum. After confirming that the descending colon and the mesentery are not twisted, colorectal anastomosis is performed intracorporeally by the double-stapling technique. Airtightness is tested by transanal injection of air while the anastomosis is checked endoscopically, and the intestinal rings are examined for secure placement. When the SRA is preserved, extracorporeal functional end-to-end anastomosis is performed. The small intestines are repositioned in front of the left mesocolon. An intracorporeal drainage tube is placed at the discretion of the surgeon and, if placed, is inserted at the bottom of the umbilicus.

27.3.10   Wound Closure

The final incision has been extended to a length comparable to the size of the specimen or the tumor. The fascia is closed with interrupted absorbable sutures. The peritoneum is not closed separately. After the fascia is closed, the wound is rinsed free of blood and cell debris with Ringer's lactate solution. An anchoring suture is tied to the rectus sheath at the bottom of the umbilicus, and subcutaneous absorbable sutures are placed. Finally, the incision is re-measured.

27.4   Tips and Tricks

The procedure is subject to instrument collision, limited in-line viewing, and inadequate counter-traction. These frustrations occur mainly if an assistant lacks skill or because of the close distance between trocars.

The gravity of the intestinal tract itself is useful for obtaining good visualization and counter-traction. At the beginning of the operation, the patient is placed in the supine position with legs spread apart for diagnostic exploration of the abdomen and detection of metastasis. The patient is then tilted to the deep Trendelenburg position and inclined to the right for dissection of the left colonic mesentery with complete lymphadenectomy. For mobilization of the splenic flexure, the operating table is moved to a head-up position and inclined to the right to the fullest extent possible.

The access device placed in the small incision is rotated to achieve the ideal operative view and triangulation and to avoid or resolve collision of the instruments. By carefully rotating the access device for the necessary angle, the operation will progress and be duly accomplished in a certain manner, minimizing the surgeon's stress.

Intracorporeal supporting devices, such as the EndoGrab Retractor (Virtual Ports), sometimes help the surgeon achieve good visualization and appropriate counter-traction. This retractor facilitates laparoscopic organ retraction to increase tissue access and visualization. It provides anterior and superior organ retraction during laparoscopic procedures and allows reduction in the number of ports and incisions. It works with particular efficiency in the management of the greater omentum. However, if the surgeon feels limited even when using such a device, an additional incision or trocar port should be placed without hesitation to complete the procedure. Conversion to open laparotomy should also be done without hesitation when deemed necessary. The indication and timing of insertion or conversion are dependent on the surgeon's judgment.

27.5 Recommendations from the Author

Conventional laparoscopic surgery is accepted as minimally invasive management in comparison to open surgery, and its application to colon cancer has increased remarkably over the last decade. However, even more minimally invasive techniques have been in demand recently. Surgeons experienced in conventional MLC are challenged to further decrease trauma and improve outcomes by reducing the number of ports and/or size of the trocars [1].

Since SLC for colon cancer was introduced by Remzi et al. [15] and Bucher et al. [16] in 2008, the feasibility of this procedure has been proven in two randomized controlled trials [10, 11] and in several case–control studies [3–9] that compared short-term outcomes between SLC and MLC. Many authors have reported that SLC offers better cosmesis with similar perioperative results, but SLC is still somewhat controversial. With regard to the management of malignant lesions, certain oncologic clearance is the most important task. The manner by which to best dissect the regional lymph nodes or remove the mesocolon in SLC remains to be more carefully evaluated.

Four case–control studies have been conducted to assess short-term outcomes of SLC with particular respect to such expected benefits as shortened operation time, length of hospital stay, reduced complications, reduced pain, and other positive outcomes [3, 4, 7, 9], but the results have been controversial. Champagne et al. [9] and Poon et al. [10] reported reduced postoperative pain associated with a shorter hospital stay for patients treated by SLC. We too have documented reduced postoperative pain. This fact suggests that the lateral port sites in the abdominal wall contribute substantially to postoperative discomfort. However, it remains unclear whether the reduced postoperative pain leads to faster postoperative recovery.

Despite the technical difficulty of SLC, all but two RCTs and other studies reported similar operation times [7, 8]. The reported median SLC operation time ranges from 83 to 225 min [17]. Standardization will make it possible to complete the procedure within an acceptable time frame, although a more careful and precise procedure with complete mesenteric excision may necessitate a longer operation.

An additional port will be required mainly to allow for appropriate transection of the rectum. Thus, applying single-site laparoscopic surgery to rectal cancer should be more deliberate at present. However, this emerging minimally invasive surgery has another benefit: the surgeon can choose to insert one or more additional trocars at any time during the procedure.

Oncologic resection with meticulous mesocolic dissection and optimal lymph node clearance may improve oncologic outcomes [18, 19]. The embryologic tissue planes must be respected to minimize the likelihood of cancer recurrence, and true central ligation of the lymphatic drainage maximizes the harvest of regional lymph nodes [20]. Standardization of CME has improved oncologic outcomes without increasing the postoperative complication or mortality rates [21].

The minimal invasiveness of SLC should be assessed and verified by detailed analysis of postoperative pain at all port sites in a future randomized controlled trial. Long-term oncologic outcomes, cost, education for SLC techniques, and the stress levels of surgeons performing SLC should be also evaluated.

References

1. Curcillo PG 2nd, Podolsky ER, King SA (2011) The road to reduced port surgery: from single big incisions to single small incisions, and beyond. World J Surg 35:1526–1531
2. Takemasa I, Sekimoto M, Ikeda M, Mizushima T, Yamamoto H, Doki Y, Mori M (2010) Video. Transumbilical single-incision laparoscopic surgery for sigmoid colon cancer. Surg Endosc 24:2321
3. Papaconstantinou HT, Thomas JS (2011) Single-incision laparoscopic colectomy for cancer: assessment of oncologic resection and short-term outcomes in a case-matched comparison with standard laparoscopy. Surgery 50:820–827
4. Lu CC, Lin SE, Chung KC, Rau KM (2012) Comparison of clinical outcome of single-incision laparoscopic surgery using a simplified access system with conventional laparoscopic surgery for malignant colorectal disease. Colorectal Dis 14:171–176
5. Chen WT, Chang SC, Chiang HC, Lo WY, Jeng LB, Wu C, Ke TW (2011) Single-incision laparoscopic versus conventional laparoscopic right hemicolectomy: a comparison of short-term surgical results. Surg Endosc 25:1887–1892
6. Ramos-Valadez DI, Ragupathi M, Nieto J, Patel CB, Miller S, Pickron TB, Haas EM (2012) Single-incision versus conventional laparoscopic sigmoid colectomy: a case-matched series. Surg Endosc 26:96–102
7. Champagne BJ, Lee EC, Leblanc F, Stein SL, Delaney CP (2011) Single-incision vs straight laparoscopic segmental colectomy: a case-controlled study. Dis Colon Rectum 54:183–186
8. Kim SJ, Ryu GO, Choi BJ, Kim JG, Lee KJ, Lee SC, Oh ST (2011) The short-term outcomes of conventional and single-port laparoscopic surgery for colorectal cancer. Ann Surg 254:933–940
9. Champagne BJ, Papaconstantinou HT, Parmar SS, Nagle DA, Young-Fadok TM, Lee EC, Delaney CP (2012) Single-incision versus standard multiport laparoscopic colectomy: a multicenter, case-controlled comparison. Ann Surg 255:66–69
10. Poon JT, Cheung CW, Fan JK, Lo OS, Law WL (2012) Single-incision versus conventional laparoscopic colectomy for colonic neoplasm: a randomized, controlled trial. Surg Endosc 26:2729–2734
11. Huscher CG, Mingoli A, Sgarzini G, Mereu A, Binda B, Brachini G, Trombetta S (2012) Standard laparoscopic versus single-incision laparoscopic colectomy for cancer: early results of a randomized prospective study. Am J Surg 204:115–120

12. Akiyoshi T, Kuroyanagi H, Oya M, Ueno M, Fujimoto Y, Konishi T, Yamaguchi T (2010) Factors affecting difficulty of laparoscopic surgery for left-sided colon cancer. Surg Endosc 24:2749–2754
13. Law WL, Fan JK, Poon JT (2010) Single incision laparoscopic left colectomy for carcinoma of distal transverse colon. Colorectal Dis 12:698–701
14. Lee SW, Milsom JW, Nach GM (2011) Single-incision versus multiport laparoscopic right and hand-assisted left colectomy: a case-matched comparison. Dis Colon Rectum 54:1355–1361
15. Remzi FH, Kirat HT, Kaouk JH, Geisler DP (2008) Single-port laparoscopy in colorectal surgery. Colorectal Dis 10:823–826
16. Bucher P, Pugin F, Morel P (2008) Single port access laparoscopic right hemicolectomy. Int J Colorectal Dis 23:1013–1016
17. Makino T, Milsom JW, Lee SW (2012) Feasibility and safety of single-incision laparoscopic colectomy: a systematic review. Ann Surg 255:667–676
18. West NP, Hohenberger W, Weber K, Perrakis A, Finan PJ, Quirke P (2010) Complete meso-colic excision with central vascular ligation produces an oncologically superior specimen compared with standard surgery for carcinoma of the colon. J Clin Oncol 28:272–278
19. West NP, Kobayashi H, Takahashi K, Perrakis A, Weber K, Hohenberger W, Sugihara K, Quirke P (2012) Understanding optimal colonic cancer surgery: comparison of Japanese D3 resection and European complete mesocolic excision with central vascular ligation. J Clin Oncol 30:1763–1769
20. Adamina M, Manwaring ML, Park KJ, Delaney CP (2012) Laparoscopic complete mesocolic excision for right colon cancer. Surg Endosc 26:2976–2980
21. Bertelsen CA, Bols B, Ingeholm P, Jansen JE, Neuenschwander AU, Vilandt J (2011) Can the quality of colonic surgery be improved by standardization of surgical technique with complete mesorectal excision? Colorectal Dis 13:1123–1129

Chapter 28
Anterior Resection of the Rectum

Masaki Fukunaga, Goutaro Katsuno, Kunihiko Nagakari, and Seiichiro Yoshikawa

Abstract Single-port laparoscopic surgery (SPLS) for colorectal cancer is a recent development in minimally invasive surgery. Although the devices and techniques for SPLS are being improved year by year, some technical difficulties remain. In this chapter, we explain how to perform SPLS for sigmoid and rectal cancer. SPLS is usually applied to patients with a relatively small tumor (less than 4 cm) and without peritonitis carcinomatosa. A vertical incision (approximately 2.5 cm in length) is made. After insertion of an atraumatic wound retractor (Alexis™ (Applied Medical, Rancho Santa Margarita, CA, USA)), which remains in place throughout the procedure, a multi-access platform (MAP) is manually inserted into the incision. In most cases, standard straight laparoscopic instruments are used. All SPLS procedures are performed with surgical techniques similar to those used in our standard laparoscopic procedures. Left-sided anastomoses are performed intracorporeally with a circular stapler. We usually divide the colon or rectum using a flexible laparoscopic linear stapler inserted through the MAP. However, when it is technically difficult to divide the rectum at the lower level, we often use the prolapsing technique to cut the rectum more confidently.

Keywords Prolapsing technique • Rectal cancer • Sigmoidal cancer • Single-port laparoscopic surgery

M. Fukunaga (✉) • G. Katsuno • K. Nagakari • S. Yoshikawa
Department of Surgery, Juntendo Urayasu Hospital, Juntendo University,
2-1-1 Tomioka, Urayasu 279-0021, Japan
e-mail: masaki-f@juntendo-urayasu.jp

T. Mori and G. Dapri (eds.), *Reduced Port Laparoscopic Surgery*,
DOI 10.1007/978-4-431-54601-6_28, © Springer Japan 2014

28.1   Introduction

Conventional laparoscopic surgery (CLS) for colon cancer has been shown to be oncologically equivalent to open surgery in large prospective randomized studies [1, 2], and CLS is accepted as standard surgery for colon cancer. In recent years, transumbilical single-port laparoscopic surgery (SPLS) has gained interest and popularity [3]. SPLS is an emerging surgical method in the pursuit of minimally invasive surgery. In this chapter, we explain how to perform SPLS for colon cancer safely and reliably.

28.2   Indications and Contraindications

SPLS is usually applied to patients with a relatively small tumor (less than 4 cm) and no peritonitis carcinomatosa. Obesity (BMI >30 kg/m^2) and extensive dilatation of the intestine are contraindications for SPLS. When we encounter difficulties that prevent us from performing SPLS safely and reliably, we usually convert SPLS to reduced-port laparoscopic surgery or CLS.

28.3   Pre-operative Evaluation

Three-dimensional computed tomography angiography is generally performed pre-operatively. Having a good grasp of vessel distribution preoperatively is very useful in planning and simulating the operation. When SPLS is planned for patients with a small tumor, preoperative endoscopic marking of the colonic lesion by tattooing and clipping is recommended.

28.4   Surgical Devices

A 30-degree 5-mm-diameter rigid laparoscope or 5-mm flexible scope is usually used. According to our experience, SPLS for colorectal cancer is feasible and safe when performed by the "parallel method" with standard straight laparoscopic instruments. Laparoscopic coagulating shears (LCS) and Ligasure™ (Covidien, New Haven, CT, USA) are useful to control intraoperative bleeding, simplifying the surgical procedure, and improving the safety and reliability of SPLS.

28.5   Set-up

28.5.1   Body Position

General anesthesia is used in the same manner as in conventional laparoscopic colectomy. The patient is first placed in the lithotomy position (Fig. 28.1a). The operating table is then tilted so that the patient is in the steep Trendelenburg position. Changing the body position as needed becomes useful for maintaining the working space in SPLS. The body position must be secured by adequate padding and snug restraints in SPLS.

28.5.2   Port Position

A single intraumbilical 25-mm incision is made, and a multi-access platform (MAP) is inserted. Nowadays, we tend to use the EZ-access™ (Hakko Co., Nagano, Japan) MAP: The umbilicus is the only point of access to the abdomen for all patients. Three 5-mm ports are placed in the EZ-access™ (Hakko) (Fig. 28.1b). According to our clinical experience, the distance between each port must be at least 2 cm so that SPLS can be performed comfortably. The operator usually grasps forceps with the left hand and LCS with the right hand. A camera assistant must work on the left side of the surgeon to reduce the incidence of interference between the operator's instruments and the camera during the surgery (Fig. 28.1a).

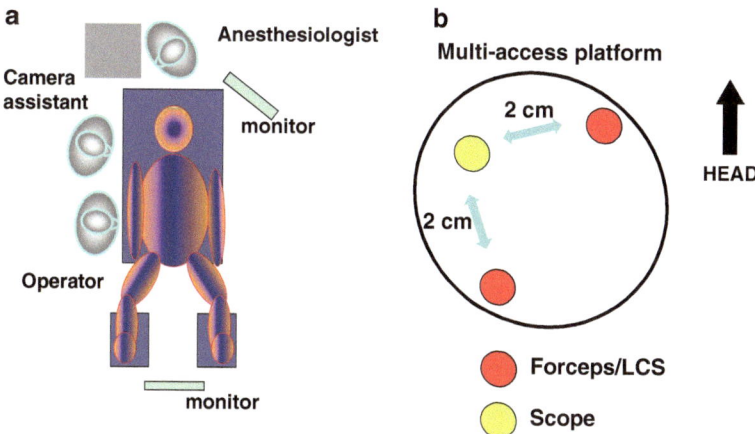

Fig. 28.1 Set-up. (**a**) Body position. (**b**) Port positions

28.6   Surgical Procedure

SPLS is principally performed with the use of standard straight laparoscopic instruments (Fig. 28.2). The tumor is exteriorized through a small umbilical incision covered with a wound protector. Anastomosis is performed laparoscopically by means of the double-stapling technique.

28.6.1   Medial-to-Lateral Approach

The working space around the inferior mesenteric artery (IMA) must first be secured by fully mobilizing the small intestine toward the cranial space. The surgeon then gently grasps and lifts the IMA ventrally using forceps held in the left hand. The left colonic mesentery and mesorectum are mobilized by a medial-to-lateral approach, keeping the superior hypogastric plexus and proper rectal fascia in view and preserving them with the aid of LCS or laparoscopic bipolar scissors held by the right hand (Fig. 28.3).

Tips for Maintaining the Working Space

In CLS, the operator concentrates only on lymph node dissection around the IMA because the assistant surgeon can maintain the working space by grasping the IMA gently and lifting it ventrally. In SPLS, however, the operator must perform lymph node dissection while securing the working space himself. Therefore, in SPLS, the operating table must be fully tilted so that the patient remains in the steep

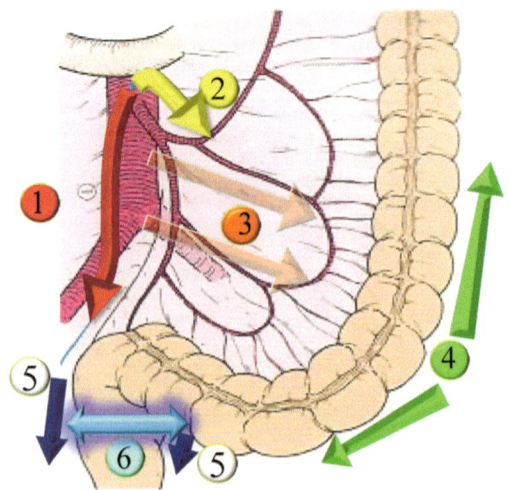

Fig. 28.2 Surgical steps

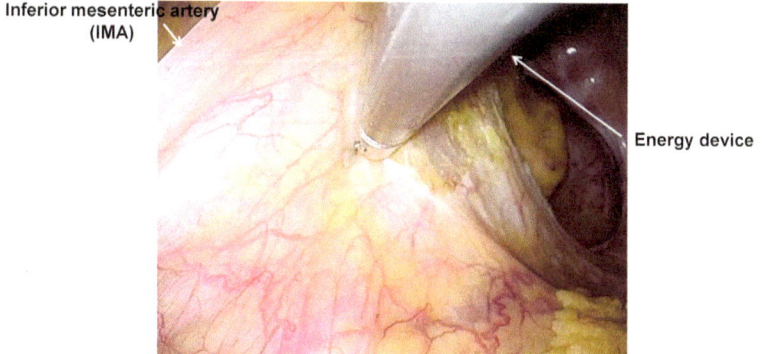

Fig. 28.3 Medial-to-lateral approach. The left colonic mesentery is mobilized by a medial-to-lateral approach, preserving the superior hypogastric plexus with the aid of LCS or laparoscopic bipolar scissors held by the right hand

Trendelenburg position. This keeps the intestines from interfering with the working space. Large gauze is also useful for maintaining the working space when it is placed at the left side of the IMA.

28.6.2 Lymph Node Dissection Around the Root of the Inferior Mesenteric Artery (IMA)

In patients with advanced-stage cancer, the root of the IMA is exposed with LCS, and the IMA is sealed and divided along with lymph node dissection with a LigaSure™ (Covidien) vessel sealer. In patients with early-stage cancer, the superior rectal artery is sealed and divided to preserve the left colic artery (Fig. 28.4). The LCS is also useful for hemostasis during lymphadenectomy.

28.6.3 Division of the Inferior Mesenteric Vein (IMV)

The IMV is sealed and divided at the level of the IMA stump with the use of a LigaSure™ (Covidien) vessel sealer (Fig. 28.5). The working space is then expanded. Great care must be exercised to prevent injury to the left colic artery because this vessel usually lies close to the IMV. Absence of bleeding contributes to maintaining a good working space and a clear laparoscopic view, especially when performing SPLS. Identifying the subperitoneal fascia is very important. This serves as a landmark for preserving the underlying ureter and gonadal vessels.

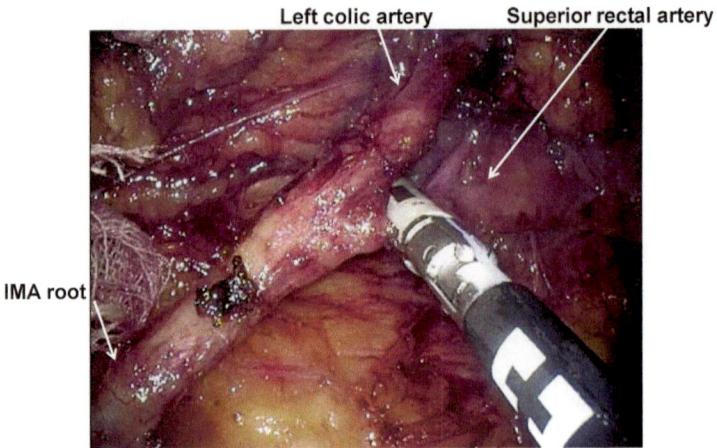

Fig. 28.4 Lymph node dissection. The superior rectal artery is sealed and divided to preserve the left colic artery in cases of early-stage cancer

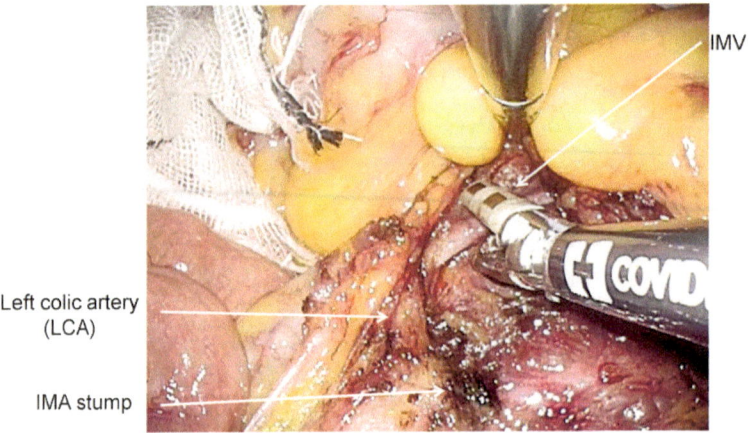

Fig. 28.5 Division of inferior mesenteric vein (IMV). The IMV is sealed and divided at the level of the IMA stump with a LigaSure™ vessel sealer (Covidien). The IMV is usually close to the LCA

28.6.4   Mobilization of the Left Colon

The operating table is fully tilted to the right. By simply incising the lateral attachment near the sigmoid-descending (SD) junction, the sigmoid colon, and the rectum, the left colon is fully mobilized.

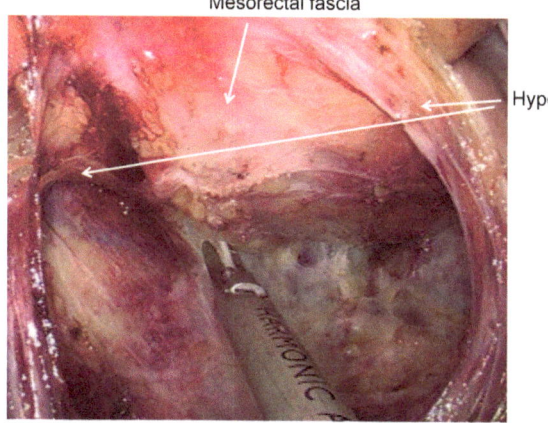

Mesorectal fascia

Hypogastric nerve

Fig. 28.6 Rectal mobilization from the retroperitoneum. The rectum must be fully mobilized from the retroperitoneum by means of sharp and blunt dissection toward the pelvic floor

28.6.5 Mobilization of the Rectum with Total Mesorectum Excision

Mobilization of the rectum while preserving the proper rectal fascia is very important. When the rectum is lifted with gauze grasped by the forceps held with the left hand, the risk of damaging the rectal fascia is reduced. The rectum must be fully resected through total mesorectum excision, which means sharp and blunt dissection toward the pelvic floor (Fig. 28.6). The better the mobilization, the more comfortable the division of the rectum.

28.6.6 Transection of the Mesorectum and Rectum

The proper rectal fascia is incised at the distal resection line with LCS (Fig. 28.7a), and the mesorectal tissue bundles are sealed thoroughly and transected with the aid of LigaSure™ (Covidien). The distal rectum is then clamped with detachable forceps, and rectal washout is performed. The rectum is then transected with an endoscopic linear stapler inserted through the MAP with no more than three cartridges (Fig. 28.7b).

Tips for Transecting the Mesorectum

The mesorectum is usually divided by inserting LCS through the umbilical site. It is difficult to correctly transect the mesorectum vertical to the rectum when cutting the

Fig. 28.7 (a) Transection of distal mesorectum. Proper rectal fascia is incised at the distal resection line with LCS. The operator needs to place the mesorectum at a vertical direction to the LCS by mobilizing the rectum deep enough into the pelvic space. (b) Transection of distal rectum. The rectum is transected with an endoscopic linear stapler inserted through the MAP with no more than three cartridges

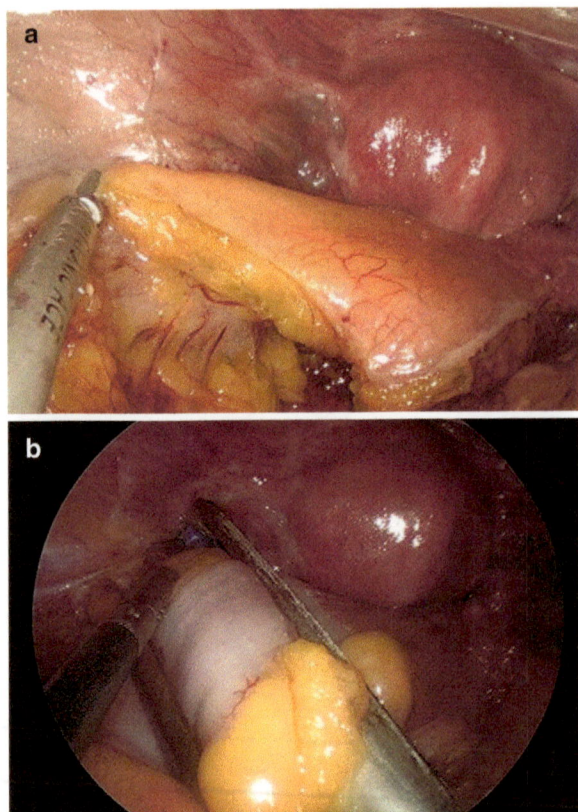

lower rectum. To overcome this difficulty, the operator needs to place the mesorectum (not the LCS!) vertical to the LCS by mobilizing the rectum deep into the pelvic space. Marking the distal incision line by LCS is also important.

28.6.7 Specimen Extraction

28.6.7.1 Extraction Through the Umbilical Wound

The surgical specimen is usually extracted through the small umbilical wound. The wound must be covered with a wound protector (Alexis™ (Applied Medical)). The colon is exteriorized, and the mesocolon is divided with Ligasure™ (Covidien). The anvil of the stapler is secured in the proximal colon. The umbilical incision may need to be lengthened slightly to accommodate extraction of a large tumor.

Fig. 28.8 Extraction through the natural orifice. (**a**) The distal rectum is gradually everted and pulled transanally out of the body. (**b**) The prolapsing technique is useful when it is technically difficult to cut the lower rectum with an endoscopic linear stapler inserted through the umbilicus

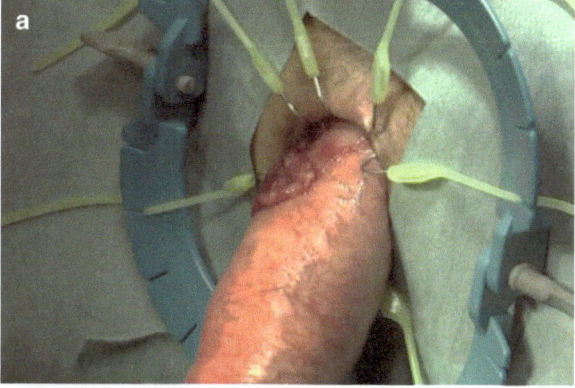

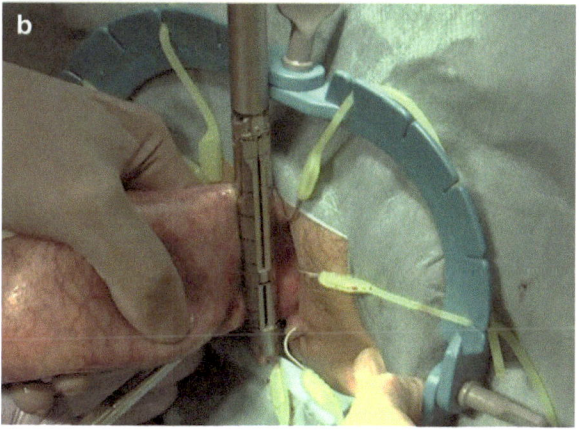

28.6.7.2 Extraction Through the Natural Orifice (Anus) by the Prolapsing Technique

The prolapsing technique is useful when cutting the lower rectum by inserting an endoscopic linear stapler through the MAP is technically difficult [4]. The first step for this procedure is to divide the mesentery intracorporeally until the bowel tube is exposed to secure an adequate proximal surgical margin. The proximal bowel is then transected with a flexible laparoscopic stapler inserted through the MAP without transecting the distal rectum. Grasping forceps are then inserted under laparoscopic observation from the anus to grab the staple line of the distal rectum safely. Finally, the distal rectum is gradually everted and pulled transanally out of the body (Fig. 28.8a). Rectal washout and wiping off are performed extracorporeally by the perineal surgeon, who uses approximately 2,000 mL of saline mixed with povidone iodine. This is followed by vertical transection of the distal bowel with a stapler (TA™ stapler with a green cartridge or Echelon™ (Ethicon, Cincinnati, OH, USA) with a gold cartridge) at a slow speed (Fig. 28.8b). The inverted rectal stump can be reinforced with stitches under direct vision. The distal end of the bowel is pushed back into the body. The anvil head is usually attached to the proximal colon extracorporeally. It can be connected to the circular stapler introduced from the anus laparoscopically.

28.6.8 Anastomosis

Intracorporeal anastomosis is performed by the double-stapling technique. All anastomoses are tested by rectal air insufflation. Generally, a drainage tube is not placed.

28.7 Conclusion

SPLS is indicated only for selected patients because SPLS is more technically difficult than CLS. It is important for surgeons to grasp the specific properties of SPLS to ensure that SPLS will be performed safely and reliably.

References

1. The Clinical Outcomes of Surgical Therapy Study Group (2004) A comparison of laparoscopically assisted and open colectomy for colon cancer. N Engl J Med 350:2050–2059
2. Jayne DG, Guillou PJ, Thorpe H, Quirke P, Copeland J, Smith AM, Heath RM, Brown JM, UK MRC CLASICC Trial Group (2007) Randomized trial of laparoscopic-assisted resection of colorectal carcinoma: 3-year results of the UK MRC CLASICC Trial Group. J Clin Oncol 21:3061–3068
3. Katsuno G, Fukunaga M, Nagakari K, Yoshikawa S, Ouchi M, Hirasaki Y (2011) Single incision laparoscopic colectomy for colon cancer: early experience with 31 cases. Dis Colon Rectum 54:705–710
4. Fukunaga M, Kidokoro A, Iba T, Sugiyama K, Fukunaga T, Nagakari K, Suda M, Yosikawa S (2005) Laparoscopy-assisted low anterior resection with a prolapsing technique for low rectal cancer. Surg Today 35:598–602

Chapter 29
Appendectomy

Noriaki Kameyama

Abstract Single-incision laparoscopic appendectomy (SILA) is an emerging technique and gaining increased attention by its superiority in cosmesis. A 2.0-cm vertical transumbilical incision is commonly used for the single-port, followed by fascial puncture method, multi-channel port method, or glove method. Appendectomy can be performed either extra- or intracorporeally. In cases of minor inflammation or interval appendectomy, the cecum can be mobilized and the appendix is divided extracorporeally. By contrast, in cases of severe inflammation, the mobilization of cecum is often difficult and the division of the appendix is performed intracorporeally. In intracorporeal appendectomy, ligation (preformed knot) is mostly used for the division of the appendix and endostapler is used for the necrotic base of the appendix. Ligasure™ (Covidien, New Haven, CT, USA) is widely used for the division of the mesoappendix. Randomized controlled trials and our retrospective analysis comparing single-incision with standard 3-port appendectomy have shown equivalent clinical outcomes among the two approaches in terms of operative time, postoperative pain, and complications. In this context, SILA can be a good option for children and young women.

Keywords Appendectomy • Single-incision laparoscopic surgery (SLS) • Single-incision laparoscopic appendectomy

N. Kameyama (✉)
Department of Surgery, International Goodwill Hospital, 1-28-1, Nishigaoka, Izumi,
Yokohama, Kanagawa, Japan
e-mail: drkameyama@yahoo.co.jp

T. Mori and G. Dapri (eds.), *Reduced Port Laparoscopic Surgery*,
DOI 10.1007/978-4-431-54601-6_29, © Springer Japan 2014

29.1 Introduction

Acute appendicitis remains the most common gastrointestinal emergency in developed countries occurring approximately 8 % of the population [1]. Laparoscopic appendectomy has been widespread since the first introduction by Semm in 1983 [2] and evidence regarding its relevance and effectiveness has already been established by multiple randomized prospective studies [3] that demonstrate the superiority of laparoscopic approach over open approach in terms of pain, morbidity, postoperative recovery, hospital stay, and cosmesis. Single-incision laparoscopic appendectomy (SILA) was first reported by Pelosi et al. [4] in 1992. This report introduced an effort to reduce multiple port access in laparoscopic appendectomy. Thereafter, the concept of reduced port laparoscopic surgery has been developed and gained its popularity to minimize the total length of skin incision and number of port access for potential benefit on pain and/or cosmesis over standard 3-port appendectomy. In SILA, single incision is made within the umbilicus, which is defined as a natural embryonic scar. In this context, this approach can be referred to as a subtype of natural orifice translumenal endoscopic surgery (NOTES) or embryonic-NOTES (e-NOTES). The umbilical scar is deepened inside the groove of the umbilicus and hardly visible after surgery.

There have been numerous reports of various techniques for SILA. This report summarizes a variety of surgical techniques systematically, reviews prospective randomized controlled studies versus standard 3-port appendectomy, and provides discussion on current status of SILA based upon evidence-based approach to justify the indication for SILA.

29.2 Indications and Contraindications

29.2.1 SILA Versus 3-Port Laparoscopic Appendectomy

SILA has become widespread in parallel with other single-incision laparoscopic surgeries such as cholecystectomy, sleeve gastrectomy, and donor nephrectomy, and been an area of active investigation. However, its true relevance was unknown that directed subsequent publication of randomized controlled trials (RCTs) comparing single-incision with standard 3-port appendectomy since 2011 (Table 29.1). Although these RCTs are scientifically well-designed, the outcomes are rather various between the trials. Based on data from these RCTs, broad consensus has been established in terms of longer operative time for SILA, equivalent complication rates, and equivalent hospital stay. However, many trials support that the difference in operative time will become negligible with experience of the surgeon who performs SILA [5]. More intriguingly, the outcomes for postoperative pain are diametrically opposite. Two trials demonstrated less pain for SILA [6, 7], while one trial revealed less pain for 3-port appendectomy [8] with the other two being no

Table 29.1 RCTs for standard 3-port appendectomy *vs.* SILA

Author	Year	Port	Appendectomy	Operative time		Pain score (VAS score)		Complications		Hospital stay (h)	
				SILA	3-port	SILA	3-port	SILA	3-port	SILA	3-port
St Peter	2011	Fascial puncture	Extracorporeal	35	30	9.6	8.5	3.30 %	1.70 %	23	22
Frutos	2013	SILS port	GIA 45 mm	38	32	2.76	3.78	4/91	4/93	19	21
Sozutek	2013	SILS port	2/0 suture	33	30	2.9	3.4	1	1	26	29
Kye	2013	Glove	Endoloop	37	38	3.22	3.9	1.96 %	1.96 %	75	117
Perez	2013	Fascial puncture	GIA 45 mm	46	34	ns	ns	1	0	40	37

significant difference for postoperative pain [5, 9]. As shown by these different outcomes, it is been controversial whether postoperative pain is less for SILA compared to standard 3-port appendectomy due to the effect of less access port sites. SILA eliminates muscular penetration, which might result in less postoperative pain; while, fascial incision is greater for SILA, which might result in more postoperative pain. It is possible that discrepancies between the trials may be due to differences in the method for umbilical port access and/or division of the appendix. SILA includes a variety of surgical techniques as stated above. For example, SILS™ port (Covidien, New Haven, CT, USA) or wound retractor protect the umbilicus from contamination while the umbilicus cannot be protected by fascial puncture method, which may impact on different outcomes in wound infection. In addition, a larger fascial incision is required for SILS™ port (Covidien) insertion compared to Alexis wound retractor™ (Applied Medical, Rancho Santa Margarita, CA, USA), which may affect the outcomes in postoperative pain. Moreover, surgical difficulty level changes depending on how to divide the appendix (stapling or ligation), which may affect on operative time.

29.2.2 SILA for Complicated Appendicitis

The difficulty in keeping instrument triangulation limits the indication of SILA in cases with a retrocecal appendix or perforated appendix. It has been shown that operative time was significantly longer with complicated appendicitis (gangrene, abscess, perforation, and/or peritonitis) [6]. In addition, retrocecal appendicitis often necessitates a second, or even a third port [10]. Therefore, it is conceivable that complicated and retrocecal appendicitis can be considered as a relative contraindication for SILA. However, Kye et al. [7] performed SILA for cases of complicated appendicitis and showed comparable results in operative time and even better results in hospital stay and recovery time to daily life in comparison with standard 3-port appendectomy. Therefore, it is possible that advance in surgical instruments for SILA and maturation in our surgical techniques to perform SILA could broaden the indication of SILA for complicated appendicitis in the near future.

29.2.3 Indications for SILA

In obese patients, it is even more difficult to keep the instrument triangulation in SILA; therefore, they do not benefit from SILA [11]. SILA for patients with a body mass index >95th percentile shows longer operative time, increased postoperative pain, and increased complication rates (wound infection and intraabdominal abscess). In addition, patients with previous lower abdominal surgery are almost inevitable to have abdominal adhesions that could limit the indication for SILA. Taken together, relative contraindications for SILA include retrocecal appendicitis, complicated appendicitis, obese patients, and past history of lower abdominal surgery. However, technical and instrumental progress in the single-port approach could expand the current indication. Given the fact that almost all the clinical outcomes are equivalent between SILA and standard 3-port appendectomy, the major advantage of SILA over standard 3-port appendectomy is focused mostly on cosmesis. In this regard, good populations that notably benefit from SILA include children and premenopausal women.

29.3 Technique

29.3.1 Patient Positioning and Room Set-up

Operation room is set up and the patient is placed in a fashion analogous to conventional 3-port laparoscopic appendectomy. Briefly, the patient is placed in the supine position with the legs together, the left arm is tucked, and a Foley catheter inserted to decompress the bladder. The surgeon and camera assistant both stand on the left of the patient facing the monitor on the right side at the patient's hip. The operating table is tilted in the Trendelenburg position with the right side up for 15–20°. To perform single-incision surgery, the laparoscope should have a co-axial, not perpendicular, light cable to avoid crowding. A 30 degree 5-mm laparoscope is often used.

29.3.2 Umbilical Port

29.3.2.1 Fascial Puncture Method (Direct Access Method)

After local anesthetic infiltration, a 2.0-cm vertical transumbilical incision is made and a subcutaneous pocket is created to expose the anterior fascia. A Veress needle is inserted to establish pneumoperitoneum and removed after insufflation. Three laparoscopic ports (one 10-mm and two 5-mm ports or three 5-mm ports) are placed by a closed access method or an optical trocar access method. The first trocar is at the base of the umbilical stalk with the second at the inferior edge along the linea alba and the third at the superior edge along the linea alba or the right hand side of the first trocar. The first trocar can be inserted without pneumoperitoneum through a small umbilical fascial defect at the base of the umbilical stalk. Three ports should be of low-profile (preferably threaded and different in length) in order to avoid clashing.

29.3.2.2 Multi-Channel Port Method (Access Device Method)

After local anesthetic infiltration, a 2.0-cm vertical transumbilical incision is made down to the peritoneum under direct vision. A multiple-entry port from various manufactures (Table 29.2) is inserted through the incision by an open access method.

Table 29.2 Multiple-entry ports	SILS™ port, Covidien, New Haven, CT, USA
	Gelport, Applied Medical, Rancho Santa Margarita, CA, USA
	Unix-X, Pnavel Systems, Brooklyn, NY, USA
	Triport, Advanced Surgical Concepts, Wicklow, Ireland
	SSLAS, Ethicon, Cincinnati, OH, USA
	X-Cone, Karl Storz-Endoskope, Tuttlingen, Germany
	OCTO port, Dalim Surgnet, Seoul, Korea
	Spider surgical system, TransEnterix, Durham, NC, USA

29.3.2.3 Glove Method (Home Made Port Method)

After local anesthetic infiltration, a 2.0-cm vertical transumbilical incision is made for Alexis wound retractor™ XS size (Applied Medical), which is inserted by an open access method and a surgical glove (size 5.5) is attached. Three low-profile laparoscopic ports (all 5-mm trocars) are inserted through the holes of the surgical glove with cut fingertips (Figs. 29.1 and 29.2).

29.3.3 Appendectomy

29.3.3.1 Extracorporeal Appendectomy

The appendix locates at the posteromedial border of the cecum and can be identified by following the anterior taenia coli to its confluence with the other two taeniae. The cecum is mobilized by incising the lateral attachment (Jackson's membrane and Lane's band) and the fusion fascia of Toldt. Complete mobilization of the appendix is confirmed by withdrawing the appendix towards the left upper quadrant. The appendix can be easily exteriorized if the instrument reaches a halfway point between the left costrochodral margin and the umbilical port. The appendix is withdrawn through the umbilicus and exteriorized to perform a conventional "open" appendectomy. If the appendix is perforated, the operating surgeon prefers to perform an intracorporeal appendectomy. Extracorporeal appendectomy is less expensive compared to intracorporeal appendectomy and can be a good alternative to expensive intracorporeal devices.

29.3.3.2 Intracorporeal Appendectomy

Exteriorization of the appendix is not always possible in cases of more inflamed appendicitis or obese patients. For such cases, the appendix must be divided intracorporeally. The identification and mobilization of appendix can be performed in the same manner as in extracorporeal appendectomy. The following appendectomy

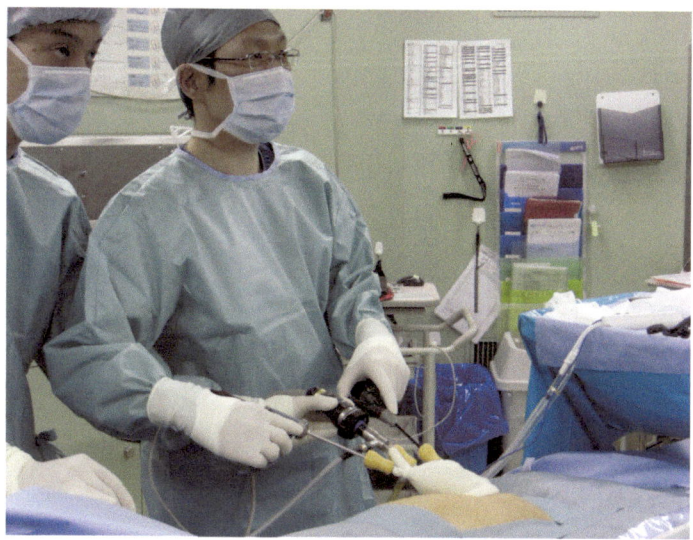

Fig. 29.1 Glove method using Alexis wound retractor™ (Applied Medical)

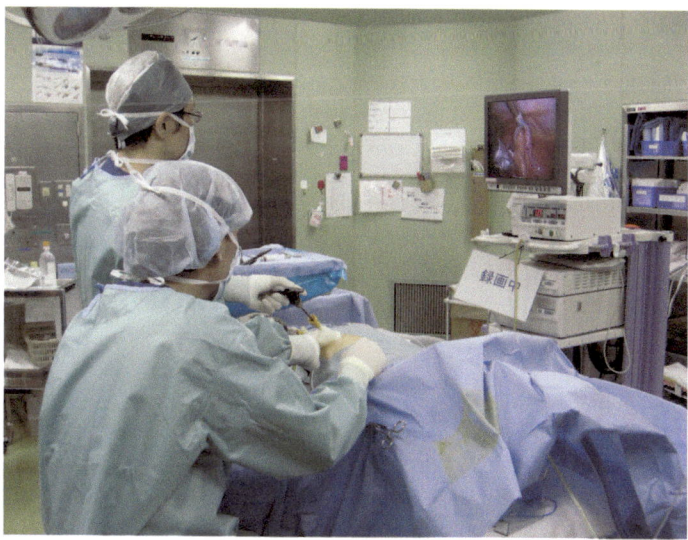

Fig. 29.2 Positioning of the surgeon and assistant

is done in a purely laparoscopic approach without exteriorizing the appendix. This method has the potential to be more technically demanding than the extracorporeal method, accounting for the higher intraoperative and postoperative complication rates, such as hemorrhage, wound infection, and intrabdominal abscess [12].

Fig. 29.3 Division of the appendix by a 45-mm endostapler

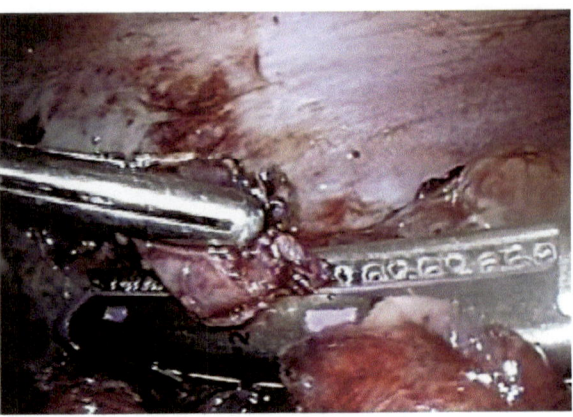

29.3.3.3 Division of the Appendix

Endoscopic Stapling

A mesoappendicular window is created at the base of the appendix. Care must be taken to avoid the avulsion of a friable appendix. The mesoappendix is transected by a 30- or 45-mm endostapler (vascular load). The appendix is then transected at its base by a 30- or 45-mm endostapler (tissue load; Fig. 29.3). Division of the appendix should be as close to the cecum as possible in order to avoid stump appendicitis. The base of the appendix and the mesoappendix are checked for any evidence of bleeding from their staple lines. If the base of the appendix is necrotic, a small portion of the cecum can be resected by the stapler. To perform endoscopic stapling technique, one of the trocars must be a 12-mm trocar for insertion of the endoscopic stapling system. A retrieval bag is inserted through the 12-mm trocar for retrieval of the resected appendix to avoid port-site contamination.

Endoscopic Ligation

A mesoappendicular window is created at the base of the appendix. A 2/0 polyglactin suture is delivered through the window and the mesoappendix is ligated with a fishermen's knot tied extracorporeally. This procedure is repeated for the appendix (Fig. 29.4), and the appendix and mesoappendix are transected by endoscopic scissors between the ligatures. The mucosa is cauterized. Double ligation is preferred for the base of appendix. A retrieval bag is inserted for retrieval of the appendix. Alternatively, the surgeon can use commercially available endoscopic ligation devices such as Endoloop Ligature™ (Ethicon (Cincinnati OH, USA); Fig. 29.5) or Surgitie Loop™ (Covidien). Endoscopic stapling rather than ligation is often preferred for a severely inflamed appendix to secure the closure of the appendix.

Fig. 29.4 Division of
the appendix by a 2/0
polyglactin suture ligation

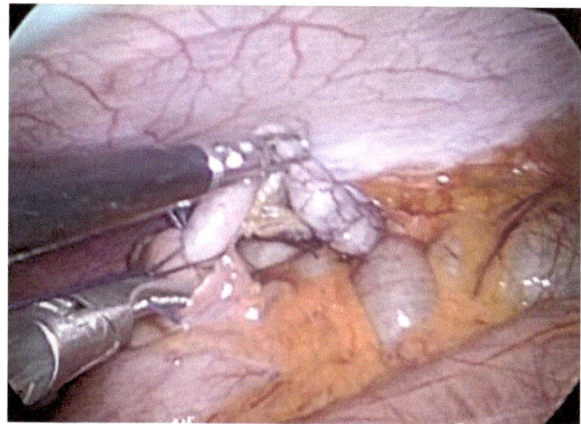

Fig. 29.5 Division of the
appendix by an Endoloop™
(Ethicon)

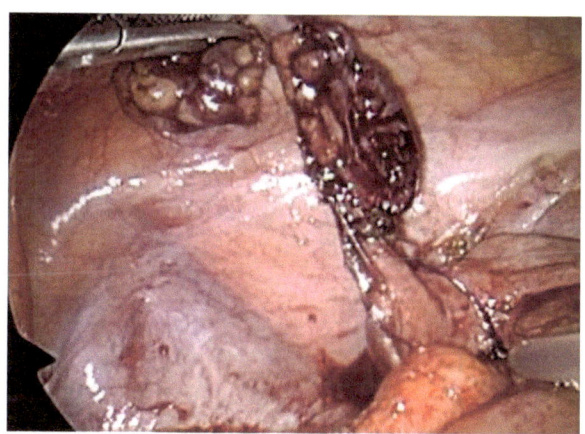

29.3.3.4   Division of the Mesoappendix

The mesoappendix and appendiceal artery can also be safely transected by an ultrasonic shears (Harmonic Scalpel™ (Ethicon)), a bipolar electrocautery (Ligasure™ (Covidien)), or an endoscopic clipping (Fig. 29.6).

29.3.4   Normograde and Retrograde Appendectomy

When performing intracorporeal appendectomy, the appendectomy can be either normograde or retrograde depending on the visibility of the tip of the appendix. Mobilization of the appendix is not a mandatory procedure before transection of the appendix. Transection of the appendix can be preceded by mobilization if the tip of the appendix is not clearly visible.

Fig. 29.6 Division of the mesoappendix by Ligasure™ (Covidien)

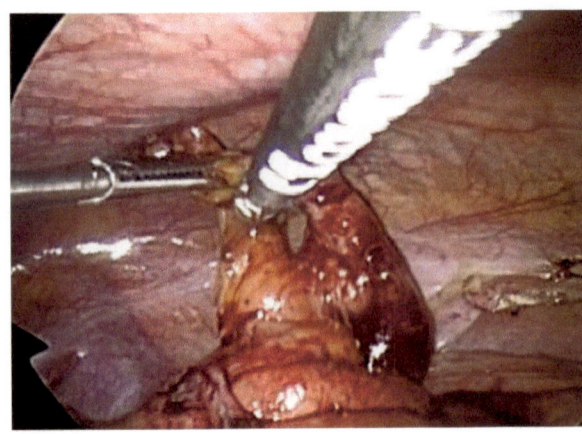

29.3.5 Single-port PLUS-ONE

It is difficult to keep the instrument triangulation in single-port surgery and an additional suspension device can be helpful to establish triangulation. The appendix is suspended by a transabdominal sling suture [10, 13, 14], a port-free endocavity retractor (EndoGrab™, Virtual Ports, Inc., Caesaera, Israel) or a supplemental miniport.

29.4 Tips and Tricks

29.4.1 Patient Position

SILA is a solo surgery, in which only two ports are available for manipulation. Therefore initial patient positioning is important in order to obtain a good view with no intestines around the appendix. We often set the patient in the left semilateral position with a vacuum mattress that can be molded to take the intestines away from the appendix. In addition, the operating table is tilted in the Trendelenburg position with the right side up for 15–20°.

29.4.2 Laparoscope

A rigid or non-flexible camera is preferred for SILA. Flexible laparoscopic instruments have a high chance of getting damaged due to instrument crowding and interference. In addition, a co-axial, not perpendicular, light cable is mandatory to avoid crowding.

29.4.3 Cross-Hand Technique

Articulating devices are not necessary to perform SILA. However, a cross-hand technique is required to perform SILA with conventional (straight) laparoscopic instruments. The surgeon may need to hold the appendix by his/her right hand and manipulate the mesoappendix with an energy device with his/her left hand, which requires a learning curve. Right-handed surgeons should train their left hand to behave as the same as their right hand.

29.5 Recommendations from the Author

29.5.1 Retrospective Analysis of Our Experience

We have introduced SILA in October 2009. Between October 2009 and April 2013, we performed 160 appendectomies at the Department of Surgery in International Goodwill Hospital. Open appendectomy (n=82) was mainly chosen for compli-cated cases such as abscess formation (46 %), gangrenous appendicitis (55 %), or diffuse peritonitis (40 %; Table 29.3). Standard 3-port appendectomy (n=7) was performed as a bridge between open and SILA and chosen for more complicated cases compared to SILA. SILA (n=71) was not selected for complicated cases but for early stages of appendicitis and female patients, including 27 cases (38 %) of interval appendectomies. Early stages of appendicitis were confirmed pathologi-cally with a high percentage of catarrhal appendicitis (31 %). Parametric values of

Table 29.3 Demographical characteristics of the patients

	Open	Standard 3-port	SILA	P
Patients	82	7	71	
Men/women	53/29	6/1	30/41	<0.05
Mean age (years)	42.8±2.3	43.9±3.7	37.7±1.9	NS
Interval appendectomy n (%)	0	0	27 (31)	
Conversion n (%)		1 (14)	3 (4)	
Abscess formation n (%)	38 (46)	3 (43)	4 (6)	<0.001
Gangrenous appendicitis n (%)	45 (55)	3 (43)	8 (11)	<0.001
Diffuse peritonitis n (%)	33 (40)	3 (43)	1 (1)	<0.001
Local peritonitis n (%)	49 (60)	4 (57)	42 (59)	NS
Pathology n (%)				
Catarrhal	4 (5)	1 (14)	22 (31)	<0.001
Phlegmonous	30 (37)	2 (29)	26 (37)	NS
Gangrenous	42 (52)	3 (43)	15 (21)	<0.001
Chronic	1 (1)	1 (14)	8 (11)	<0.05

Table 29.4 Surgical
technique for SILA

	SILA (n=71)
Intra-/Extracorporeal appendectomy	
Intra-	39
Extra-	32
Division of the appendix	
Endoloop	25
Endostapler	4
Ligation	10
Division of the mesoappendix	
Ligasure	37
Ligation	3

Table 29.5 Operative and postoperative results (n=160)

	Open (n=82)	Standard 3-port (n=7)	SILA (n=71)	P
Operative time (min)	81±5	74±5	65±3	<0.01
Blood loss (mL)	90±23	0±0	8±6	<0.01
Total doses of analgesics	4.2±0.3	3.7±0.7	2.4±0.2	<0.001
Oral intake (days)	3.8±0.5	3.0±0.7	1.7±0.1	<0.001
Hospital stay (days)	8.1±0.7	7.4±2.3	4.0±0.2	<0.001
Complications n (%)				
Wound infection	8 (10)	0 (0)	0 (0)	<0.05
Ileus	3 (4)	2 (29)	0 (0)	NS
Fecal fistula	2 (2)	0 (0)	0 (0)	NS

the three groups were analyzed retrospectively and compared with a one-way analysis of variance (ANOVA) followed by Newman–Keuls post-hoc test for pairwise comparisons. All the P values listed in the following tables were open vs. SILA. Values are expressed as means ± SEM.

SILA was performed both intra- and extra-corporeally with almost the same degree (Table 29.4). Division of appendix was mostly performed by Endoloop™ (Ethicon), and mesoappendix by Ligasure™ (Covidien). Division can be substituted by simple ligation with a 2/0 polyglactin suture, which results in a marked reduction in operative cost. Endostapler was used for the division of a gangrenous base of the appendix. A supplemental miniport was required for only four cases and the other 67 cases (94 %) were performed by pure single-port surgery.

The mean operative time and blood loss were less in the SILA group (Table 29.5). Total doses of analgesics and wound infection were also less in the SILA group. Furthermore, the time of starting oral intake was shorter in the SILA group, which resulted in shorter hospital stay.

29.5.2 Recommendations from the Authors

This analysis is obviously retrospective. Complex cases were allocated for open surgery with early cases, being allocated for single-port surgery. Therefore it is not fair to compare these two approaches from our results. However, it may be conceivable to conclude that SILA reduces operative time, pain, and postoperative complications, contributing to its less invasiveness and superiority among other approaches. We speculate that the less invasiveness of SILA outweighs its surgical difficulty especially for early cases including interval appendectomy cases.

References

1. Sauerland S, Lefering R, Neugebauer EA (2004) Laparoscopic versus open surgery for suspected appendicitis. Cochrane Database Syst Rev CD001546
2. Semm K (1983) Endoscopic appendectomy. Endoscopy 15:59–64
3. Katkhouda N, Mason RJ, Towfigh S et al (2005) Laparoscopic versus open appendectomy: a prospective randomized double-blind study. Ann Surg 242:439–448, discussion 448–450
4. Pelosi MA, Pelosi MA 3rd (1992) Laparoscopic appendectomy using a single umbilical puncture (minilaparoscopy). J Reprod Med 37:588–594
5. Sozutek A, Colak T, Dirlik M et al (2013) A prospective randomized comparison of single-port laparoscopic procedure with open and standard 3-port laparoscopic procedures in the treatment of acute appendicitis. Surg Laparosc Endosc Percutan Tech 23:74–78
6. Frutos MD, Abrisqueta J, Lujan J et al (2013) Randomized prospective study to compare laparoscopic appendectomy versus umbilical single-incision appendectomy. Ann Surg 257:413–418
7. Kye BH, Lee J, Kim W et al (2013) Comparative study between single-incision and three-port laparoscopic appendectomy: a prospective randomized trial. J Laparoendosc Adv Surg Tech A 23:431–436
8. St Peter SD, Adibe OO, Juang D et al (2011) Single incision versus standard 3-port laparoscopic appendectomy: a prospective randomized trial. Ann Surg 254:586–590
9. Perez EA, Piper H, Burkhalter LS et al (2013) Single-incision laparoscopic surgery in children: a randomized control trial of acute appendicitis. Surg Endosc 27:1367–1371
10. Ates O, Hakguder G, Olguner M et al (2007) Single-port laparoscopic appendectomy conducted intracorporeally with the aid of a transabdominal sling suture. J Pediatr Surg 42:1071–1074
11. Iqbal CW, Ostlie DJ (2012) The minimally invasive approach to appendectomy: is less better? Eur J Pediatr Surg 22:201–206
12. Rehman H, Ahmed I (2011) Technical approaches to single port/incision laparoscopic appendicectomy: a literature review. Ann R Coll Surg Engl 93:508–513
13. Akgur FM, Olguner M, Hakguder G et al (2010) Appendectomy conducted with single port incisionless-intracorporeal conventional equipment-endoscopic surgery. J Pediatr Surg 45:1061–1063
14. Lee SY, Lee HM, Hsieh CS et al (2011) Transumbilical laparoscopic appendectomy for acute appendicitis: a reliable one-port procedure. Surg Endosc 25:1115–1120

Chapter 30
Incisional and Ventral Hernia Repair

Norihito Wada, Toshiharu Furukawa, and Yuko Kitagawa

Abstract Ventral hernia is a common type of abdominal hernia. There are three types of ventral hernia: incisional hernia, spigelian hernia, and epigastric hernia. Traditionally, hernia repairs have been performed as open procedures. In the last decade, laparoscopic hernia repair has become popular. Laparoscopic surgery allows for a smaller incision, which results in less post-operative pain and less risk of incisional hernia. Decreases in the size and number of trocars should be considered if outcomes similar to those of traditional laparoscopic technique can be obtained. The indication for laparoscopic ventral hernia is a hernia with a minimum defect size of 3 cm. In cases of simultaneous contamination, the use of mesh is basically contraindicated. An inability to tolerate general anesthesia and uncontrolled coagulopathy are also contraindications. A small incision of 2–3 cm is made on the hernia bulge along the previous surgical scar. A silicone wound protector is used, and a silicone cap for use of several trocars is set. At least two trocars of 5-mm are needed to introduce the laparoscope and a tacker for mesh fixation. After complete detachment of all adhesions below the surgical scar, all incisional hernias must be evaluated, including small fascial defects. The mesh should be larger than the hernia defect with a margin of at least 3 cm in all directions. The silicone cap is opened, and the mesh is easily introduced through the wound protector and spread flat with the knitted side up. Lifting stitches are caught by a suture passer and fixed to the abdominal wall. With the use of fixation tacks, the edge of the mesh is circumferentially fixed to the abdominal wall.

Keywords Adhesiolysis • Incisional hernia • Ventral hernia • Mesh repair • Reduced port laparoscopic surgery

N. Wada (✉) • T. Furukawa • Y. Kitagawa
Department of Surgery, School of Medicine, Keio University,
35 Shinanomachi, Shinjuku-ku, Tokyo 160-8582, Japan
e-mail: nori-kkr@umin.ac.jp

T. Mori and G. Dapri (eds.), *Reduced Port Laparoscopic Surgery*,
DOI 10.1007/978-4-431-54601-6_30, © Springer Japan 2014

30.1 Introduction

The ventral hernia is a common type of abdominal hernia that accounts for approximately 10 % of all hernias. There are three types of ventral hernia: the incisional hernia, spigelian hernia, and epigastric hernia. Of these three types, the incisional hernia is the most common. An incisional hernia develops in an estimated 10–15 % of laparotomy incisions [1]. In the United States alone, approximately 400,000–500,000 incisional hernias arise from 4 to 5 million laparotomies performed annually [2].

Traditionally, hernia repairs have been performed as open procedures. Recurrence rates after open suture repair of incisional hernias are between 31 and 49 %, according to large-scale studies involving more than 100 cases [3]. With the introduction of mesh repair and component separation techniques, the recurrence rate has decreased dramatically. A recent meta-analysis showed the recurrence rate to be as low as 5 % [4]. Over the last decade, laparoscopic hernia repair has become popular. Good visualization of the entire incision scar ensures complete coverage of the hernia orifice, even in cases of a small subclinical hernia. Laparoscopic surgery, in comparison to open surgery, allows for a small incision, which results in less postoperative pain and less likely development of an incisional hernia, although the in-hospital costs are greater [4–7]. Laparoscopic ventral hernia repair can be offered by surgeons proficient in advanced laparoscopic techniques [8].

Conventional laparoscopic hernia repair usually requires a trocar for the camera, along with two to four trocars placed contralaterally on the sides of the abdomen for dissection and mesh placement. At least one of these trocars must be more than 10-mm for introduction of the mesh. Current laparoscopic procedures tend to reduce the number and size of the ports; thus, there are many reports of reduced port laparoscopic hernia repair (RPLHR). A decrease in the number and size of the trocars should be considered if outcomes similar to those of traditional laparoscopic hernia repair can be obtained.

30.2 Indications and Contraindications (Table 30.1)

Closing the hernia orifice even under local anesthesia can treat small ventral hernias. This method is, of course, less invasive than laparoscopic mesh repair. An Italian group [9] reported the indication for laparoscopic ventral hernia to be a hernia with a minimum defect of 3 cm (Fig. 30.1). The site of the defect does not seem to influence the indications/contraindications [9]. In cases of simultaneous contamination, due for example to bowel injury or intestinal strangulation, use of prosthesis is basically contraindicated. Uncontrolled coagulopathy is a contraindication for laparoscopic hernia surgery, and because the procedure is usually performed under general anesthesia, inability to tolerate general anesthesia is also a contraindication. Old age itself is not a contraindication for this procedure [10], and obese patients are good candidates for laparoscopic ventral hernia repair, too [11].

Table 30.1 Indications and contraindications for laparoscopic hernia repair

Indications
Hernia with a minimum defect size of 3 cm
Symptomatic hernia
Contraindications
Bowel injury
Intestinal strangulation
Intolerance to general anesthesia
Uncontrolled coagulopathy

Fig. 30.1 A typical incisional hernia indicated for reduced-port laparoscopic hernia repair

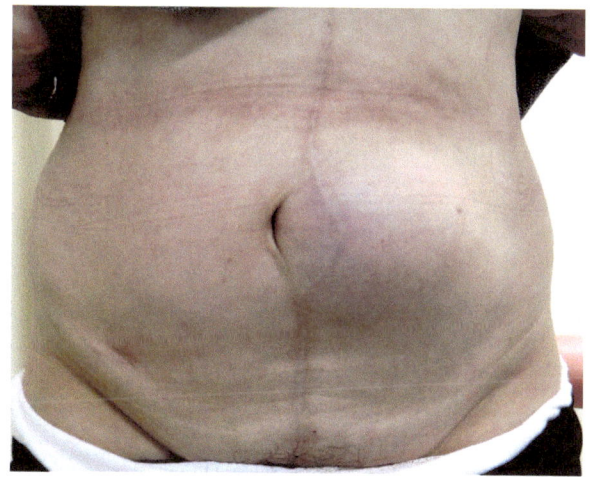

The indications and contraindications are basically the same for both conventional and RPLHR.

The advantages and disadvantages of RPLHR should be considered. The obvious advantage of fewer ports is better cosmesis, although equivalence in terms of clinical outcome is not well established. Informed consent must be obtained from patients in a careful manner.

30.3 Technique

The patient is placed in a supine position. Hair surrounding the incisional area is removed, and the skin surface is prepared in a routine manner. The region is covered with sterile drapes. To ensure adequate overlap of the prosthetic mesh, more than 10 cm should be added to the maximum measurements of the fascial defect in all directions.

Fig. 30.2 Appearance of
the surgical scar soon after
reduced-port laparoscopic
hernia repair

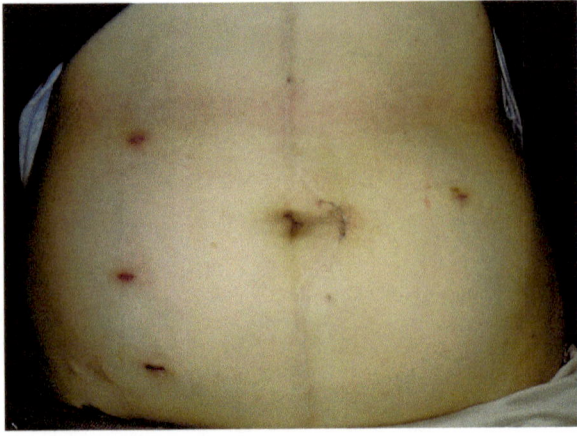

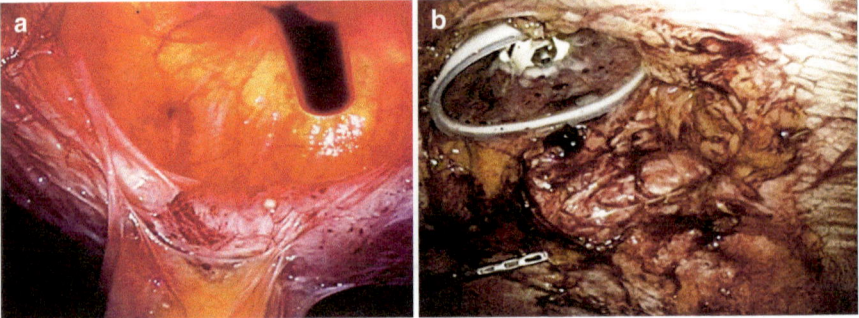

Fig. 30.3 The largest port through which the surgical sponges and mesh for hernia repair are
introduced. This incision is made within the fascial defect

A small incision of 2–3 cm is made on the hernia bulge along the previous surgical scar (Fig. 30.2). This incision is used for the first trocar and for the port to introduce surgical sponges and the mesh for the hernia repair (Fig. 30.3). The
subcutaneous tissue is carefully dissected down to the abdominal cavity. Once the
hernia sac is opened, the abdominal contents are placed back in the abdomen.
If severe adhesions around the hernia sac are observed, dissection 2 cm from the
edge of the incision line is enough to place the first port. A silicone wound protector
(Lap Protector™ (Hakko Co., Nagano, Japan)) is used, and a silicone cap (EZ
Access™ (Hakko)) designed for the use of several trocars is set. There are other
methods of initial trocar placement [12]. The best technique is the one with which
the surgeon is most experienced and comfortable. After 10-mmHg pneumoperitoneum is established, a 5-mm trocar is inserted at least 4 cm away from the fascial
edge, usually in the lateral abdomen. At least two trocars of 5-mm are necessary to
introduce the laparoscope and a tacker for fixation of the mesh. These two trocars

Fig. 30.4 All incisional hernias must be evaluated, including small fascial defects

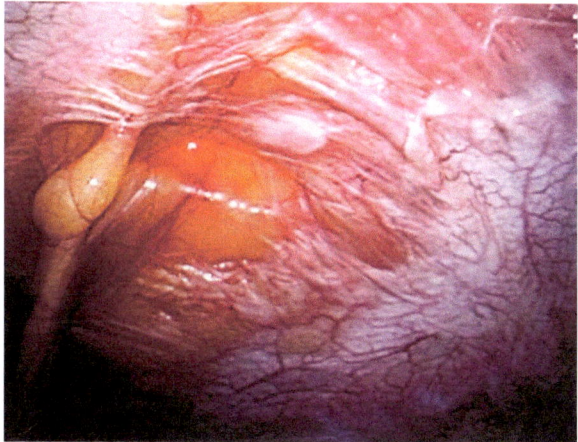

may be placed in a single-port. However, the longer incision may be a risk factor for development of an incisional hernia. Therefore, reducing the size of the ports rather than the number of ports would be preferable in this setting. If the planned trocar site cannot be visualized laparoscopically due to intraperitoneal adhesion, adhesiolysis is carried out from the first port with the use of several trocars.

After complete detachment of all adhesions below the surgical scar, all incisional hernias must be evaluated, including small fascial defects (Fig. 30.4). Some surgeons prefer to close the edge of the fascial defect laparoscopically [13, 14]. The clinical merits of this technique are not well clarified. If the fascial defect is closed in patients with a large central defect, the "tension free" concept will be abandoned, and the risk of rupture of the closed hernia orifice and recurrence of the hernia may increase. However, the risk of seroma formation and mesh migration into the cavity will be minimized [15]. The mesh should be larger than the hernia defect with a margin of at least 3 cm in all directions. Some reports indicate that the overlap should be at least 5 cm. Indeed, the optimal amount of overlap depends on the size and the anatomical site of the hernia orifice.

Many prosthetic materials are now available for ventral hernia repair [16, 17]. We usually use Parietex™ Composite mesh (Covidien, New Haven, CT, USA), which has a reabsorbable collagen barrier on one side to limit visceral attachments and a polyester knit structure on the other [18]. The mesh is introduced through the largest port or a 12-mm trocar. With our procedure, the EZ Access™ silicone cap (Hakko) is opened, and the mesh is easily introduced through the wound protector and spread flat with the knitted side up. Pneumoperitoneum is re-established, and the collagen-covered surface is confirmed to be facing the viscera. After the mesh is successfully spread, the incision with the Lap Protector™ (Hakko) is closed. In patients with a relatively small hernia orifice, fascial separation is approximated before skin closure. Lifting stitches, which are connected to the edge of the mesh, are caught by a suture passer (EndoClose™ (Covidien)) and firmly fixed to the

Fig. 30.5 The edge of the
mesh is circumferentially
fixed to the abdominal wall
with fixation tackers

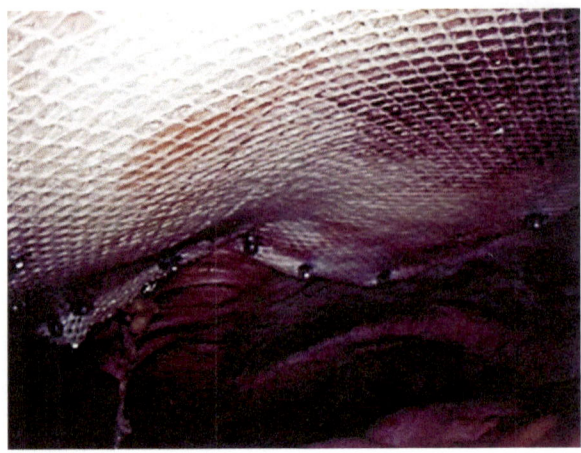

abdominal wall. With the use of fixation tacks [2], the edge of the mesh is
circumferentially fixed to the abdominal wall (Fig. 30.5). Opinions vary on the
method of mesh fixation, whether with a single or double crown of tacks, with or
without defect closure [19]. We do not use the double crown configuration or defect
closure routinely, although strong evidence supporting mesh fixation is lacking.
A port site is carefully closed if the incision is longer than 5 mm. This is done to
avoid development of an incisional hernia.

30.4   Tips and Tricks

To introduce the mesh into the abdominal cavity, a port of at least 12-mm in diameter is needed. This is a potential site of future incisional hernia. With our procedure, the largest incision through which prosthesis is inserted is made within the
hernia defect and finally covered with the mesh prosthesis. One of the major advantages of RPLHR is improved cosmesis. Our method is reasonable in this respect
because the longest incision is made on the previous surgical scar. All other ports
are 5 mm or less in diameter.

For mesh fixation with a tacking device, a certain distance from the trocar to the
edge of the mesh must be maintained to obtain an effective tacking angle. Therefore,
at least two ports 5-mm in diameter should be placed, one on each side of the hernia.
This limitation means that surgery performed through multiple small ports is preferable to that performed through a larger single-port. True RPLHR is possible for
selected patients. The longer incision, however, may become a risk factor for an
additional incisional hernia. Careful fascial closure of the large port site is essential.
We usually place a port within the hernia bulge where the mesh will cover the incision. Other ports used for adhesiolysis and mesh fixation should be 5-mm at most.

Use of a bladeless optical trocar as the first trocar is encouraged if the patient is obese [11]. Of course, the trocar site should be away from the previous surgical incision under which substantial adhesion is anticipated.

Many types of prosthesis are available for incisional hernia repair [16]. The mesh for IPOM (Intraperitoneal Onlay Mesh) repair is the gold standard. Some types of mesh have a memory coil ring, which facilitates the self-spreading function. However, these prostheses require a larger port for introduction into the intraperitoneal cavity and may be unsuitable for RPLHR.

30.5 Recommendations from the Author

In summary, laparoscopic hernia repair performed through small multiple ports is superior to that performed through a larger single-port in reduced port settings. If a long incision is covered with mesh, the risk of incisional hernia may be decreased. A long incision should be made on the previous surgical scar for the sake of cosmesis. The mesh prosthesis should be larger than the hernia defect with a margin of at least 3 cm in all directions. Depending on the size and location of the hernia orifice, a longer overlap should be considered. All adhesions on the abdominal wall should be removed for precise diagnosis of a small hernia and optimal mesh spreading.

RPLHR may be most feasible. Successful single-port laparoscopic surgeries have been reported in recent years [20–22]. Advances in the development of materials, devices, and techniques for prosthetic placement would further improve outcomes in the repair of abdominal wall incisional hernias [23]. A clinical study that involved a small group of patients showed promising clinical utility [24]. We need strong clinical evidence that RPLHR is not only feasible but also suitable for providing good patient outcomes.

References

1. Kingsnorth A, LeBlanc K (2003) Hernias: inguinal and incisional. Lancet 362(9395): 1561–1571. doi:10.1016/S0140-6736(03)14746-0
2. Sajid MS, Parampalli U, McFall MR (2013) A meta-analysis comparing tacker mesh fixation with suture mesh fixation in laparoscopic incisional and ventral hernia repair. Hernia 17(2):159–166. doi:10.1007/s10029-012-1017-z
3. Munro A, Cassar K (2002) Surgical treatment of incisional hernia. Br J Surg 89(5):534–545. doi:10.1046/j.1365-2168.2002.02083.x
4. Sauerland S, Walgenbach M, Habermalz B, Seiler CM, Miserez M (2011) Laparoscopic versus open surgical techniques for ventral or incisional hernia repair. Cochrane Database Syst Rev (3):CD007781. doi:10.1002/14651858.CD007781.pub2
5. Eker HH, Hansson BM, Buunen M, Janssen IM, Pierik RE, Hop WC, Bonjer HJ, Jeekel J, Lange JF (2013) Laparoscopic vs. open incisional hernia repair: a randomized clinical trial. JAMA Surg 148(3):259–263. doi:10.1001/jamasurg.2013.1466

6. Colavita PD, Tsirline VB, Belyansky I, Walters AL, Lincourt AE, Sing RF, Heniford BT (2012) Prospective, long-term comparison of quality of life in laparoscopic versus open ventral hernia repair. Ann Surg 256(5):714–722. doi:10.1097/SLA.0b013e3182734130, discussion 722–713

7. Hwang CS, Wichterman KA, Alfrey EJ (2009) Laparoscopic ventral hernia repair is safer than open repair: analysis of the NSQIP data. J Surg Res 156(2):213–216. doi:10.1016/j.jss.2009.03.061

8. Pham CT, Perera CL, Watkin DS, Maddern GJ (2009) Laparoscopic ventral hernia repair: a systematic review. Surg Endosc 23(1):4–15. doi:10.1007/s00464-008-0182-8

9. Cuccurullo D, Piccoli M, Agresta F, Magnone S, Corcione F, Stancanelli V, Melotti G (2013) Laparoscopic ventral incisional hernia repair: evidence-based guidelines of the first Italian Consensus Conference. Hernia 17(5):557–566. doi:10.1007/s10029-013-1055-1

10. Polavarapu HV, Kurian AA, Josloff R (2012) Laparoscopic ventral hernia repair in the elderly: does the type of hernia matter? Hernia 16(4):425–429. doi:10.1007/s10029-012-0932-3

11. Lee J, Mabardy A, Kermani R, Lopez M, Pecquex N, McCluney A (2013) Laparoscopic vs open ventral hernia repair in the era of obesity. JAMA Surg 148(8):723–726. doi:10.1001/jamasurg.2013.1395

12. Melvin WS, Renton D (2011) Laparoscopic ventral hernia repair. World J Surg 35(7):1496–1499. doi:10.1007/s00268-011-1028-4

13. Liang MK, Subramanian A, Awad SS (2012) Laparoscopic transcutaneous closure of central defects in laparoscopic incisional hernia repair. Surg Laparosc Endosc Percutan Tech 22(2):e66–e70. doi:10.1097/SLE.0b013e3182471fd2

14. Rea R, Falco P, Izzo D, Leongito M, Amato B (2012) Laparocopic ventral hernia repair with primary transparietal closure of the hernial defect. BMC Surg 12(Suppl 1):S33. doi:10.1186/1471-2482-12-S1-S33

15. Chelala E, Thoma M, Tatete B, Lemye AC, Dessily M, Alle JL (2007) The suturing concept for laparoscopic mesh fixation in ventral and incisional hernia repair: mid-term analysis of 400 cases. Surg Endosc 21(3):391–395. doi:10.1007/s00464-006-9014-x

16. Shankaran V, Weber DJ, Reed RL 2nd, Luchette FA (2011) A review of available prosthetics for ventral hernia repair. Ann Surg 253(1):16–26. doi:10.1097/SLA.0b013e3181f9b6e6

17. Primus FE, Harris HW (2013) A critical review of biologic mesh use in ventral hernia repairs under contaminated conditions. Hernia 17(1):21–30. doi:10.1007/s10029-012-1037-8

18. Rosen MJ (2009) Polyester-based mesh for ventral hernia repair: is it safe? Am J Surg 197(3):353–359. doi:10.1016/j.amjsurg.2008.11.003

19. Muysoms F, Vander Mijnsbrugge G, Pletinckx P, Boldo E, Jacobs I, Michiels M, Ceulemans R (2013) Randomized clinical trial of mesh fixation with "double crown" versus "sutures and tackers" in laparoscopic ventral hernia repair. Hernia 17(5):603–612. doi:10.1007/s10029-013-1084-9

20. Podolsky ER, Mouhlas A, Wu AS, Poor AE, Curcillo PG 2nd (2010) Single Port Access (SPA) laparoscopic ventral hernia repair: initial report of 30 cases. Surg Endosc 24(7):1557–1561. doi:10.1007/s00464-009-0810-y

21. Bucher P, Pugin F, Morel P (2011) Single-port access prosthetic repair for primary and incisional ventral hernia: toward less parietal trauma. Surg Endosc 25(6):1921–1925. doi:10.1007/s00464-010-1488-x

22. Bower CE, Love KM (2011) Single incision laparoscopic ventral hernia repair. JSLS 15(2):165–168. doi:10.4293/108680811X13071180406475

23. Turner PL, Park AE (2008) Laparoscopic repair of ventral incisional hernias: pros and cons. Surg Clin North Am 88(1):85–100, viii. doi:10.1016/j.suc.2007.11.003

24. Gronvold LB, Spasojevic M, Nesgaard JM, Ignjatovic D (2012) Single-incision laparoscopic versus conventional laparoscopic ventral hernia repair: a comparison of short-term surgical results. Surg Laparosc Endosc Percutan Tech 22(4):354–357. doi:10.1097/SLE.0b013e318257cefc

Chapter 31
Inguinal Hernia Repair: TEP

Goro Kaneda and Masaya Kitamura

Abstract We started to perform single-incision laparoscopic surgery (SLS) for total extraperitoneal pre-peritoneal repair (Single-TEP) since 2009 for the adult groin hernia. In this paper we introduce our Single-TEP techniques and its results. From August 2009 through October 2010, we performed Single-TEP in 52 patients diagnosed with inguinal hernia. The group consisted of 43 men and 9 women, including four with bilateral hernia and three with recurrence. For surgeons who are knowledgeable in inguinal anatomy and well-versed in laparoscopic surgical techniques, this procedure can be implemented safely and can be as effective as conventional TEP.

Keywords Laparoscopic hernia repair • Reduced port laparoscopic surgery • SLS • Surgical treatment for inguinal hernia • TEP

31.1 Introduction

We have used total extraperitoneal pre-peritoneal repair (TEP) since 2008 for the surgical repair of inguinal hernia, paying particular attention to the membrane structure of the groin. This technique allows dissection of the pre-peritoneal space without the use of balloon dilation, and it also allows us to conduct the surgery under direct visualization [1]. We use SLS for total extraperitoneal pre-peritoneal repair (Single-TEP). Our surgical techniques and results are described below.

G. Kaneda (✉) • M. Kitamura
Department of Surgery, National Hospital Organization, Sagamihara Hospital,
18-1 Sakuradai, Sagamihara City, Kanagawa 252-0392, Japan
e-mail: g-kaneda@sagamihara-hosp.gr.jp

T. Mori and G. Dapri (eds.), *Reduced Port Laparoscopic Surgery*,
DOI 10.1007/978-4-431-54601-6_31, © Springer Japan 2014

31.2 Preoperative Preparation

Preoperative examinations required for general anesthesia are conducted on an outpatient basis. If those preoperative examinations reveal no problems, the surgery is generally conducted on the day of the admission. The patient stays in the hospital that night and discharges on the following day.

31.3 Set-up (Table 31.1)

31.3.1 Patient Positioning (Fig. 31.1)

The patient is placed in a supine position, arms tucked at the sides, head down at an angle of 20–30° (Trendelenburg position). For Single-TEP, the surgeon stands closer to the patient's head than for standard TEP, so the surgical procedures are facilitated if the patient's arms are kept close to the sides.

31.3.2 Instruments and Mesh

The instruments used for this operation include a 5-mm, 30-degree oblique view laparoscope (Olympus Medical, Tokyo, Japan), standard straight forceps and laparoscopic coagulating shears or electro-cautery. It is difficult to maneuver roticulator forceps in the restricted working space in the pre-peritoneum. An insufflation

Table 31.1 Our operative set-up

Set-up	Notes
Patient's positioning	Patient in the supine position, arms tucked at the sides, head down at an angle of 20–30°
Narrow laparoscopic muscle hook (KS Hook)	8×80-mm muscle hook developed by our department to gently dissect the rectus abdominis from the posterior rectus sheath.
Camera	Olympus, 5-mm, 30° laparoscope.
Forceps	We use forceps designed for standard laparoscopic surgery. This is because roticulator forceps are difficult to maneuver in the restricted working space within the preperitoneum.
Insufflator	We use an insufflation pressure of 8 mmHg
Laparoscopic coagulating shears or electric scalpel	Standard type
Mesh	We use a 12×10-cm or larger mesh
Mesh delivery system	Mesh is rolled into a plastic cylinder and inserted into the preperitoneal space
Absorbable clips	These are used to secure the mesh

Fig. 31.1 Intraoperative scene of actual set-up

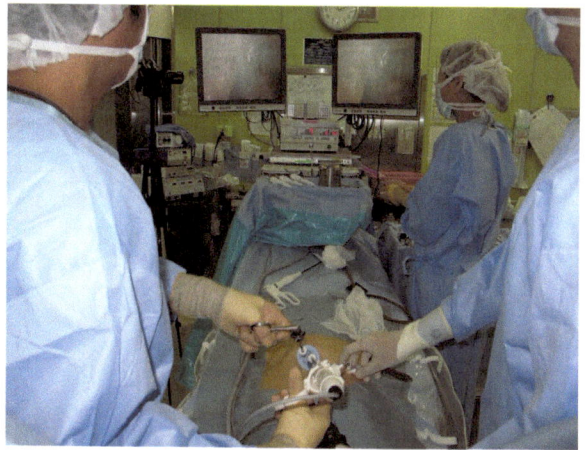

Fig. 31.2 Narrow laparoscopic muscle hook (KS Hook (Takasago))

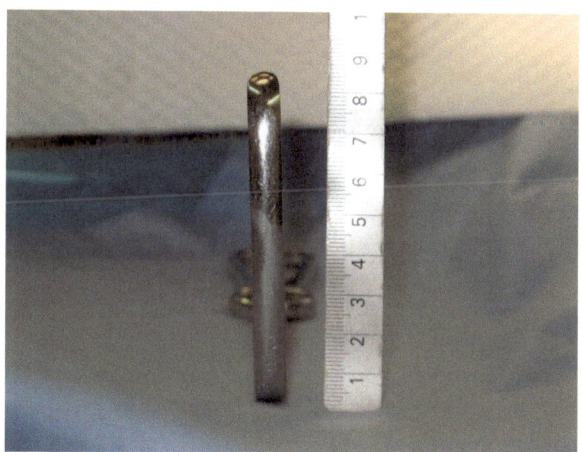

pressure of 8 mmHg is maintained, the same as that used for standard laparoscopic surgery. Careful monitoring is required to avoid an insufflation pressure above 15 mmHg, which can cause subcutaneous emphysema. An 8×80 mm retractor, developed in our department is used to gently dissect the rectus abdominis from the posterior rectal sheath. (KS Hook, Takasago Medical Industry Co., Ltd., Japan (Fig. 31.2). A 12×10-cm or larger mesh is routinely used [2] (Microval Mesh JG, MicroVal SA, France). The mesh is rolled into a plastic cylinder and inserted into the pre-peritoneal space (Mesh Delivery System) (Fig. 31.3). The aim of this maneuver is to prevent damage to the inferior epigastric vessels and the transverse fascia during mesh insertion. Absorbable clips are applied to secure the mesh.

Fig. 31.3 Mesh delivery
system

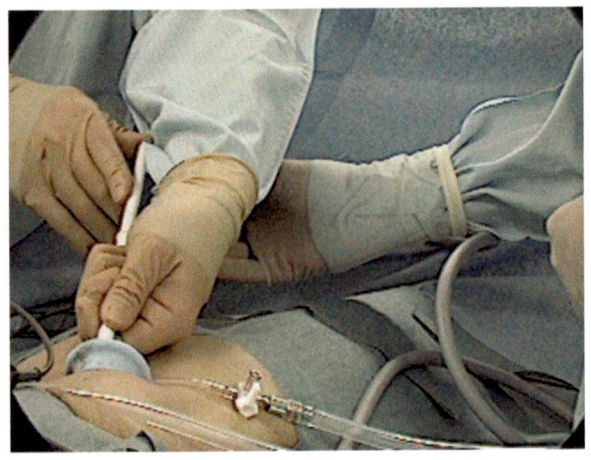

31.4   Indications

This technique can be used on any type of hernia, with the exception of huge,
nonreducible, scrotal hernias. Preferred indications are recurrent hernias, mainly
after conventional repairs, with the advantage of avoiding anterior scar tissue, bilateral hernia where both sides can be approached through the same access, and hernias
with massive destruction of the posterior abdominal wall (a defect diameter greater
than 3 cm or pantaloon hernias). Contraindicated included the patients under treatment with anticoagulants.

Two methods of approach are available:

1. Multi-trocar approach. Insertion of three trocars through a single incision.
2. Multi-channel approach. Use of a commercially available multi-channel access
   port.

In our department, standard practice is to use the multi-channel approach because
it facilitates trocar insertion into the pre-peritoneum and insufflation.

Hints for device operation and expanding the surgical field are as follows.

Single-TEP is conducted in the pre-peritoneal area, where the working space is
more restricted than in standard single-incision intra-abdominal laparoscopic surgery. Because the forceps have only limited left-right movement, dissection must be
in a combination up-down and back-forward movement, regardless of the method,
namely the cross method or the parallel method, is used. It is also important to prevent the forceps from interfering with the camera. The first priority is to maintain
the field of vision, so forceps movement should be adjusted as necessary to avoid
interference.

31.5   Surgical Techniques (Multi-channel Approach)

31.5.1   Skin Incision

To minimize the risk of surgical wound infection and mesh infection, a 2.5-cm subumbilical arcuate incision rather than a transumbilical incision is employed.

31.5.2   Inguinal Dissection

The superficial layer of the pre-peritoneal fascia (between the transverse fascia and the superficial pre-peritoneal fascia) (Figs. 31.4 and 31.5) is dissected using a KS hook. An incision is made in the white line, and access is initiated through the para-rectus abdominis. After through manual dissection between the rectus abdominis and posterior rectus sheath, a 5-mm multi-channel port (SILS™ port (Covidien,

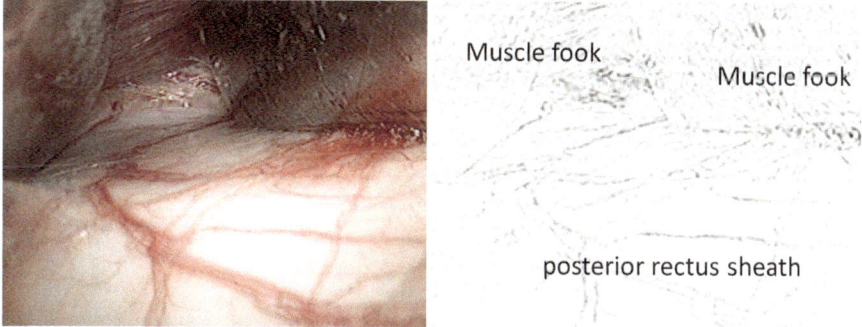

Fig. 31.4 Separation between the posterior rectus muscle sheath and rectus muscle

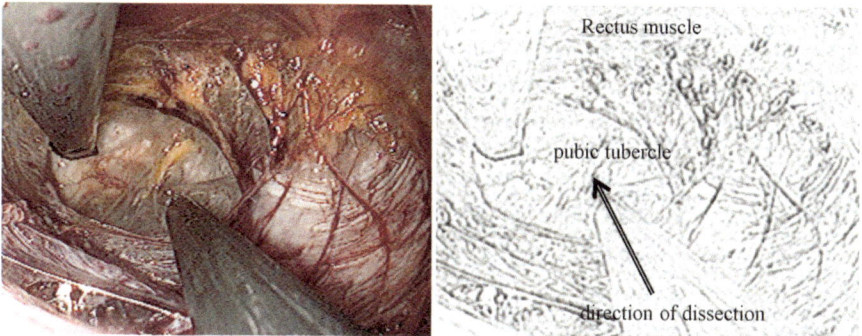

Fig. 31.5 Inguinal dissection: we dissect the superficial layer of the pre-peritoneal fascia using a KS hook

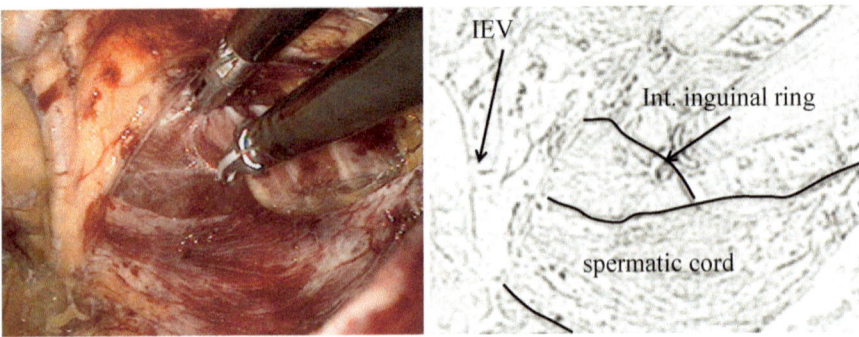

Fig. 31.6 Deep layer of the pre-peritoneal fascia (between the superficial and deep layers of the pre-peritoneal fascia)

New Haven, CT, USA)) is inserted in the pre-peritoneal space. Care must be taken to avoid bleeding and damage to the abdominal wall. Insufflation is then started, without the use of balloon dilation. A 30°, 5-mm scope is inserted and the superficial layer of the pre-peritoneal fascia is dissected to the pubic bone, until the pubic tubercle is clearly seen under direct visualization. The area should be thoroughly dissected medially to the pubic tubercle and laterally to the inferior epigastric vessels (IEVs) in order to create a sufficient working space.

31.5.3 Lateral Inguinal Dissection

Deep layer of the pre-peritoneal fascia (between the superficial and deep layers of the pre-peritoneal fascia) (Fig. 31.6).

The laparoscope camera is adjusted slightly laterally and angled upward. For lateral inguinal dissection, care must be taken to spare one additional layer in the peritoneal cavity (the deepest layer of the pre-peritoneal fascia), paying close attention to the integrity of the membrane structure. The IEV is used as a landmark but is not completely exposed. Alternatively, lateral dissection may be sometimes employed, with one layer of the IEV membrane spared. As lateral dissection proceeds, a point near the origin of the landmark IEV is approached where the outer edge of the internal inguinal ring has been depressed by folding of the pre-peritoneal fascia. Dissection from this point toward the flank reduces the risk of damage to the peritoneum and facilitates dissection of the deep layer of pre-peritoneal fascia without any confusion about which portions of the inguinal structure to dissect.

31.5.4 Parietalization (Fig. 31.7)

The spermatic cord is dissected from the outside inward and carefully parietalized, preserving the spermatic sheath (the deep layer of the pre-peritoneal fascia on the

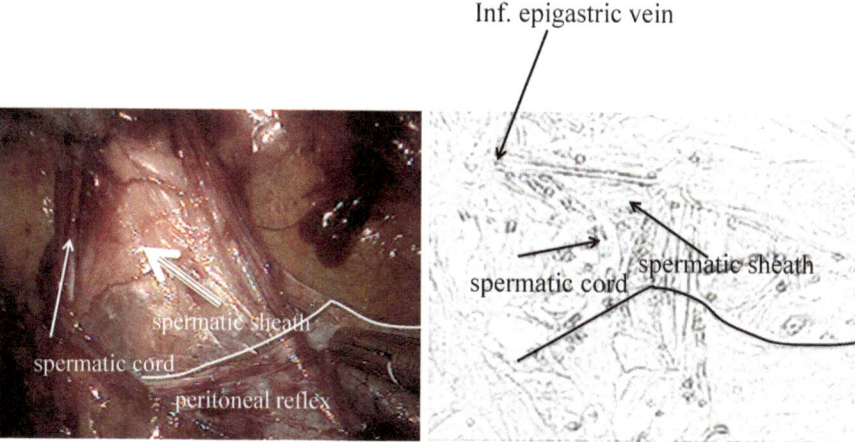

Fig. 31.7 Parietalization: The spermatic cord is dissected from the outside inward and carefully parietalized, preserving the spermatic sheath

posterior wall side of the spermatic cord) as much as possible, and thorough dissection is continued up to the peritoneal reflection. If the sac has been torn, we use an Endloop™ (Covidien) to close the peritoneal margin with a double ligature. At this point, grasping forceps can be used to grasp the peritoneal margin, and the forceps axis can be rotated to twist and occlude the peritoneum.

31.5.5   Mesh Insertion

A mesh is inserted using the mesh delivery system described above.

31.5.6   Mesh Fixation (Fig. 31.8)

For an external inguinal hernia, AbsorbaTack™ (Covidien) is generally used to anchor the mesh at three points: at the pubic bone, on the lower abdominal midline, and lateral to the inferior epigastric vessels. For an internal inguinal hernia, an additional tack is usually applied between the pubic bone and the lower abdominal midline, for a total of four anchor points.

31.5.7   Closure

After closing the anterior sheath of the rectus abdominis, surgery is concluded by closing the subumbilical incision with subcuticular suture (Fig. 31.9).

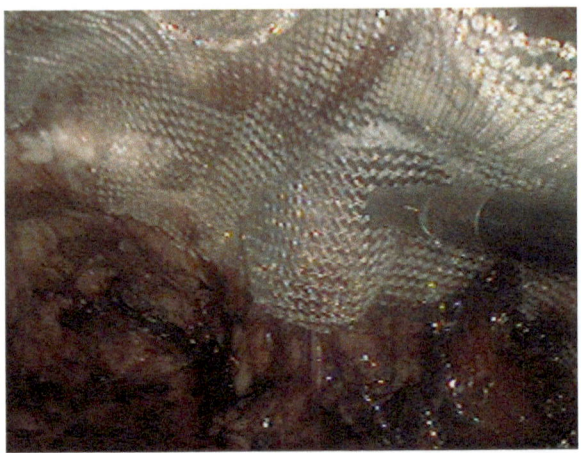

Fig. 31.8 Mesh insertion and fixation

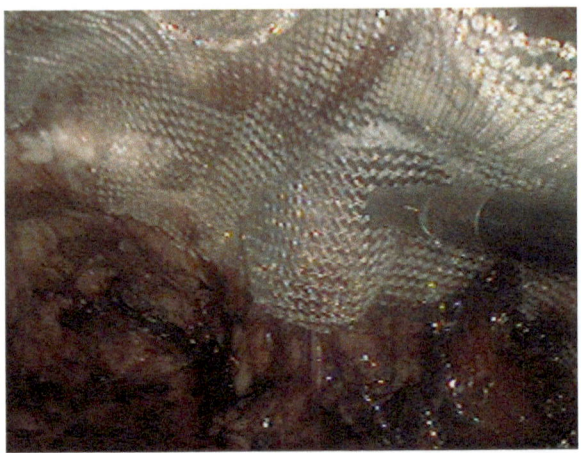

Fig. 31.9 Postoperative view of abdomen with 2 cm single incision

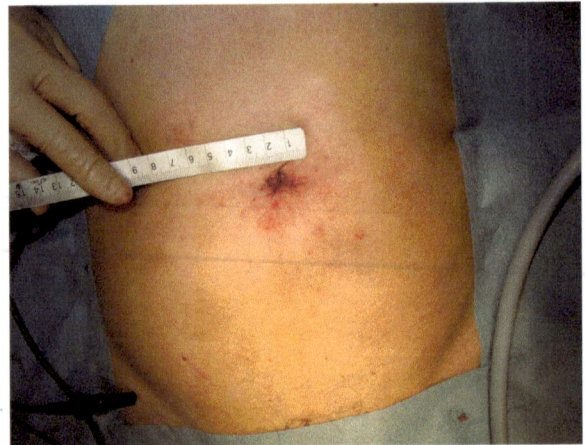

31.6   Conclusion

From August 2009 through October 2010, we performed Single-TEP in 52 patients diagnosed with inguinal hernia. The group consisted of 43 men and 9 women, including 4 with bilateral hernia and 3 with recurrence. Intraoperative diagnoses, under the categories defined by the Japanese Hernia Society (http://www.med. teikyo-u.ac.jp/~surgery2/hernia/page4/page4.html), were as follows: type 1 (external inguinal hernia) in 28 cases, type 2 (internal inguinal hernia) in 13 cases, type 3 (femoral hernia) in 2 cases, type 4 (complex hernia), in ten cases, and type 5 (unclassified) in two cases (including recurrence). All hernias were operable, regardless the type. The multi-trocar approach was used in seven cases and the multi-channel port approach in 45 cases. Mean operation time was 81.7 ± 27.1 min (50–153 min). In two instances in which the multi-trocar approach is attempted, trocar insertion into the pre-peritoneal space was unsuccessful; the procedure is converted to 2-port laparoscopy. For Single-TEP, trocar insertion into the pre-peritoneal space must be confirmed and pneumoperitoneum is required. As a result, a multi-channel SILS™ port (Covidien) is currently the standard practice.

We have described here our use of Single-TEP surgical techniques. For surgeons who are knowledgeable in inguinal anatomy and well versed in laparoscopic surgical techniques, this procedure can be implemented safely and can be as effective as conventional TEP.

31.7   Recommendation from the Authors

Single-TEP can be used safely if the surgeon is sufficiently knowledgeable of inguinal anatomy and proficient in laparoscopic surgical techniques. Urgent need exists for review of the indications and advantages of single-port laparoscopy and for the preparation of additional educational methods to adapt surgical techniques so that this procedure will be both safe and reliable. At present, this technique must be learned under the direction of an experienced surgeon. Further advances in educational techniques will make this procedure safer and more widely accessible [3–5].

References

1. Kitamura M et al (2011) TEP (totally extraperitoneal preperitoneal repair) without dialation baloon (in Japanese). JSES. Nihon Naishikyo Gakkaishi 16:51–56
2. Guidelines for Endoscopic Surgery (2008) Guidelines for the surgical repair of inguinal hernia by endoscopic surgery in Naishikyo Geka Shinryo Gaidorain. Guidelines for Endoscopic Surgery, pp 101–113 (in Japanese)
3. Cugera JF et al (2008) First case of single incision laparoscopic surgery for totally extraperitoneal inguinal hernia repair. Acta Clin Croat 47:249–252
4. Surgit O (2010) Single-incision laparoscopic surgery for total extraperitoneal repair of inguinal hernia in 23 patients. Surg Laparosc Endosc Percutan Tech 20:114–118
5. He K et al (2011) Single incicsion laparoscopic totally extraperitoneal inguinal hernia repair. Hernia 15(4):451–453

Chapter 32
Inguinal Hernia Repair: TAPP

Salvador Morales-Conde, Isaias Alarcón, and María Socas

Abstract Inguinal hernias are very common, with a lifetime risk of 27 % for men and 3 % for women. Hernia repair is one of the most common procedures performed worldwide. Currently, laparoscopic inguinal hernia repair is not only widely accepted, but in many cases, especially with recurrent hernia or bilateral inguinal hernia, this approach has become a method of choice.

The existing trend to minimize the invasiveness of surgical procedures, combined with an attempt to achieve the best therapeutic effects and cosmesis, resulted in single-incision laparoscopic surgery (SLS). It now represents the next step in the advancement of mini-invasive surgery, as it is an innovation, which allows reduced intraoperative trauma and provides superior cosmetic results.

Keywords Inguinal hernia • Single-port laparoscopy • TAPP

32.1 Introduction

Since the laparoscopic approach to inguinal hernia repair was described in the early 1990s, this technique has spread widely and experienced substantial changes. Currently, laparoscopic inguinal hernia procedures are performed either through a transabdominal approach (trans-abdominal preperitoneal: TAPP) or a totally extraperitoneal endoscopic approach (TEP). The most common indications are recurrent hernia, bilateral hernia and, as a patient choice, in unilateral primary hernia. There are two main reasons why laparoscopic inguinal hernia repair has become popular worldwide. First, laparoscopy has allowed placement of a large piece of mesh behind the defect where, according to Laplace's Law, the same forces that cause the

S. Morales-Conde (✉) • I. Alarcón • M. Socas
Unit of Innovation in Minimally Invasive Surgery, Department of General and Digestive Surgery, University Hospital "Virgen del Rocío", Sevilla, Spain
e-mail: smoralesc@gmail.com

T. Mori and G. Dapri (eds.), *Reduced Port Laparoscopic Surgery*,
DOI 10.1007/978-4-431-54601-6_32, © Springer Japan 2014

hernia are used to reinforce the repair. Second, the associated benefits of minimally invasive surgery, such as less postoperative pain, a shorter recovery period, early return to daily activities and work, and better cosmetic results.

Recently, SLS has become a natural step toward to an even less minimally invasive surgery. The potential benefits are associated with less trocar incisions, improved patient recovery and the avoidance of injuries related to the sharp introducers used for traditional 3-ports laparoscopic inguinal hernia repair. The single-port (SP) introduced via a single incision allows the deployment of 3-ports with blunt introducers, hence negating the risks of potential catastrophic bowel or vascular punctures. The first case report by Filipovic-Cugura et al. in 2009 paved the way for its application in this laparoscopic surgical procedure [1]. However, SLS has its unique challenges, mainly the relative loss of [2–4], which must be overcome before it can be popularized.

32.2 Indications and Contraindications

SP devices are designed to be placed through an incision of 1.8–2.5 cm. Within our working group, the indications for SLS are those procedures requiring an incision for removal of a specimen, such us colonic surgery, spleen, adrenal glands, etc., or for the introduction of a material, such us meshes during ventral hernia repair, gastric banding, or those which require an incision for the introduction of the balloon used for dissecting the preperitoneal spaces during a TEP.

Moreover, in those functional procedures, such as antireflux surgery, in those in which the specimen to be removed is small, such us appendectomies, or in those in which the material to be introduced in the abdominal cavity enters through a 5-mm trocar, mini-laparoscopy is a major indication.

For the reasons previously mentioned, TAPP could be considered an indication for mini-laparoscopy in cases where a light-weight mesh is to be used, since these meshes could be introduced through a 5-mm trocar. But, on the other hand, heavy-weight meshes need a 10-mm trocar to be introduced into the abdominal cavity, making the SP approach an alternative to conventional multiport surgery.

Regardless of the aspects previously discussed, the SP approach would be a clear indication for inguinal hernia repair using the principles of TAPP in cases of concomitant surgery, such as during a laparoscopic cholecystectomy together with an inguinal hernia repair, or in patients who are diagnosed with both an umbilical and an inguinal hernia, since the SP devices would be placed into the defect of the umbilical hernia, which would be repaired at the end of procedure, once the inguinal hernia has been repaired.

On the other hand, the use of SLS in females is a very good indication, since they usually present small hernias involving an easier dissection of the peritoneal flap and less maneuvers to reduce the hernia sac. In these patients, the cosmetic results are excellent with a high degree of satisfaction.

Finally, there are no real contraindications for this type of approach, being the same as those that may exist for conventional laparoscopic approach. However, the difficult cases for conventional laparoscopic surgery, including large hernias and particularly the inguino-scrotal ones, are not the best cases for this new type of SP approach, since the capacity for traction of tissue in reducing the hernia sac is diminished by the existing instruments, becoming a very complex surgery. A conventional laparoscopic approach is advisable for these cases.

32.3   Technique

A 1.5–2.5 cm transverse trans-umbilical skin incision is made at the center aspect of the umbilicus. The SP device is then placed through the incision (Fig. 32.1) and the abdomen is insufflated up to 14 mmHg of pressure. We have used two type of SP devices, the SILS™ port (Covidien, New Haven, CT, USA), with two orifices of 5-mm and one of 12-mm, and the Tri-port plus® (Olympus, Tokyo, Japan). The SILS™ port (Covidien) is placed using a pair of Kocher clamp (Figs. 32.1 and 32.2) at the inferior edge with the gas insufflator hose being distal, with the surgeon's left hand retracting the rectus upward. The TriPort plus® (Olympus) is placed using its applicator device. The elastic properties of the SP devices and its ports with valve prevent loss of pneumoperitoneum. A 5-mm 30° scope (Olympus) is used for the surgery (Fig. 32.3a, b).

At this stage, we place the patient 10–15° head down. The principles of TAPP repairs are the same and must be followed to avoid injuries to bladder, vessels, nerves, and vas deferens. The maneuvers to identify the anatomical structures of the area and to dissect of the hernia sac are performed with a flexible grasper (Roticulator Endodissect/grasp (Covidien)) in the left hand, through one of the 5-mm orifice, using the other 5-mm orifice to introduce different conventional straight

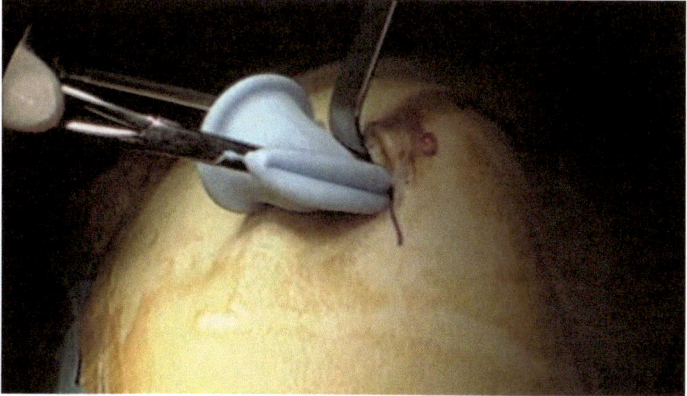

Fig. 32.1 The single trocar device (SILS™ port (Covidien)) is introduced in place

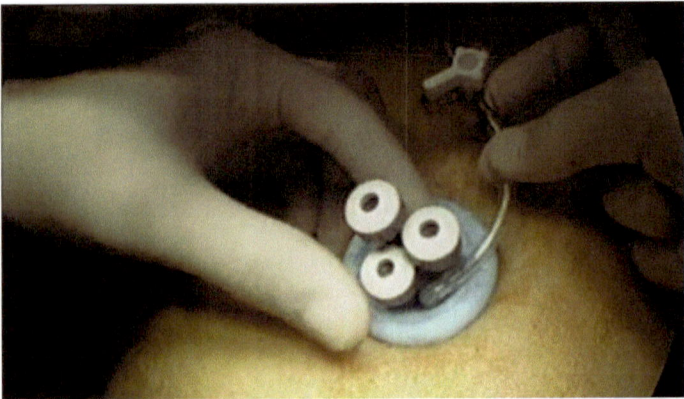

Fig. 32.2 The SILS™ port (Covidien) is used with three 5-mm working channels: one for a roticulator grasper in the left hand of the surgeon, one for the 5-mm optic and the last one to introduce different standard laparoscopic straight instruments, such as the endoscopic graspers, and the endoscopic scissors and dissectors with electrocautery. The abdominal cavity is insufflated up to 14 mmHg of pressure through the port device

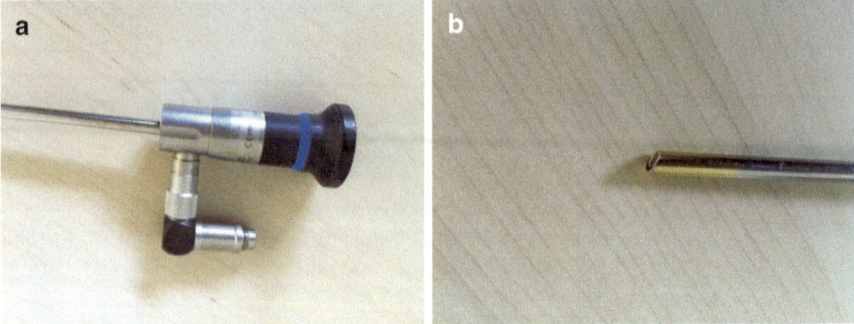

Fig. 32.3 (**a**, **b**) 5-mm 30° scope with the angle for the light source

instruments, such as the endoscopic graspers, scissors and dissector with electrocautery. We consider that this combination of instruments avoids surgery with surgeon's hands crossed, thus decreasing the consequent learning curve of this procedure. The dissection proceeds then just the same as for conventional endoscopic TAPP repair: a flap of the peritoneum is created with the endoscopic scissor 2-cm above the superior edge of the hernia (Figs. 32.4 and 32.5), the symphysis pubis is identified and dissected free of areolar tissues and the bladder, the inferior epigastric vessels are then identified, and the lateral space is then dissected and continued medially until the cord structures are identified. An indirect sac and its accompanying lipoma of the cord are reduced with sufficient proximal dissection of

Fig. 32.4 The roticulater grasper grasps the peritoneum 2-cm above the superior edge of the hernia

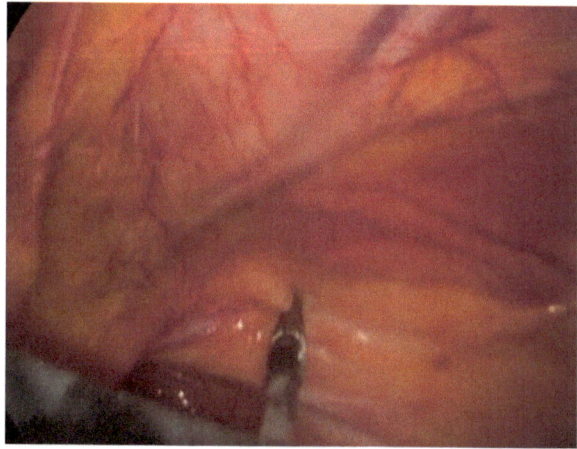

Fig. 32.5 A flap of the peritoneum is created with the endoscopic scissors with electrocautery

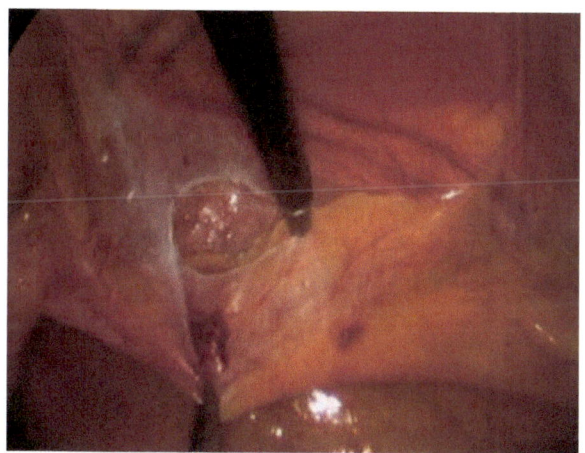

the peritoneal reflection to allow the inferior edge of the mesh to lie well clear of it. This dissection then continues medially and any direct sac is reduced.

Once the sac is reduced, one of the 5-mm ports is replaced for a 12-mm port in the device in order to introduce the mesh, replacing the 5-mm port to continue the surgery. An anatomical pre-shaped mesh (3DMax Mesh®, Bard Davol Inc., Warwick RI, USA) is introduced through the 10–12 mm orifice of the SP devices and placed covering all the weak areas of the inguinal region (Fig. 32.6a, b). The mesh is correctly expanded. Although the mesh could be left in place without any fixation, fibrin glue (Tissucol®, Baxter, Vienna, Austria) is used in most of the cases, avoiding mechanical fixation in order to decrease postoperative pain. The peritoneal flap is closed, avoiding the mesh being exposed to the bowel (Fig. 32.7), using a

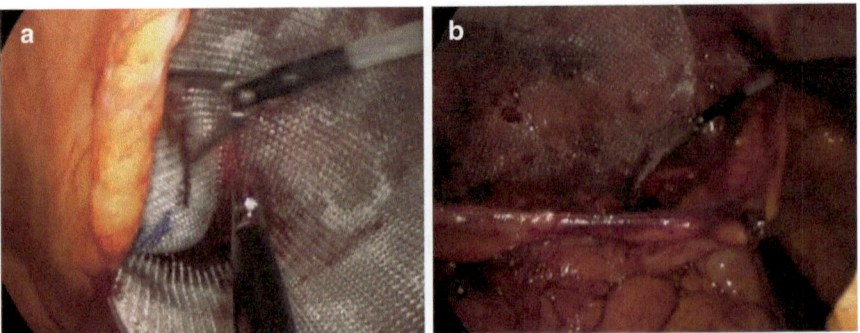

Fig. 32.6 (**a**, **b**). The mesh is expanded. A three-dimensional, anatomically curved mesh is used since this prosthesis facilitates its placement

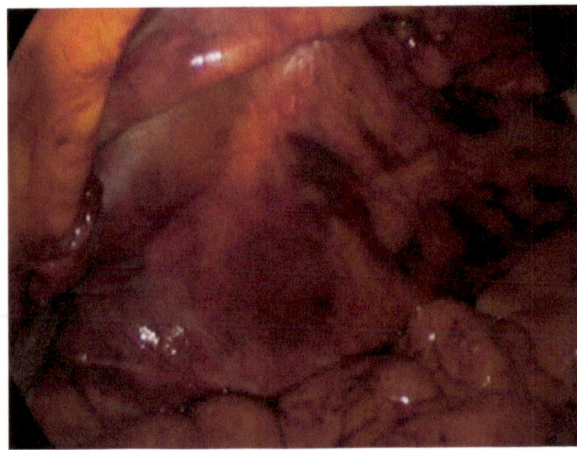

Fig. 32.7 The flap of the peritoneum is closed, avoiding the mesh being exposed to the bowel

conventional running suture, tacks or new closure devices, such us V-loc® (Covidien). This last new device is a revolutionary technology that eliminates the need to tie knots, so the incision can be closed up to 50 % faster without compromising strength and security. Finally, the fascia is closed with interrupted sutures and the skin is also closed.

32.4   Tips and Tricks

Minimally invasive surgery aims to provide an effective treatment of surgical diseases while decreasing access related morbidity. Theoretically, the advantages of SLS include that the procedure can be performed through the same incision where the specimen is removed. Abdominal wall surgery does not require the removal of a specimen, but includes the need to insert a prosthetic material into the abdominal cavity, or into the preperitoneal space, making this approach as a possible indication for SLS.

SP access surgery is the result of the continuous search for increasingly less invasive approaches, which enables the introduction of several instruments. Nevertheless, previous literature evidence reports conflict among instruments when operating in such a confined space making it appear to be a highly-complex technique New specialized instruments, either bent or articulated, have been developed. Flexible graspers (Roticulator Endodissect/grasp (Covidien)) prove to be useful in dissection and traction maneuvers during this approach in order to decrease clashing of the instruments and eliminating the need for surgeons to perform the surgery with the two hands crossed. We believe that our procedure, with one roticulator instrument on the left hand, that allows the exposition of the operative field, and the use of conventional straight laparoscopic instruments on the right one, helps to decrease the learning curve. But, since the space of the inguinal area is very small some authors prefer to use two straight conventional laparoscopic instruments [5], of different length in order to decrease clashing, than the roticulator or pre-bent instruments.

Another aspect to be considered is the type of scope to be used. Because all three instruments are in the same port, severe and disheartening clashing of these will occur, especially if a normal 10-mm scope is used. For this reason, a 5-mm scope is highly recommended.

Mesh placement could be particularly challenging and time-consuming during conventional TAPP, being considered one of the most difficult steps of this procedure, especially when being performed by SLS. For this reason, it is also recommended to use a pre-shaped mesh in order to facilitate the maneuverability, which will reduce surgical time and decrease the learning curve. The use of a 5-mm optic will also facilitate this step of the surgery since the prosthetic material can be introduced under direct vision through the 10–12 mm orifice of the SP device.

Finally, closing the peritoneal flap is another challenge of this procedure. Different authors have suggested performing this maneuvers using [6], although pain could increase. A reasonable alternative is the use of the new running suture known as V-loc® (Covidien), that eliminates the need to tie knots, so incisions can be closed up faster without compromising strength and security.

32.5 Recommendations from the Authors

Minimally invasive surgery aims to provide effective treatment of surgical diseases while decreasing access related morbidity. SLS is the result of the continuous search for increasingly less invasive approaches, although it appears to be a highly complex technique. New specialized instruments, either bent or articulated, are being developed and will facilitate the surgery. Indications for laparoscopic TAPP inguinal hernia repair need to be established, being important to be avoided in large scrotal hernias for this type of approach. The best indications are in cases of concomitant surgery (such us cholecystectomy and inguinal hernia or umbilical and inguinal hernias), small direct hernias, and for females.

Further studies are needed to determine if TAPP inguinal hernia repair is an indication for the SLS approach for mini-laparoscopy, since this surgery could be performed with one 3-mm [7] or two 5-mm trocars [8], since new low-weight polypropylene mesh can be introduced through a 5-mm trocar. The main difference with SP TEP repair is that during this preperitoneal repair a 2-cm incision is still needed to introduce the balloon dissector and could be replaced by the SP device, while this incision is not needed during the laparoscopic TAPP repair.

In the authors' opinion, in experienced hands, SLS can be extended safely to laparoscopic TAPP repair of inguinal hernias. Although, we have to take into consideration, the inherent learning curve of SLS as a technically demanding [9, 10]. Prospective randomized studies comparing SLS and conventional multiport laparoscopic TAPP are needed to evaluate the advantages of SLS beyond cosmetics.

References

1. Cugura JF, Kirac I, Kulis T et al (2008) First case of single incision laparoscopic surgery for totally extraperitoneal hernia repair. Acta Clin Croat 47:249–252
2. Kucuk C (2011) Single-incision laparoscopic transabdominal preperitoneal herniorrhaphy for recurrent inguinal hernias: preliminary surgical results. Surg Endosc 25:3228–3234
3. Rahman SH, John BJ (2010) Single-incision laparoscopic trans-abdominal pre-peritoneal mesh hernia repair: a feasible approach. Hernia 14:329–331
4. Goo TT, Goel R, Lawenko M, Lomanto D (2010) Laparoscopic transabdominal preperitoneal (TAPP) hernia repair via a single port. Surg Laparosc Endosc Percutan Tech 20:389–390
5. Yilmaz H, Alptekin H (2013) Single-incision laparoscopic transabdominal preperitoneal herniorrhaphy for bilateral inguinal hernias using conventional instruments. Surg Laparosc Endosc Percutan Tech 23(3):320–323
6. Pesta W, Kurpiewski W, Luba M, Szynkarczuk R, Grabysa R (2012) Single incision laparoscopic surgery transabdominal pre-peritoneal hernia repair – case report. Wideochir Inne Tech Malo Inwazyjne 7(2):137–139
7. Lee YS, Kim JH, Hong TH, Lee IK, Oh ST, Kim JG, Badakhanian R (2011) Transumbilical single-port laparoscopic transabdominal preperitoneal repair of inguinal hernia: initial experience of single institute. Surg Laparosc Endosc Percutan Tech 21(3):199–202
8. Brinkmann L, Lorenz D (2011) Minilaparoscopic surgery: alternative or supplement to single-port surgery? Chirurg 82(5):419–424
9. Roy P, De A (2010) Single-incision laparoscopic TAPP mesh hernioplasty using conventional instruments: an evolving technique. Langenbecks Arch Surg 395(8):1157–1160
10. Macdonald ER, Ahmed I (2010) "Scarless" laparoscopic TAPP inguinal hernia repair using a single port. Surgeon 8(3):179–181

Chapter 33
Adjustable Gastric Banding for Obesity

Rami E. Lutfi

Abstract Bariatric surgery has been leading the field of reduced port laparoscopic surgery. Adjustable gastric banding (AGB) is ideal for this technology due to its simplicity and attraction to the younger and lighter bariatric patients; who are most interested in cosmesis and having no visible scars.

The ergonomic challenge caused by having different instruments come through a single incision (umbilicus) could be overcome by using specialized articulating, flexible, or curved instruments and laparoscopes. These modifications allow for maintaining the triangulation principle, and preserving the working space needed for instruments to move with ease allowing safe and efficient completion of advanced laparoscopic tasks.

We present our technique using curved instruments and flexible tip laparoscope for AGB placement through a single umbilical incision. A step by step description of the operation is provided along with intra-operative images.

Reduced port placement of AGB is as safe and as effective as traditional laparoscopy with possible decrease in postop pain and definite superior cosmetic results. It should be offered to appropriate patients as an alternative to traditional multi port laparoscopy. This could drive obese patients who are hesitant due to fear of abdominal scars and pain, to come forward and seek a surgical solution to their obesity.

Keywords Flexible tip • Lapband • Reduced port laparoscopic surgery • Single-incision laparoscopic surgery (SLS)

R.E. Lutfi (✉)
Clinical Assistant Professor of Surgery, University of Illinois at Chicago,
2913 North Commonwealth Avenue Suite 400, Chicago, IL 60657, USA
e-mail: rami.lutfi@gmail.com

T. Mori and G. Dapri (eds.), *Reduced Port Laparoscopic Surgery*,
DOI 10.1007/978-4-431-54601-6_33, © Springer Japan 2014

33.1   Introduction

The evolution of gastric banding surgery lends itself to continuously minimizing the invasiveness of the operation ending in scarless placement of the band.

The first band was an adjustable silicone band developed by Dr. Szinicz and Schnapka [1] and placed around the top of a rabbit stomach in 1982. In 1986, Dr. Kusmak of New Jersey placed the first adjustable silicone gastric band (ASGB) in human using laparotomy [2]. The need for laparotomy to place the band, prevented wide acceptance of this operation despite the many advantages of adjustability and restriction it provided.

Laparoscopic placement of gastric band was not possible until the BioEnterics Lap-Band (Inamed Health, Santa Barbara, CA, USA) was developed and offered the laparoscopic adjustable gastric band (LAGB). The Lap-Band system was first placed in September 1993 by Dr. Belachew in Belgium [3].

The laparoscopic application made this operation simple and safe. Therefore, it quickly became one of the most popular bariatric operations worldwide, and currently, many chose this operation for the ability to have it done without any visible scar using reduced port laparoscopic surgery (RPLS) technique.

Placing the LAGB went through many technical modifications before it was optimized and standardized. The initial technique known, as the *perigastric* technique, was associated with a high slippage rate. Thus it was later modified to the *pars flaccida* technique [4], in which, the band is placed at a higher position, away from the body of the stomach higher position and without opening the lesser sac or clearing the lesser curve. This technique made band placement simple, safe, reproducible, easily teachable, and more importantly decreased the slippage rate.

While *pars flaccida* technique is fairly standard, the instruments used and the trocar placement varied amongst surgeons based on preference without any data to support one method or another.

In general, a camera port, liver retractor, and 3 or 4 "working" trocars are used with at least one large 15-mm trocar to pass the band. The total number of incisions comes to 5–6, which equals the number of incisions needed to perform the more complex bariatric operations such as the gastric bypass or sleeve gastrectomy (that do not even require a large 15-mm trocar).

For that reason, we believe that this simple operation should be able to be completed in simpler manner using fewer instruments through fewer incisions.

The need for that shift in technique towards scarless band placement comes from the market shift for banding towards the less obese and adolescents. Two groups that would care most about cosmetic results compared to the rest of bariatric population.

For the less obese with body mass index (BMI) 30–34 kg/m^2, the FDA in 2011 approved band placement. As for the morbidly obese adolescents who may not come forward due to fear of scarring and permanent anatomical changes, banding is considered the procedure of choice due to its reversibility. Fielding et al. [5] showed excellent durable results in a group of 41 adolescents who had no operative or 60-day morbidity or mortality, with estimated excess weight loss of 70 %, which was maintained at 5 years follow up. This led to the FDA-approved trial in the US, which showed promising early results but has not been completed [6].

Since early reports of single site LAGB [7, 8], many showed the safety and equivalency of this technique to traditional placement of the band, and some showed decreased postoperative pain and faster recovery [9]. While there is general consensus on the increased technical challenge of this operation, our group and others showed that the learning curve is in fact relatively short [10, 11].

Below, we describe our technique for RPLS LapBand placement. This technique could be applied to different band brands with minor technical changes depending on their specific design.

33.2 Patient Selection

Once patients hear about the "scarless" option, most will desire to have it and some will demand it! Exclusion criteria depend on surgeon preference and experience.

As our experience evolved and improved, we now feel comfortable doing this operation on patients weighing up to 300 pounds or with BMI up to 50 kg/m². In the super obese population, we feel the advantage of reduced port surgery does not justify the significant increase in technical challenge posed by the massive visceral fat and liver size. We also prefer avoiding this technique once patient's height go over 5′8″ and that's strictly related to available instruments and reach from the point of entry being the umbilicus. Outside these general guidelines, surgeons may alter their decision based on general body habitus (central obesity, apple versus pear shape obesity), gender (male tend to have more central obesity and higher riding diaphragm adding more technical challenge), and race (tendency towards increased visceral fat in Caucasians).

The same contraindications to conventional placement of LAGB apply to this operation. While laparoscopic cholecystectomy should not add significant challenge, any other operation through the midline (involving the umbilicus) or upper abdominal scars (open cholecystectomy) should be considered a contraindication to RPLS.

Realistic goals should be set. This operation after all is offered mainly for the cosmetic advantage. Patients with existing scars, elderly and super obese are not best candidate for it.

33.3 Technique

33.3.1 Patient Positioning

The surgeon stands either between the legs or on the patient's right side.

Standing between the legs has the advantage of having a direct line between the surgeon, the instruments entry point (umbilicus) and the target (hiatus). This decreases the ergonomic challenge and thus hands fatigue. However, to stand between the legs, patient has to be on a "split leg" table (expensive and not readily available), or patient would have to be placed in lithotomy position (adds significant time to protect pressure points in the morbidly obese, and limits the ability for safe steep reverse Trendelenburg position).

For these reasons, we prefer to stand on patient right side, and the assistant stands on the left side holding the camera and the liver retractor (if used).

We place a foot-board in all bariatric operations and place the patient in a moderate reverse Trendelenburg position about 30°. We secure the legs at the ankle level and thighs with wide tape and Velcro strap. The monitors are placed cephalad over the shoulders.

33.3.2 Port Placement

Despite some reports about decreased postoperative pain, it is agreed upon that the main advantage of RPLS remains a cosmetic one. To achieve the cosmetic advantage, the port should always be placed through the umbilicus to hide the scar.

In super obese patients the pannus becomes significantly larger and the umbilicus starts shifting down getting further away from the xiphoid and the hiatus. This poses significant increase in technical challenge. To avoid the struggle, some surgeons would then make the incision superior to the umbilicus. We believe that if a large scar has to be made in mid abdomen to place the RPLS port, it wound defeats the purpose and traditional laparoscopy would be the better option.

We start by everting the umbilicus with sharp towel clips and bring up its center. This is sometimes challenging in larger patients, but in most, can be done. I prefer to clean it again with betadine as the initial prep may not reach down deep.

The incision is 2.5 cm made longitudinally just lateral (towards patient right) to the stalk. It is important to leave the stalk naturally attached, for best cosmetic reason (Fig. 33.1). We incise the fascia at the midline for about 2.5 cm.

Access remains controversial. Some surgeons place many trocars through different fascial incisions (while using a single skin incision). We believe the incident of umbilical hernia may be increased by making adjacent holes leaving thin strips of intact fascia in between (personal opinion without any supporting data). In addition, ergonomic challenge may increase with many trocars clashing in a small space (a problem that could be decreased by using low profile trocars). We prefer using a single multi-channel port through a single fascial opening. Many commercial products are available and discussed in different chapter; each has its advantages and disadvantages. We personally use the TriPort® (Olympus, Tokyo, Japan), which has three openings (one 12-mm, two 5-mm, and two small opening for insufflation and deflation of gas). Orientation of the port should be thought of carefully since improper orientation leads to instrument clashing and increased ergonomic difficulties.

Figure 33.2 shows the Triport® (Olympus) with the proper orientation with the camera placed through the inferior port. We keep the 12-mm port to the surgeon's right hand and would use it to pass needles or larger suturing devices (if desired by

Fig. 33.1 Longitudinal
incision through the
umbilicus after lifting its
center with towel clips

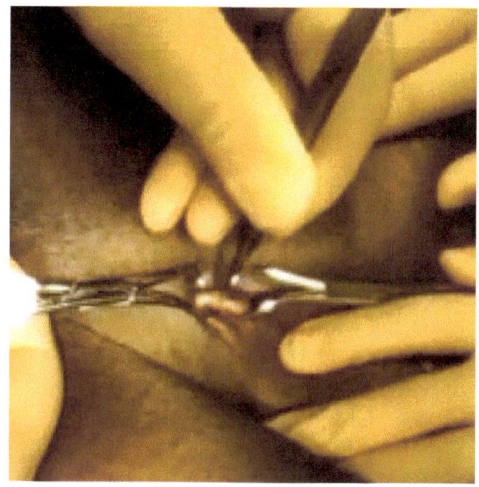

Fig. 33.2 TriPort (Olympus)
in the proper orientation.
Inferior 5-mm port is used for
the flexible tip laparoscope,
superior 12-mm port is used
for grasper or passing a
needle or 100 mm suturing
device, the *superior 5-mm*
port is for electrocautery or a
grasper

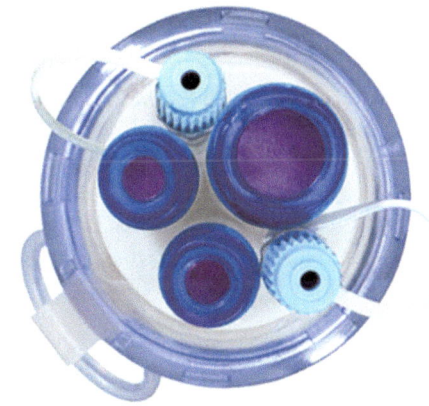

the surgeon), while the other 5-mm is kept superiorly and to the patient right side
and is used by the surgeon left hand for retraction and electrocautery (to clear the
left crus and later make an opening over the right crus for tunneling).

33.3.3 Band Placement

It is important to remember to place the band prior to tunneling as the working port
in the only access to the peritoneal cavity. We typically start the operation by lifting
the liver and inspect the perigastric fat, we then decide size of the band. Two sizes
are current available: AP standard and AP large; if in doubt, we place the larger size.

Once the band is chosen and prepared, we place it in the peritoneal cavity and try to leave it in the upper abdomen so it is easier to get later after placing the patient in reverse Trendelenburg.

33.3.4 Liver Retraction

This is probably the most controversial step. Some surgeons are able to perform this operation without a liver retractor. This helps decreasing the number of instruments passed through the umbilicus, or avoid making another incision (depending on type of retraction).

The majority of surgeons believe that proper retraction of the liver and excellent exposure of the hiatus is essential for proper placement of the band. We tend to follow this principle and feel strongly that this operation should not be done unless it is performed at the same standard as traditional laparoscopy.

The liver must be retracted well and the hiatus should be well exposed to rule out a hiatal hernia as missing one leads to adverse outcome.

Liver retraction could be achieved in three different ways:

– *Second epigastric incision and placement of a retractor* (formal liver retractor or smaller instrument through a smaller incision). The advantage is avoiding an added instrument in the umbilical port (sparing the use of one channel and decreasing instrument jam). The disadvantage is leaving additional scar.
– *Retraction instrument placed through the umbilical port.* This would avoid the added epigastric scar and make the operation truly "scarless", but would occupy one of the channels and further limit the actual working space (increase ergonomic challenge).
– *Intra-corporeal methods.* Using a virtual retractor to suspend the left lobe of the liver either by using hooks to the peritoneum or by placing sutures between the abdominal wall and the hiatus or crus to suspend the lateral left lobe. This method avoids the need for additional incision or additional instrument for retraction. However, placing these devices or sutures is often time consuming, has a significant learning curve, and often does not provide optimal exposure.

We went through many of these methods and always believed that the liver must be well retracted. Eventually, we decided to retract the liver using a small caliber trans-cutaneous instrument and we use the 2.3-mm wide MiniLap® Alligator (Stryker, Kalamazoo, MI, USA) with a sharp tip that can go through a stab without the need for a formal incision (Fig. 33.3). This provides a quick retraction and excellent hiatal exposure to see any subtle hiatal hernia (Fig. 33.4) without leaving a visible scar.

Fig. 33.3 2.3-mm rigid instrument to retract the liver. Shown is the sharp tip that allows passing it through a tiny stab at the skin to avoid visible scar

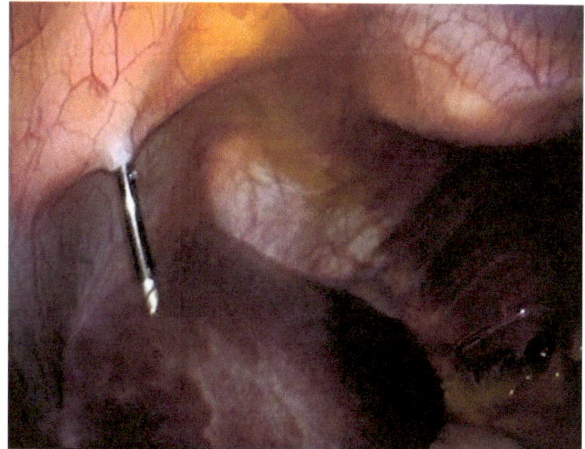

Fig. 33.4 Excellent exposure is paramount to detect small hiatal hernia and perform the operation well

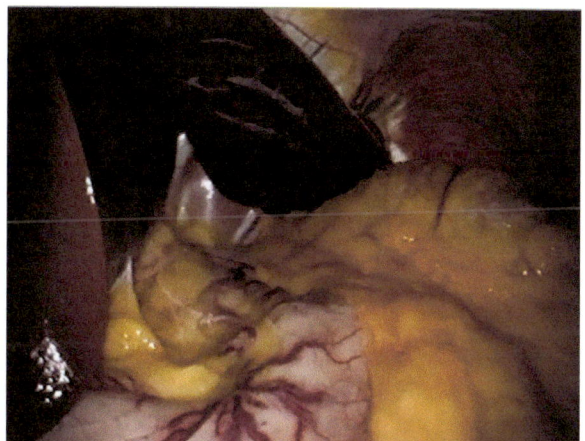

33.3.5   Instruments

The rate-limiting step in evolution of single-site laparoscopic surgery (SSLS) remains the visualization and instrumentation. Adoption of RPLS has gone through two phases. The initial one was rapid adoption that came quick but also faded quick. The second phase was a slower, more careful adoption and this is where we are now. Surgeons initially jumped quickly on the idea of performing "scarless surgery" and many got into it without proper planning and without any modification in instruments or technique. These surgeons simply moved all their conventional "straight, rigid" instruments and scopes to have them all come through a small incision in the umbilicus. This led to the "Sword Fighting" phenomena, where parallel instruments clash in a very limited space that makes it impossible for them to manipulate or dissect tissues.

Fig. 33.5 Using a flexible tip laparoscope and curved instruments moves the triangulation to inside the abdomen and avoid instruments clash

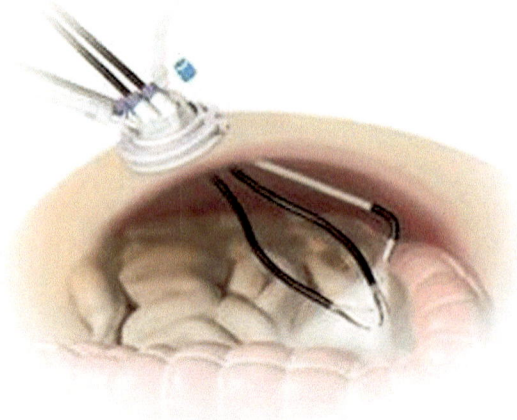

These instruments also clashed against the laparoscope adding significant visual impairment. This caused surgeon frustration and jeopardized the safety of the operations causing most to abandon RPLS. The few who continued to have interest were those true innovators who felt the need for using different instruments while keeping the principles of traditional laparoscopy. Triangulation remains essential for exposure and good dissection and should be maintained. It just had to be moved from the abdominal wall to the peritoneal cavity. This necessitates the shift from using straight rigid instruments to reticulating, bent, or curved ones. For better visualization, a flexible tip laparoscope is highly preferred. This would allow instruments to come into the abdomen through a small opening (umbilicus), spread apart in the abdominal cavity, and then come back together towards the target to perform dissection.

Many available commercial products provide this concept. These are discussed elsewhere. Reticulating instruments are common, but often force surgeons to cross their hands adding additional ergonomic challenge.

We prefer to use curved instruments. These are rigid instruments with two curves: One extracorporial at the side of the handle (to separate surgeon's hands and give them space to work), and the other intracorporial towards the tip (to allow space for the tips to be moved freely for tissues manipulation and dissection). The main advantage over reticulating instruments is preserving the orientation and avoiding the need for surgeons to cross their hands.

In the same logic of triangulation and preserving wide working space, we strongly feel the need for a flexible tip laparoscope. This allows the shaft of the scope to be directed away from the target (giving the surgeon space to work), while the flexible tip (the actual lens) is re-directed towards the target providing a steady and excellent focus on the area of interest without competing for working space (Figs. 33.5 and 33.6).

Figures 33.7 and 33.8 show the assistant holding the laparoscope against the right thigh leaving working space for surgeon's hands. This allows the operating surgeon to move his hands comfortably and without ergonomic challenge.

Fig. 33.6 Moving the "triangulation" from the abdominal wall to the peritoneal cavity. Notice the scope shaft being away from the target, while its flexible tip is redirected to look down on the target. The curve of the instruments allows freedom of movement and avoids "Sword Fighting"

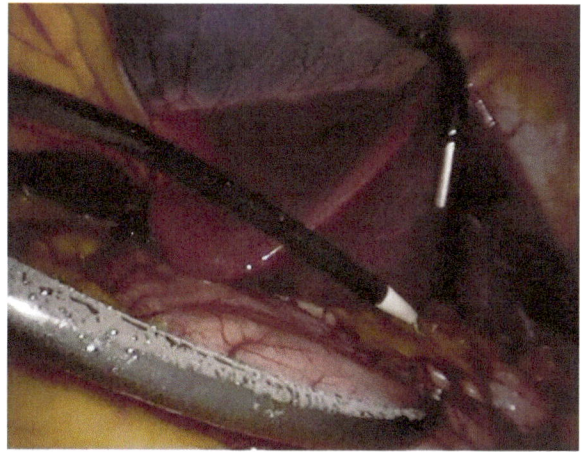

Fig. 33.7 Laparoscope is held against the right thigh by the assistant, who also holds the liver retractor

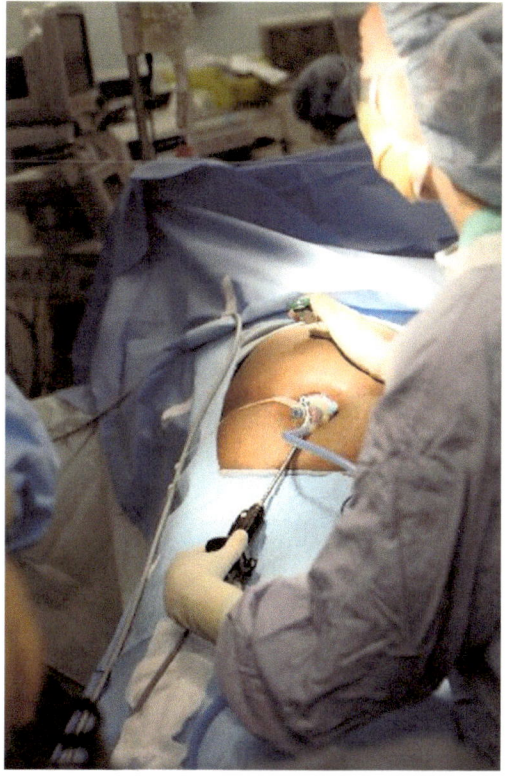

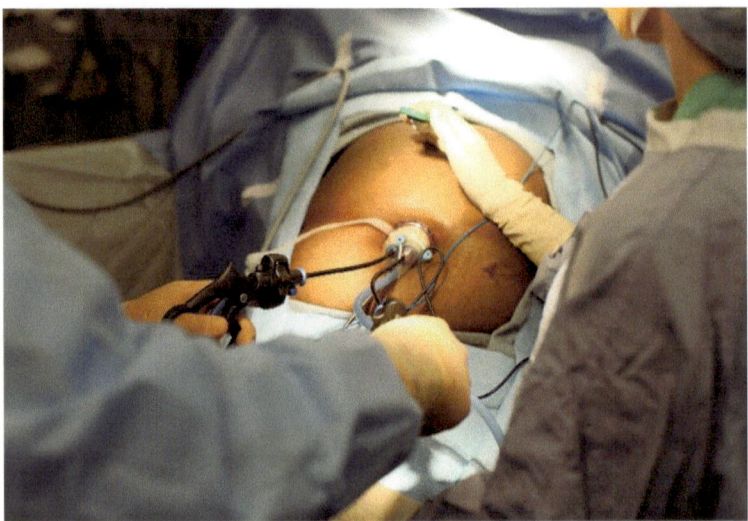

Fig. 33.8 Assistant's hand and scope are away from surgeon's hands. The curved handles separate the two operating hands giving freedom of movement and decreasing the ergonomic challenge

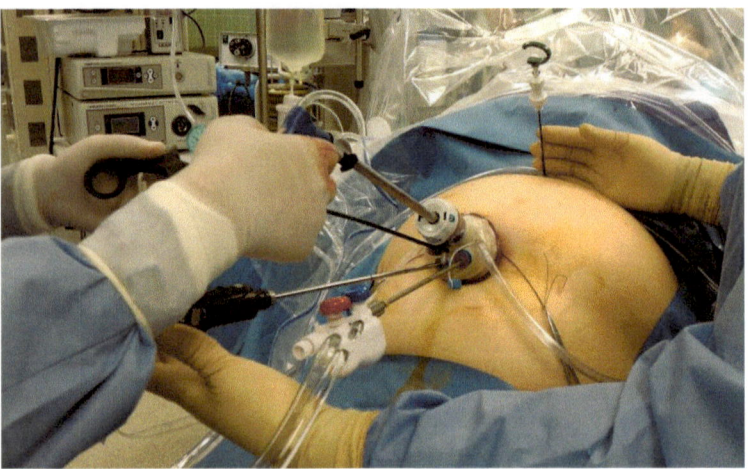

Fig. 33.9 Preserving working space while placing four instruments through a small incision (for sleeve gastrectomy in this case). The flexible tip of the camera and the curve of the instruments allow that separation

Figure 33.9 illustrates the ergonomics in a more complex sleeve gastrectomy case. It shows the surgeon standing on the right side while the assistant on the left side holding the camera (below and away from surgeon's hands) and the small liver retractor. The laparoscope comes from below the instruments, and ends up (in the peritoneal cavity) above them with the tip articulated down to look at the operative field (as shown in the previous figure). Notice the surgeon's hands are separated

Fig. 33.10 Right handed grasper is used to grab and retract the fundus to allow the left hand to clear the left crus

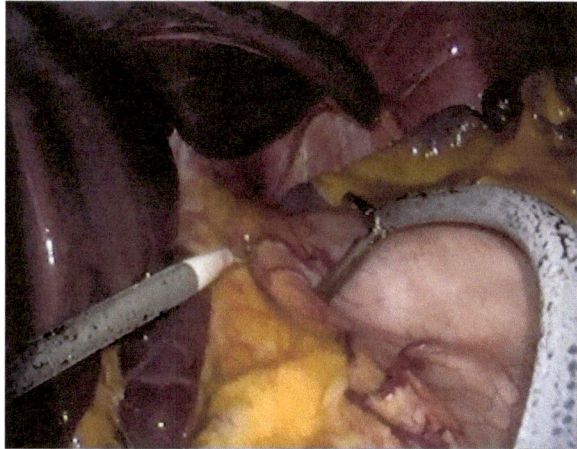

Fig. 33.11 Left crus is well exposed by retracting the fundus, and easily cleared using a hook. Notice the comfort of moving in the space as the tips are coming from different directions while the instruments enter the abdomen through a small single small incision (triangulation concept is preserved and moved intracorporeally)

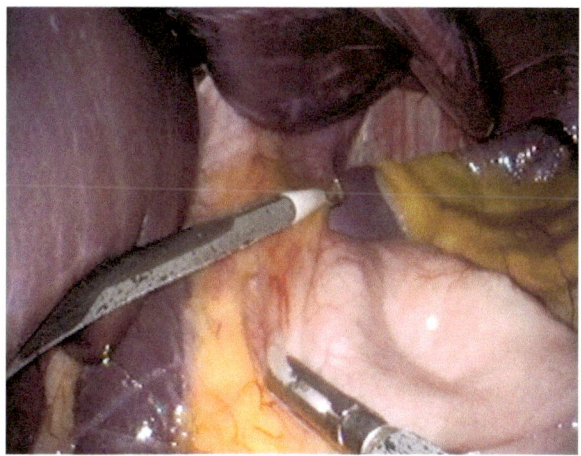

with comfortable distance from each other's and from the laparoscope. Shown is a different port with four channels where a suction device can be added.

Below are the steps of the operation performed using the above described principles and instruments:

- **Clearing the Left Crus**
  Using a right handed gasper and left handed hook cautery, the fundus is pulled straight caudally and the peritoneum over the left crus is divided (Figs. 33.10, 33.11, and 33.12).
- **Hiatal Hernia Repair** (if present)
  As we discussed earlier, optimal hiatal exposure is critical, and repair hiatal hernia is essential for optimal results. We incise the sac with my cautery then bluntly

Fig. 33.12 Clearance of the left crus. The curve makes the instrument seem to be coming from the patient right side as in traditional laparoscopy, while in fact it is coming through the midline (umbilicus)

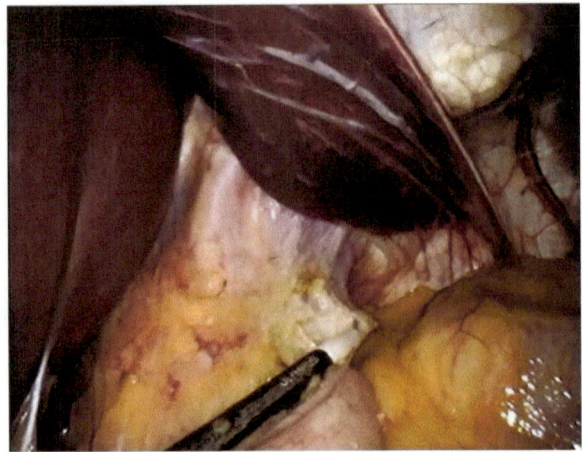

Fig. 33.13 Dividing the peritoneal attachments to the left crus in preparation to incise the hernia sac

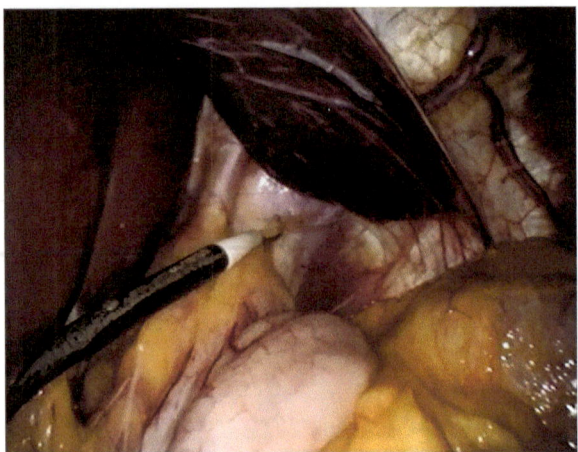

dissect the hiatus using our right handed grasper until we enter the hiatal space. This is an avascular plane and should be simple to penetrate once the sac is incised (Figs. 33.13, 33.14, 33.15, and 33.16).

We close these small hernias anteriorly to avoid posterior dissection (in order to maintain the principles of the *pars flaccida* technique) (Fig. 33.17).

We tend not to place bands in patients with large hiatal hernias requiring posterior repair with mesh.

– **Tunneling**

Without instrument exchange, we apply lateral traction to the lesser curvature using the right hand grasper to place the avascular gastrohepatic ligament under tension. We then divide it with the left hand hook cautery (the liver provides the contralateral traction) (Fig. 33.18).

Fig. 33.14 Blunt dissection leads into the hiatal space after the hernia sac is incised

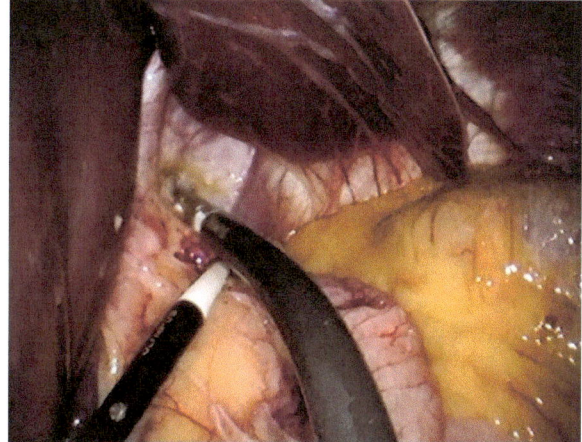

Fig. 33.15 Incising the rest of the hernia sac

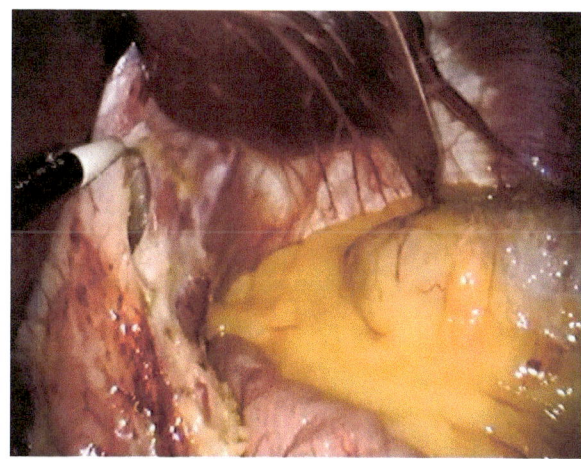

Fig. 33.16 Clearing the medial aspect of the crus in preparation to suture and close the hiatal defect

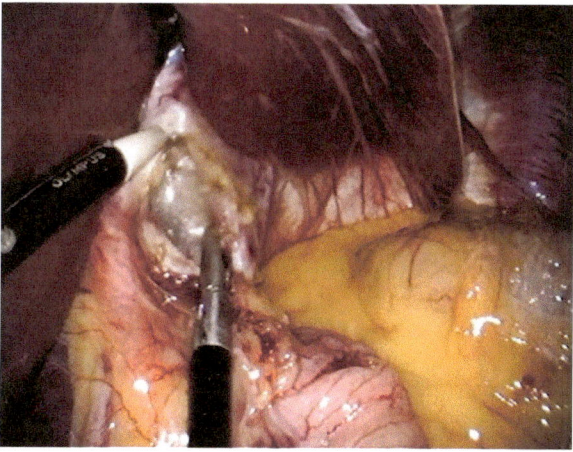

Fig. 33.17 Anterior repair
of the hiatal hernia

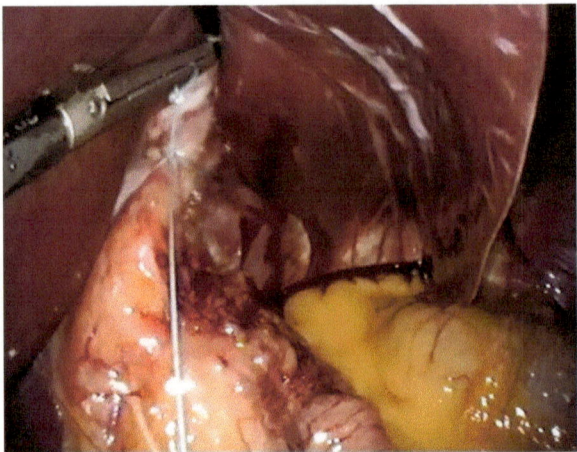

Fig. 33.18 Incising the
gastro-hepatic ligament

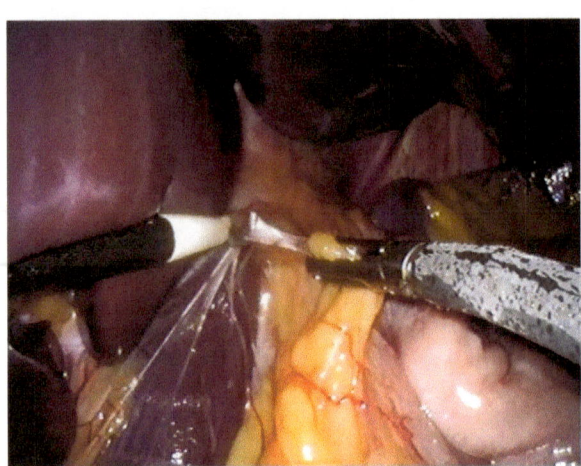

Optimal exposure of the right crus is critical for safety before tunneling is attempted. If good exposure is impossible, trocars should be added at this point for proper retraction and exposure, and the procedure should be converted to traditional laparoscopy. The flexible tip of the laparoscope is advantageous in providing exposure especially in cases of enlarged fatty or floppy liver (Fig. 33.19).

We use the right-handed grasper to elevate the fat over the right crus. This gives an excellent visualization in preparation to performing the tunnel (Fig. 33.20). Using the hook, a small (few millimeters) cut is made just below the middle of the right crus (Fig. 33.21). At this point, we make the first instrument exchange and we take a left-handed blunt tip grasper instead of the hook (which we will not use anymore). We use this instrument to make the tunnel by carefully advancing its tip towards the previously dissected angle of His. The curve makes

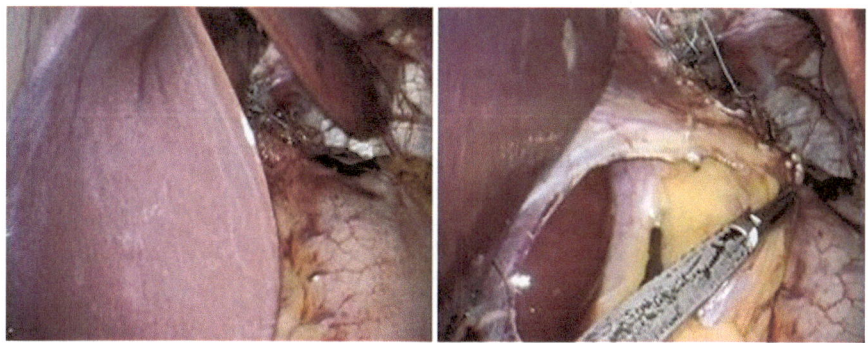

Fig. 33.19 Exposure of the right crus around a floppy liver

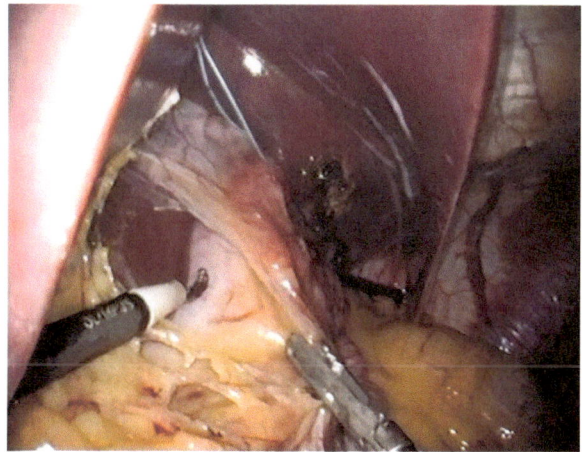

Fig. 33.20 Lateral retraction of the fat over the right crus presents the crus in preparation for the tunnel

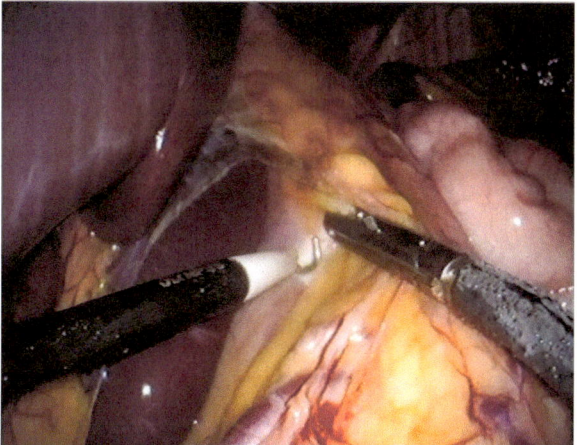

Fig. 33.21 Limited opening of the peritoneum in preparation of the tunnel. Notice the ergonomic ease despite the instruments coming in together through the umbilicus

Fig. 33.22 Starting the tunnel

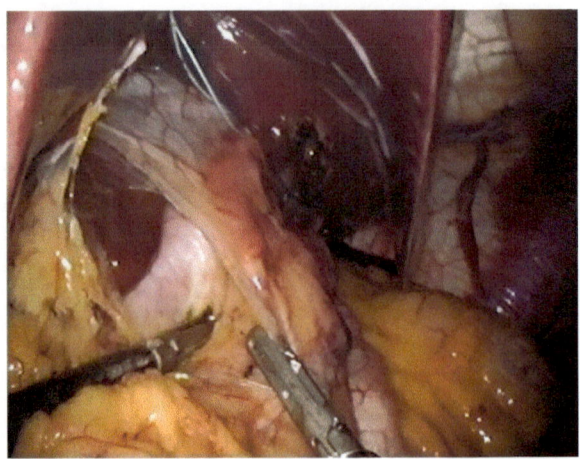

Fig. 33.23 Tunneling. Notice how the curve helps directing the instrument in the correct direction towards the Angle of His

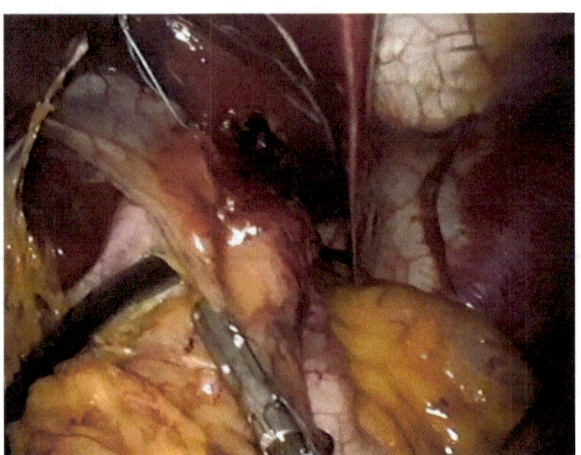

this a natural advancement. It is important not to push hard and to be able to see the tip through transparent tissues before pushing it through (in order to avoid posterior gastric wall injury) (Figs. 33.22, 33.23, and 33.24).

This step is where we see the curved instruments being most advantageous. The direction of the curve allows for an easy and natural tunneling directed to the angle of His despite the instrument entering through the umbilicus (Fig. 33.25).

– **Placing the Band**

At this point, the tail of the band (already placed in the abdomen) is handed to the left handed grasper and pulled through the tunnel and the band is locked in place (Fig. 33.26).

At this stage, we find it easier to pull and leave the tubing end out to help with locking the band, and with later retraction for suturing (as long as the port used will not leak significant gas while the tubing is out) (Fig. 33.27).

Fig. 33.24 Tunnel completed

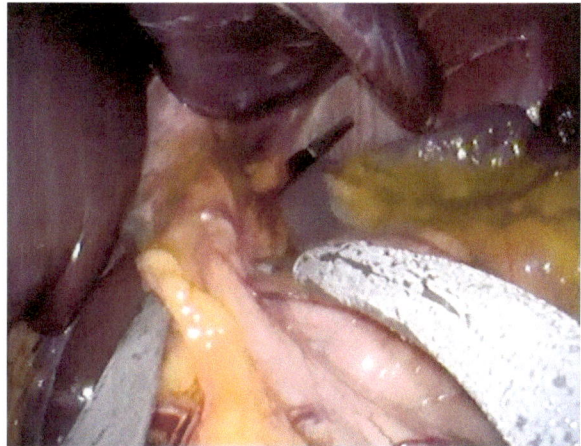

Fig. 33.25 Notice how the curve allows an instrument coming from the midline to easily create a right to left tunnel

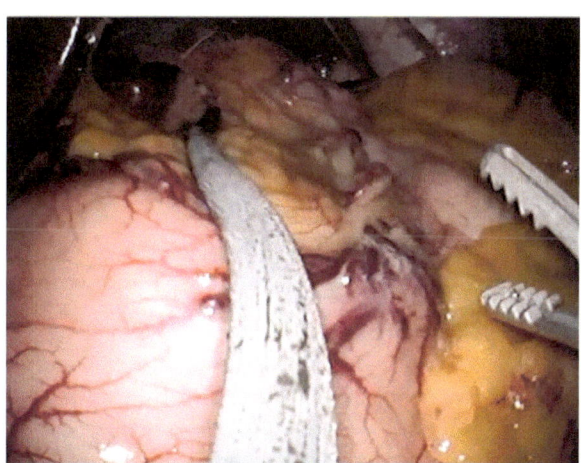

Fig. 33.26 Locking the band. The curves allow for easy movement of the graspers and thus, easy handling and locking of the band

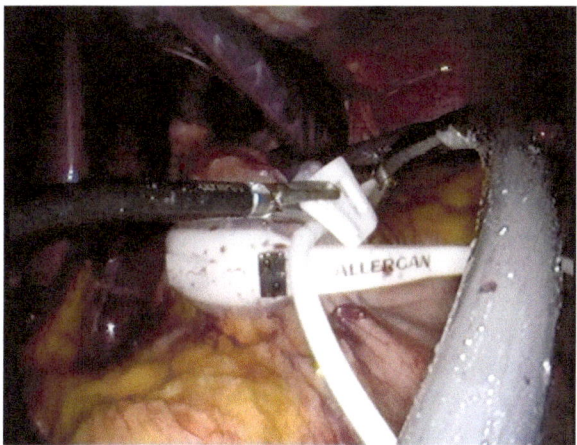

Fig. 33.27 Pulling on the tubing provides good retraction for easier locking the band and suturing the stomach

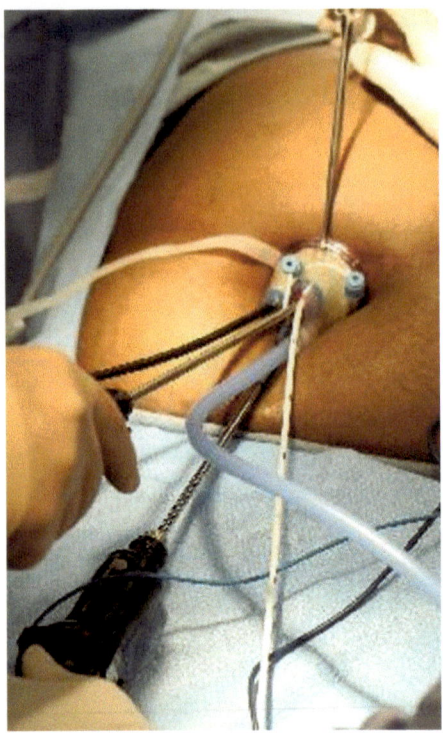

To fix the band in place, a running or interrupted non-absorbable suture is used to perform anterior gastro-gastric plication over the anterior body of the band. We personally use a running Ethibond® suture (Ethicon) with 3 bites on each side and tie it to itself. This makes it faster and helps avoiding time consuming excessive instruments exchange.

We typically perform suturing using a regular laparoscopic needle holder assisted by a curved instrument (Figs. 33.28, 33.29, 33.30, and 33.31), although other suturing devices can be used to make this task an easier (although more expensive) one (Fig. 33.32).

As in traditional laparoscopy, we believe that adding an inferior stitch may play a role in decreasing the incidence of slippage and we always do it (Fig. 33.33).

– **Placing the Port**

After completion of band placement, the gas is emptied and the port is removed and the tubing is brought out.

Placing the band port differs among surgeon. We strongly warn against leaving the port implanted in the umbilicus as this is too painful for adjustment and carries high risk of infection. We also like to avoid passing the tubing through the umbilical fascia as this would prevent proper closure of the umbilical defect, and will cause problem should patients undergo future laparoscopy when unfamiliar surgeons go through the umbilicus and encounter the tube.

Fig. 33.28 Suturing using a needle holder and grasper

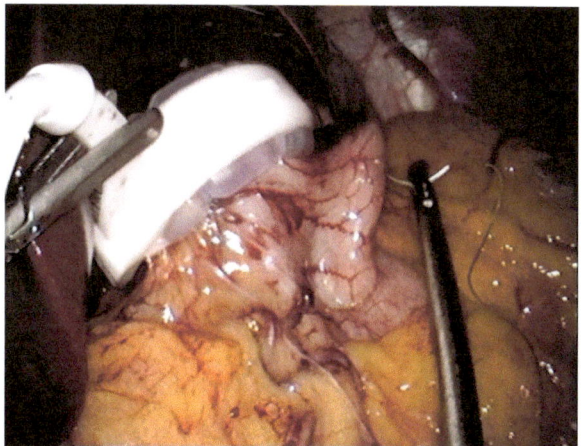

Fig. 33.29 Gastro-gastric placation

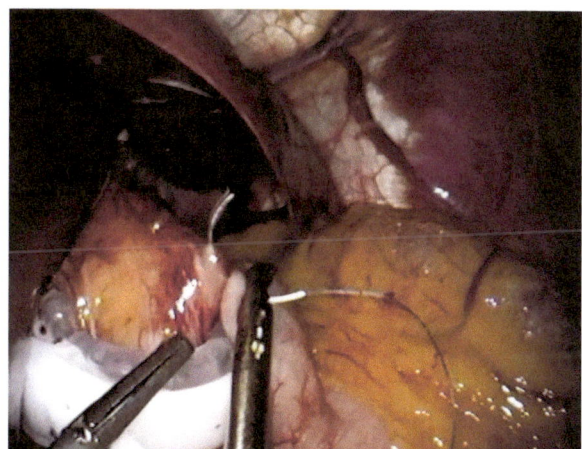

Fig. 33.30 Notice the ability to perform advanced tasks like suturing despite having both instruments coming together through a small incision

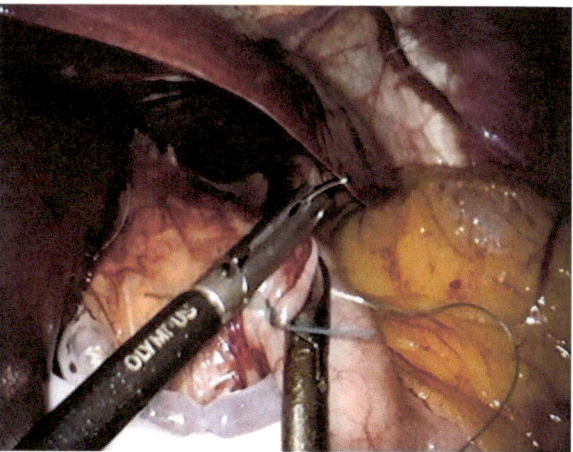

Fig. 33.31 Running suture
line is used to perform the
plication and fix the band in
place

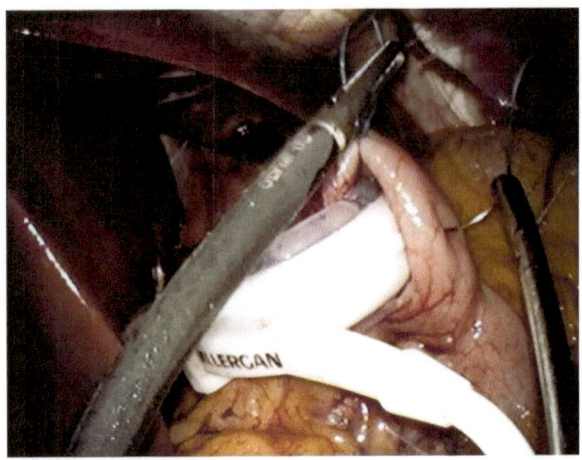

Fig. 33.32 Using suturing
devices, adds cost but can
facilitate suturing in single
site surgery

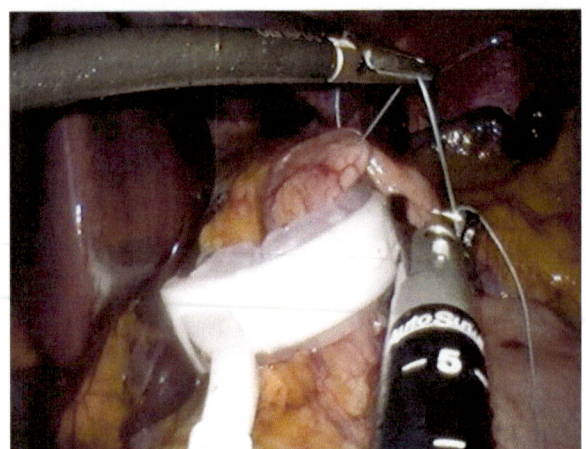

Fig. 33.33 Inferior
"anti-slip" stitch

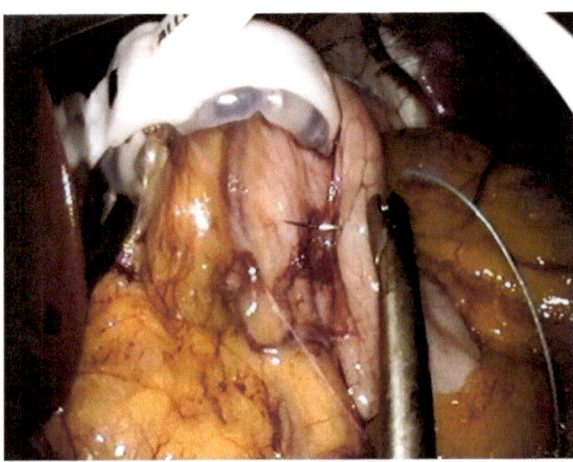

Fig. 33.34 Blunt finger dissection through the umbilical incision is used to create a pocket in the left upper abdominal wall (same location as in traditional multi-port laparoscopy)

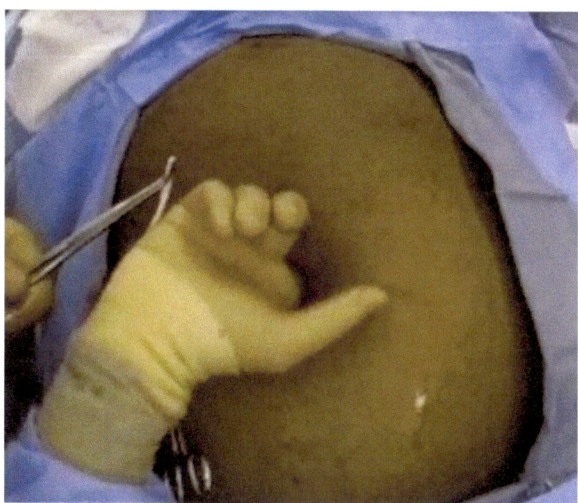

In our practice the port is placed in the same upper left location whether the operation is done using traditional laparoscopy or SLS. This makes the adjustment for our ancillary staff easier as they always know where the port would be.

A pocket is made with blunt finger dissection through the umbilical incision towards the left upper quadrant. The tubing tip is then passed using a right angle through the left rectus muscle 4 cm above and to the left of the umbilicus (after feeling for and ensuring the absence of any adherent bowel in that area) (Figs. 33.34 and 33.35).

It is our practice in traditional LAGB placement to suture the port to a polypropylene mesh to make it adherent to the fascia instead of suturing the actual port directly to the fascia. The technique came handy when we switched to SLS as the port is placed deep in the left upper abdominal wall pocket through the tiny umbilical incision making it impossible to suture (Fig. 33.36).

– **Closure**

We close the fascia with three figure-of-eight absorbable sutures.

Leaving the stalk of the umbilicus intact at the beginning of the procedure helps bringing the skin edges together easily for closure and provide better cosmetic results (Fig. 33.37). This also allows for the final closure to be done using simple interrupted subcuticular stitches leaving a non-visible deep scar (Figs. 33.38 and 33.39).

Due to the deep incision and likely drainage, we pack the umbilicus with cotton balls after painting the area with antibiotic ointment and cover with occlusive dressings. We then aspirate the air to provide a strong seal with negative pressure (Fig. 33.40).

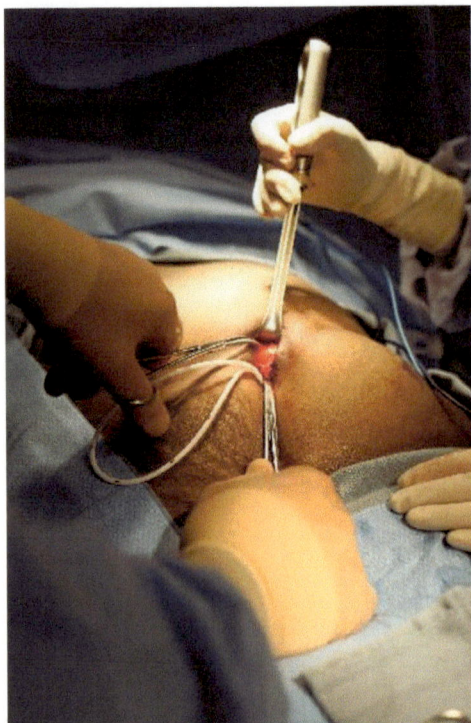

Fig. 33.35 The tubing is passed using right angle through the left rectus is order to connect with the port. Neither the LAGB port nor the tubing remain in the umbilical area

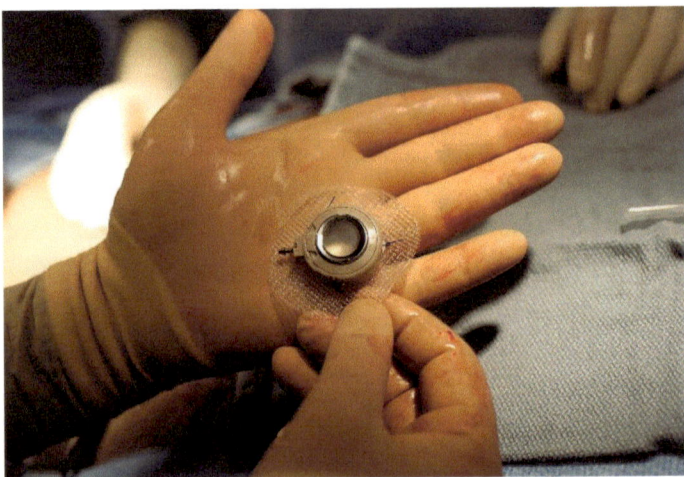

Fig. 33.36 The port is sutured to a polypropylene mesh to make it adherent to the fascia to prevent port flips. This is especially useful in single site surgery as suturing the port to the fascia in the deep left upper quadrant pocket through the small umbilical incision is not technically feasible

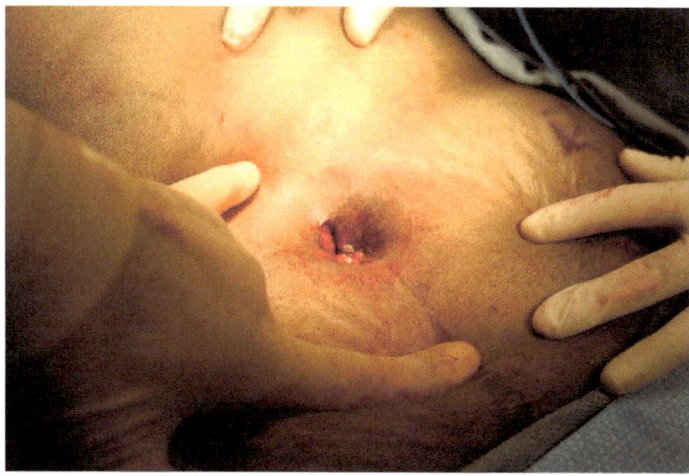

Fig. 33.37 The skin edges come together nicely because the umbilical stalk is left intact

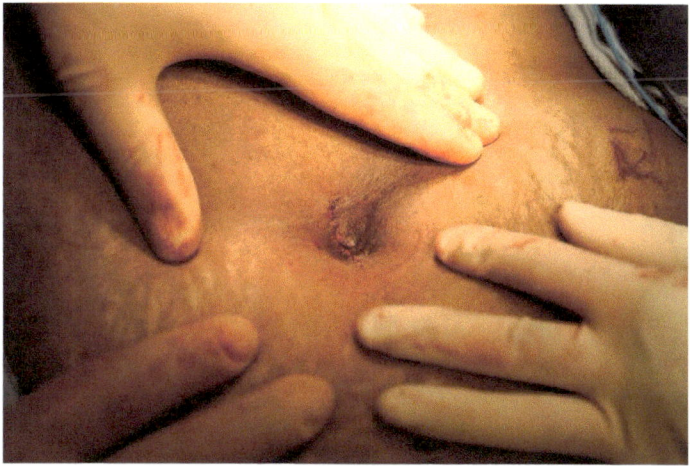

Fig. 33.38 Simple approximation is enough to close the wound and bring back the natural look of the umbilicus. The future scar ends up deep and not visible

33.4   Conclusion

Surgery is an evolving field, and RPLS seems to be part of the natural evolution of laparoscopy. Placing a gastric band using this technique is feasible with relatively short learning curve. For weight loss surgery, this technology may be of particular

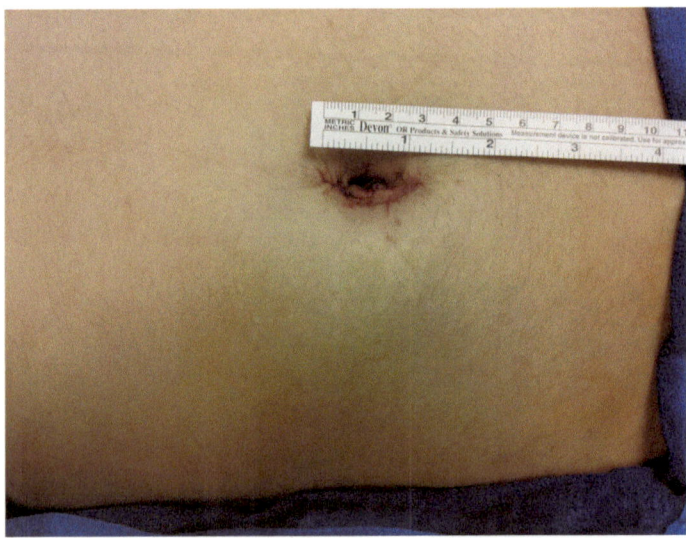

Fig. 33.39 Incision is about 2.5 cm

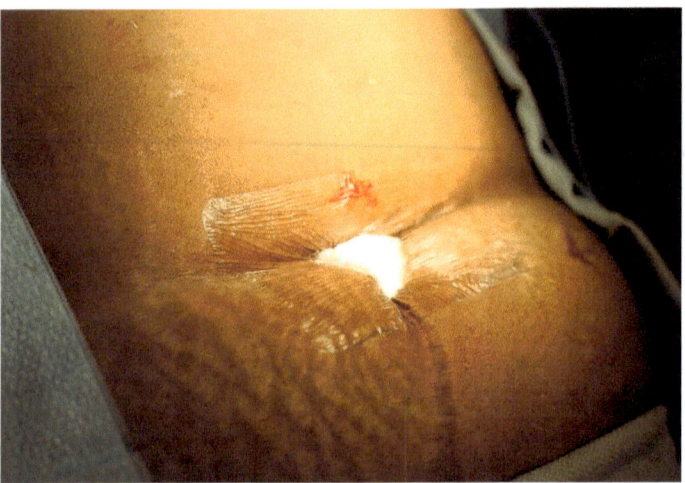

Fig. 33.40 Negative pressure dressings keep wound dry in the deep umbilicus decreasing wound complications

value as pain and scarring may be what hold many obese patients from coming for surgical consultation. Minimizing pain and eliminating scarring can motivate these struggling patients to finally consider bariatric surgery as it is the only long term effective treatment for their morbid obesity.

References

1. Szinicz G, Schnapka G (1982) A new method in the surgical treatment of disease. Acta Chir Aust Suppl 43
2. Kuzmak LI, Yap IS, McGuire L, Dixon JS, Young MP (1990) Surgery for morbid obesity. Using an inflatable gastric band. AORN J 51:1307–1324
3. Belachew M, Legrand MJ, Vincent V (2001) History of Lap-Band: from dream to reality. Obes Surg 11:297–302
4. Fielding GA, Allen JW (2002) A step-by-step guide to placement of the LAP-BAND adjustable gastric banding system. Am J Surg 184(6B):26S–30S
5. Fielding GA, Duncombe JE (2005) Laparoscopic adjustable gastric banding in severely obese adolescents. Surg Obes Relat Dis 1(4):399–405, discussion 405–407
6. Holterman AX, Browne A, Dillard BE 3rd, Tussing L, Gorodner V, Stahl C, Browne N, Labott S, Herdegen J, Guzman G, Rink A, Nwaffo I, Galvani C, Horgan S, Holterman M (2007) Short-term outcome in the first 10 morbidly obese adolescent patients in the FDA-approved trial for laparoscopic adjustable gastric banding. J Pediatr Gastroenterol Nutr 45(4):465–473
7. Nguyen NT, Hinojosa MW, Smith BR, Reavis KM (2008) Single laparoscopic incision transabdominal (SLIT) surgery-adjustable gastric banding: a novel minimally invasive surgical approach. Obes Surg 18(12):1628–1631
8. Saber AA, El-Ghazaly TH (2009) Early experience with single-access transumbilical adjustable laparoscopic gastric banding. Obes Surg 19(10):1442–1446
9. Raman SR, Franco D, Holover S, Garber S (2011) Does transumbilical single incision laparoscopic adjustable gastric banding result in decreased pain medicine use? A case-matched study. Surg Obes Relat Dis 7(2):129–133
10. Gawart M, Dupitron S, Lutfi R (2012) Laparoendoscopic single-site gastric bands versus standard multiport gastric bands: a comparison of technical learning curve measured by surgical time. Am J Surg 203(3):327–329
11. Galvani CA, Gallo AS, Gorodner MV (2012) Single-incision and dual-incision laparoscopic adjustable gastric band: evaluation of initial experience. Surg Obes Relat Dis 8(2):194–200

Chapter 34
Roux-en-Y Gastric Bypass for Obesity

Chih Kun Huang and Anirudh Vij

Abstract The incidence of morbid obesity is increasing worldwide, and bariatric surgery has proven to be the only effective therapy. Roux-en-Y gastric bypass (RYGB) is regarded as the gold standard bariatric procedure that has stood the test of time. The surgical technique has undergone considerable evolution, and recently, the laparoscopic approach (LRYGB) has become widely popular due to its numerous advantages. The concept of minimal invasiveness with an excellent cosmetic outcome has spurred the recent development of the reduced port and single incision laparoscopic approach. This was initially attempted for basic surgical procedures like cholecystectomy but now has expanded to bariatric surgery as well. Performing LRYGB with a single incision is technically demanding due to loss of triangulation and crowding of trocars and instruments both within and outside the abdomen. This could be partly overcome with the use of commercially available single-incision port devices, low profile trocars, flexible scopes, and curved instruments. The single-incision trans-umbilical (SITU) technique of LRYGB developed innovations like the omega umbilicoplasty, which allows multiple conventional trocars to be placed within the umbilical incision, and the liver suspension tape for retraction of the liver which enables the surgery without specialised instruments. Though comparative studies showed that the SITU-LRYGB had a longer operative time than the conventional technique, it was equally safe and efficacious, with a better cosmetic outcome and wound satisfaction. Future expansion of this approach is expected with further advancements in medical technology.

Keywords Bariatric surgery • Obesity • Reduced port laparoscopy • Roux-en-Y gastric bypass

C.K. Huang (✉) • A. Vij
E Da Hospital, Bariatric and Metabolic International Surgery Centre, Kaohsuing, Taiwan
e-mail: dr.ckhuang@hotmail.com

T. Mori and G. Dapri (eds.), *Reduced Port Laparoscopic Surgery*,
DOI 10.1007/978-4-431-54601-6_34, © Springer Japan 2014

34.1   Introduction

Obesity is a condition characterised by excessive accumulation of body fat that adversely affects health and decreases life expectancy [1, 2]. A more metric definition is body weight exceeding the ideal body weight by 20 % or a body mass index (BMI = Weight (kg)/[Height (m)]^2) of more than 30 kg/m^2. Obesity is currently reaching epidemic proportions in many developed countries of the world and is thought to be a multi-factorial aetiology including genetic, environmental, dietary as well as cultural and psycho-social factors.

Body weight exceeding the ideal by 100 % or a BMI of more than 40 kg/m^2 is defined as "morbid obesity". It is associated with adverse effects on almost all the organ systems and can dramatically decrease the life expectancy and the quality of life. The most prevalent associated diseases include degenerative joint disease, hypertension, type 2 diabetes mellitus, obstructive sleep apnea, asthma, right heart failure, arrhythmias, venous ulcers, infertility, stress urinary incontinence, pseudo-tumor cerebri, depression, and increased incidence of various cancers [3]. Besides these medical ailments, morbidly obese patients are subject to social stigmatization, prejudice, and discrimination, contributing to a high incidence of psychological problems like poor self-image and depression.

Medical therapy for obesity aims to reduce body weight through a combination of decreased caloric intake by dieting and increased energy expenditure through exercise. However, these measures are largely unsuccessful in achieving a sustained and meaningful weight loss as demonstrated in several large prospective studies, especially in morbid obesity [4, 5]. Pharmacological therapy using drugs may induce modest weight loss, but the effects are temporary with a prompt relapse in weight gain once the drug is discontinued [6].

34.2   Evolution of Bariatric Surgery

34.2.1   Open Bariatric Surgery

The term "bariatric surgery" is coined from the Greek word "baros" meaning weight and refers to surgical procedures performed to reduce body weight [7]. It has been proved to be the only effective treatment for morbid obesity. In 1991, the National Institute of Health (NIH) consensus established the guidelines for bariatric surgery for patients with BMI > 35 kg/m^2 with severe obesity-related comorbidity, as well as patients with BMI > 40 kg/m^2 with or without comorbidity [8]. Jejuno-ilelal bypass was perhaps the first bariatric procedure designed to lose weight by bypassing most of the small intestine, but it was associated with a high morbidity and a significant mortality rate. Many patients eventually had to undergo reversal of the procedure

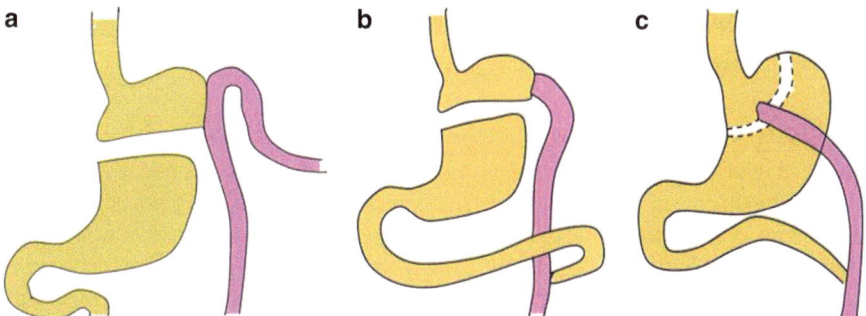

Fig. 34.1 Evolution of Roux-en-Y gastric bypass. (**a**) Mason and Ito (1966), (**b**) Griffin modification (1977), (**c**) Torres (1980)

due to its severe side effects, and it was finally abandoned [9]. The development of the first gastric bypass procedure has been credited to Mason and Ito in 1966 [10]. Their procedure involved horizontal transection of the stomach with a retrocolic loop gastrojejunostomy. They later refined the surgery by calibrating the gastric pouch and adjusting the diameter of the gastrojejunostomy to improve the effects on weight loss [10, 11]. Griffen in 1977 modified the original operation by replacing the loop with a Roux-en-gastrojejunostomy, thus reducing the incidence of bile reflux and marginal ulceration and improving the quality of life for the patient [12]. Torres further amended it by creating a small pouch based on the lesser curvature and excluding the fundus which generated the current type of Roux-en-Y gastric bypass (RYGB) [13] (Fig. 34.1).

34.2.2 Laparoscopic Bariatric Surgery

Morbidly obese patients are at high risk of cardiopulmonary and wound-related complications when receiving laparotomy surgery and are proven to benefit from a minimally invasive approach [14]. The first laparoscopic RYGB (LRYGB) was performed by Wittgrove and Clark in 1994 [15]. The laparoscopic approach facilitates the popularity of RYGB due to the general benefits such as decreased pain, superior cosmesis, shorter postoperative stay, an earlier return to activity, and a reduction in the perceived magnitude of the procedure [16]. This brought about the bariatric revolution in the late 1990s, and since then, the number of bariatric procedures performed worldwide has increased exponentially [17]. Presently, LRYGB is the most commonly performed bariatric procedure worldwide and has been established as the "gold standard" due to its long term effects on weight loss and remission of obesity-related comorbidities [18].

34.2.3 Reduced Port Laparoscopy and Single-Incision Laparoscopy

Conventional laparoscopic bariatric surgery generally makes use of 5–7 trocars distributed over the abdomen and may be associated with a pigmentation scar and variable cosmetic outcome, especially among dark-skinned patients. This may not be acceptable in certain subsets of the population, particularly among young females who form a substantial proportion of the bariatric surgeon's practice. The desire for superior cosmetic outcome from surgery brought about the development of natural orifice trans-lumenal endoscopic surgery (NOTES), reduced port laparoscopy (RPL), and single-incision laparoscopy (SLS) [19]. Recently, SLS has become more popular because it avoids the risk of visceral perforation from NOTES and is more comfortable for the surgeon due to the familiarity of the instrumentation and operating technique. There have been some series reports from various surgical procedures using this technique, such as cholecystectomy [20, 21], appendectomy [22], colectomy [23], and also bariatric surgeries [24, 25]. Initially, RPL and SLS were both implicated in adjustable gastric banding and sleeve gastrectomy as these procedures involved making a large incision for the introduction of the band and specimen extraction, respectively [24, 25]. With rapid progression, the technique was extrapolated to perform LRYGB. The first case of RYGB by the single incision transumbilical (SITU) laparoscopic approach was reported in 2009 by our group [27]. We made use of several innovations like the omega umbilicoplasty for trocar placement, liver suspension tape for retraction, and stay suture for traction on the jejunostoma during closure. This made it possible to complete the procedure successfully in all patients without additional trocars or specialised instrumentation. Other groups like Tacchino et al. performed the single incision RYGB using the commercially available Triport device (Advanced Surgical Concepts, Wicklow, Ireland) and "double loop technique" for gastro enteric anastomosis. Fernandez et al. reported performing the surgery with a GelPOINT (Applied Medical, Rancho Santa Margarita, CA, USA) and a totally handsewn gastrojejunal anastomosis but required an additional 5 mm trocar in the left flank. Saber et al. published their experience of performing a 3-trocar LRYGB successfully in 16 morbidly obese patients [26]. They made use of conventional trocars (2 umbilical and 1 in right upper quadrant) and long instruments but required placement of the Nathanson liver retractor and a 5 mm flexible laparoscope for endovision. Lee et al. similarly performed a transumbilical two-site LRYGB, placing two ports within the umbilical incision and another one in the left lateral abdominal wall, and compared their results with the conventional technique.

Here we describe our technique for SITU-LRYGB.

34.3 Technique

The patient is placed in the supine position with appropriate padding of the pressure points and strapped to the table to avoid slipping during the extremes of position. The arms are abducted laterally. The surgeon stands on the right

Fig. 34.2 Operation set-up

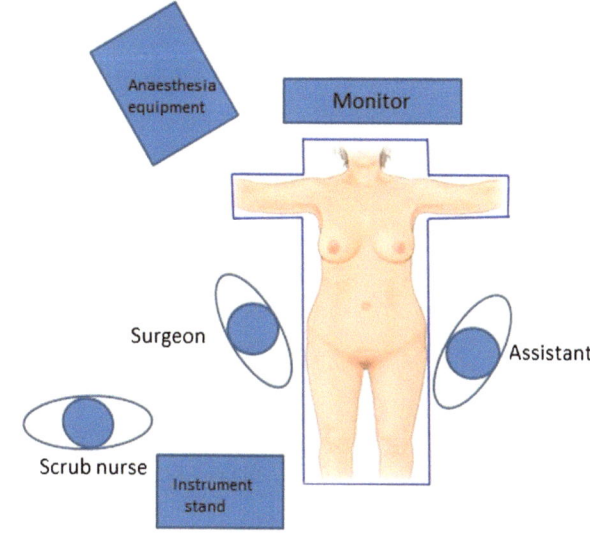

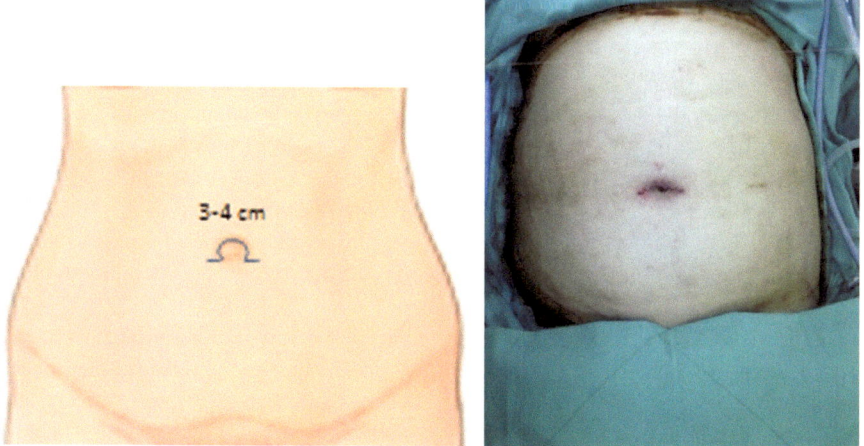

Fig. 34.3 Incision and port placement for SITU-LRYGB

side of the patient and the camera assistant on the left while the scrub nurse is behind the surgeon (Fig. 34.2). The incision is 4–6 cm transverse curvilinear (omega incision) [31] located at the superior border of the umbilicus and deepened up to the linea alba (Fig. 34.3). The subcutaneous fat is partly dissected to create the space for trocar placement. After creation of pneumoperitoneum, a 12-mm trocar is inserted at the 12 o' clock position in the centre of the incision. Two other trocars (5 mm and 10 mm) are then placed under vision laterally in the bilateral 'arms' of the incision at the 4 o' clock and 7 o' clock positions (Fig. 34.4).

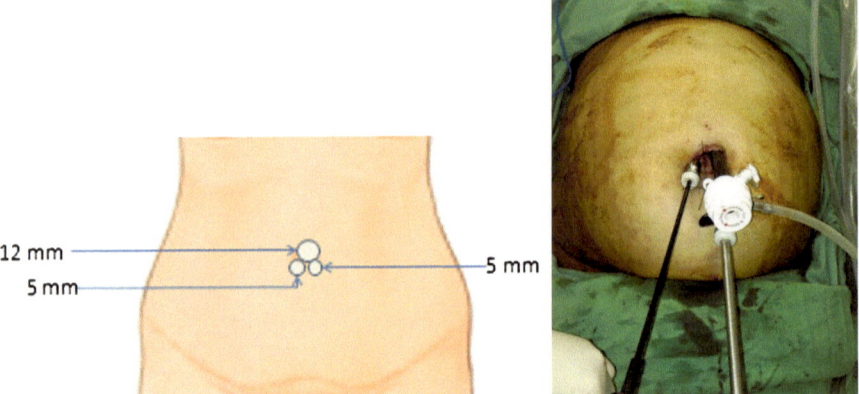

Fig. 34.4 Port placement for SITU-LRYGB

A 10-mm, 30° long scope (45 cm) is employed for endovision which is placed through the right lateral trocar, while the two working instruments are placed through the central and left trocars. During the initial learning phase, we advise making a longer (6 cm) incision, allowing a sufficient space for manipulation between the trocars. The incision can then be reduced to 4 cm as the surgeon gains experience. The trocars are not placed perpendicularly but slightly obliquely, aiming towards the hiatus in order to avoid torque during instrument manipulation.

The liver suspension tape [31] is prepared by cutting a 6 cm portion of Jackson–Pratt drain near the drainage hole. The drainage tube is then pierced with 2-0 Prolene suture (Monofilament Polypropylene Suture W8400™ (Ethicon, Cincinnati, OH, USA), according to the diameter of the hole. Needles are left in both sides for further liver puncture. The tube is placed inside the peritoneal cavity for retraction of the left lobe of the liver and for a clear view of the angle of His, the crura, and the gastroesophageal junction. Two or three tapes may be required, depending upon the bulkiness of the liver and the view obtained.

The dissection starts at the lesser curvature just below the first branch of the left gastric vessel. The tissue is cut using ultrasonic shears, and the retrogastric tunnel is entered. A 30 cc gastric pouch is created using laparoscopic linear staplers. The proximal jejunum is traced from the ligament of Treitz, and a length of 100 cm is measured. An enterotomy is created and a laparoscopic linear stapler is used to create 2 cm gastrojejunostomy which is placed in the antecolic and antegastric position. The proximal jejunum is then transected using a laparoscopic linear stapler adjacent to the gastrojejunostomy. One hundred centimeter of Roux limb is measured and side-to-side jejunojejunal anastomosis is performed using a laparoscopic linear stapler at this point. The entry holes of the staplers are closed by intracorporeal continuous suturing using a 3-0 absorbable suture. The mesenteric, as well as the Petersen, defects are closed by continuous intracorporeal suturing with 2-0 non-absorbable sutures. The liver suspension tape is removed, and the puncture hole of the liver is cauterized for hemostasis.

After removing the trocars, all three fascial defects are closed individually with 2-0 Vicryl sutures. In cases of a long umbilical skin incision, the subcutaneous fat and the skin at the angles are removed, and an umbilicoplasty is performed. The final wound is circular and buried within the umbilicus. With increased experience, the initial skin incision made is smaller and an umbilicoplasty is unnecessary.

34.4 Surgical Results

The operation time reported has generally been longer than that of the conventional laparoscopic approach, mostly attributed to the technical difficulties encountered during the procedure. However, none of the groups reported any intra-operative or early postoperative complications related to the surgical technique. Problems related to loss of triangulation were managed by placement of an extra 5-mm trocar, as seen in 18 of 100 patients undergoing two-site LRYGB. Because of the surgeons' sufficient experience, there was no need of conversion to conventional LRYGB or open procedure in any of the published reports. The two largest series compared their results with conventional LRYGB. The length of postoperative hospital stay, postoperative complications, and excess weight loss up to 12 months was not significantly different between the two groups. Although the SITU-LRYGB group in our study required more morphine administration for post-operative pain control, it did not reach statistical significance. There may be an increased risk of seroma formation due to wide dissection of the subcutaneous tissue, and the patients generally need to care for their wound for a longer time compared to conventional multiport laparoscopy [28]. Finally, the wound satisfaction score at 3 months was significantly higher for the SITU group, suggesting that they were more satisfied with the cosmetic outcome of the surgery.

34.5 Pitfalls and Their Management

34.5.1 Trocar Placement

The surgery may be performed using the commercially available single-port devices or conventional trocars [27–32]. The former devices provide less sufficient space between the instruments and hence necessitate the use of curved or articulating instruments [30, 32]. Because of their large size, they require the creation of an equivalent fascial defect which, if not closed properly, can increase the risk of incisional hernia. Moreover, these devices add considerable cost to the procedure. In SITU method, placement of all three operating trocars within a small umbilical incision would cause excessive crowding and hamper manipulation. This could be overcome by the technique we developed, omega umbilcoplasty [31]. The initial umbilical incision was around 6 cm in length along the superior border of the umbilicus, allowing for comfortable placement of the three trocars with a gap of 4 cm between each trocar. The instrument clashing was overcome by using low profile trocars and instruments of different lengths, allowing adequate space between the surgeon's hands. The trocars are all angled to the area of interest and not perpendicular to the abdominal wall, reducing the torque and shoulder strain for the surgeon.

The initial dissection of the subcutaneous space for trocar placement weakens the grip of the abdominal wall on the trocars and may result in gas leakage. The repeated instrument exchanges and excessive torque forces add to this problem and enlarge the existing fascial defect, necessitating the use of threaded trocars or skin suture for anchoring the ports. It is preferable to use a 30 ° 10 mm long telescope for creating good endovision. The light cable of the telescope is a frequent cause of interference. This is counteracted by using a light cable adapter that allows the light source to exit at an acute angle from the scope. Some authors have used semi-flexible scopes with integrated light and camera cables to make the procedure more comfortable, albeit at a higher cost.

34.5.2   Liver Retraction

Liver retraction is essential in bariatric surgery to perform dissection near the hiatus as the left lobe is usually bulky and friable and usually obscures this area if there is insufficient exposure. Earlier reports described the use of the conventional Nathanson liver retractor during RPL-RYGB [26]. Tacchino et al. performed the surgery without using any form of the liver retraction and managed to use the articulating stapler to push up the left liver lobe during pouch creation [30]. With this technique, the mean length of the gastric pouch was as large as 8 cm to avoid the technical difficulties that would have been encountered by big left liver, during the creation of a pouch and the subsequent higher gastrojejunal anastomosis. The liver suspension tape [31] that we developed can be easily prepared before the procedure, and multiple tapes can be used in the situation when one is not enough to retract liver well. The concern about the safety of liver suspension and its effect on postoperative liver function has been allayed by a prospective randomized trial wherein the three different methods of liver retraction were compared with respect to the time required for placement, postoperative pain, and liver function tests. Surprisingly, we found that the Nathanson liver retractor caused more pain and liver dysfunction compared to our liver suspension techniques [33].

34.5.3   Instruments and Surgical Technique

The successful performance of SITU-LRYGB requires that the dissection and anastomosis be confined to a single abdominal quadrant. Long instruments and harmonic shears (43 cm) are required to reach hiatus. Several authors have reported the use of articulating instruments like the endograsp for creating artificial triangulation within the abdomen. However, this requires crossing of the surgeon's hands, creating confusion and sword fighting during the procedure. The success of using straight instruments mostly depends on the surgical steps we performed. After creating the pouch, we brought the uncut loop of jejunum to the gastric pouch for creation of the gastrojejunal anastomosis. Some authors then measure the foot of the Roux limb, create the jejunojejunostomy, and transect between the two anastomoses to finally separate the biliary and alimentary limbs [30]. In our technique, we transected the biliary limb after gastrojejunal anastomoses to avoid excessive tension. In both approaches, the entire manipulation and suturing is confined to the supracolic compartment and avoids excessive torque forces and change of position to the infracolic region which would make this step extremely difficult. We used instruments with curved opposing tips to create angles required for intracorporeal looping and knot tying. A to-and-fro movement of the instruments helps create loops especially using a monofilament suture material with a strong memory.

34.5.3.1 Fascial Closure

Closing of the fascial defects is important, as some studies have documented an increased rate of incisional hernias following single incision laparoscopy [34]. We recommend routinely closing all three defects under vision in SITU technique to prevent this complication.

34.5.3.2 Limitations and Contra-Indications for SLS Bariatric

LRYGB using the SLS technique has its limitations. We do not recommend this technique for very tall patients (>180 cm), those with a long xiphisternum-to-umbilicus distance (>25 cm), super obese (BMI > 50 kg/m^2) patients, and those with a pendulous abdomen. There is increased difficulty of approaching the hiatal area from the umbilicus, even with long instruments, in tall patients and those with a long torso. Super obese patients have excessive visceral and mesenteric fat, making dissection and manipulation particularly difficult. The patients with a pendulous abdomen and lax skin usually require a plastic procedure after bariatric surgery when they have lost a sufficient amount of weight. Thus, these patients do not benefit from the cosmetic advantage provided by the initial operation.

34.6 Recommendations and Conclusions

We first recommend that the surgeon should perform the surgery with a reduced number of ports, as proposed by Saber [26]. This helps the surgeon become familiarized with the operation technique without the help of a conventional liver retractor and the countertraction provided by the assistant. After this is mastered, the ports can be placed closer together to execute the manipulation and suturing with smaller angles. After this stage, the SLS technique may be attempted, but there should be a low threshold for placement of additional trocars in the initial few cases so as not to compromise the safety of the procedure.

SLS offers a virtually 'scar-less' surgery, particularly through the transumbilical approach. Although it is more challenging technically with a significantly longer operative time compared to the conventional surgery, it has shown better postoperative outcomes regarding wound satisfaction. It requires greater expertise and experience before it can be attempted successfully.

References

1. Calle EE, Thun MJ, Petrelli JM et al (1999) Body mass index and mortality in a prospective cohort of U.S. adults. N Engl J Med 341:1097–1105
2. Haslam DW, James WP (2005) "Obesity". Lancet 366(9492):1197–1209
3. Garfinkel L (1985) Overweight and cancer. Ann Intern Med 1103:1034
4. Sjöström L, Lindroos AK, Peltonen M, Swedish Obese Subjects Study Scientific Group et al (2004) Lifestyle, diabetes and cardiovascular risk factors 10 years after bariatric surgery. N Engl J Med 351(26):2683–2693
5. Maggard MA, Shugarman LR, Suttorp M et al (2005) Meta-analysis: surgical treatment of obesity. Ann Intern Med 142(7):547–559
6. Hainer V, Hainerová IA (2012) Do we need anti-obesity drugs? Diabetes Metab Res Rev Suppl 2:8–20
7. Collins English Dictionary – Complete & Unabridged, 10th edn. HarperCollins Publishers, Glasgow, UK
8. National Institutes of Health (1991) Gastrointestinal surgery for severe obesity; consensus development conference panel. Ann Intern Med 115:956–961
9. Griffen WO Jr, Bivins BA, Bell RM et al (1983) The decline and fall of jejunoileal bypass. Surg Gynecol Obstet 157:301–308
10. Mason EE, Ito C (1967) Gastric bypass in obesity. Surg Clin North Am 47:1345–1351
11. Mason EE, Printen KJ, Hartford CE et al (1975) Optimizing results of gastric bypass. Ann Surg 182:405–414
12. Griffen WO, Young VL, Stevenson CC (1977) A prospective comparison of gastric and jejunoileal bypass procedures for morbid obesity. Ann Surg 186:500–509
13. Torres JC, Oca CF, Garrison RN (1983) Gastric bypass Roux-en-Y gastrojejunostomy from the lesser curvature. South Med J 76:1217
14. Schauer PR, Ikramuddin S, Gourash W et al (2000) Outcomes after laparoscopic Roux-en-Y gastric bypass for morbid obesity. Ann Surg 232:515–529
15. Wittgrove AC, Clark GW, Tremblay LJ (1994) Laparoscopic gastric bypass, Roux-en-Y: preliminary report of five cases. Obes Surg 4:353–357
16. Tian HL, Tian JH, Yang KH et al (2011) The effects of laparoscopic vs. open gastric bypass for morbid obesity: a systematic review and meta-analysis of randomized controlled trials. Obes Rev 12:254–260
17. Buchwald H, Williams SE (2004) Bariatric surgery worldwide 2003. Obes Surg 14(9):1157–1164
18. Sugerman HJ, Kellum JM, Engle KM et al (1992) Gastric bypass for treating severe obesity. Am J Clin Nutr 55:560S–566S

19. Kalloo AN, Singh VK, Jagannath SB et al (2004) Flexible transgastric peritoneoscopy: a novel approach to diagnostic and therapeutic interventions in the peritoneal cavity. Gastrointest Endosc 60:114–117
20. Hall TC, Dennison AR, Bilku DK (2012) Single-incision laparoscopic cholecystectomy: a systematic review. Arch Surg 147(7):657–666
21. Tacchino R, Greco F, Matera D (2009) Single-incision laparoscopic cholecystectomy: surgery without a visible scar. Surg Endosc 23(4):896–899
22. Rehman H, Mathews T, Ahmed I (2012) A review of minimally invasive single-port/incision laparoscopic appendectomy. J Laparoendosc Adv Surg Tech A 22(7):641–646
23. Fung AK, Aly EH (2012) Systematic review of single-incision laparoscopic colonic surgery. Br J Surg 99(10):1353–1364
24. Saber AA, Elgamal MH, Itawi EA et al (2008) Single incision laparoscopic sleeve gastrectomy (SILS): a novel technique. Obes Surg 18(10):1338–1342
25. Nguyen NT, Hinojosa MW, Smith BR et al (2008) Single laparoscopic incision transabdominal (SLIT) surgery-adjustable gastric banding: a novel minimally invasive surgical approach. Obes Surg 18:1628–1631
26. Saber A, Elgamal MH, Tarek H et al (2010) Three trocar laparoscopic Roux-en-y gastric bypass: a novel technique en route to the single-incision laparoscopic approach. Int J Surg 8:131–134
27. Huang CK, Houng JY, Chiang CJ et al (2009) Single incision transumbilical laparoscopic Roux-en-Y gastric bypass: a first case report. Obes Surg 19(12):1711–1715
28. Huang CK, Lo CH, Houng JY et al (2012) Surgical results of single-incision transumbilical laparoscopic Roux-en-Y gastric bypass. Surg Obes Relat Dis 8(2):201–207
29. Lee WJ, Chen JC, Yao WC et al (2012) Transumbilical 2-site laparoscopic Roux-en-Y gastric bypass: initial results of 100 cases and comparison with traditional laparoscopic technique. Surg Obes Relat Dis 8(2):208–213. doi:10.1016/j.soard.2010.12.004
30. Tacchino RM, Greco F, Matera D et al (2010) Single-incision laparoscopic gastric bypass for morbid obesity. Obes Surg 20(8):1154–1160
31. Huang CK, Tsai JC, Lo CH et al (2011) Preliminary surgical results of single-incision transumbilical laparoscopic bariatric surgery. Obes Surg 21(3):391–396
32. Fernández JI, Ovalle C, Farias C (2013) Transumbilical laparoscopic Roux-en-Y gastric bypass with hand-sewn gastrojejunal anastomosis. Obes Surg 10:140–144. doi:10.1007/s11695-012-0804-z
33. Goel R, Shabbir A, Tai CM (2013) Randomized controlled trial comparing three methods of liver retraction in laparoscopic Roux-en-Y gastric bypass. Surg Endosc 27(2):679–684
34. Alptekin H, Yilmaz H, Acar F et al (2012) Incisional hernia rate may increase after single-port cholecystectomy. J Laparoendosc Adv Surg Tech A 22(8):731–737

Chapter 35
Sleeve Gastrectomy for Obesity

Kazunori Kasama and Yosuke Seki

Abstract Obesity is a rising problem not only in Western countries but also in Asia. Bariatric surgery is not a cosmetic surgery, but some patients, especially young females, tend to want to avoid telling friends they have undergone bariatric surgery. Thus, cosmetic concerns are an important aspect of bariatric surgery for such patients. The fact that TANKO/reduced port (RP) bariatric surgery is the most common of advanced laparoscopic procedures is still not known in Japan. Bariatric surgery demands advanced skills because the surgical field is narrow, intra-abdominal fat is significant, and manipulation of the instruments is limited by the thickness of the subcutaneous fat. Some bariatric surgeons may oppose TANKO bariatric surgery. To ensure both safety and good cosmesis, we prefer RP surgery rather than strict observance of TANKO.

Keywords Bariatric surgery • Liver retraction • Reduced port laparoscopic surgery

35.1 Introduction to the Technique

Obesity is a rising problem not only in Western countries but also in Asia. The number of bariatric surgeries in Asia is increasing in line with patient demand. Candidates for bariatric surgery are younger than candidates for cancer surgeries, and female patients are predominant. Bariatric surgery is not cosmetic surgery, but some patients, especially young females, tend to want to avoid telling friends that they have undergone bariatric surgery. Thus, cosmesis is an important aspect of bariatric surgery for such patients.

K. Kasama (✉) • Y. Seki
Weight Loss and Metabolic Surgery Center, Yotsuya Medical Cube, Tokyo, Japan
e-mail: Kasama@mcube.jp

T. Mori and G. Dapri (eds.), *Reduced Port Laparoscopic Surgery*,
DOI 10.1007/978-4-431-54601-6_35, © Springer Japan 2014

TANKO procedures were developed from laparoscopic cholecystectomy, just as laparoscopic surgery itself arose from cholecystectomy, and TANKO procedures account for the majority of cholecystectomies. Over 350,000 bariatric procedures are performed annually worldwide, but the fact that TANKO/reduced port (RP) bariatric surgery is the most common of advanced laparoscopic procedures is still not known in Japan.

Bariatric surgery demands advanced skills because the surgical field is narrow, intra-abdominal fat is significant, and manipulation of instruments is limited due to the thickness of the subcutaneous fat. Some bariatric surgeons may oppose TANKO bariatric surgery because conventional laparoscopic bariatric surgery itself is difficult; making the procedure even more complex seems unwise to some. There are also claims that the trend is "business driven."

35.1.1 TANKO Bariatric Surgery Worldwide

The major bariatric procedures performed worldwide are described below.

The TANKO procedures (Fig. 35.1) performed, starting with the simplest, include laparoscopic adjustable gastric banding (LAGB) [1, 2], which is thought to be the least technically demanding of the TANKO procedures, followed by laparoscopic sleeve gastrectomy (LSG) [3, 4]. Some surgeons now perform laparoscopic Roux-en-Y gastric bypass (LRYGB) [5, 6] and laparoscopic biliopancreatic diversion (LBPD) [7], both of which include anastomosis creation.

1. TANKO laparoscopic adjustable gastric banding (LAGB)
   TANKO LAGB seems to be the least technically demanding of the TANKO bariatric surgeries. LAGB requires an adjustable port beneath the skin, so a 3-cm skin incision is mandatory. Some surgeons use that skin incision for a TANKO approach [1]. Some use an intraumbilical approach [2] with the interest of cosmesis. There is, however, the possibility of infection in the umbilical area because the adjustable port is a foreign body. Care must be taken to avoid infection. If infection occurs, the adjustable port should be removed immediately.

2. TANKO laparoscopic sleeve gastrectomy (LSG)
   The number of LSGs performed in Japan and worldwide has been increasing recently and is now second to the number of LRYGBs performed worldwide. The most common TANKO bariatric surgery performed worldwide may be LSG. There are two possible approaches for TANKO LSG. One is from above the umbilicus, and the other is from the umbilicus itself. Of course, from the standpoint of cosmesis, the umbilical approach is better. Usually, morbidly obese patients are very large, and the distance from the umbilicus to the xiphoid is too great to reach the upper part of the stomach during the procedure, so some surgeons perform TANKO LSG from above the umbilicus. The only real advantage of TANKO is better cosmesis, so we think the umbilical approach is the only meaningful one. Patient selection is important when considering TANKO bariatric surgery.

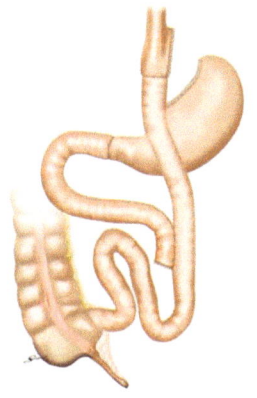

Laparoscopic Roux en Y Gastric Bypass
(LRYGB)

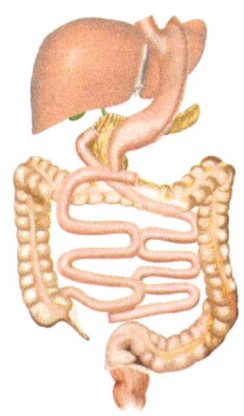

Laparoscopic Biliopancreatic Diversion
(LPBD)

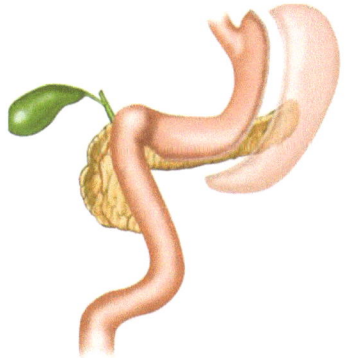

Laparoscopic Sleeve Gastrectomy
(LSG)

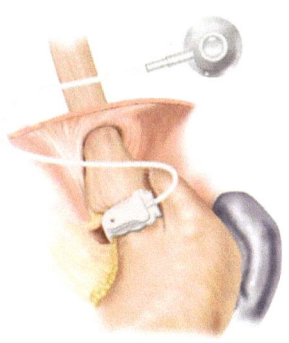

Laparoscopic Adjustable Gastric Banding
(LAGB)

Fig. 35.1 Bariatric Procedures

We use the RP approach instead of TANKO in consideration of patient safety, as discussed below.

3. TANKO laparoscopic Roux-en-Y gastric bypass (LRYGB)
    LRYGB is a complex procedure that requires two anastomoses. As far as we know, only a few surgeons perform this procedure [5–7]. Some surgeons use the RP approach.

    Huang reported the first case of TANKO LRYGB, which was performed via the skin near the umbilicus incision, as shown in Fig. 35.2 [5]

4. TANKO laparoscopic biliopancreatic diversion (LBPD)
    LBPD is the most effective procedure for morbid obesity, but it performed less frequently than LRYGB. Only a few surgeons perform TANKO LBPD [8].

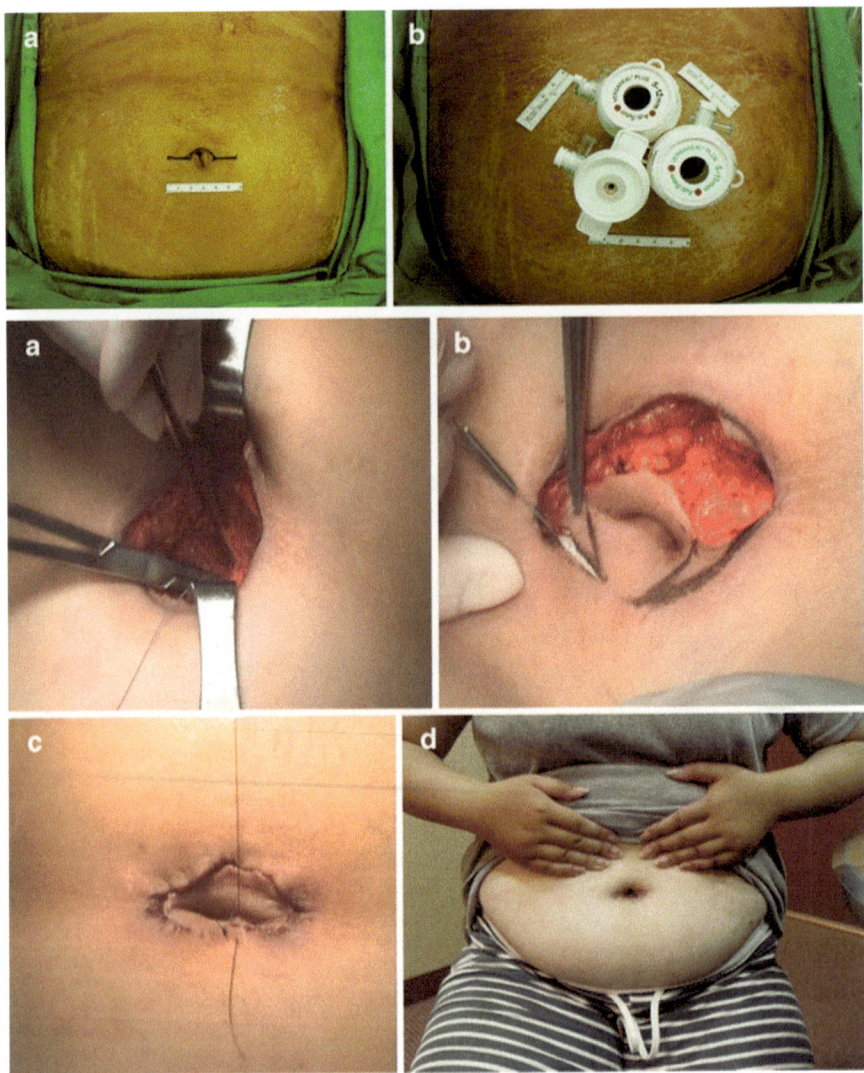

Fig. 35.2 *Upper*: (**a**) Omega shape incision and (**b**) trocar placements. *Lower*: (**a**) Fascia closure, (**b**) Trimming of skin, (**c**) Skin closure, (**d**) Scar (see Huang et al. [9])

35.1.2 *Objections to TANKO Bariatric Surgery*

Bariatric surgery is not easy because the patients treated are morbidly obese. Such patients have significant intra-abdominal fat and a liver enlarged by fatty liver disease; the working space is narrow. These characteristics make exposure of the surgical field difficult and increase the possibility of bleeding and other risks in comparison to the risks conferred by other surgeries.

Traction and counter-traction, triangulation, and surgical exposure are mandatory for safe surgery. The TANKO approach, in comparison to the conventional laparoscopic approach, is disadvantageous in terms of safety because it lacks these features. This is why a number of well-established bariatric surgeons are hesitant to introduce the TANKO approach.

35.1.3 Our Method

Our principal goals for TANKO/RP surgery are as follows:

1. to give proper consideration to cosmesis
2. to achieve the same results that conventional laparoscopic surgery achieved in terms of quality of life and long-term outcomes
3. to provide a safety level equivalent to that of conventional laparoscopic surgery.

We need not to be bound to a certain number of holes. We must maintain safety but strive for the cosmesis realized by "invisible" scars. Some surgeons take cosmesis too lighty, but cosmetic results have a long-term life effect, especially for younger patients, so we pay careful attention to this matter.

The TANKO/RP approach should yield the same outcome as conventional laparoscopic surgery. We need to perform the same procedure in the abdominal cavity, and we cannot shortcut any safety measures, even in TANKO/PR.

We prefer to perform RP surgery by the umbilical approach using a TANKO platform, adding a 5-mm port on the left side and 2-mm K-wire for liver retraction.

35.2 Indications and Contraindications

We perform LSG as an RP procedure only.

Indications for RP LSG at our institute are as follows:

1. female sex and a BMI less than 40 (for an acceptable amount of intra-abdominal fat)
2. patient height of less than 165 cm (for acceptable distance from umbilicus to the upper part of the stomach)
3. preoperative weight reduction achieved through a very low calorie diet. This is usually considered mandatory in the lead-up to bariatric surgery.

Contraindications for an RP LSG at our institute are as follows:

1. contraindications for bariatric surgery in general
2. patient height of more than 170 cm (reaching the upper part of stomach from the umbilicus is impossible, however, it depends on the length of the instruments.)

3. too much intra-abdominal fat (which usually means a BMI 40–45 kg/m^2 or more
    and male)

35.3   Description of the Technique and Tips and Tricks

35.3.1   Set-up

The patient is placed in the French position, and the surgeon stands between the
patient's legs. An assistant stands on the right side of the patient.

35.3.2   Approach

We first employed a multiport approach with one 12-mm port and two 5-mm ports,
but this method sometimes results in a loss of air-tightness in the abdominal cavity
and poses difficulty during surgery. We have recently started using the TANKO
platform or EZ Access (Hakko, Tokyo, Japan) or other single-incision access
system.

Before insertion of the TANKO platform, a Silicon Disk for liver protection is
inserted in the abdominal cavity through an umbilical incision. One 5-mm port is
placed 5 cm below the left costal margin. Laparoscopic coagulating scissors (LCS)
and a needle driver can be used thorough this port, and the procedure is carried out
in much the same way as conventional LSG (Fig. 35.3a).

35.3.3   Exposure of the Surgical Field: Liver Retraction

The Silicon Disk and 2-mm K-wire are used for retracting the liver; the K-wire is
held with a gasper holder (Fig. 35.4). This method allows for an invisible scar and
retraction of the liver without injury.

35.3.4   Manipulation

Two or three ports are inserted from the TANKO platform, and a 5-mm camera is
operated from the platform. A grasper, which is introduced through the umbilical
port, and LCS, which is introduced through the left subcostal port, are used to dissect the vessels on the greater curvature from a point 4 cm proximal to the pyloric

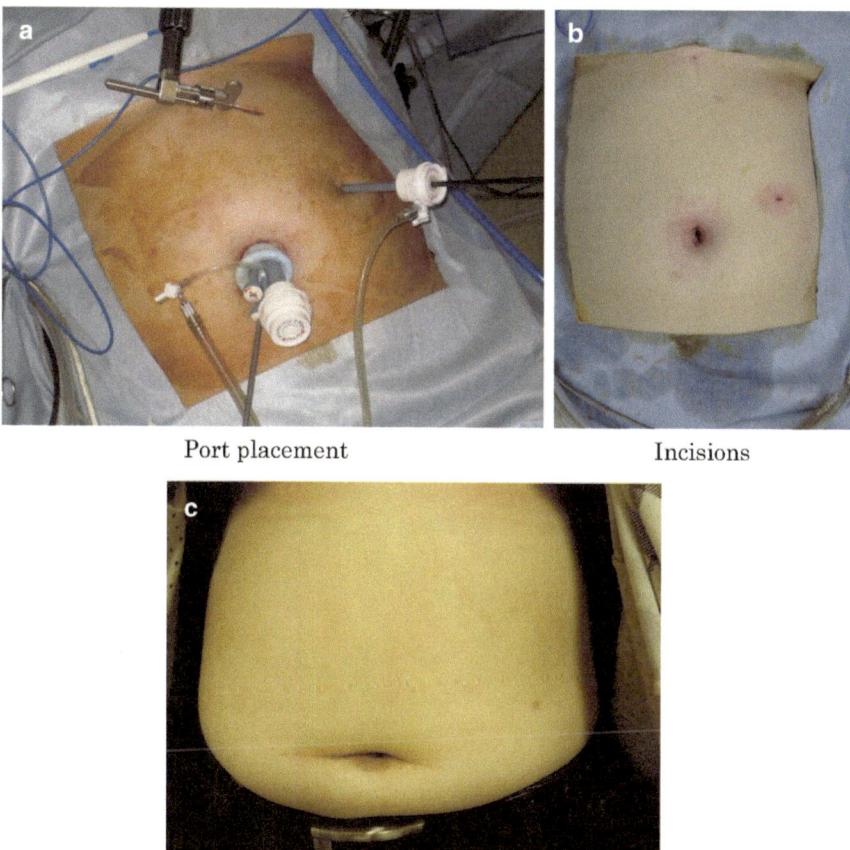

Port placement   Incisions

Scar at 1month post ope.

Fig. 35.3 Reduced Port Sleeve Gastrectomy: (**a**) Port placement, (**b**) incisions, and (**c**) scar at 1 month post ope

ring to the angle of His. A 12-mm port is then inserted from the TANKO platform, and a stapler is inserted via this port.

A 36-Fr. orogastric bougie is inserted by an anesthesiologist, and dissection of the stomach is performed with linear staplers along the bougie. Usually, the first stapler cartridge is green, the second gold, and the third blue, with the blue staples used at the end of the sleeve. A roticulated stapler is needed depending on the portion of the stomach being stapled. Reinforcement of all staple lines by hand-sewn imbrication is recommended to prevent bleeding or leakage. For this suturing, triangulation of the instruments is important to make the procedure easy and secure. A drain is not usually placed.

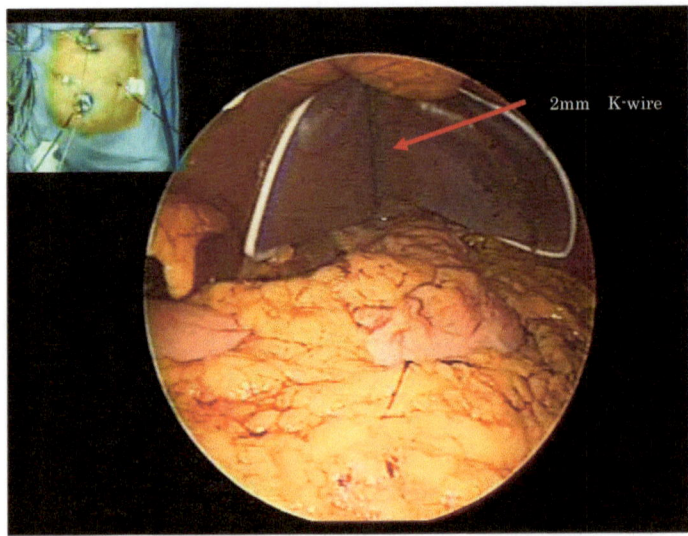

Fig. 35.4 Liver retraction with K-wire

35.3.5   Scars and Results

Scars as they appear immediately after the surgery and 1 month later are shown in Fig. 35.3b, c. The weight loss results are similar to those currently achieved with conventional LSG.

35.4   Recommendations from the Author

As bariatric surgery itself poses greater risk than other procedures dose because of patients' co-morbidities, we must think of safety first, rather than cosmetics. Only experts in laparoscopic bariatric surgery should perform TANKO and RP bariatric procedures.

35.5   Conclusion

TANKO bariatric surgery remains controversial.

To ensure both safety and good cosmetic results, we prefer performing RP bariatric surgery rather than strict TANKO bariatric surgery.

References

1. Teixeira J, McGill K, Binenbaum S, Forrester G (2009) Laparoscopic single-site surgery for placement of an adjustable gastric band: initial experience. Surg Endosc 23:1409–1414
2. Tacchino RM, Greco F, Matera D (2009) Laparoscopic gastric banding without visible scar: a short series with intraumbilical SILS. Obes Surg 19:500–503
3. Reavis KM, Hinojosa MW, Smith BR, Nguyen NT (2008) Single-laparoscopic incision trans-abdominal surgery sleeve gastrectomy. Obes Surg 18:487–496
4. Saber AA, Elgamal MH, Itawi EA, Rao AJ (2008) Single-incision laparoscopic sleeve gastrec-tomy (SILS): a novel technique. Obes Surg 18:1338–1342
5. Huang CK, Houng JY, Chiang CJ, Chen YS, Lee PH (2009) Single-incision transumbilical laparoscopic Roux-en-Y gastric bypass: a first case report. Obes Surg 19:1711–1715
6. Saber AA, El-Ghazaly TH, Minnick D (2009) Single port access transumbilical laparoscopic Roux-en-Y gastric bypass using the SILS Port: first reported case. Surg Innov 16:343–347
7. Tacchino RM, Greco F, Matera D, Diflumeri G (2010) Single-incision laparoscopic gastric bypass for morbid obesity. Obes Surg 20:1154–1160
8. Tacchino RM, Greco F, Matera D (2010) Single-incision laparoscopic biliopancreatic diver-sion. Surg Obes Relat Dis 6:444–445
9. Huang CK, Tsai JC, Lo CH, Houng JY, Chen YS, Chi SC, Lee PH (2011) Preliminary surgical results of single-incision transumbilical laparoscopic bariatric surgery. Obes Surg 21:391–396

Chapter 36
Gastric Plication for Obesity

Lawrence E. Tabone, Eugene P. Ceppa, and Dana Portenier

Abstract Laparoscopic adjustable gastric banding (LAGB) is an established primary bariatric procedure. However, LAGB is associated with lower expected weight loss when compared to other primary bariatric procedures, and this is cited as the primary limitation of LAGB as a weight loss procedure. Greater curvature plication has been used in both bariatric and non-bariatric procedures with limited morbidity and comparable short-term weight loss to sleeve gastrectomy and gastric bypass. We describe the combination of LAGB and greater curvature plication as a single and novel bariatric procedure. In addition, this procedure can be performed through single-incision laparoscopic surgery (SLS).

LAGB with greater curvature plication was performed with video recording. Still photographs were acquired from the high definition video in order to summarize and depict our step-by-step efficient approach.

LAGB with greater curvature gastric plication is a feasible and simple procedure that can be performed through a SLS approach. This chapter outlines the procedure and highlights key points of operative technique. In addition, we review the literature in regards to gastric plication. Randomized controlled trials comparing these procedures are needed and likely to occur in the near future.

Keywords Bariatric procedures • Gastric plication • Obesity • Weight loss surgery

L.E. Tabone
Department of Surgery, Duke University Medical Center, Durham, NC, USA

E.P. Ceppa
Department of Surgery, Indiana University, Indianapolis, IN, USA

D. Portenier (✉)
Department of Surgery, Duke University Medical Center, Durham, NC, USA

Duke Center for Metabolic and Weight Loss Surgery,
407 Crutchfield Road, Durham, NC 27704, USA
e-mail: dana.portenier@duke.edu

T. Mori and G. Dapri (eds.), *Reduced Port Laparoscopic Surgery*,
DOI 10.1007/978-4-431-54601-6_36, © Springer Japan 2014

36.1   Introduction

Current primary bariatric procedures are varied in both method and success in accomplishing the reduction of excess weight and the resolution of medical comorbid conditions. Each primary procedure has unique aspects that lead to both beneficial and detrimental effects. When the optimal surgical approach to a problem remains unknown, we often see a common surgical theme where multiple techniques/methods exist. Weight loss surgery has a long past with evolving techniques searching for the optimal method to induce sustained weight loss and comorbidity reduction with minimal risk profile [1]. Gastric plication is the latest procedure in this search to spark cautious wide spread interest within the weight loss community.

In its purest form gastric plication involves folding/invaginating the stomach on itself to reduce the overall gastric volume. The technique of gastric plication was described as early as 1911 [2] and animal studies in 2006 indicate plications utility in weight loss [3]. The first laparoscopic clinical use of gastric plication came from Iran [4], adopted to overcome the economic cost of modern day weight loss procedures, which entail costly placement of a device or surgical stapling.

Recently several authors have attempted laparoscopic greater curvature gastric plication as a primary method for weight loss with salient short-term data comparable to combined procedures [4, 5]. These authors have found excellent short-term weight loss outcomes with weight loss velocity comparable to laparoscopic sleeve gastrectomy (LSG) and laparoscopic Roux-en-Y gastric bypass (LRYGB). However, the greatest potential disadvantage is the lack of long-term data with unknown durability. Technically, this method is similar by way of reliance upon suture for sustained mucosal-mucosal apposition to pyloric exclusion for which the trauma literature demonstrates eventual re-cannulation of the duodenum [6]. Extrapolation of this finding would suggest that a potential exists for the plication to become undone causing a loss of gastric restriction. Similarly most techniques in plication involve greater curvature gastric plication, creating a "sleeve like" stomach configuration where the greater curve is invaginated rather than resected. The significant rate of postoperative nausea after plication suggests the immediate surgical process of plication creates significant mucosal edema creating a situation where initial sizing of the "sleeve like" gastric lumen may vary significantly after the initial edema subsides. Recent reports show LSG size increases significantly over time [7], if plication follows this same pattern it may result in questionable durability.

A recent case report describes laparoscopic adjustable gastric banding (LAGB) combined with gastric plication (Fig. 36.1) as a novel technique for maximizing the advantages of gastric plication (better rate and extent of weight loss) and LAGB (excellent safety profile and established durability) while minimizing the disadvantages of both procedures (unknown durability, poor rate and extent of weight loss) [8]. We believe that this procedure holds tremendous potential for the bariatric population, and we support the hypothesis that combining LAGB with plicated sleeve gastroplasty (PSG) should allow for greater overall weight loss with greater weight loss velocity. We hypothesize that the addition of a plication to the gastric band will increase gastric emptying of the stomach as seen in sleeve gastrectomy triggering

Fig. 36.1 LAGB with PSG.
The band is placed around
the upper part of the stomach
to form a small gastric pouch.
The fundus of the stomach is
plicated to reduce gastric
volume

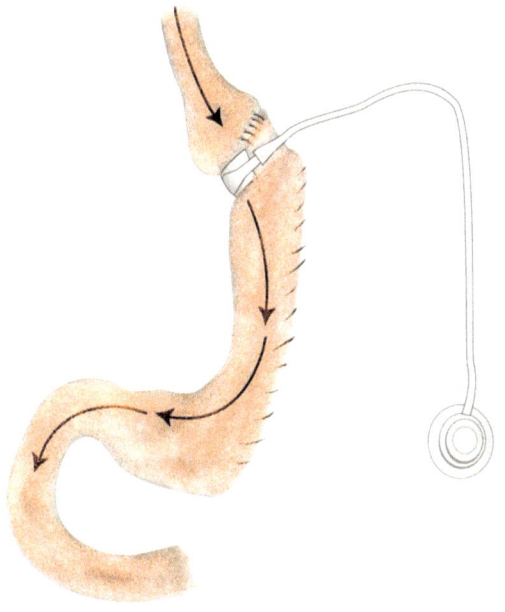

the hormonal [e.g., increased glucagon-like peptide-1 (GLP-1) and peptide YY (PYY)] effects of gastric bypass and sleeve gastrectomy [9]. Furthermore, LAGB complements PSG by providing proven durability, while the PSG complements LAGB by reducing potential complications such as band slippage [10].

Gastric plication can be done as a standalone procedure or in combination with LAGB. Although unproven, we believe that gastric plication in combination with LAGB is likely to provide longer weight loss durability. It can also be done below the band or all the way up the stomach with a band placed over the top of the plication. We have chosen to place a band by traditional methods and plicate below in order to capitalize upon the published durability of the band [11]. The gastric plication can be done as an anterior plication or as a greater curvature plication. Greater curvature plication has been shown to have a greater weight loss potential [5] and therefore is our preferred technique. We describe the steps used to perform a LAGB with PSG. The use of gastric plication for weight loss surgery is still considered investigational by the American Society for Metabolic and Bariatric Surgery (ASMBS) and their recommendation is that such procedures should be done with Institutional Review Board (IRB) approval [12].

36.2   Indications and Contraindications

Because LAGB with PSG is a novel technique, we recommend that the operation be done under the approval of an IRB. We believe that the procedure will be an effective operation for treating morbid obesity and its related comorbidities.

The intention of the operation is to augment the weight loss seen in LAGB. Indications for the procedure would include the indications for metabolic surgery in general, body mass index (BMI) greater than 35 kg/m^2 or a BMI of 30 kg/m^2 with comorbidities associated with obesity including hypertension, diabetes, obstructive sleep apnea.

The benefit of this operation over other metabolic surgeries is that no bowel anastomosis or gastrointestinal resection is performed. Patients at high risk for resection line or anastomotic leaks are likely to benefit from this operative approach over LRYGB or LSG. This patient population includes those who are immunosuppressed or have inflammatory bowel disease.

Another benefit of the operation is the ability to "reverse the operation" and essentially restore the anatomy to its original configuration. The LAGB can be removed and the PSG can be reversed by removing the plication sutures. This is a benefit over LSG or LRYGB that cannot be easily reversed. LAGB with PSG is also indicated in patients with previous abdominal operations that may have reduced bowel length or significant bowel adhesions that may make LRYGB difficult or contraindicated.

We would avoid offering this operation to patients who have had a history of gastric cancer or are at increased risk for gastric cancer. After the PSG there is a significant amount of stomach that cannot be inspected by endoscopy and this could potentially lead to a delayed diagnosis for gastric cancer. These patients are likely to be better served by LSG or LRYGB with resection of the gastric remnant.

36.3   Technique

36.3.1   Step 1: Operative Set-up

The patient is placed in the supine position with both arms tucked at the patient's side. The bed is placed in steep reverse Trendelenburg to allow for eventual exposure of the esophageal hiatus. The assistant stands on the patient's left side while the operative surgeon is positioned on the patient's right side.

36.3.2   Step 2: Access to the Abdomen

The procedure can be done either using a multiport laparoscopic approach or through a SILS™ port (Covidien, New Haven, CT, USA). For the multiport laparoscopic approach we place a 5-mm port just superior and to the left of the umbilicus to be used as a camera port utilizing a 5-mm 30° laparoscope. The assistant is on the left side of the patient and the assistant port is placed along the left anterior axillary line in the subcostal region, 5-mm port. The working ports are a 15-mm port in the midclavicular line half-way between the subcostal margin and the umbilicus. This port is eventually used to introduce the adjustable gastric band. And a 5-mm

Fig. 36.2 Multiport
placement for LAGB. A
Nathanson retractor can be
used in cases where the left
lobe of the liver obscures the
proximal stomach

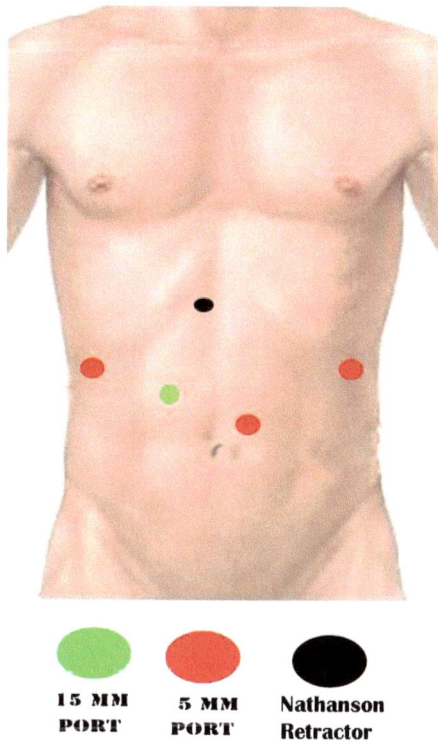

| 15 MM | 5 MM | Nathanson |
| PORT | PORT | Retractor |

port in the right anterior axillary line in the subcostal space serves as the second
working port (Fig. 36.2). A Nathanson liver retractor is placed in the subxiphoid
space to retract the left lobe of the liver.

To perform the procedure through a single incision we use a SILS™ port
(Covidien) at the umbilicus. Through the SILS™ port (Covidien) we place three
trocars. One trocar is used for a 5-mm articulating laparoscope while the other two
trocars are used for the operative instruments. These trocars vary between 5-mm to
15-mm depending on the step being performed in the procedure. It is helpful to
select a SILS™ port (Covidien) that allows for the upsizing and downsizing of trocars while maintaining pneumoperitoneum.

36.3.3   Step 3: Placement of the Adjustable Gastric
Band (AGB)

AGBs are placed via the accepted pars flaccida technique described by O'brien and
colleagues [13] with a few exceptions pointed out below. As usual the retro-gastric
tunnel is created from the infero-medial base of the right crus of the diaphragm and
extended to the angle of His as marked by the consistently found left inferior phrenic

Fig. 36.3 The band is
plicated in place by
approximating the cardia of
the stomach to the fundus
over the band with non-
absorbable sutures

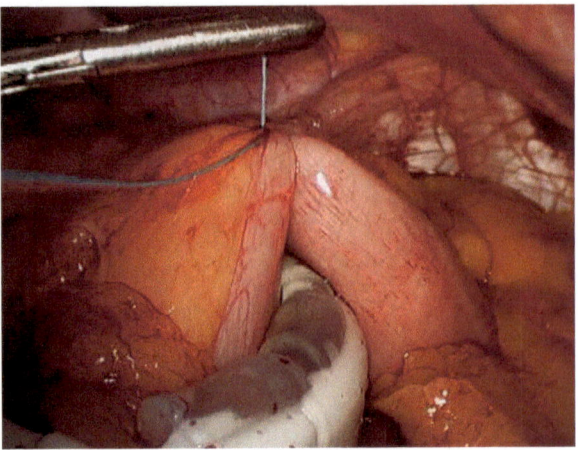

vein. We advocate the use of an articulating grasper to avoid potential injuries to the posterior gastric wall. The band tubing and buckle are coupled, but left unlocked (which is a deviation from the traditionally described technique) in order to facilitate passage of an endoscope. Typical gastro-gastric plication is then performed between the fundus and cardia of the stomach. The most cephalad aspect of the fundus is plicated with 2–3 interrupted, non-absorbable sutures in order to create a loose gastric tunnel (Fig. 36.3).

36.3.4   Step 4: Gastroscopy

A standard gastroscope (29Fr equivalent) is advanced through the pyloric channel and positioned along the lesser gastric curvature. The gastroscope serves as both a calibration tube as well as a means to evaluate the gastric lumen upon completion of the greater curvature plication (Fig. 36.4). The use of a calibration tube (bougie) is not universally performed by varying surgeons (Table 36.1) for gastric plication. We find that an endoscope helps to prevent over narrowing of the gastric lumen that can lead to obstruction.

36.3.5   Step 5: Identification of the Pylorus

The pylorus is typically identified laparoscopically, but the endoscope may be employed if necessary. A point 8 cm proximal to the pylorus, along the greater curvature, is marked as the distal extent of the plication (Fig. 36.5).

Fig. 36.4 Endoscopic
evaluation of the gastric
lumen after plication to
confirm a uniform tubular
narrowing of the lumen

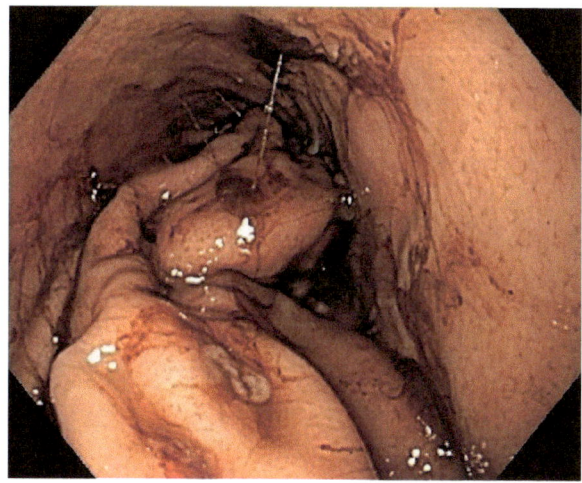

Table 36.1 Variation in published techniques for plicated sleeve gastroplasty

Study (first author)	Year	Plication	Approach	Method	Patients	Bougie	Distance from pylorus (cm)
Talebpour [4]	2007	Greater curvature	Laparoscopic	Suture	100	None	3
Huang [8]	2011	Greater curvature	Laparoscopic	Suture	1	38 Fr	3
Ramos [14]	2010	Greater curvature	Laparoscopic	Suture	42	32 Fr	0
Brethauer [5]	2011	Anterior Greater curvature	Laparoscopic	Suture	9 6	None	4

Bougie size measured in French (Fr) units

36.3.6   Step 6: Mobilization of the Greater Curvature

A bipolar or ultrasonic dissector is used to mobilize the greater curvature of the stomach. Care is taken to avoid thermal injury to the gastric wall since this will not be resected. The dissection is started 8 cm from the pylorus and continued proximally to the inferior aspect of the band (Fig. 36.6). Adhesions encountered in the lesser sac are divided to fully mobilize the posterior stomach. No dissection is performed posterior or superior to the level of the band in order preserve its natural path through the pars flaccida plane, which is outside the lesser sac avoiding posterior slippages of the band.

Fig. 36.5 The plication is carried distally to approximately 8 cm from the pylorus. Standard graspers are used to measure the distance from the pylorus

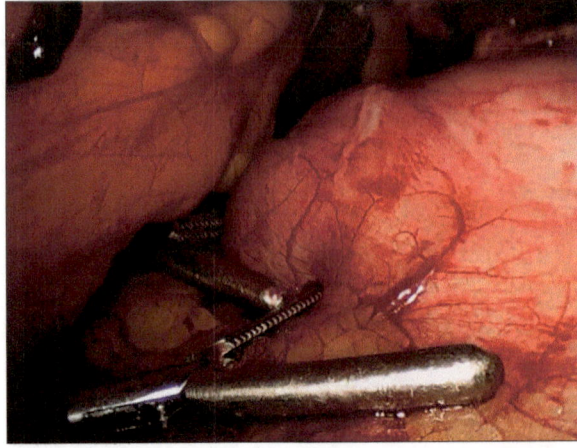

Fig. 36.6 The greater curvature of the stomach is mobilized by dividing the short gastrics with an ultrasonic dissector

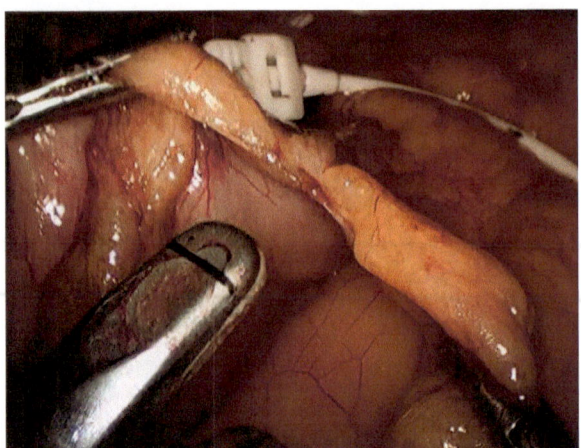

36.3.7   Step 7: Alignment of the Greater Curvature Plication

The greater curvature plication (GCP) is initially formed by the placement of 3–4 alignment sutures. The first suture is placed 2 cm inferior to the band to help avoid obstruction of the band from the invaginated stomach. A full-thickness non-absorbable suture is placed 2 cm lateral to the posterior branches of the left gastric arcade (Fig. 36.7), and secured to a corresponding location along the anterior aspect of the stomach. Initial creation of the gastric tube is achieved by imbricating the greater curvature while securing the knot. The goal is to obtain serosal apposition of the anterior and posterior gastric walls while avoiding ischemia. This is repeated several times along the length of the stomach but no further than 8 cm proximal to the pylorus (Fig. 36.8). Frequent checks are made to ensure the gastroscope remains along the lesser curve throughout the plication.

Fig. 36.7 The greater curvature plication is started approximately 2 cm inferior to the band

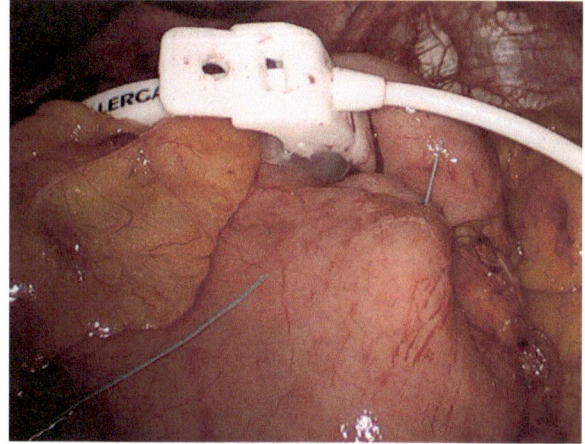

Fig. 36.8 The plication is carried down the greater curvature of the stomach and stopped approximately 8 cm from the pylorus. The plication is done with nonabsorbable sutures

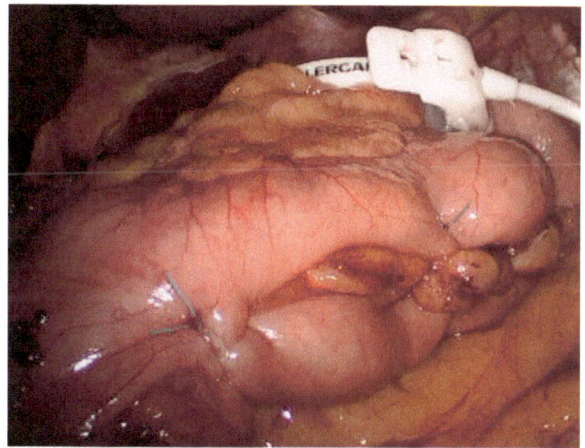

36.3.8 Step 8: Completion of the GCP

A running, non-absorbable, full-thickness suture is performed along the outer aspect of the plication (Fig. 36.9) and continued to the antrum, 8 cm from the pylorus (Fig. 36.10). The initial bite of the running suture incorporates any redundant fundus of the stomach in order to prevent postoperative dilation of this fundic region over time. The running suture incorporates the mobilized aspect of the greater curvature in order to collapse the intra-luminal fold. We avoid the tendency to further imbricate the stomach and create a smaller gastric lumen. This is most critical at the incisura angularis.

Fig. 36.9 A second running plication stitch is performed going back along the greater curvature to secure the plication and increase the amount of gastric luminal restriction

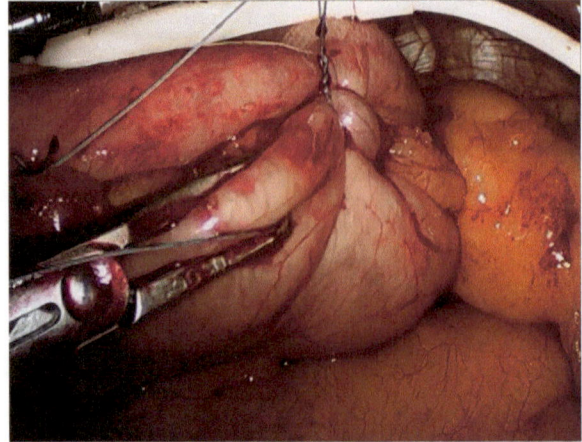

Fig. 36.10 The second running plication stitch is carried down to approximately 8 cm proximal to the pylorus

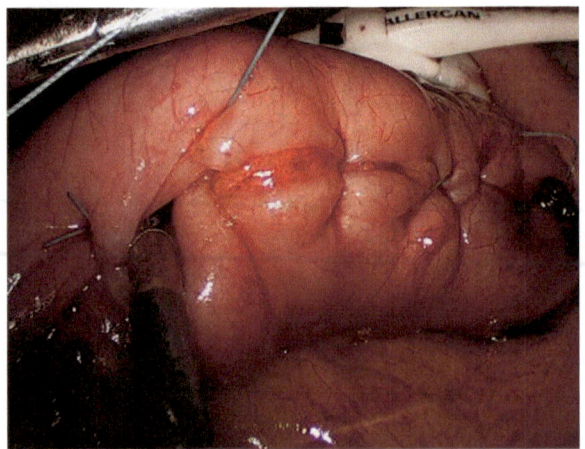

36.3.9   Step 9: Final Gastroscopic Evaluation

Upon completion of the GCP, a final intraluminal and laparoscopic evaluation (Fig. 36.11) of the distended gastric tube is performed. Endoscopically, it is imperative to ensure a patent lumen. The crescent-shaped mucosal fold is clearly demonstrated opposite the lesser curve (Fig. 36.4). Upon laparoscopic evaluation, one often notes dilatation of the proximal fundus adjacent and inferior to the AGB. If present the redundant fundus is further pexied with a u-stitch to the proximal gastric plication.

Fig. 36.11 The completed plication results in a symmetrical gastric tube

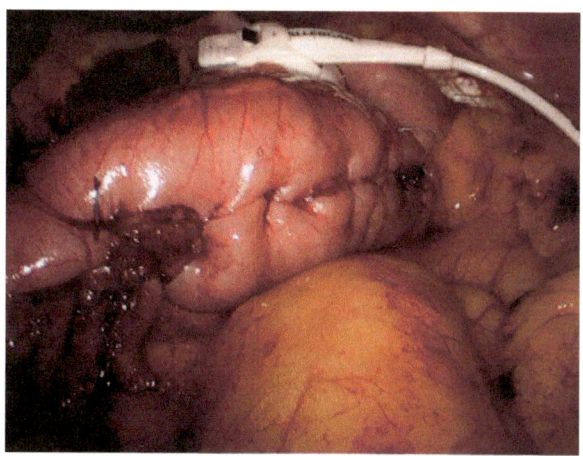

36.3.10   Step 10: AGB Port Placement

The endoscope is withdrawn and the AGB is locked into position. The silastic tubing is exteriorized via the right mid-abdominal 15-mm port and secured to the injection port. The port is secured to the anterior rectus fascia.

36.3.11   Step11: Confirmation of Port Placement

The placement of the band is confirmed on barium swallow X-ray (Fig. 36.12).

36.4   Tips and Tricks

LAGB with PSG can be performed with SLS. It is unknown if SLS results in decreased postoperative pain, faster recovery time, or decreased wound infection when performed for gastric plication. There is an apparent cosmetic benefit when gastric plication is done with a SLS approach. A unique benefit for bariatric SLS is confidentiality, where a SLS approach can completely hide the scars from the operation. And no signs of surgery are apparent even when the patient's abdomen is exposed.

Not every patient will benefit or be a candidate for a SLS approach. We have found that proper patient selection for SLS is often the key to success. The cosmetic benefit of SLS is most realized when the port is placed in the umbilicus. In the obese population, not every patient has the body habitus to allow for umbilical port access.

Fig. 36.12 A barium upper gastrointestinal study performed post-operatively shows the band in place with free flowing contrast through a narrowed gastric lumen

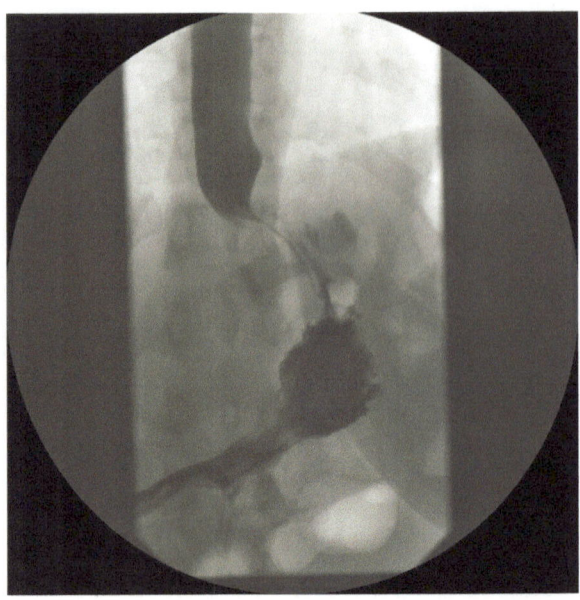

Fig. 36.13 Multiport laparoscopy allows for triangulation onto a single point of interest

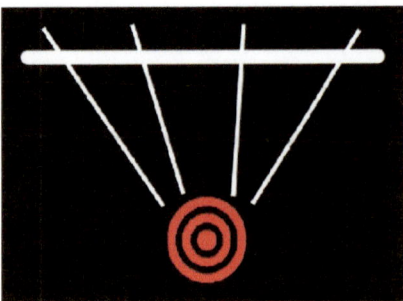

As the patient is placed in steep reverse Trendelenburg for the procedure the umbilicus can be displaced caudally and the distance from the umbilicus to the esophageal hiatus may exceed the length of most laparoscopic instruments. To identify this potential pitfall before operation, preoperatively we have the patient stand and measure the distance from the xiphoid to the umbilicus. If this distance from the xiphoid to umbilicus in the standing position is greater than 25 cm than it is highly unlikely that the procedure can be performed through a single incision at the umbilicus.

SLS requires overcoming the challenges of instrument crowding and collision. Standard multiport laparoscopy allows for triangulation of the instruments onto the site of interest (Fig. 36.13). SLS can create crowding of instruments, paradoxical motion for the operative surgeon, and instrument collision (Fig. 36.14). Special instrumentation is needed to overcome these challenges. To perform LAGB with PSG through a SILS™ port (Covidien), three trocars will need to be placed through

Fig. 36.14 SLS with standard straight shaft instruments requires crossing of the instruments to converge on a single point of interest

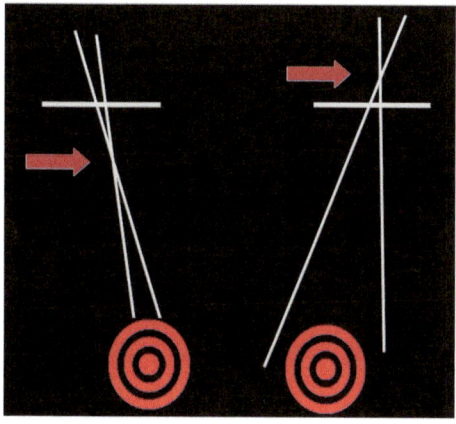

Fig. 36.15 Commercially available SILS™ port devices (Covidien)

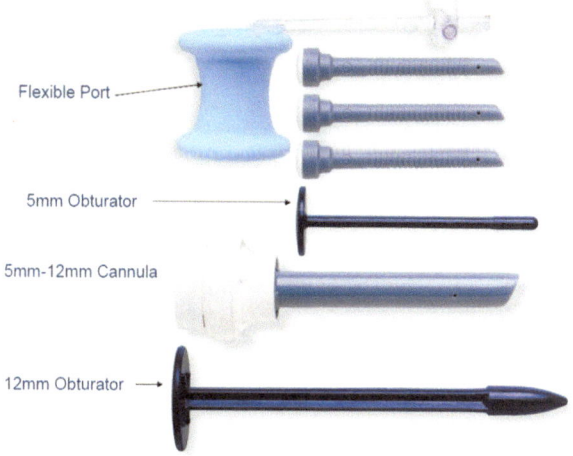

Flexible Port

5mm Obturator

5mm-12mm Cannula

12mm Obturator

the port. To avoid collision with the camera and to obtain the best image it is essential to have a 5-mm flexible tip laparoscope. Both Stryker® (Kalamazoo, MI, USA) and Olympus® produce a product that is suitable for this application.

Multiple SLS port devices are available on the market. We prefer to use the SILS™ port (Covidien) (Fig. 36.15). The port allows for multiple interchangeable trocars to be placed through the port. The trocars can range from 5-mm to 15-mm cannulas. The individual trocars can be upsized from 5-mm to 12-mm or 15-mm cannulas during the operation at different steps then downsized back to 5-mm trocars without causing significant air leaks or loss of pneumoperitoneum. The ability to add, upsize, and downsize trocars through a single-port throughout the operation is greatly beneficial. One difficulty that we have found in using the SILS™ port (Covidien) is that the low profile of the port in an obese patient can cause the port to

Fig. 36.16 The challenge with commercially available SLS port devices includes port retraction below the surface of the skin

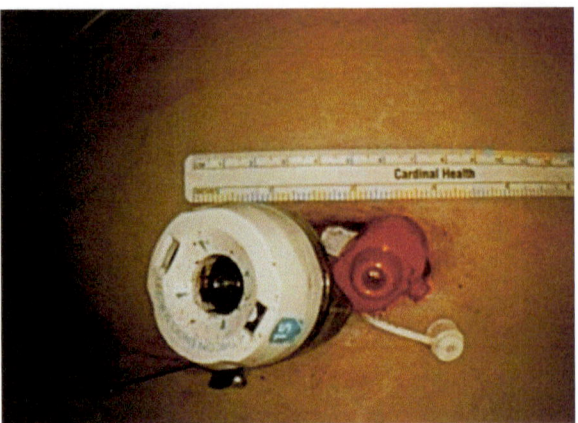

Fig. 36.17 The use of a wound protector to avoid SLS port retraction below the surface of the skin

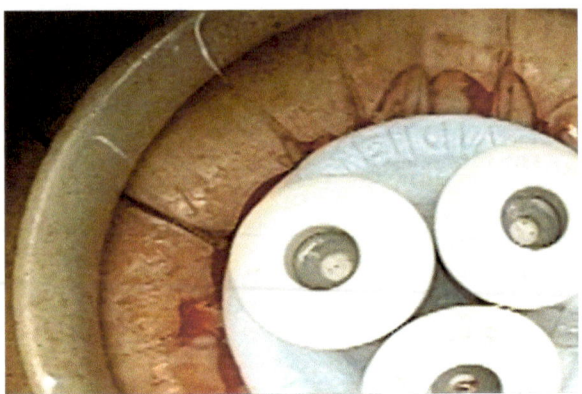

sink below the level of the skin (Fig. 36.16). To overcome this challenge we have found that using a medium sized wound protector compresses the abdominal wall (skin, adipose tissue, and fascia) and prevents the port from sinking below the level of the skin (Fig. 36.17).

Upon placing the SILS™ port (Covidien), it is helpful to place figure-of-eight fascial sutures at the beginning of the operation to be tied at the end of the operation for fascial closure. These sutures are best placed at the beginning of the operation before abdominal wall torque from the SILS™ port (Covidien) distorts the anatomy making fascial closure more difficult. Also these untied figure of eight sutures can be wrapped around the SILS™ port (Covidien) to resolve any air leaks during the operation.

Using at least one articulating instrument helps overcome the challenge of inline instrument placement in SLS. There are several articulating instruments on the market. We have found that most if not all articulating instruments have a degree of torque in the shaft when the instrument is articulated. This can make fine dissection difficult. We recommend using one articulating instrument for retraction along with a standard straight laparoscopic instrument for dissection.

One of the most challenging steps in SLS gastric plication is suturing. We have found that using a barbed suture (V-Loc™ (Covidien) or Angiotech Pharmaceuticals The Quill™ (Vancouver BC, Canada)) can greatly help overcome these challenges. These barbed sutures avoid the need for knot tying which can be difficult in a SLS. The barbed sutures also have the added benefit of maintaining tension on the approximated tissue avoiding the need for an instrument dedicated to applying tension on the suture. Another instrument that we employ for SLS suturing is the SILS™ stitch (Covidien) articulating suturing device. This device functions as an articulating EndoStitch™. The SILS™ stitch (Covidien) articulating suturing device can also function as an articulating band passer, which helps to position the AGB.

A large floppy left lobe of the liver can obscure the view of the esophageal hiatus and make dissection difficult. With multiport laparoscopy we will use a Nathanson liver retractor to alleviate this problem; SLS requires other approaches to overcome this challenge. To overcome this challenge we have used intra-abdominal tissue retracting systems including EndoGrab™ (Virtual Ports Ltd., Caesaera, Israel) and EndoLift™ (Virtual Ports Ltd., Caesaera, Israel). If intra-abdominal tissue-retracting systems are not available, using a pledged stitch can serve the same function.

A unique challenge encountered in some patients is a fat pad located at the pars flaccida that obscures the view needed for dissection. We have used the EndoStitch™ (Covidien) to create a pulley system to retract this fat pad. This is done by passing the suture through the fat pad and tying a slip knot then passing the suture through the abdominal peritoneum at the angle needed for retraction then leaving the suture long and pulling it out of the SILS™ port (Covidien). The assistant can then apply tension to the suture to retract the fat pad. This is not needed on most cases, but when the fat pad is obscuring the view this technique can be helpful.

If the operation is not progressing in the SLS approach then we recommend inserting additional ports. When inserting additional ports we proceed with port placement similar to our multiport laparoscopic approach (Fig. 36.2). The camera and one dissecting instrument can remain at the SILS™ port (Covidien). A second and third 5-mm trocar can be inserted in the right and left anterior axillary line in the subcostal region. If the left lobe of the liver is not being retracted correctly then a Nathanson retractor can be inserted in the subxiphoid region.

36.5 Recommendations from the Author

The field of metabolic and weight loss surgery has evolved over the last several decades. Treatments ranging from the ileojejunal bypass to the vertical banded gastroplasty to endoluminal therapies have come and gone. Currently there are well proven operations like the LRYGB that have been shown to improve the quality of life and significantly reduce comorbidities. It is important to have the appropriate review process in place when introducing new procedures like the PSG. We believe that this operation will likely have a permanent place in metabolic and weight loss surgery. And recommend that it be investigated further under the review of IRB committees.

LAGB with PSG can be done either through a multiport or SLS approach. We recommend first performing PSG with a multiport approach. After an initial multiport experience has been gained, we would recommend introducing the SLS approach in a less technically challenging patient population, which are usually patients with a BMI of 30–35 kg/m² who have had no previous foregut operations. With the proper experience and patience a SLS approach can be performed for most patients. When struggling to complete a SLS procedure it is helpful to place an additional 5-mm trocar in the left upper quadrant to allow help from an assistant. Gaining the technical skills needed for SLS is often a stepwise approach of moving from multiport laparoscopy to reduced port laparoscopy and eventually to SLS.

References

1. Baker MT (2011) The history and evolution of bariatric surgical procedures. Surg Clin North Am 91(6):1181–1201
2. Testut L, Jacob O (1911) Tratado de Anatomia Topografica con aplicaciones medicoquirurgicas. Salvat Editores, Barcelona, Print
3. Fusco PE, Poggetti RS, Younes RN et al (2006) Evaluation of gastric greater curvature invagination for weight loss in rats. Obes Surg 16:172–177
4. Talebpour M, Amoli BS (2007) Laparoscopic total gastric vertical plication in morbid obesity. J Laparoendosc Adv Surg Tech A 17(6):793–798
5. Brethauer SA, Harris JL, Kroh M et al (2011) Laparoscopic gastric plication for treatment of severe obesity. Surg Obes Relat Dis 7(1):15–22
6. Carrillo EH, Richardson JD, Miller FB (1996) Evolution in the management of duodenal injuries. J Trauma 40(6):1037–1045
7. Baumann T, Grueneberger J, Pache G et al (2011) Three-dimensional stomach analysis with computed tomography after laparoscopic sleeve gastrectomy: sleeve dilation and thoracic migration. Surg Endosc 25:2323–2329
8. Huang CK, Asim S, Lo CH (2011) Augmenting weight loss after laparoscopic adjustable gastric banding by laparoscopic gastric plication. Surg Obes Relat Dis 7(2):235–236
9. Ramon JM, Salvans S, Crous X et al (2012) Effects of Roux-en-Y gastric bypass vs sleeve gastrectomy on glucose and gut hormones: a prospective randomized trial. J Gastrointest Surg 16:1116–1122
10. Hussain A, Mahmood H, El-Hasani S (2010) Gastric plication can reduce slippage rate after laparoscopic gastric banding. J Soc Laparoendo Surg 14(2):221–227
11. O'Brien PE, MacDonald L, Anderson M et al (2013) Long-term outcomes after bariatric surgery fifteen-year follow-up of adjustable gastric banding and a systematic review of the bariatric surgical literature. Ann Surg 257:87–94
12. Clinical Issues Committee (2011) ASMBS policy statement on gastric plication. Surg Obes Relat Dis 7(3):262–264
13. O'Brien PE, Dixon JP, Laurie C et al (2005) A prospective randomized trial of placement of the laparoscopic adjustable gastric band: comparison of the perigastric and pars flaccida pathways. Obes Surg 15(6):820–826
14. Ramos A, Galvao NM, Galvao M et al (2010) Laparoscopic greater curvature plication: initial results of an alternative restrictive bariatric procedure. Obes Surg 20(7):913–918

Chapter 37
Malabsorptive and Mixed Procedures for Obesity

Roberto M. Tacchino

Abstract Laparoscopic bariatric surgery has been introduced since 1992 and is today the gold standard approach for obesity surgery.

Single-incision laparoscopy (SIL) has been developed with the aim of further reducing the invasiveness of traditional laparoscopy.

The approach through a single intra-umbilical incision was implemented to perform advanced bariatric procedures such as gastric bypass and biliopancreatic diversion.

High technical skill is required for manipulating, measuring, and suturing the bowel with articulated instruments, however emerging technology has contributed to the feasibility of SIL.

Minimally invasive techniques have become an integral part of general surgery and proved to be a safe and feasible when compared with multiple ports approach.

Cosmesis scores and patient satisfaction showed a preference of patients for SIL. Further benefit is the positive feedback of this approach on the surgical technique. The need to minimize the manipulation of organs and tissues has led to better understanding of mechanism of action of the different procedures and to a simplification of the surgical steps. This represents a general benefit to laparoscopic surgery.

We discuss the general approach, the technical details ad the benefit of SIL in malabsorptive and mixed procedures.

Keywords Bariatric surgery • Biliopancreatic diversion • Minigastric bypass • SIL • Single-incision • Single loop gastric bypass

R.M. Tacchino (✉)
Department of Surgery, Catholic University SH, Rome, Italy

Badana Clinic, Mouwasat Hospital, Dammam, Saudi Arabia
e-mail: roberto.tacchino@yahoo.it

T. Mori and G. Dapri (eds.), *Reduced Port Laparoscopic Surgery*,
DOI 10.1007/978-4-431-54601-6_37, © Springer Japan 2014

37.1 Introduction

Single-incision laparoscopy (SIL) has been improved during the last 5 years.

Access Port

The advent of the trocar with multiple accesses, such as OCTOport™ (Covidien, New Haven, CT, USA), TriPort™ (Olympus, Tokyo, Japan) and Octoport™ (Dalim Surgnet, Seoul, South Korea) has significantly reduced the inconvenience of using multiple trocars through a single incision. In that developmental phase, loss of pneumoperitoneum when replacing the instruments, particularly those of large bore such as EndoStitch™ (Covidien) and the staplers, significantly reduced the quality of vision which, when too compromised, in fact made it impossible to continue with the intervention with the necessary safety.

Triangulation

The fundamental principle of SIL is the crossing of instruments in the navel where they enter the abdominal cavity. Thanks to the use of at least one articulated or curved instrument, paired with another instrument, either straight or articulated, it is possible to recreate a triangulation similar to that of traditional laparoscopy.

As a consequence the instrument held with the right hand is to be operated to the left on the screen and vice-versa [1].

Telescope

The use of a long shaft 30-degree and 5-mm camera is mandatory to reduce to a minimum not only the obstruction, but also to facilitate its movement during the course of the intervention and in order to reduce clashing of the instruments, particularly outside the abdomen.

The use of a camera with articulated head (EndoEYE™ (Olympus)) furthermore reduces the need for these movements and offers optimal visual angles, thus avoiding conflict with surgical instruments: it therefore should be regarded as a very useful instrument for this type of intervention [2].

Exposure

With regard to bariatric surgery, the need to expose the gastroesophageal junction, to perform anastomosis and suture has posed specific problems: some steps need to be modified so that, for example, the use of a liver retractor would not be necessary [2, 3].

Patients' Selection

When new surgical techniques are adopted, selecting suitable patients is recommended. Although defining certain parameters may be simple, like distance from the xyphoid, in practice it might not be enough.

Relative contraindications, also in relation to the surgeon's level of experience, such as a previous laparotomy or a previous laparoscopy, for which the navel was used as the access point, should be taken into account. In both cases, the difficulty of access or of positioning of the trocar in the peritoneal cavity should be verified. In fact, SIL lacks the possibility of a provisional access for the camera at a point far from the navel or in any case of suspected adhesions, so that lysis can be performed to facilitate access.

In SIL, the thickness of the abdominal wall is another feature to take into account as the port may not be sufficiently long to completely pass through it and therefore there might be a tendency to slide out, causing loss of the pneumoperitoneum and risk of damage when introducing the instrument.

A further consideration when selecting suitable patients is the position of the navel. The distance of the abdomen and hence the final position of the navel is difficult to determine in many cases and it may be reasonably far from the initial position in the case of a large flaccid abdomen. In addition to that, the final distance at which the surgeon operates, such as the distance of the gastroesophageal junction from the navel, also depends on the patient's height and physical build.

The possibility, even at present, of having dedicated and extra-long instruments available must be part of these preoperative evaluations, although intra-operative evaluation remains crucial.

Benefits

SIL is now known in many centers worldwide. Several publications report different acronyms and describe various technical variations reflecting the creativity and originality of the surgeons who first introduced this method but at present few randomized, controlled trials have been completed [4]. For this reason, it is not possible to state with certainty which are the real benefits of this "new" surgery [5], although a reduction of complications associated with the introduction of the trocar, such as bleeding and incisional hernias can be assumed and, of course, an advantage from the cosmetic point of view that makes the method extremely attractive to the patient. The absence of a final visible scar, accounts not only for an aesthetic result but also has some psychological benefits: we know that many patients perceive surgery as a failure to control their own habits and do not want their friends and relatives know that they had been operated on. Indeed, we perceived a high level of satisfaction in the obese patients, which underwent SIL bariatric [2, 4, 6].

Although for matters regarding cholecystectomy there are now several published works [7, 8] and a substantial amount of case studies, in the field of bariatric surgery, SIL technology is gaining ground more slowly since it is extremely complex.

Hence the need for a larger learning curve and specific training in bariatric surgery centers that are already carrying out these interventions; at present, however, being the privilege of a few.

Thus, as after the introduction of laparoscopy, an initial increase of specific surgical complications have been observed, it is easy to foresee a similar trend after the spread of SIL technology, although the difference between the two techniques is probably smaller than that of "open" surgery and laparoscopy.

What has so far facilitated the spread of this technique on a large scale is the possibility of "conversion" from SIL to traditional laparoscopy, which is easily achievable in the event of difficulties and limited to the introduction of one or two additional trocars, a simple maneuver, without the consequences of laparotomy, not only from the surgical point of view but also from the psychological point of view of the patient and surgeon, the so-called reduced port laparoscopic surgery (RPLS). This is a great advantage for its diffusion compared to other innovative techniques such as natural orifice transluminal endoscopic surgery (NOTES), combined with the fact that a SIL intervention can also be performed with the help of fewer specific instruments than classic laparoscopy.

37.1.1 Limited Absorption and Mixed Procedures

All different types of surgery have been successfully completed by SIL: adjustable gastric banding, Roux-en-Y gastric bypass (RYGB), minigastric bypass (MGB), biliopancreatic diversion (BPD), and sleeve gastrectomy (SG) [1, 2, 9, 10]. We are going to discuss more in detail the procedures that are based partially or totally on limited absorption.

We prefer the term limited absorption to "malabsorption" as the latter entails a concept of disease. Malapsorption exists in gastrointestinal disease where either the physiological or anatomical functioning has been altered by a specific derangement. In the case of bariatric surgery we believe it is more appropriate to speak of limited absorption as none of the organs or functions involved is diseased. In these procedures the bowel is perfectly normal, rather its length, or the segment that is allowed to absorb food, are modified.

We should also specify that we are talking about limiting the absorption of macronutrients: calories. Absorption of micronutrients, such as vitamins or mineral salts, could be limited with different mechanisms also in other non-malabsorptive procedures.

According to the above definitions the two procedures that entail limited absorption are the MGB and the BPD.

37.1.2 MGB

The MGB has also been named single loop gastric bypass, one anastomosis gastric bypass, and omega loop gastric bypass.

It consists in creating a narrow and long gastric pouch from the cardias to the angulus on the stomach's lesser curvature. The shape and size of this pouch is very similar to that of a SG. Normally it is calibrated along a 12-mm outer diameter orogastric tube. This pouch is then anastomosed in a Billroth II manner to the jejunum

Fig. 37.1 No visible scar

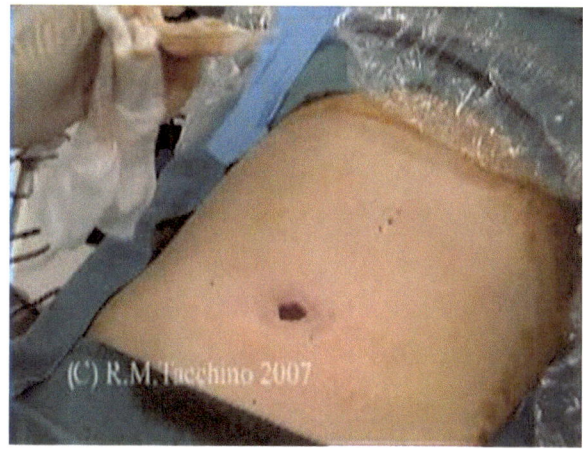

at a distance from the Treitz ligament of 200-cm. The afferent loop is sutured to the lateral aspect of the pouch to prevent food from entering the biliary limb.

The length of this biliary limb can be adjusted, either at the time of primary surgery either as revisional surgery, to change the level of absorption and thus the weight of stabilization of the patient.

On the other hand the size of the pouch can be enlarged to reduce the degree of restriction we want to give to the patient.

These two parameters give to the procedure a great flexibility, easy adjustability and make total reversal very simple.

Introducing the Port

In order to totally hide the scar after surgery (Fig. 37.1), the umbilicus is completely everted (Fig. 37.2) and an Ellis clamp is affix at its base so as to demarcate the cut that will be about 12-mm. At this level the fascia and the skin are very close to each other so it's easy to gain access to the peritoneal cavity with an open technique. The port is prepared, loading the plastic ring on the introduction device that is insert into the peritoneal cavity by making counter-traction with two forceps. The ring slides in the peritoneal cavity and the introducer is retracted; by pulling on the device, the inner ring is joined to the abdominal wall and the outer ring is joined to the skin: in this way you can adjust this kind of access to wall thickness (Fig. 37.3).

Surgical Procedure

The first step of MGB is the creation of the gastric pouch of about 10-cm in length, measured from the angle of His. A perigastric dissection is carried out with the use of Ligasure Blunt Tip® (Covidien) coupled to a Endo Grasp Roticulator® (Covidien) that keeps traction on the stomach. These instruments cross each other at the navel allowing the creation of triangulation to exert traction and counter traction so

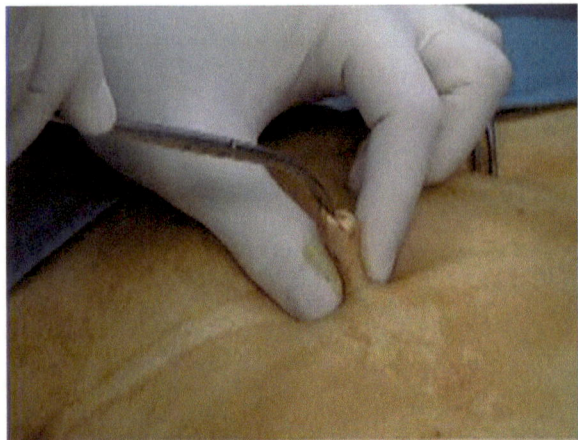

Fig. 37.2 Eversion of the umbilicus

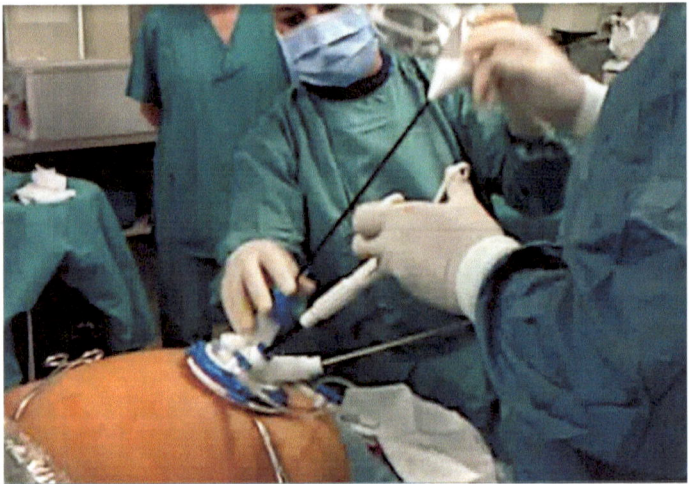

Fig. 37.3 Port in place

typical of traditional laparoscopy. In this case the main trunk of the left gastric artery and the branches of the vagus nerve (the Latarjet) are preserved. Once the opening is made a 45-mm blue or purple cartridge EndoGIA® (Covidien) is fired and the first transverse section of the stomach is done (Fig. 37.4). During these maneuvers the instruments are crossed at the level of the port, so the stomach is maintained in tension by an Endo Grasp Roticulator® (Covidien), which appears into the right side of the screen but is controlled by the left hand of the surgeon. A 13-mm (outer diameter) orogastric probe is brought forward filling the pouch and is used for calibration; the stapler is applied as close as possible to the probe to ensure the small volume of the pouch. The stomach is transacted vertically (Fig. 37.5).

Fig. 37.4 Horizontal
transverse section of stomach

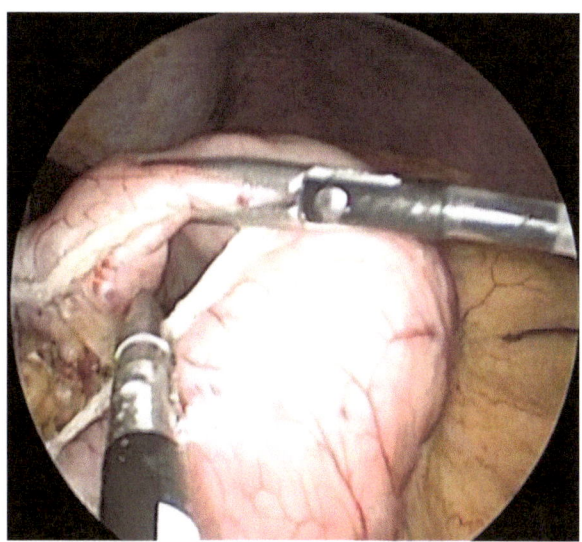

Fig. 37.5 Vertical stapling
along calibration orogastric
tube

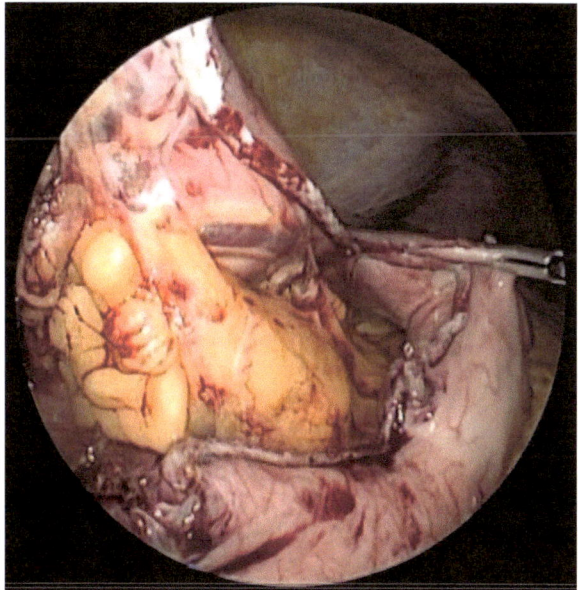

Retraction of the left lobe of the liver was achieved with a transfix stitch, applied on the right crus and suspended from outside (Fig. 37.6). It is therefore unnecessary to use any dedicated tool. Several (3–5) applications of 60-mm blue or purple cartridges EndoGIA® (Covidien) are necessary to join the angle of His. Before completely dividing the pouch from the stomach you should find some short vessels that may need to be coagulated before inserting the stapler (Fig. 37.7). Moreover, this

Fig. 37.6 Liver retraction

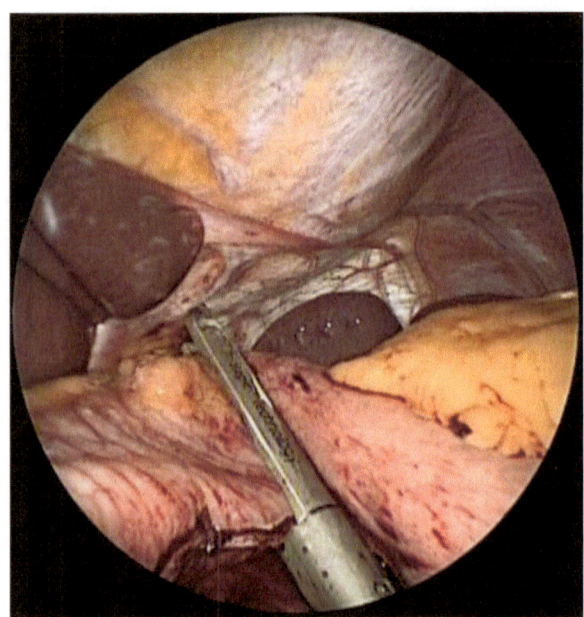

Fig. 37.7 Ensure complete division

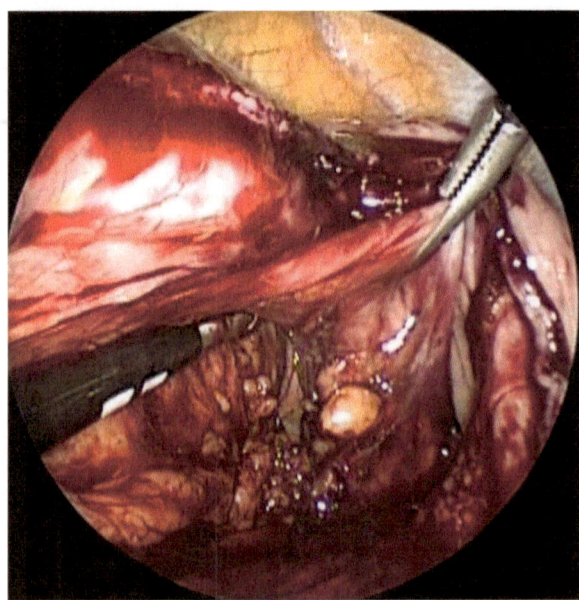

dissection allows for certainty of the separation of the pouch from the stomach. The pouch is made narrow and long, similar to the one done in sleeve gastrectomy. This method allows you to stay away from esophagus and helps when performing the gastroenteric anastomosis by decreasing the distance, and thus the tension, between

Fig. 37.8 Small bowel
measurement

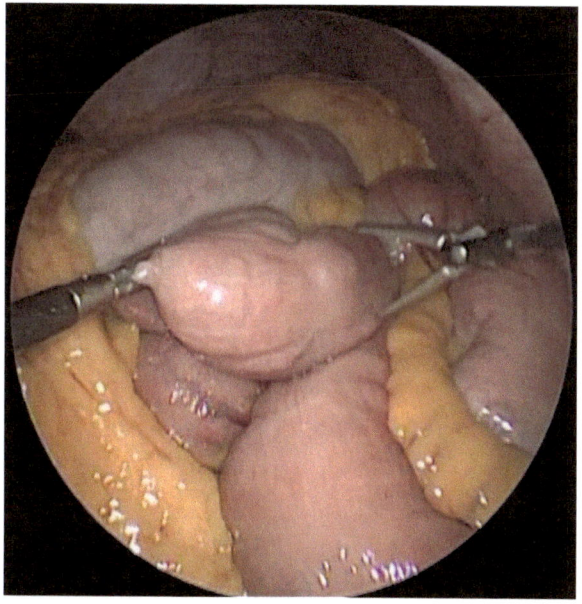

the pouch itself and the intestine. Once the pouch is completed, the gastrotomy is opened. The hole is made on a free portion of the pocket, away from the rhymes of suture to avoid ischemia, on either the front or rear wall. The orogastric tube is withdrawn by 10-cm to avoid being accidentally caught in the coming anastomosis. The hole is enlarged with a small bowel clamp to facilitate the future introduction of the stapler. In this case you use regular scissors and straight clamp coupled with an articulated grasper. In the almost horizontal position, you perform the measurement of the bowel (Fig. 37.8): the omentum is shifted upward and to the left of the screen, the mesocolon is put under tension by pulling on an epiploic appendix in proximity of the left colic flexure, where it is thin enough and relaxed enough to allow easy exposure the ligament of Treitz. The biliary limb is measured up to 200-cm from the Treitz's ligament. After the enterotomy is done (Fig. 37.9) an articulated 30-mm blue cartridge EndoGIA® (Covidien) (anvil) is introduced into the bowel, and then the stapler is closed and approaches the gastric pouch: the direction of the joint is changed and the head of the stapler is rotated by 180°. At this point the cartridge of the stapler presents itself ready in proximity to the gastrotomy. The patient is put back into an anti-Trendelemburg position and using both the stapler and an articulated grasper the pouch is retrieved. The pouch is pulled down and the gastroenteric anastomosis is performed (Fig. 37.10). Its wedge shape facilitates the insertion of the cartridge in the stomach. The service opening is closed with a hand-made suture carried out with the Endostitch® (Covidien) (Fig. 37.11): it consists of an initial extra mucous layer and a second serosal layer in polysorbate 2/0. The anastomosis is checked with the methylene-blue test while two clamps close both the afferent and efferent loops. The last step of the procedure is the creation of an anti-reflux mechanism (Fig. 37.12): the firsts 5- to 6-cm of the afferent loop are

Fig. 37.9 Enterotomy

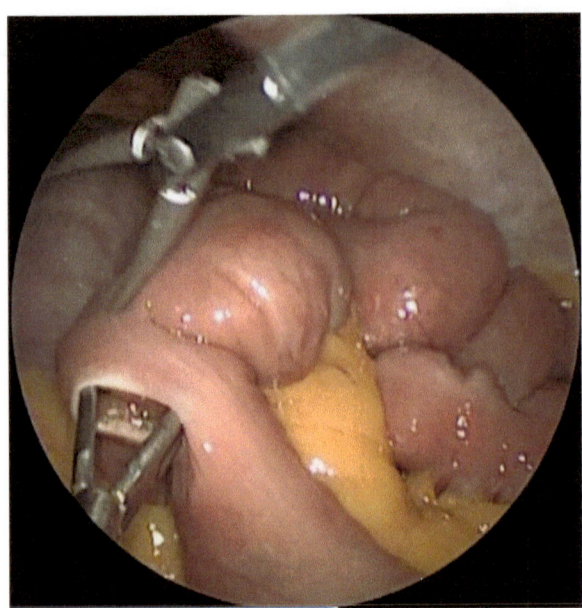

Fig. 37.10 Gastroenteric
anastomosis

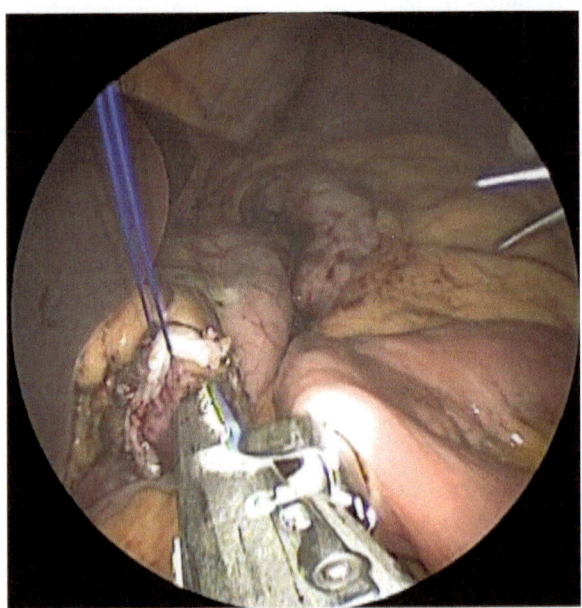

sutured to the pouch vertically, and so provide a preferential way for food and liquid
progressing toward the alimentary/efferent limb and thus reduce the risk of reflux of
bile into the pouch.

A last stitch will fix the efferent limb to the antrum (Fig. 37.13).

Fig. 37.11 Closing of the service opening

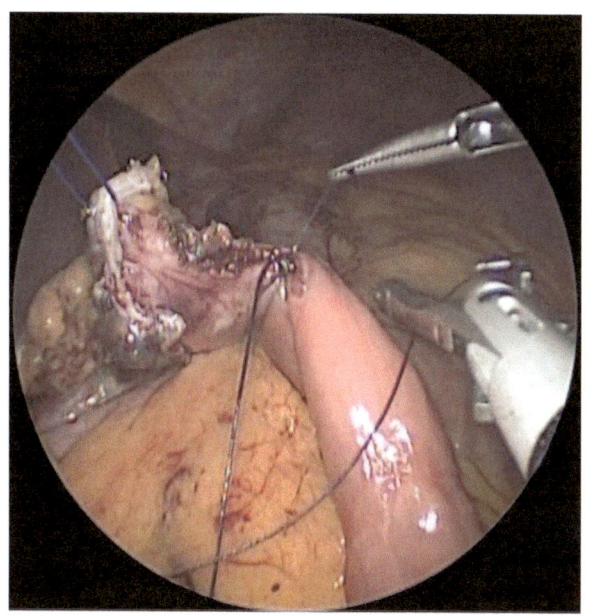

Fig. 37.12 Afferent loop sutured to the gastic pouch

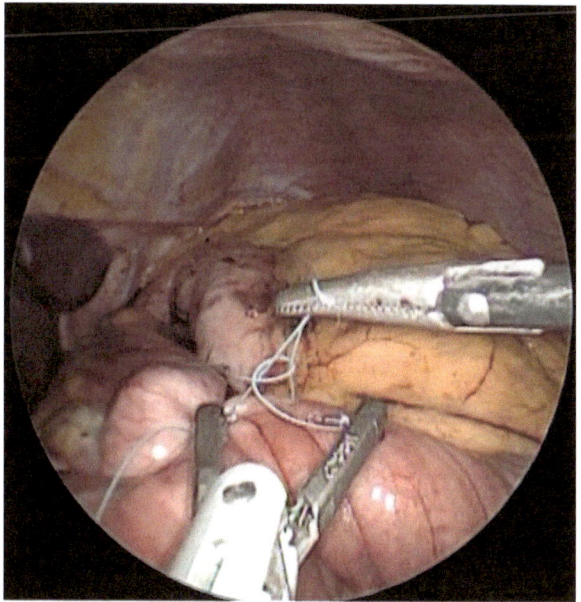

Fig. 37.13 Efferent loop
sutured to the gastric antrum

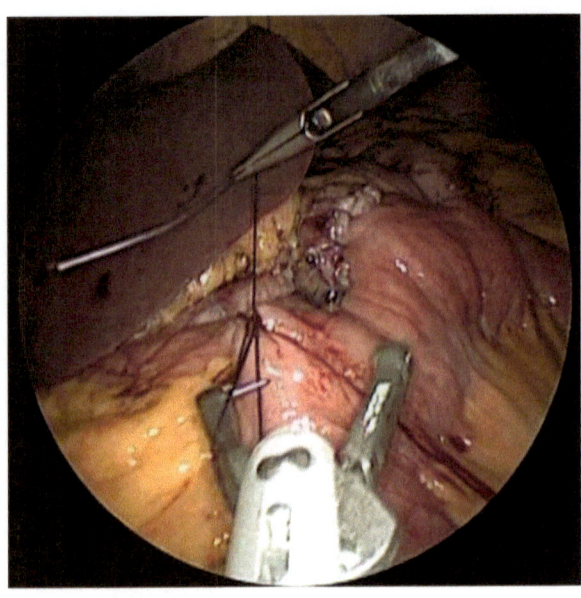

Roux-en-Y Conversion

A Roux-en-Y reconstruction may be accomplished, if necessary, in an easy way
after the gastroenteric anastomosis is done, with the "double loop" technique: at
about 10-cm from the gastroenteric anastomosis along the biliary limb an enterotomy is made for the next entero-enteric anastomosis. The second loop (alimentary
limb) is measured starting from the gastroentero anastomosis just completed toward
the ileocecal valve and the enteroenteric anastomosis is performed. With this technique the surgical field of view is very restricted and the movements are minimized
thus facilitating the implementation of the intervention and reducing the risk of
twisting the mesentery. The last step of the intervention is the interruption of continuity between the two anastomosis to create the Roux-en-Y: a passage into the
mesentery near the intestinal wall is made without using coagulation, being careful
not to cause vascular damage to prevent ischemia; a 60-mm white cartridge
EndoGIA® (Covidien) is inserted in the passage created and the stapler is fired.

No drainage was left in place. The operation ends with the evacuation of the
pneumoperitoneum and the removal of the port. The fascia is closed with an absorbable suture and the navel is reinstated in its original position [2].

37.1.3 BPD

The BPD as originally described by Scopinaro [11] has in the years undergone several modifications that however have not altered the fundamental working principle:
limited absorption of fat and carbohydrates.

The typical procedure consists in creating a large gastric pouch, with a volume between 300 and 500 mL, such that it will not in any manner limit food intake. This is to mean that there should not be any permanent restriction and that part of the digestive capacities of the stomach is maintained. The distal gastric remnant can be removed, as originally described, or preserved, as many authors, including us, prefer [12–14]. The advantage of not resecting the stomach is the full reversibility, less surgical trauma and earlier recovery. The potential, but not proven, risk is an increase in marginal ulcers.

The reconstruction of the alimentary tract is performed as a Roux-en-Y with an alimentary limb of 200–250 cm and a common limb of 50-cm.

Several authors have modified these limb lenghts. If you elongate the "total" alimentary limb (distance between the stomach and the ileocecal valve) you reduce the risk of protein malnutrition, but you compromise the weight loss result. The need for a Roux-en-Y reconstruction can also be questioned. A Billroth II at 300-cm from the ileocecal valve is feasible, safe and effective. We will discuss this further after description of the technique.

Surgical Technique

Patient is placed in supine position with the left arm abducted and right arm along the body. The laparoscopic tower is placed in proximity of the left patient's shoulder. Surgeon operated at right side of the patient while the assistant kept the camera, standing on the left side. We choose to perform an intra-umbilical incision as described for the others bariatric procedures in order to have the scar completely hidden at the end of intervention. Access to the abdominal cavity is obtained with an open technique; the port is deployed in the opening and used for all instrument insertion and for insufflation of the abdomen. The intervention starts with the dissection at the level of the lesser curvature of the stomach that is carried out at about 10-cm from the gastroesophageal junction. An articulated Endograsp® (Covidien) kept the stomach under traction and dissection is performed with Ligasure Blunt Tip® (Covidien): these instruments are crossed each other allowing to create a triangulation to exert the necessary traction and counter. Once the opening is made the stomach is transacted transversally with four applications of articulated 60-mm blue cartridge EndoGIA® (Covidien). Before dividing completely the stomach accurate hemostasis of the gastroepiploic vessels is obtained with repeated application of Ligasure®. The gastric pouch volume is about 350 mL. A gastrotomy is opened on the anterior surface of the stomach pouch near the lesser curvature and the hole is enlarged with a small bowel clamp to facilitate the future introduction of the stapler. In this case we use straight scissors and straight clamp coupled with an articulated grasper. The surgeon moves on the left side of the patient near the cameraman and the patient is put in almost horizontal position; the omentum is shifted upward and to the right hypocondrium and the ileocecal valve is identified; two enterotomies are opened at 50- and 250-cm from the ileocecal valve. Measurement of the bowel is done coupling a straight small bowel clamp with the articulated endograsp and enterotomies is opened with coagulating scissor and marked with a stitch.

Fig. 37.14 Gastroenteric
anastomosis

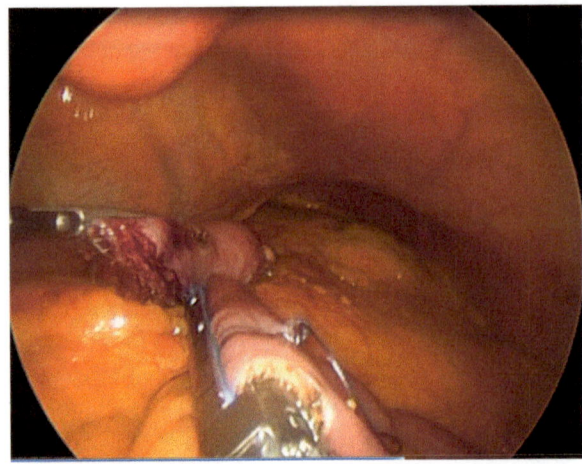

Fig. 37.15 Retrieval of the
point at 50-cm from
ileocecal valve

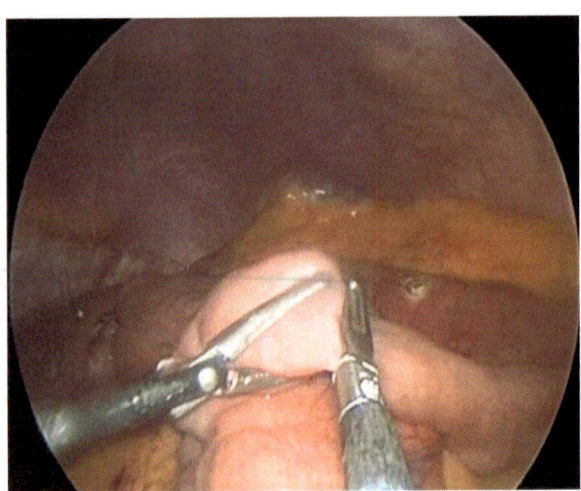

The gastroenteric anastomosis is performed immediately using an articulated
45-mm blue EndoGIA® (Covidien) (Fig. 37.14): the patient is put back into an anti-
Trendelemburg position and the gastric remnant is retrieved with the grasper; the
anvil is placed in the jejunum at 250-cm from the ileocecal valve, then the stapler is
closed, shifted up and approached the gastric pouch while the direction of the joint
was changed presenting the cartridge of the stapler in proximity of the gastrotomy.
The service hole is closed with a double layer hand-made suture carried out with the
Endostitch® (Covidien). At about 10-cm from the gastroenteric anastomosis along
the afferent limb another enterotomy is made for the next enteroenteric anastomosis
with the point at 50-cm from ileocecal valve that is found easily on the efferent limb
(Fig. 37.15). We use an articulated 60-mm white cartridge EndoGIA® (Covidien) to
achieve the enteroenteric anastomosis and the final closure of the gap is performed

Fig. 37.16 Enteroenteric anastomosis

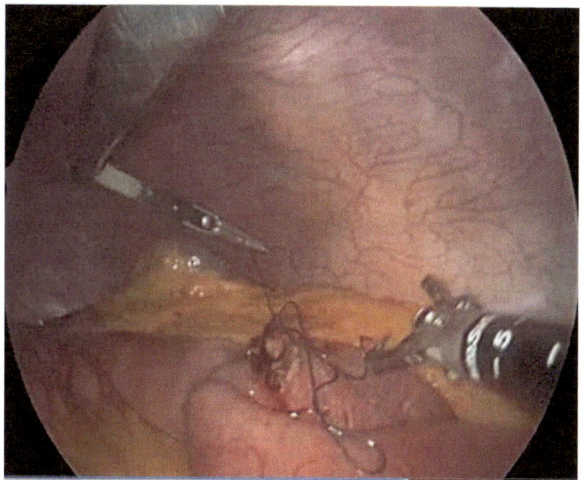

Fig. 37.17 Creation of the Roux-en-Y

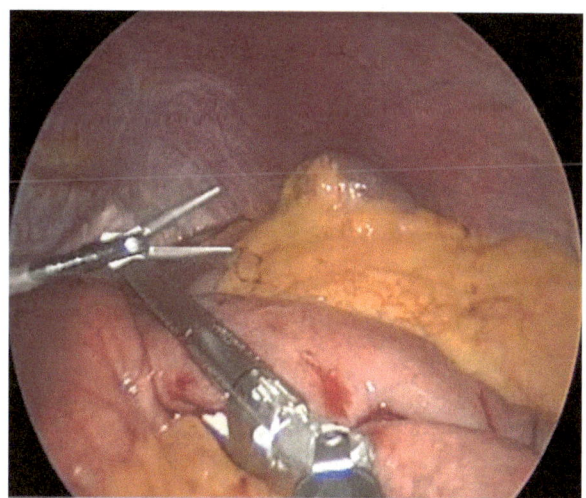

with a double layer hand-made polysorbate 2/0 suture (Fig. 37.16). The last step of the procedure consists in the interruption of the continuity between the two anastomosis to create the Roux-en-Y with an articulated 60-mm white cartridge EndoGIA® (Covidien) (Fig. 37.17). The patency and the tightness of the gastroenteric anastomosis are tested with methylene blue. No drainage is left in place. The operation ends with the evacuation of the pneumoperitoneum and the removal of Triport® (Olympus). The fascia is closed with an absorbable suture and the navel is reinstated in its original position [9].

37.1.4   Learning from SIL

Several lessons can be learned from the SIL experience.

The first aspect is about the access. While practicing SIL you realize that any procedure can be carried on with only three ports, one for the camera and two for the operating instruments. This has beneficial consequences. It is only one surgeon who is manipulating the tissues and organs thus minimizing the trauma and more important the risk of damage by improper maneuvers of the assistant. The assistant is concentrated in holding the camera still. You learn that to give good vision to the operating surgeon the most important thing for the camera-man is to stand still and stay out of the way of the operating field, to such a point that he can be substituted by a mechanical camera holder, asking to the assistant only minor adjustments.

As you are using only three accesses when you go back, for any reason, to standard laparoscopy you will still use three ports. You will not look anymore for an access to introduce a liver retractor that has been proven unnecessary. Thus also in multiple port laparoscopic surgery you will reduce the number of ports with a benefit for the patient.

The second aspect concerns the surgical technique. Every step is reduced to the essential movements. No effort and time is spent to do "tricks" that we used to think important. And then the surgery becomes simple and fast.

Finally, but more important, you learn that may be we had a lot of prejudice about certain types of surgical approaches. We have come to re-evaluate the Billroth II reconstruction as opposed to the Roux-en-Y. Building up experience with the MGB we were more and more convinced that one of the criticism, biliary reflux, was totally overrated. With the proper technique, pouch size, shape and length of bowel limbs, Billroth II technique is not only safe but also largely superior to Roux-en-Y [15]. The pouch size can be adapted from 15 to 20 mL to a large size of 300–350 mL (Fig. 37.18). This way we can decide the degree of food intake restriction to give to the patient. As a consequence we can adapt the bowel lengths (Figs. 37.19 and 37.20) to add more or less limitation to absorption.

The different bariatric procedures that we have today, RYGB, MGB, BPD, as a matter of fact differ for the size of the pouch, the length of the biliary, common and alimentary limb. The Billroth II reconstruction preserves the physiological effect of these adjustments while maintaining a more physiological intestinal transit. This has become evident from the greatly reduced incidence of dumping, hypoglycemia after MGB.

Last but not least we stress the importance of the easy adjustability and reversibility of such approach.

All this we learned from SIL, an approach that required some collateral thinking and freedom from prejudice.

We hope that the future will give more and more attention to RPLS always with the intent of offering the patient better care.

Fig. 37.18 Pouch sizes

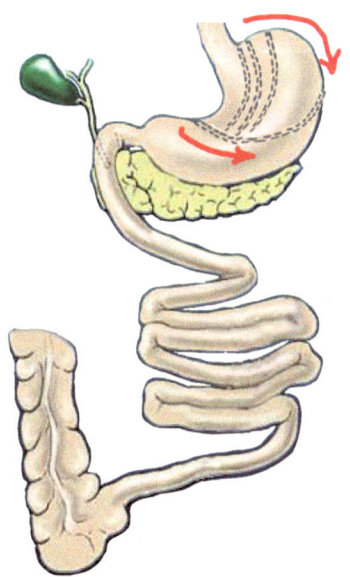

Fig. 37.19 Intestinal lengths

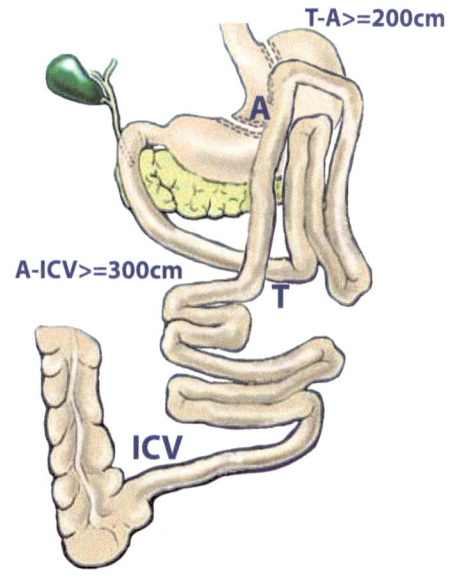

Fig. 37.20 Billroth II MGB
with large pouch (300 mL)
and short alimentary limb
(300 cm). Functional
equivalent of a BPD

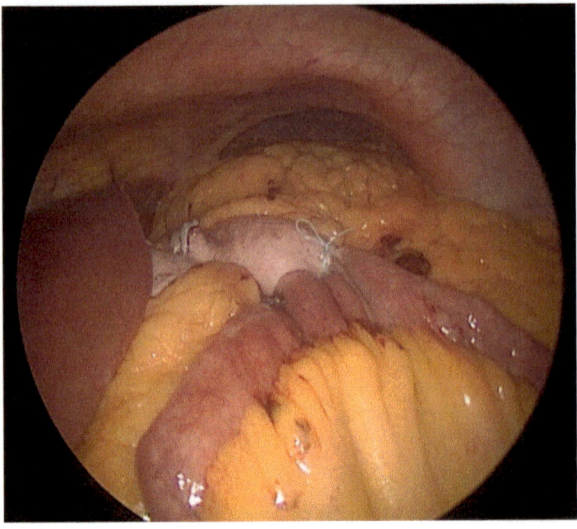

References

1. Tacchino R, Greco F, Matera D (2010) Laparoscopic gastric banding without visible scar: a short series with intraumbilical SILS. Obes Surg 20(2):236–239. doi:10.1007/s11695-009-9908-5, Epub 2009 Jul 15
2. Tacchino R, Greco F, Matera D, Diflumeri G (2010) Single-incision laparoscopic gastric bypass for morbid obesity. Obes Surg 20(8):1154–1160
3. Tacchino R, Greco F, Matera D (2008) Single-incision laparoscopic cholecystectomy: surgery without a visible scar. Surg Endosc 23:896–899
4. Marks JM, Phillips MS, Tacchino R, Roberts K, Onders R et al (2013) Single-incision laparoscopic cholecystectomy is associated with improved cosmesis scoring at the cost of significantly higher hernia rates: 1-year results of a prospective randomized, multicenter, single-blinded trial of traditional multiport laparoscopic cholecystectomy vs single-incision laparoscopic cholecystectomy. J Am Coll Surg 216(6):1037–1047
5. Agarwal BB, Chintamani, Ali K, Goyal K, Mahajan KC (2012) Innovations in endosurgery-journey into the past of the future: to ride the SILS bandwagon or not? Indian J Surg 74(3):234–241. doi: 10.1007/s12262-012-0583-8, Epub 2012 Jun 21
6. Steinemann DC, Raptis DA, Lurje G, Oberkofler CE, Wyss R, Zehnder A, Lesurtel M, Vonlanthen R, Clavien PA, Breitenstein S (2011) Cosmesis and body image after single-port laparoscopic or conventional laparoscopic cholecystectomy: a multicenter double blinded randomised controlled trial (SPOCC-trial). BMC Surg 11:24. doi:10.1186/1471-2482-11-24
7. Trastulli S, Cirocchi R, Desiderio J, Guarino S, Santoro A, Parisi A, Noya G, Boselli C (2013) Systematic review and meta-analysis of randomized clinical trials comparing single-incision versus conventional laparoscopic cholecystectomy. Br J Surg 100(2):191–208. doi:10.1002/bjs.8937, Epub 2012 Nov 12
8. Chamberlain RS, Sakpal SV (2009) A comprehensive review of single-incision laparoscopic surgery (SILS) and natural orifice transluminal endoscopic surgery (NOTES) techniques for cholecystectomy. J Gastrointest Surg 13(9):1733–1740
9. Tacchino R, Greco F, Matera D (2010) Single-incision laparoscopic biliopancreatic diversion. Surg Obes Relat Dis 6(4):444–445

10. Saber AA, Elgamal MH, Itawi EA, Rao AJ (2008) Single incision laparoscopic sleeve gastrectomy (SILS): a novel technique. Obes Surg 18(10):1338–1342. doi:10.1007/s11695-008-9646-0, Epub 2008 Aug
11. Scopinaro N, Giannetta E, Civalleri D et al (1979) Bilio-pancreatic by-pass for obesity: II. Initial experience in man. Br J Surg 66:613–620
12. Resa JJ, Solano J, Fatás JA et al (2004) Laparoscopic biliopancreatic diversion with distal gastric preservation: technique and three-year followup. J Laparoendosc Adv Surg Tech A 14(3):131–134
13. Larrad-Jimenez A, Diaz-Guerra CSC, de Cuadros Borrajo P et al (2007) Short-, mild- and long-term results of Larrad biliopancreatic diversion. Obes Surg 17:202–210
14. Crea N, Pata G, Di Betta E, Greco F, Casella C, Vilardi A, Mittempergher F (2011) Long-term results of biliopancreatic diversion with or without gastric preservation for morbid obesity. Obes Surg 21(2):139–145. doi:10.1007/s11695-010-0333-6
15. Sánchez-Pernaute A, Rubio MA, Pérez Aguirre E, Barabash A, Cabrerizo L, Torres A (2012) Single-anastomosis duodenoileal bypass with sleeve gastrectomy: metabolic improvement and weight loss in first 100 patients. Surg Obes Relat Dis 9(5):731–735, Epub ahead of print

Chapter 38
Revisional Obesity Surgery

Alan A. Saber, Jason M. Saber, and Angie A. Saber

Abstract There is a growing trend towards surgical techniques that minimize abdominal wall trauma. This will expand the benefits of traditional laparoscopic surgery with less pain, less scarring, less injury to tissues, shorter hospital stay, quicker return to normal physical activities, and better cosmetic outcome. This facilitates the development of a new concept: reduced port laparoscopic surgery (RPLS) with a decrease in either the number of ports or the size of ports, or a combination of both. After our extensive experience with primary bariatric RPLS, we started exploring revisional procedures. In this chapter we will discuss the operative strategy, technical challenges, and step-by-step description of revisional obesity RPLS and transversus abdominus plan block (TAP block).

Keywords Reduced port laparoscopic surgery • Revisional surgery • Sleeve gastrectomy

38.1 Introduction

There is a growing trend towards surgical techniques that minimize abdominal wall trauma. This will expand the benefits of traditional laparoscopic surgery with less pain, less scarring, less injury to tissues, shorter hospital stay, quicker return to normal physical activities, and better cosmetic outcome.

A.A. Saber (✉)
Chief of Minimally Invasive Surgery, Director of Bariatric Surgery, The Brooklyn
Hospital Center, Weill Cornell Medical College, New York, NY, USA

J.M. Saber
Pace University, New York, NY, USA

A.A. Saber
Rutgers University, New Brunswick, NJ, USA

T. Mori and G. Dapri (eds.), *Reduced Port Laparoscopic Surgery*,
DOI 10.1007/978-4-431-54601-6_38, © Springer Japan 2014

This facilitates the development of a new concept: reduced port laparoscopic surgery (RPLS) with a decrease in either the number of ports or the size of ports, or a combination of both. The application of this approach has expanded to bariatric surgery. Since our initial description of the single-incision laparoscopic surgery (SLS) sleeve gastrectomy (SG) in 2008 [1], we have applied the same principle to a wide variety of both bariatric and non-bariatric procedures [1–6]. After our extensive experience with RPL primary bariatric RPLS, we started exploring revisional procedures, mainly the revision of the adjustable gastric band (AGB) to SG. In this chapter we will discuss the technical challenges and step-by-step description of revisional obesity RPLS.

38.2 Operative Strategy and Technical Considerations

The feasibility of RPLS is enhanced when tailored according to each patient's body habitus. In patients with a relatively low body mass index (BMI), peripheral obesity, a small liver, and a short umbilicus–xiphoid distance, we proceeded with transumbilical SLS. In addition to the cosmetic advantages of a hidden intraumbilical single incision, the umbilicus provides a safe zone for abdominal access, while minimizing the torque effect of an obese patient's thick abdominal wall.

38.3 Technical and Physical Challenges in SLS Approach

38.3.1 Lost Triangulation and Trocar Placement Strategy

Achieving adequate triangulation is a basic principle of traditional laparoscopic surgery.

Trocars can be directed from multiple points of entry, guiding instruments towards the target organ, where adequate manipulation can be achieved (Fig. 38.1a).

Operating through a single incision with only rigid instruments would be challenging, because the surgeon would either implement a parallel positioning of instruments (Fig. 38.1b) or a 'crossing' arrangement (Fig. 38.1c). In the parallel technique, both instruments emerge through the umbilicus; thus, controlling both instruments outside the abdomen would pose a challenge because the surgeon's hands would be at such close proximity. On the other hand, in the crossing arrangement, there would be a considerably more comfortable range of movement on the outside; however, on the inside, the left hand controls the right instrument, and vice versa, posing a challenge for first-time SLS adopters. As the overall flexibility of the instruments increases, triangulation issues can be overcome without sacrificing external maneuverability.

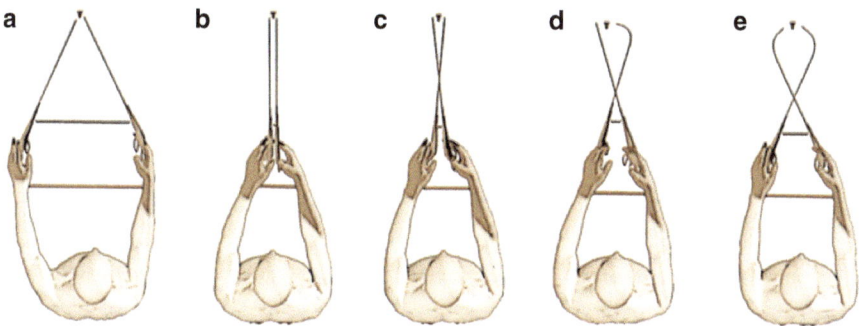

Fig. 38.1 Conflict of instrumentation and triangulation in single incision laparoscopic surgery and trocar reduction. With Permission from [6]

Flexible instruments have articulating shafts, steering the tip of the instrument toward the target organ and restoring lost triangulation. Thus, combining flexible and rigid instruments has resulted in a more comfortable configuration (Fig. 38.1d, e), increasing maneuverability and the feasibility of advanced surgical procedures using SLS. Recently, curved laparoscopic instruments have been introduced to the field of SLS to restore triangulation and minimize fighting between instruments and laparoscope.

38.3.2 Conflict of Instruments

Multiple instruments inserted at close proximity through a common port of entry produce an undesirable limitation of movement both inside and outside. Many advanced procedures involve switching instruments more often, potentially compromising the pneumoperitoneum. These challenges have led to the development of multi-channel ports to avoid the clinching of laparoscopic instruments diverting from a common point.

If multichannel ports are not available, it is necessary to insert 3 trocars through the same umbilical skin incision but with different fascial incisions at different levels in a triangular fashion. Using a flexible tip scope minimizes the external conflict of instruments because its cable exits through the back end of the instrument, keeping it away from the operative field.

38.3.3 Abdominal Wall 'Torque Effect'

Utilizing the umbilicus (the thinnest part of the abdominal wall) minimizes the torque effect on trocars inserted at such close proximity, providing a wider range of motion for the instruments and trocars in different directions. However, if incisions are made further away from the umbilicus, the 'torque effect' on trocars increases with the increasing thickness of the point of abdominal access, counteracting the movement of trocars and decreasing maneuverability.

38.3.4 Umbilical Recession

In super obese patients a receded umbilicus can reduce the feasibility of the transumbilical approach, favoring an epigastric placement of trocars to ensure that the gastroesophageal junction is within comfortable reach of the laparoscopic instruments.

38.3.5 Retraction of Large Liver

Bariatric patients have a higher incidence of fatty liver, potentially obscuring the operative field and presenting a challenge for the SLS approach. Liver retraction can be achieved by using internal retraction (i.e. sutures), using external retraction (i.e. subxiphoid, transumbilical liver retractor), or using the mobilized portion of the stomach.

38.4 Operative Technique for RPL Revision of AGB to SG

The patient is placed in the supine position. The surgeon stands either on the patient's right side or between the legs of the patient, with the assistant on the left side.

Both the location of the single incision and the method of liver retraction are tailored according to the operative strategy discussed in the previous section. If the subcutaneous port is in the vicinity of the umbilicus, we choose a transumbilical approach GelPOINT (Applied Medical, Rancho Santa Margarita, CA, USA) placement to conduct the procedure, and at the end to remove the subcutaneous port.

The deepest point in the umbilical scar is pulled up using Kocker graspers while applying subtle pressure on the abdominal wall to tent up the umbilical scar. A 2.5-cm intraumbilical skin incision is created and deepened to the linea alba. A fascial opening up to a length of 3-cm is established. This large facial incision minimizes fighting between instruments and laparoscope. The GelPOINT (Applied Medical) is placed. Three 10-mm trocars are introduced through the GelPOINT (Applied Medical) (Fig. 38.2). The pneumoperitoneum is initiated to a pressure of 15 mmHg. A long 45-degree 5-mm laparoscope with L connection is inserted.

Using a 5-mm LigaSure (Covidien, New Haven, CT, USA) and 5-mm flexible grasper, the greater curvature of the stomach is retracted (Fig. 38.3) and mobilized (Fig. 38.4), beginning from a point 6-cm proximal to the pylorus, staying close to

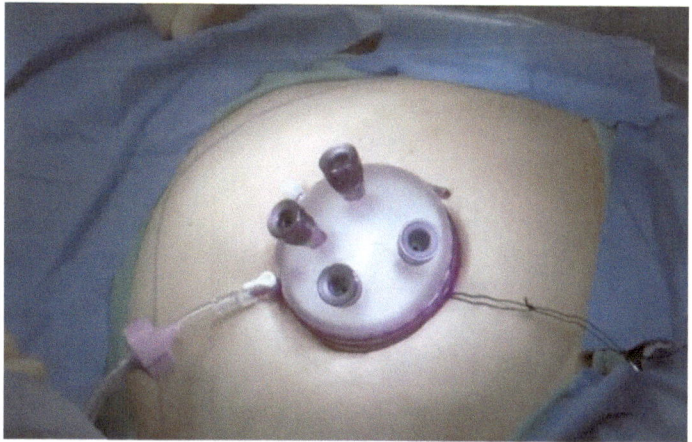

Fig. 38.2 GelPOINT (Applied Medical) inserted in the umbilicus

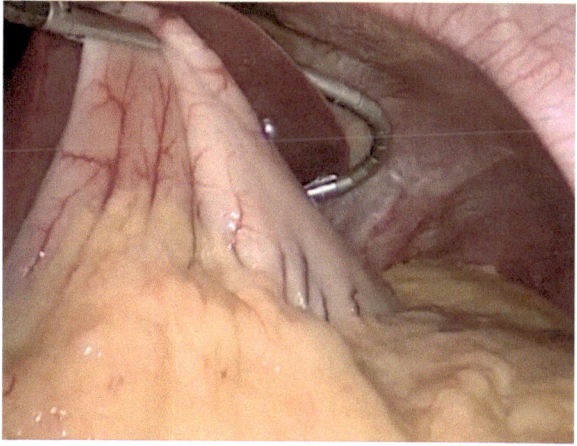

Fig. 38.3 Retraction of the greater curvature of the stomach

the wall of the stomach, all the way up the greater curvature to the angle of His, dividing both gastrocolic and gastrosplenic ligaments. This is followed by liver retraction with a flexible liver retractor inserted through the GelPOINT (Applied Medical).

The fibrous capsule over the AGB is taken down (Fig. 38.5). The AGB is then used as a retractor and eventually cut (Fig. 38.6). The gastrogastric plication is taken down with laparoscopic scissors. In the case of dense adhesions at the gastrogastric plication, a linear stapler is used to take down the plication instead.

Fig. 38.4 Mobilization of
the greater curvature of the
stomach with Ligasure
(Covidien)

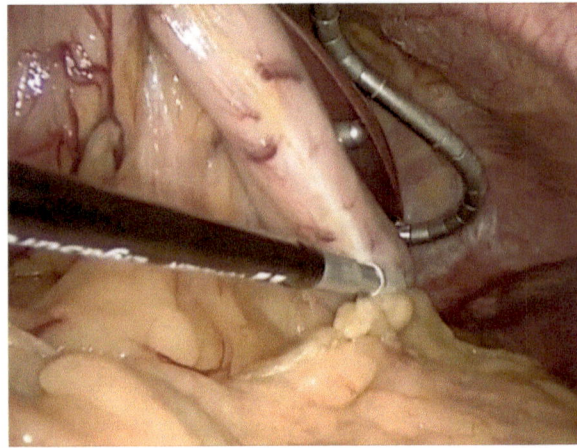

Fig. 38.5 Taking down the
fibrous capsule around the
AGB

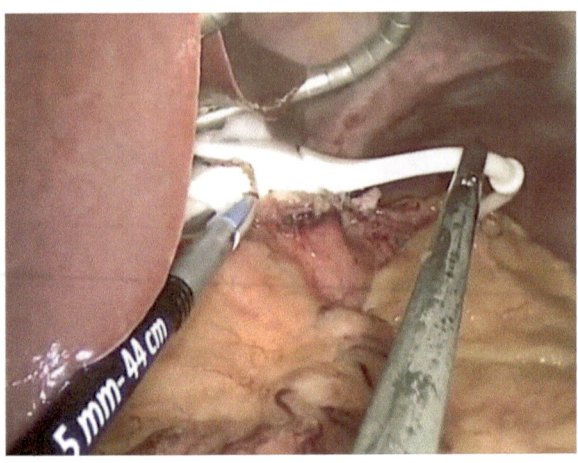

It is important to identify and mobilize the angle of His, with exposure of the left crus of the diaphragm, to facilitate complete resection of the fundus. Retrogastric adhesions are taken down with the LigaSure (Covidien). This allows complete mobilization of the stomach, eliminates any redundant posterior wall of the SG, and excludes the fundus from the SG.

Once the stomach is completely mobilized, a 34F oro-gastric tube is inserted orally into the pylorus and placed against the lesser curvature. This calibrates the size of the SG, prevents constriction at the gastroesophageal junction and incisura angularis, and provides a uniform shape to the entire stomach.

The gastric transection is started at a point 6-cm proximal to the pylorus, leaving the antrum intact and preserving gastric emptying. A long laparoscopic roticulating 60 mm XL Endo-GIA stapler (Covidien) with green cartridge 4.8-mm staples and synthetic absorbable buttressing material is inserted through the 15-mm trocar in a

Fig. 38.6 Cutting the AGB

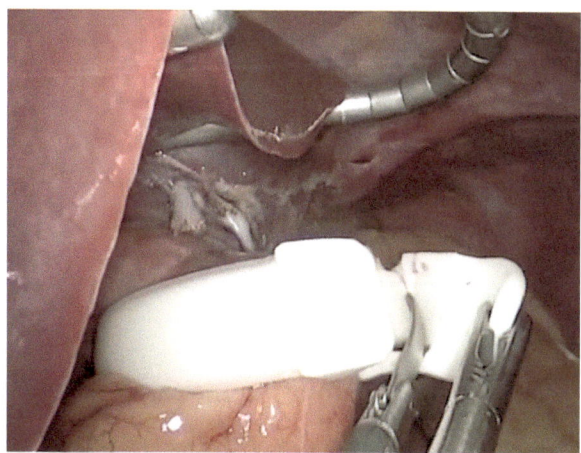

Fig. 38.7 Gastric stapling along 34 French orogastric tube

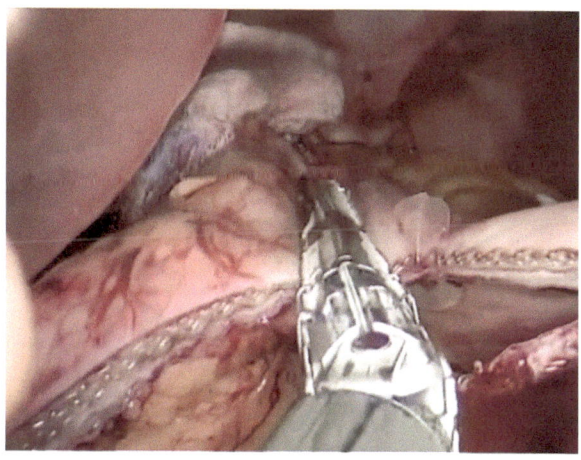

cephalad direction (Fig. 38.7). The stapler is fired consecutively along the length of the orogastric tube until the angle of His is reached. Care must be taken not to narrow the stomach at the incisura angularis. It is important to inspect the stomach anteriorly and posteriorly to ensure there is no redundant posterior gastric wall. Approximately 80 % of the stomach is separated. The entire staple line is inspected for bleeding and tested for leakage. Insufflating air under saline and infusing methylene blue into the remaining stomach tests the integrity of the staple line. The resected stomach is extracted along with the GelPOINT (Applied Medical) without the need for an Endobag (Fig. 38.8). The band port is removed through the umbilical incision (Fig. 38.9). The fascial defect of the port site is closed with a figure-of-eight 2-0 nonabsorbable suture to prevent port site hernia formation. The skin incision is closed with 4-0 absorbable suture in a subcuticular fashion (Fig. 38.10).

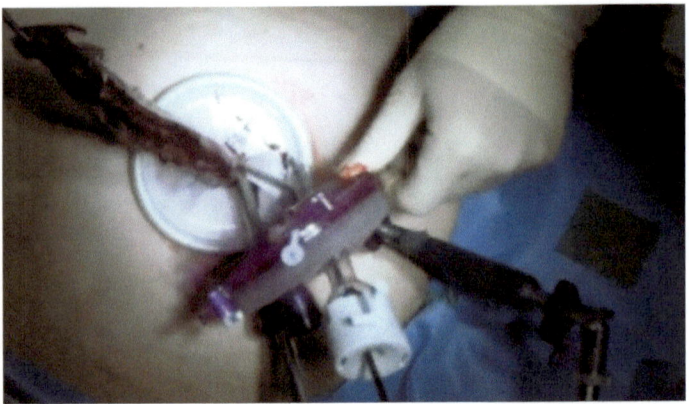

Fig. 38.8 Removal of SG specimen

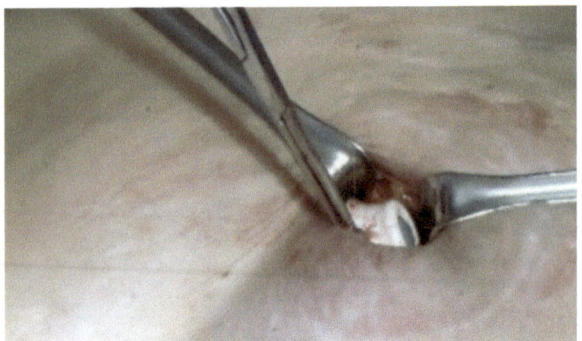

Fig. 38.9 Removal of band port through the umbilical incision

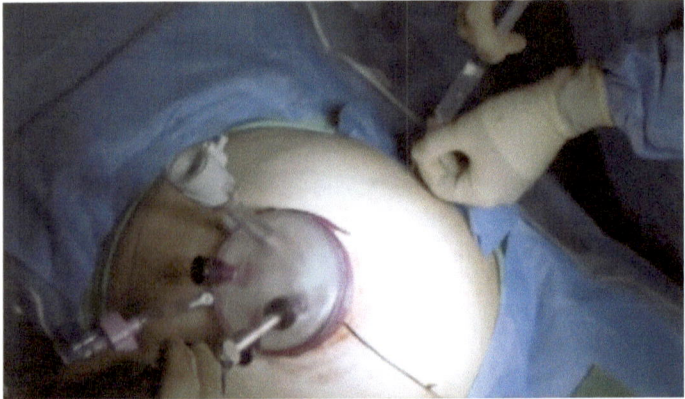

Fig. 38.10 Laparoscopic-guided TAP block

38.4.1   *Transversus Abdominus Plan Block (TAP block)*

The SLS approach involves a single incision, as opposed to multiple tiny incisions scattered all over the abdomen in standard laparoscopic operation. We take advantage of this situation by selectively blocking the nerves supplying the periumblical area. This is achieved by either ultrasound or laparoscopic-guided transversus abdominis plane (TAP) block (Fig. 38.10). In our experience, if the block is performed correctly, the SLS incision stays relatively pain-free, allowing subsequent reduction of the requirement for pain medications and a faster recovery for the patient.

38.5   Comment

- In expert hands, revisional obesity RPLS is a safe and feasible option in selected patients.
- The approach is particularly attractive for procedures that require a 2–3 cm incision to retrieve or insert the AGB and the port as in AGB, or to retrieve a big specimen as in SG. The use of a single-port device would be helpful in that task.
- In our experience, the SLS approach has many potential advantages over the conventional laparoscopic approach, including less postoperative pain, less need for analgesia, and a shorter hospital stay. In addition, it improves cosmesis and body image, an important outcome to consider in the bariatric population where there is a predominance of young women.
- The SLS approach has outcomes similar to those of its conventional multiport counterpart in terms of morbidity, mortality, reoperation, readmission, weight loss, and comorbidity improvement.
- However, some technical challenges are encountered during SLS bariatric procedures, including lost triangulation, conflict of instruments, umbilical recession, and fatty large liver. These could be overcome by using long flexible instruments, a flexible tip scope, multichannel access ports, and a liver retractor.
- If any difficulties are encountered during the procedure, do not hesitate to add more trocars to achieve the same operative goal.

References

1. Saber AA, Elgamal MH, Rao AJ. Single Incision laparoscopic sleeve gastrectomy: A Novel Technique. Obes Surg. (2008) 18:1338–1342
2. Saber AA, El-Ghazaly TH, Elian A, Dewoolkar AV, Slayton SA (2010) Single-incision laparoscopic sleeve gastrectomy versus conventional multiport laparoscopic sleeve gastrectomy: technical considerations and strategic modifications. Surg Obesity Relat Dis 6(6):658–664

3. Saber AA, El-Ghazaly TH, Elian A, Dewoolkar AV (2010) Single-incision laparoscopic placement of adjustable gastric band versus conventional multiport laparoscopic gastric banding: a comparative study. Am Surg 76(12):1328–1332
4. Saber AA, El-Ghazaly TH, Elian A (2009) Single-incision transumbilical laparoscopic sleeve gastrectomy. J Laparoendosc Adv Surg Tech A 19(6):755–758
5. Saber AA, El-Ghazaly TH (2009) Early experience with single-access transumbilical laparoscopic adjustable gastric banding. Obes Surg 19(10):1442–1446
6. Saber AA (2010) Single incision laparoscopic surgery and trocar reduction strategies for bariatric procedures. In: Deitel M, Gagner M, Dixon JB, Himpens J, Madan AK (eds) Handbook of obesity surgery. FD-Communications Inc, Toronto, pp 190–197

Chapter 39
Two or Combined Procedures

David Lomanto and Guowei Kim

Abstract With widespread acceptance of laparoscopic surgery, efforts are aimed to minimize further surgical trauma. The last decade has seen a few novel approaches, such as mini-laparoscopy, needlescopic surgery, natural orifice translumenal endoscopic surgery (NOTES), and single-port endo-laparoscopic surgery (SPES). The latter two methods are the most recent surgical innovations that have heralded the trend toward scarless and less invasive surgery. While current clinical application of NOTES requires significant improvement in technique and technology, SPES can be performed with the refinement of existing laparoscopic instruments and is gaining popularity among surgeons and patients. SPES was first performed and reported as early as 1992 by Pelosi, which were single-puncture laparoscopic appendectomy and hysterectomy. Since then, many case reports and case series have emerged in the fields of gastrointestinal, urological, and gynecological surgery using the reduced port technique. In this chapter we will review and discuss the prevailing controversies in SPES for combined surgical procedures. For the purpose of this chapter, we will use the term SPES, even though there are several accepted definitions and no agreement among the surgical community regarding the best term.

Keywords Combined surgical procedures • Single-port laparoscopic surgery • Reduced port laparoscopic surgery • Digestive surgery • Laparoscopic surgery

D. Lomanto (✉) • G. Kim
Minimally Invasive Surgical Centre, Department of Surgery, National University Health System, YLL School of Medicine, National University of Singapore, Singapore, Singapore
e-mail: davide_lomanto@nuhs.edu.sg

T. Mori and G. Dapri (eds.), *Reduced Port Laparoscopic Surgery*,
DOI 10.1007/978-4-431-54601-6_39, © Springer Japan 2014

39.1 Introduction

While procedures using combined laparoscopic surgical techniques have been reported since 1991 [1–4], the use of a single-port or single-incision approach has only recently been reported for cholecystectomies, appendectomies, ovarian cystectomies, hernia repairs, splenectomies, salpingectomies and varicocelectomies via a transumbilical single-port [5–10]. The use of reduced port laparoscopic surgery (RPLS) or even single-port endo-laparoscopic surgery (SPES) technique has been gaining popularity and its use is becoming increasingly more common for patients who have dual or multiple intra-abdominal pathologies [11–15].

The possible advantages of RPLS or SPES can be attributed to a reduction in hospital admissions and amount of general anesthesia given to patients. There is better perceived cosmesis for certain procedures with dramatically fewer ports/scars. The reduced number of ports also minimizes the risks associated with port insertion. In addition, recent studies show at least equivalent pain level, operative duration and complication rates when comparing conventional laparoscopic surgery to RPLS / SPES [4–7].

The obvious disadvantages of performing RPLS or SPES include increased cost with the use of single-port devices, but the main constraints lie in ergonomics, such as compromised exposure, inadequate retraction, conflict between the instruments and lack of triangulation. There is also a steep learning curve to overcome as surgeons first have to master conventional laparoscopic surgery and basic laparoscopic techniques before attempting RPLS or SPES and using alternative techniques to overcome the difficulties [16, 17]. A concern has arisen over the potential for increased risk of port site hernia, as most single-port devices require a slightly larger incision than usual ports. For example, an incision of 22/25-mm is suggested for the use of the SILS™ device (Covidien, New Haven, CT, USA), and an incision of 25/30-mm is suggested for GelPort (Applied Medical, Rancho Santa Margarita, CA, USA), while a smaller 14/18-mm incision is necessary to introduce the LESS (Olympus, Tokyo, Japan) device. To avoid the occurrence of port site hernia, an appropriate device should be carefully selected according to the procedure, the number of instruments required, the organ targeted and the size of the specimen to be extracted. An appropriate device, combined with a figure eight suture for the fascia closure, will certainly keep at bay the increased risk of hernia.

39.1.1 Indications

No standard guidelines have been set regarding when to perform RPLS or SPES for combined procedures. The choice to use such techniques should remain primarily with the surgeon. Multiple factors may influence the surgeon's choice, such as level of experience and skills and knowledge of the individual pathologies. Each procedure should be assessed to determine its suitability for RPLS or SPES individually first. For example, a cholecystectomy or ovarian cystectomy would be feasible, as both procedures can be easily performed with SPES techniques. On the other end of the spectrum, ultra-low anterior resection would likely be unsuitable for RPLS or SPES.

RPLS or SPES would be appropriate for patients in whom there would be multiple port sites for procedures in pathologies in different quadrants of the abdomen. For example, a laparoscopic cholecystectomy would require 2-3 working ports and one peri-umbilical camera port. A left transperitoneal adrenalectomy would require three working ports. Performing both procedures with the same setting using the SPES technique would drastically reduce the number of ports required, but technical challenges should be considered.

39.1.2 Contraindications

Like all variants of laparoscopic surgery, the standard contraindications to laparoscopic surgery apply. Indeed, patients selected for RPLS or SPES should be medically able to tolerate prolonged anesthesia times and a longer duration of pneumoperitoneum.

When performing RPLS or SPES, it is mandatory to carefully select suitable patients. A history of previous laparotomy or laparoscopy, both of which use the umbilicus as access, may cause difficult entry for the single-port device. Abdominal wall thickness with regards to obese patients would pose a problem, as the single-port device may not be long enough to traverse the abdominal wall completely.

Thought must be given to each procedure and the influence that it can have on the other procedure if done concurrently. The type of surgery performed with regards to wound classification is paramount. Ideally, clean surgeries involving the use of implants should not be performed concurrently with contaminated or potentially dirty surgeries. It would be disastrous to perform mesh repair of a ventral hernia following a cholecystectomy for acute cholecystitis with hydrops!

39.2 Technique

There is no fixed technique for performing RPLS or SPES for two or combined procedures. Instead, certain considerations have to be taken prior to surgery. Preoperative planning is paramount. Generally, if the procedures involve two or more quadrants, the umbilical area is the best choice for insertion of the device. This is became it is such placement equidistant from all parts of the abdomen. This is especially so far procedures on the upper right and lower left quadrant in opposite allows reaching the target organ by simply switching the instruments and the camera. It is important in this case to have an integrated operating theatre where the surgical monitors are mounted on a revolving arm and can be deployed in a more ergonomic view without moving the camera trolley or the patient (Fig. 39.1).

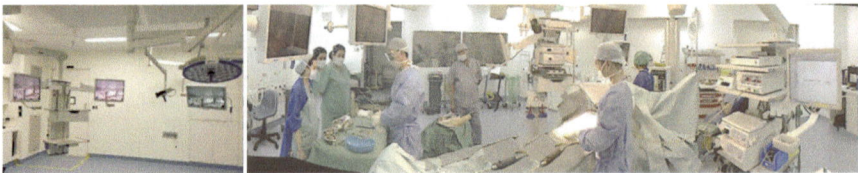

Fig. 39.1 A view of minimally invasive surgery integrated operating theatres in our institution

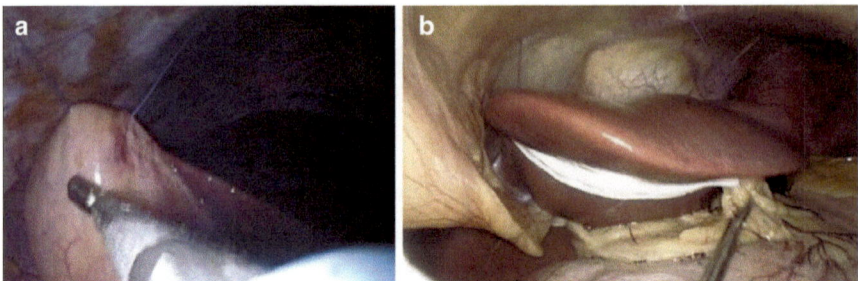

Fig. 39.2 (**a**, **b**) Two different utilizations of percutaneous suture for organ retraction

39.2.1   Instruments/Equipment

There is a large range of products available for the surgeon to utilize. Flexible, articulated, or pre-bent instruments are generally recommended to help achieve triangulation during surgical procedures. A combination of both straight and articulated or pre-bent instruments may facilitate the maneuvers and reduce conflict among instruments. It important to choose an appropriate telescope to reduce clashing; in our experience, the EndoEYE 5-mm 30° (Olympus) is one of the most comfortable options. Other alternatives include a long 10-mm 30° telescope similar to the one used in bariatric surgery, or a telescope with a flexible tip (EndoEYE Flex HD (Olympus)). For advanced procedures and when required, the use of energy-sealing devices is recommended. Today, there are several devices using different types of energy for sealing and cutting vessels up to 7-mm, ranging from ultrasonic waves to HF bipolar diathermy, or even a combination of both. By using an energy-sealing device, tissue can be dissected and transected with minimal traction as compared to using conventional diathermy. Lastly, percutaneous suture for retraction can be a useful strategy to improve retraction and surgical exposure. One or two percutaneous non-absorbable sutures can offer additional benefits when a reduced number of ports affects the technique (Fig. 39.2a, b).

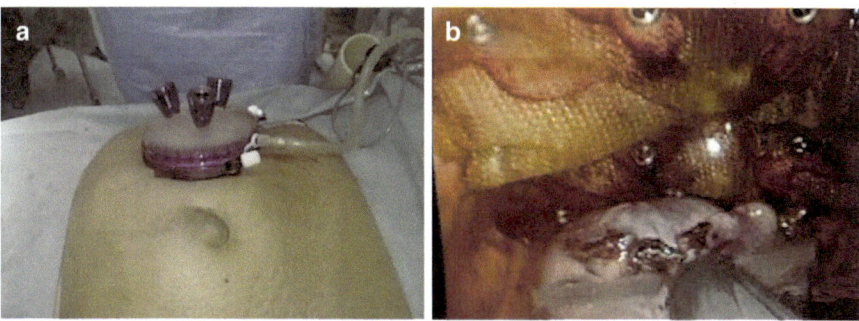

Fig. 39.3 (**a, b**) Port position and intraoperative view of SPES ventral hernia repair and oophorectomy

39.2.2 Port Placement

Prior to placing the port, thought should be given to the target pathology with regards to the working area within the abdomen. Many procedures can be performed via a single peri-umbilical port. For example, a left trans-peritoneal adrenalectomy and cholecystectomy are feasible if performed via a peri-umbilical port, whereas a ventral peri-umbilical hernia repair with an ovarian cystectomy would require the port being placed in the lower quadrant or flanks (Fig. 39.3a, b).

Adjustment of the port may be required in certain situations. For example, a totally extra-peritoneal inguinal hernia repair can be first performed extra-peritoneally, with the port being placed first in the pre-peritoneal space, and adjustments being made later to advance it intra-peritoneally for the second procedure, such as cholecystectomy.

39.3 Tips and Tricks (Compared to Multi Trocar Laparoscopy)

It is paramount to understand that there is no standard technique when performing RPLS or SPES for multiple procedures. A certain degree of creativity is required to accommodate the multitude of procedures.

Proper port placement is the corner stone for this technique, as improper port placement would result in almost certain conversion to conventional laparoscopic techniques/open surgery.

Proper thought into which procedure should be performed first is important as well. It would be logical to perform the more medically pressing procedure first. Should major difficulties arise with the first procedure, postponement of the second procedure can be considered.

There should be no hesitation to revert to conventional laparoscopic surgery or to insert additional ports should the need arise, as patient safety is paramount.

39.4 Recommendations from the Author

RPLS or SPES for two or combined procedures is only for advanced laparoscopic surgeons who have surmounted the learning curve in SPES.

Every patient should be counseled about the procedure and made aware of the pros and cons, including all treatment modalities and the extra cost involved in the use of expensive instrumentation. The risk of reversion to conventional surgery or conversion to open or non-completion of one procedure should also be explained to the patient pre-operatively.

References

 1. Pelosi MA, Pelosi MA 3rd (1992) Laparoscopic appendectomy using a single umbilical puncture (minilaparoscopy). J Reprod Med 37:588–594
 2. Pelosi MA, Pelosi MA 3rd (1992) Laparoscopic supracervical hysterectomy using a single-umbilical puncture (mini-laparoscopy). J Reprod Med 37:777–784
 3. Bailey RW, Flowers JL, Graham SM, Zucker KA (1991) Combined laparoscopic cholecystectomy and selective vagotomy. Surg Laparosc Endosc 1(1):45–49
 4. Lopez-Martinez RA, Raina S (1993) Laparoscopic cholecystectomy combined with ventral hernia repair. J Laparoendosc Surg 3(6):561–562
 5. Trastulli S, Cirocchi R, Desiderio J et al (2013) Systematic review and meta-analysis of randomized clinical trials comparing single-incision versus conventional laparoscopic cholecystectomy. Br J Surg 100(2):191–208
 6. Fung AK, Aly EH (2012) Systematic review of single incision laparoscopic colonic surgery. Br J Surg 99(10):1353–1364
 7. Seo IY, Lee JW, Rim JS (2011) Laparoendoscopic single-site radical nephrectomy: a comparison with conventional laparoscopy. J Endourol 25:465–469
 8. Rehman H, Mathews T, Ahmed I (2012) A review of minimally invasive single port/incision laparoscopic appendectomy. J Laparoendosc Adv Surg Tech A 22(7):641–646
 9. Goo TT, Goel R, Lawenko M, Lomanto D (2010) Laparoscopic transabdominal preperitoneal (TAPP) hernia repair via a single port. Surg Laparosc Endosc Percutan Tech 20(6): 389–390
10. Goo TT, Agarwal A, Goel R, Tan CT, Lomanto D, Cheah WK (2011) Single-port access adrenalectomy: our initial experience. J Laparoendosc Adv Surg Tech A 21:815–819, Epub 2011 Sept 29
11. Ghidirim GHP, Gladun EV, Danch AV et al (1996) Combined laparoscopic treatment of polycystic ovary disease and gallstones. J Am Assoc Gynecol Laparosc 3:S15
12. Lee JS, Hong TH, Park BJ et al (2012) Transumbilical single port laparoscopic surgery for the treatment of concomitant disease. Minimally Invasive Therapy Early Online, 1–6
13. Hart S, Ross S, Rosemurgy A (2010) Laparoendoscopic single-site combined cholecystectomy and hysterectomy. J Minim Invasive Gynecol 17(6):798–801

14. Lee JS, Hong TH, Park BJ, Kim JJ (2013) Transumbilical single port laparoscopic surgery for the treatment of concomitant disease. Minim Invasive Ther Allied Technol 22(3):181–186
15. Kim G, Lomanto D, Lawenko MM et al (2013) Single-port endo-laparoscopic surgery in combined abdominal procedures. Asian J Endosc Surg 6(3):209–213
16. Goel R, Lomanto D (2012) Controversies in single port surgery. Surg Laparosc Endosc Percutan Tech 22(5):380–382
17. Tang B, Hou S, Cuschieri SA (2012) Ergonomics and technologies for single port laparoscopic surgery. Minim Invasive Ther Allied Technol 21(1):46–54

Chapter 40
Urology

Takatsugu Okegawa and Kikuo Nutahara

Abstract This paper reports our experience with single-port retroperitoneal laparoscopic nephrectomy (SPRLN). From April 2010 to March 2013, 20 retroperitoneal approach surgeries for the treatment of patients with localized renal cell carcinoma were performed.

Patients were placed in the full lateral position with slight flexion under general anesthesia. Access to the retroperitoneum was obtained with the Hasson technique through a 2.5-cm skin incision at the tip of the 12th rib. A balloon dissector (PDB; Covidien, New Haven, CT, USA) was inflated in the retroperitoneum outside Gerota's fascia to create the working space. The SILS™ port (Covidien) or GelPOINT (Applied Medical, Rancho Santa Margarita CA, USA) was then placed in this incision. The first 5-mm port for the flexible laparoscope (Olympus Surgical, Tokyo, Japan) was inserted into this single-port. Using the instruments with articulation, laparoscopic surgery was performed by the retroperitoneal technique.

When the SPRLN group was retrospectively compared with the group who had undergone standard retroperitoneal laparoscopic nephrectomy, no significant difference was noted with respect to operation time, time to resume oral intake, catheter removal, or duration of postoperative hospital stay. A significant difference in favor of the SPRLN group was found with respect to the visual analog pain scale score at discharge. Although our results of SPRLN indicate that the technique is feasible with advanced techniques and optimal instrumentation, further studies are needed to determine the future direction of the technique and the extent of its clinical application.

Keywords Laparoscopic retroperitoneal surgery • Scarless surgery • Single-port laparoscopic nephrectomy • Single-port laparoscopic nephroureterectomy

T. Okegawa (✉) • K. Nutahara
Department of Urology, Kyorin University School of Medicine,
6-20-2 Shinkawa, Mitaka, Tokyo 181-8611, Japan
e-mail: toke@ks.kyorin-u.ac.jp

T. Mori and G. Dapri (eds.), *Reduced Port Laparoscopic Surgery*,
DOI 10.1007/978-4-431-54601-6_40, © Springer Japan 2014

40.1   Introduction

Standard laparoscopic surgery requires three to six ports for any given operation [1]. Single-port laparoscopic surgery (SPLS), however, represents the latest innovation in the field of laparoscopic surgery and continues to increase among urologists [2–6]. Although most surgeries could be performed transumbilically within the field of urology, several reports have shown the benefits of retroperitoneal approach [7–11]. This approach for more direct access to the posterior to the axis kidney and is possible to perform on patients who have undergone previous transperitoneal approach surgery, as well as standard retroperitoneal laparoscopic surgery. This type of surgery is, however, limited because only a small working space is obtained and the bendable laparoscopic instruments need to be used.

40.2   Single-Port Retroperitoneal Laparoscopic Surgical Methods

Patients were placed in the lateral position with slight flexion under general anesthesia. Access to the retroperitoneum was obtained with the Hasson technique through a 2.5-cm skin incision at the tip of the 12th rib. A balloon dissector (PDB; Covidien, New Haven, CT, USA) was inflated in the retroperitoneum outside Gerota's fascia to create the working space. The SILS™ (Single Incision Laparoscopic Surgery) port (Covidien) or GelPOINT (Applied Medical, Rancho Santa Margarita CA, USA) was then placed in this incision (Fig. 40.1). The first 5-mm port for the flexible laparoscope (Olympus Surgical, Tokyo, Japan) was inserted into the port. A 5-mm laparoscope was inserted into the port to ensure adequate access to the retroperitoneum was established. A second 5-mm working port was placed inferiorly to the camera port under laparoscopic observation. Using the instruments with articulation, laparoscopic surgery was performed by the retroperitoneal technique in all cases (Fig. 40.1).

The renal hilum was approached initially, and the renal artery and vein were sequentially controlled with clip-ligation (Hem-o-lok, McMedical, Tokyo, Japan). When L- and XL-type clip-ligation is necessary, the 5-mm port is temporarily changed to a 12-mm port (Fig. 40.2). For patients undergoing nephrectomy, concomitant adrenalectomy was performed in patients with an upper pole tumor or with radiographic evidence of adrenal involvement.

40.3   Learning Curve

Total operative times for the 20 single-port retroperitoneal laparoscopic nephrectomies (SPRLN) are demonstrated in Fig. 40.2. Operative time gradually decreased in about the first 5 cases and remained stable in the next 15 cases.

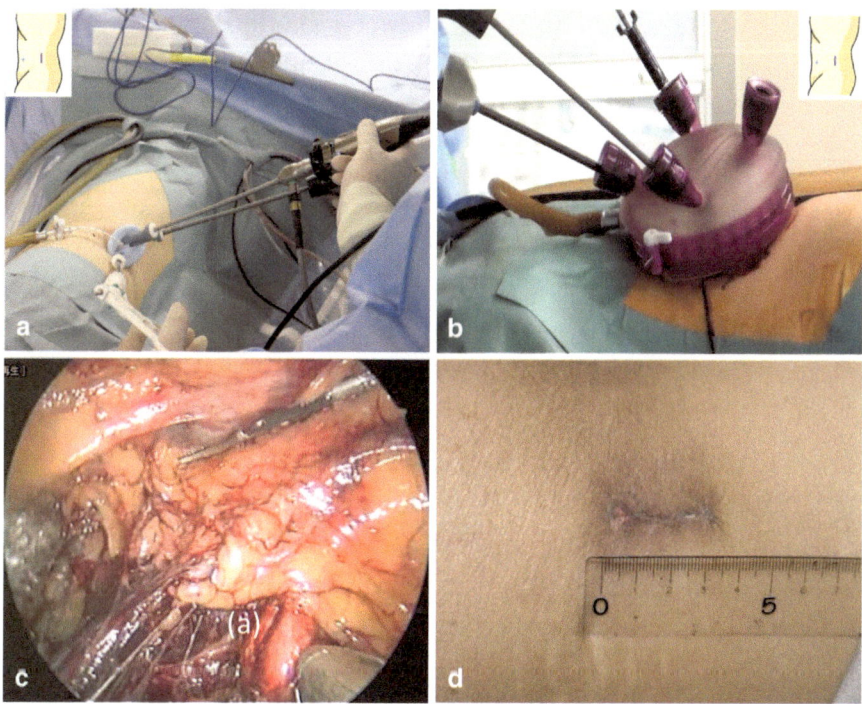

Fig. 40.1 (**a**) SILS™ port (Covidien) and laparoscope positioning during single-port left retroperitoneal laparoscopic surgery. (**b**) GelPOINT (Applied Medical) and laparoscope positioning during single-port left retroperitoneal laparoscopic surgery. (**c**) Intraoperative view. Using a flexible laparoscopic instrument (Covidien), laparoscopic surgery was performed by the retroperitoneal technique in all cases. (*a*): the left renal artery. (**d**) The wound (3.5 cm) 1 month after surgery

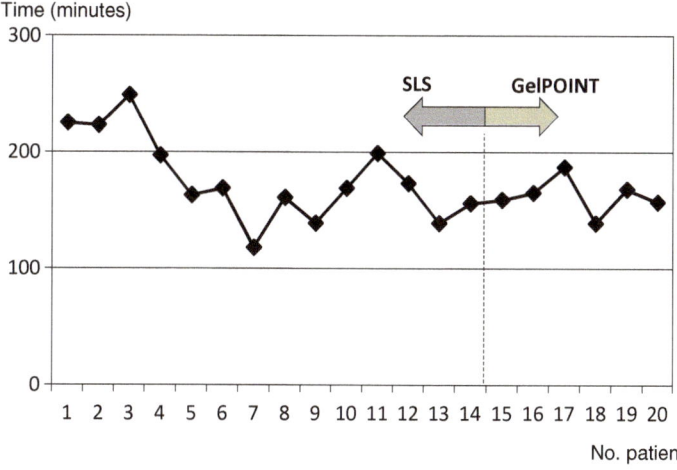

Fig. 40.2 Learning curve

40.4   Comparative Outcomes Between Single-Port and Standard Retroperitoneal Laparoscopic Radical Nephrectomy

Twenty patients with renal cell carcinoma entered our SPRLN, and 12 patients with renal cell carcinoma entered our standard retroperitoneal laparoscopic nephrectomy (SRLN) between April 2010 and March 2013.

The intra- and early postoperative data are summarized in Table 40.1. Three patients undergoing nephrectomy had previously undergone open intra-abdominal procedures. SPRLN was completed in all patients without conversion to standard laparoscopy or open surgery. No intraoperative or acute postoperative complications occurred.

Patients who had undergone SRLN by the same surgeon were identified (Table 40.1). When the SPRLN group was retrospectively compared with the group who had undergone SRLN, no significant difference was noted with respect to age, BMI, operation time, time to resume oral intake, catheter removal, or duration of postoperative hospital stay (p>0.05). EBL in the SPRLN group was significantly less than that of SRLN (p=0.027). A significant difference in favor of SPRLN group was noted with respect to the VAPS score at discharge (p=0.016).

Table 40.1 Demographic and comparative outcomes between single-port and standard retroperitoneal laparoscopic surgery

	Single-port laparoscopic nephrectomy (n=20)	Standard laparoscopic nephrectomy (n=14)	p
Mean age	66.2 (52–81)	67.8 (59–79)	0.142
Sex (males/females)	11/9	9/5	0.259
Mean BMI (kg/m²)	21.5 (19.8–29.6)	23.0 (23.1–27.5)	0.279
Operative side (right/left)	3/17	5/9	0.555
Mean OR time (min)	253.0 (158–485)	245.0 (176–268)	0.141
Mean EBL (mL)	101.5 (3–198)	166.8 (56–369)	0.027
No. blood transfusions	0	0	
Mean start to eat (days)	3.1 (3–5)	3.5 (3–6)	0.385
Mean Foley catheter removal (days)	3.6 (2–6)	3.4 (2–6)	0.267
Mean hospital stay (days)	11.4 (7–15)	13.5 (9–13)	0.241
Mean VAPS at discharge	1.5/10	2.4/10	0.016
Complications	–	–	
T stage			
T1	9 (45.0 %)	9 (64.3 %)	0.544
T2	1 (55.0 %)	5 (35.7 %)	
N stage			
N0 (%)	11 (100)	12 (100)	
Histological subtype			
Clear cell type (%)	19 (95.0)	11 (92.9)	
Chromophobe type (%)	1 (5.0)	1 (7.1)	

Table 40.2 Single-port retroperitoneal laparoscopic radical nephrectomy

Author (ref. no.)	Year	Journal	Number of cases	Port
Msezane et al. [13]	2009	BJU Int	36	Original
Ryu et al. [14]	2009	J Endourol	3	Alexis wound retractor
Chung et al. [15]	2011	World J Surg Oncol	6	Alexis wound retractor
Chueh et al. [16]	2011	BJ U Int	6	GelPOINT
Nomura et al. [17]	2011	Case Report Med	1	GelPOINT
Chen et al. [18]	2012	J Endourol	16	Original
Li et al. [19]	2012	Nan Fang Yi Ke	22	Original
Dong et al. [20]	2012	Surg Innov	29	Original
Present study [21]	2012	Int J Urol	20	SILS™ port, GelPOINT

40.5   Discussion

The first report of SPLS within the field of urology was reported by Rane et al. in abstract form at the 2007 World Congress of Endourology [2]. Desai et al. [7] reported the initial 100 patients (nephrectomy, nephroureterectomy, pyeloplasty, prostatectomy, etc.) who underwent SPLS. Desai et al. [7] and White et al. [8] concluded that SPLS is feasible, offers improved cosmesis, and may offer decreased pain.

In the future, a comparative series between conventional laparoscopic surgery and SPLS should be reported in the urological field [9–11]. Whereas most series performed SPLS transumbilically [9–11], preliminary reports of the retroperitoneal approach were found in the literature, including our study of SPRLN in 20 patients [12–14]. In our opinion, the use of a bendable grasper in the non-dominant hand is needed and a standard straight laparoscopic instrument can be used in the dominant hand. When compared with SRLN, except for a bendable grasper, SPRLN is relatively similar to a one-handed operation. The results of our study showed no difference in EBL, operation time, time to resume oral intake, catheter removal, or duration of postoperative hospital stay, but did note subjective improvement in VAS scores at discharge in SPRLN, because the specimen may be removed through the flank incision with or without extension of the wound. In addition to our findings, White et al. have shown that single-port retroperitoneal laparoscopic surgery is feasible and offers comparable surgical outcomes and pain control with standard retroperitoneal laparoscopic surgery [12]. Furthermore, several reports have shown that single-port retroperitoneal laparoscopic surgery is technically feasible and safe (Table 40.2) [13–20].

40.6   Conclusions

Although the SPRLN in this study may have reduced postoperative pain, prospective comparison between SPRLN and SRLN is needed to more clearly define its role, including oncological outcome.

References

1. Clayman RV, Kavoussi LR, Soper NJ et al (1991) Laparoscopic nephrectomy. N Engl J Med 324:1370–1371
2. Rane A, Kommu S, Eddy B et al (2007) Clinical evaluation of a novel laparoscopicport (R-port) and revolution of the single laparoscopic port procedure (SliPP). J Endourol 21(Suppl 1):A22–A23
3. Raman JD, Cadeddu JA, Rao P et al (2008) Single-incision laparoscopic surgery: initial urological experience and comparison with natural-orifice transluminal endoscopic surgery. BJU Int 101:493–496
4. Desai MM, Rao PP, Aron M, Pascal-Haber G, Desai MR, Mishra S, Kaouk JH, Gill IS (2008) Scarless single port transumbilical nephrectomy and pyeloplasty: first clinical report. BJU Int 101(1):83–88
5. Eisenberg MS, Cadeddu JA, Desai MM (2010) Laparoendoscopic single-site surgery in urology. Curr Opin Urol 20(2):141–147
6. Autorino R, Stein RJ, Lima E, Damiano R, Khanna R, Haber GP, White MA, Kaouk JH (2010) Current status and future perspectives in laparoendoscopic single-site and natural orifice transluminal endoscopic urological surgery. Int J Urol 17(5):410–431
7. Desai MM, Berger AK, Brandina R, Aron M, Irwin BH, Canes D, Desai MR, Rao PP, Sotelo R, Stein R, Gill IS (2009) Laparoendoscopic single-site surgery: initial hundred patients. Urology 74(4):805–812
8. White WM, Haber GP, Goel RK, Crouzet S, Stein RJ, Kaouk JH (2009) Single-port urological surgery: single-center experience with the first 100 cases. Urology 74(4):801–804
9. Raman JD, Bagrodia A, Cadeddu JA (2009) Single-incision, umbilical laparoscopic versus conventional laparoscopic nephrectomy: a comparison of perioperative outcomes and short-term measures of convalescence. Eur Urol 55(5):1198–1204
10. Raybourn JH 3rd, Rane A, Sundaram CP (2010) Laparoendoscopic single-site surgery for nephrectomy as a feasible alternative to traditional laparoscopy. Urology 75(1):100–103
11. Park YH, Park JH, Jeong CW, Kim HH (2010) Comparison of laparoendoscopic single-site radical nephrectomy with conventional laparoscopic radical nephrectomy for localized renal-cell carcinoma. J Endourol 24(6):997–1003
12. White WM, Goel RK, Kaouk JH (2009) Single-port laparoscopic retroperitoneal surgery: initial operative experience and comparative outcomes. Urology 73(6):1279–1282
13. Msezane LP, Mushtaq I, Gundeti MS (2009) An update on experience with the single-instrument port laparoscopic nephrectomy. BJU Int 103(10):1406–1408
14. Ryu DS, Park WJ, Oh TH (2009) Retroperitoneal laparoendoscopic single-site surgery in urology: initial experience. J Endourol 23(11):1857–1862
15. Chung SD, Huang CY, Tsai YC, Chueh SC, Hung SF, Wang SM, Liao CH, Yu HJ (2011) Retroperitoneoscopic laparo-endoscopic single-site radical nephrectomy (RLESS-RN): initial experience with a homemade port. World J Surg Oncol 9:138
16. Chueh SC, Sankari BR, Chung SD, Jones JS (2011) Feasibility and safety of retroperitoneoscopic laparoendoscopic single-site nephrectomy: technique and early outcomes. BJU Int 108(11):1879–1885
17. Nomura T, Sato F, Takahashi M, Sumino Y, Mimata H (2011) Laparoendoscopic single-site (LESS) retroperitoneal radical nephrectomy in a patient with renal cell carcinoma receiving hemodialysis. Case Rep Med 2011:506032
18. Chen Z, Chen X, Luo YC, He Y, Li NN, Xie CQ, Lai C (2012) Retroperitoneal laparoendoscopic single-site simple nephrectomy: initial experience. J Endourol 26(6):647–651

19. Li H, Xu A, Xu K, Chen B, Liu C, Zheng S, Xu Y, Fang P, Guo K, Lin Y, Zhu R (2012) Single-port laparoscopic surgery for radical nephrectomy: report of 22 cases. Nan Fang Yi Ke Da Xue Xue Bao 32(2):274–276
20. Dong J, Zu Q, Shi L, Gao J, Song T, Li H, Sun S, Zhang X, Cai W (2012) Retroperitoneal laparoendoscopic single-site radical nephrectomy using a low-cost, self-made device: initial experience with 29 cases. Surg Inov 20(4):403–410
21. Okegawa T, Itaya N, Hara H, Nutahara K, Higashihara E (2012) Initial operative experience of single-port retroperitoneal laparoscopic nephrectomy. Int J Urol 19(8):778–782

Chapter 41
Gynecology

Iwaho Kikuchi, Jun Kumakiri, Juichiro Saito, Yuki Ujihira, and Satoru Takeda

Abstract Laparoscopic surgery, which leaves small scars, is esthetic and minimally invasive. Recently, reduced port laparoscopic surgery (RPLS) including single-port laparoscopic surgery (SPLS), which further minimizes the invasiveness, has been attracting attention. In the field of gynecology, in particular, since all patients are female, the esthetic aspects should be given special consideration.

The laparoscope was first used for observation of the abdominal cavity. In the field of gynecology, the laparoscope was often used to confirm tubal patency and adhesions of the tubes to surrounding tissues, and to perform tests for infertility. Laparoscopic surgery was first performed for an appendectomy in 1981 by Semm, a gynecologist in Germany who developed an automatic pneumoperitoneum apparatus and later performed laparoscopic cholecystectomy. Initially, laparoscopic surgery was commonly performed using three ports: a port for the scope at the umbilicus, and one each in the right and left inguinal regions. However, if a surgeon wanted to use two pairs of forceps for adhesiolysis, sutures, etc., another port could be added.

RPLS represents an attempt to minimize the invasiveness of laparoscopic surgery by reducing the usual number of four ports, including the additional port placed to achieve better manipulability.

This chapter aims to describe the current status, characteristics, and problems of RPLS and SPLS in gynecology, as well as discuss unique surgical procedures based on these characteristics.

I. Kikuchi (✉)
Department of Obstetrics and Gynecology, Faculty of Medicine,
Juntendo University, Tokyo, Japan

Department of Obstetrics and Gynecology, School of Medicine,
Juntendo University, Hongo 2-1-1, Bunkyo-ku, Tokyo 113-8421, Japan
e-mail: kikuchiban@hotmail.com

J. Kumakiri • J. Saito • Y. Ujihira • S. Takeda
Department of Obstetrics and Gynecology, Faculty of Medicine,
Juntendo University, Tokyo, Japan

T. Mori and G. Dapri (eds.), *Reduced Port Laparoscopic Surgery*,
DOI 10.1007/978-4-431-54601-6_41, © Springer Japan 2014

Keywords 2-port • Hysterectomy • Laparoscopy • Myomectomy • Ovarian cystectomy • Ovary and oocyte cryopreservation • Promontorium fixation • Reduced port laparoscopic surgery • Salpingo oophorectomy • Single-incision laparoscopic surgery

41.1 Introduction

Laparoscopic surgery, which leaves small scars, is esthetic and minimally invasive [1]. Recently, "single-port laparoscopic surgery (SPLS)", which further minimizes the invasiveness, has been gaining attention [2–6] for its use of only one incision, resulting in a single surgical wound at the umbilicus. The invasiveness of the technique is even less than that of laparoscopic surgery, which usually requires three or four ports (incisions) [7]. However, SPLS has its limitations; therefore, one or two incisions for auxiliary forceps may be added without insisting on using a single incision, as the aim of laparoscopic surgery is to achieve minimal invasiveness in comparison to the conventional procedure. Thus, the technique has come to be referred to as reduced port laparoscopic surgery (RPLS).

In the field of gynecology, in particular, since all patients are female, the esthetic aspects should be given special consideration. As described later, vaginal surgery satisfies esthetic considerations in terms of natural orifice translumenal endoscopic surgery (NOTES). In gynecological surgery, there might have been similar concepts in the past [8].

This chapter aims to describe the current status, characteristics, and problems of RPLS in gynecology, as well as to discuss unique surgical procedures based on these characteristics.

41.2 History of the Endoscope and Introduction of RPLS

41.2.1 History of Laparoscopy

Laparoscopy was first used for observation of the peritoneal cavity. In the field of gynecology, the laparoscope was often used to confirm tubal patency and adhesions of the tubes to surrounding tissues, and to perform tests for infertility. Furthermore, in the case of ectopic pregnancy, such as tubal pregnancy, a definitive diagnosis can be made by laparoscopy, and the laparoscopic procedure can be converted to laparotomy if closer observation of the peritoneal cavity and surgery are deemed necessary.

Laparoscopic surgery was first performed for an appendectomy in 1981 by Semm, a gynecologist in Germany who developed an automatic pneumoperitoneum apparatus [9] and later performed laparoscopic cholecystectomy. In other words, laparoscopic surgery was begun by a gynecologic surgeon for several possible reasons:

(1) esthetic approaches are sought in this field as the patients were female; (2) laparoscopic surgery is applicable to a wide range of relatively benign tumors; (3) laparoscopy is commonly performed as described above; and (4) there was vaginal surgery which is a technique based on the concept of NOTES [10].

Initially, laparoscopic surgery was performed using three ports: a port for the scope at the umbilicus, and one each in the right and left inguinal regions. However, if a surgeon wanted to use two pairs of forceps for adhesiolysis, sutures, etc., another port could be added. Especially in the field of gynecology, where some procedures, such as uterine myomectomy, require many sutures, the addition of ports might be necessary for expansion of the indications. It can be speculated that the spontaneous addition of ports might have contributed to expansion of the indications. Although a unified arrangement of the ports has been established and the arrangement varies among institutions, placement of ports at the umbilicus and the right and left inguinal regions is common, to a large extent, among institutions. This seems to increase the reasonability of our speculation.

At our institution, an additional port is placed at the left side of the umbilicus (Fig. 41.1). This allows the surgeon standing on the left side of the patient to use his/her arms freely. The addition of this port dramatically improved the manipulability of forceps, as if "the start of bipedal walking freed both hands." Consequently, the indications for laparoscopic surgery were expanded. A similar paradigm shift must have occurred all over the world, contributing to an explosive increase in the adoption of laparoscopic surgery.

41.2.2 Addition of Ports for Improving Manipulability and the Rationale of RPLS that Opposes Such Additions

The concept of RPLS conflicts with the history described above. RPLS represents an attempt to minimize the invasiveness of laparoscopic surgery by reducing the conventional number of four ports, including the additional port placed to achieve better manipulability. There is a concern that the manipulability may be increasingly sacrificed as the number of ports is reduced from four to three, and eventually to one. Some may consider this concept as representing "backward evolution." In RPLS, which aims to reduce the number of surgical wounds, several trocars are inserted from the same incision to minimize the reduction in manipulability without affecting the number of manipulating forceps and scopes that can be used. Thus, this technique has many limitations that differ from those of conventional laparoscopic surgery. For example, the mobility of each device is impaired by the close proximity of the ends of the forceps and scopes, the trocar housing (head of the extracorporeal part), and the insertion of the devices from a single incision. Furthermore, the field of view is small because of the limited mobility of the scopes. Thus, it is undeniable that RPLS requires special techniques and skills that are substantially different from those of conventional laparoscopic surgery. Safety and reliability are critical, and only surgeons with a full understanding of these points should apply RPLS.

Fig. 41.1 The port that was added to obtain higher multiusability

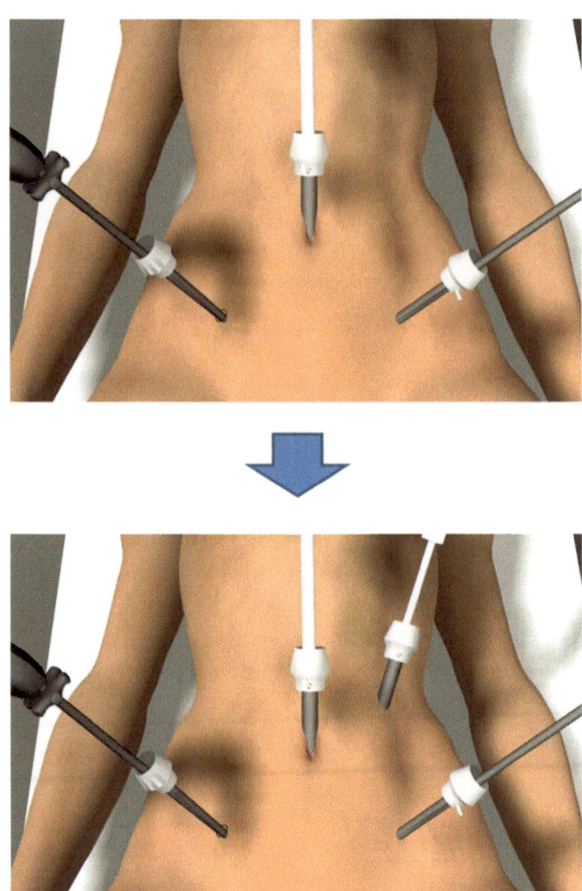

41.3   Current Status of RPLS in the Field of Gynecologic Surgery

SPLS was introduced in our department in March 2009. At first, it was applied to salpingectomy and salpingo-oophorectomy, which are based on the direct puncture technique and appear relatively easy in terms of the skill level required. When expansion of the indications was considered later, 2-port laparoscopic surgery was set as if the space between conventional 4-port laparoscopic surgery and SPLS was to be filled in consideration of the specific limitations of SPLS surgery described above [11].

In its early stages, SPLS was applied only to salpingo-oophorectomy and salpingectomy, which require fewer sutures. However, the indications have been expanded to include uterine myomectomy, total hysterectomy, promontory colposuspension, etc., by using the techniques described below. The following sections describe the actual surgical procedures.

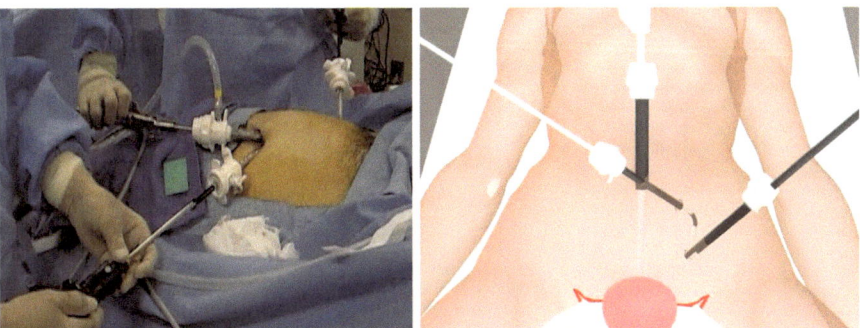

Fig. 41.2 Perioperative photograph and computer-graphics image of 2-port laparoscopic surgery [12]

41.3.1 Two-Port Laparoscopic Surgery

Figure 41.2 shows computer-graphics images of 2-port laparoscopic surgery. In 2-port laparoscopic surgery, the umbilicus is directly punctured with trocars for inserting the scope and manipulating forceps, and a 5-mm trocar is inserted via an incision made in the left inguinal region. The 5-mm port in the inguinal region can also be used for an incision for the insertion of a drain. When difficulty is encountered, incisions for the insertion of trocars are made at the same locations as in conventional 4-port laparoscopic surgery, so that trocars can be added in up to four ports in the same manner as in the conventional technique. Thus, even though up-conversion from SPLS to 2-port laparoscopic surgery and then to conventional 4-port laparoscopic surgery may be implemented, the location of the surgical wounds will consequently be the same as that in conventional surgery. When considering the burden on the patients, their satisfaction level, or the collateral for safety in the case of difficult surgery, the above points seem useful [11].

In 2-port laparoscopic surgery, the addition of an incision for trocars for SPLS allows auxiliary forceps to be inserted from a site different from that for the manipulating forceps and scope, allowing for surgery to be performed almost as easily as conventional laparoscopic surgery. Suturing, which is slightly difficult in SPLS, is simple, and 2-port laparoscopic surgery can be applied to myomectomy. Moreover, in both SPLS and 2-port laparoscopic surgery, attempts are being made to secure a good view while avoiding interference among the forceps and scopes by using flexible scopes manufactured by Olympus (Tokyo, Japan).

41.3.1.1 Uterine Myomectomy (2-Port)

Uterine myomectomy using the above 2-port laparoscopic technique is described here. Although it is performed in the same manner as the conventional 4-port laparoscopic technique, the forceps to be used by an assistant are unavailable. Because the surgery is performed with only a pair of forceps used by the surgeon, a few special techniques described below may be employed.

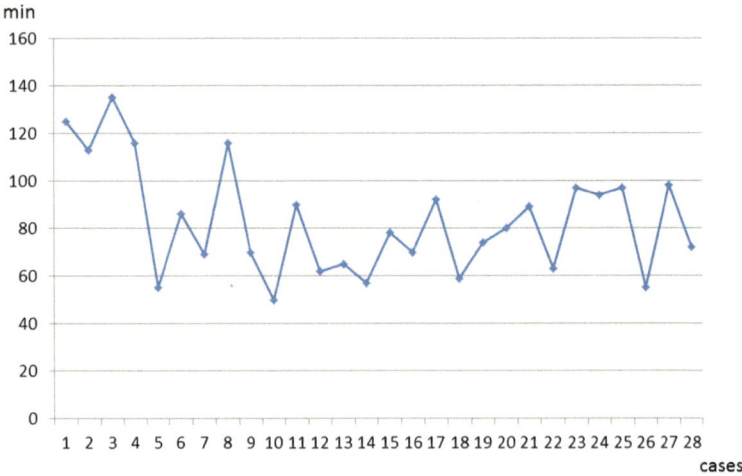

Fig. 41.3 This graph shows that the required operating time had stabilized within approximately 8 cases [15]

Securing a Good View Using a Flexible Scope

As described above, a flexible scope is used to avoid interference among devices that are inserted through trocars placed through a single incision. This is the same in SPLS. In the 2-port laparoscopic technique, a 12-mm trocar is placed at the umbilicus using the closed technique, and the scope is inserted. Under observation, a 5-mm trocar is placed in the inguinal region, and the scope is then placed in the 5-mm trocar. Under observation via the umbilical port, another 5-mm trocar is placed to intersect with the 12-mm trocar. Pneumoperitoneum leakage can be prevented by shifting the puncture site of the peritoneum. A flexible scope is inserted through the 5-mm trocar at the umbilicus. The view is secured as shown in Fig. 41.2, and surgery is performed. The forceps inserted from the trocar placed in the left inguinal region allow 2-port laparoscopic surgery to be performed in almost the same manner as that in conventional surgery.

41.3.1.2 Learning Curve in Acquiring the 2-Port Laparoscopic Technique

When 2-port laparoscopic surgery was introduced, the time needed to acquire the 2-port laparoscopic technique was examined for a single surgeon. The operation time decreased to a plateau with experience gained in approximately 8 cases (Fig. 41.3). Thus, the 2-port laparoscopic technique is fairly easy to acquire [12].

However, this technique also has its drawbacks. Because the surgery is performed with devices inserted via trocars placed at the umbilicus, there is no difference between sides. Although the posterior wall of the uterus and the Pouch of

Douglas can be approached, the approach is somewhat difficult due to the distance between the entry site and the organs. Furthermore, because forceps inserted from the umbilicus make vertical contact with the posterior wall of the uterus during surgery, suturing is difficult. Thus, surgeons must be careful when performing either 2-port laparoscopic surgery or SPLS, which is described below, for a fibroid on the posterior uterine wall.

41.3.2 Single-Port Laparoscopic Surgery (SPLS)

While RPLS includes procedures using the direct puncture technique or various retractors, this section discusses SPLS. In the same manner as 2-port laparoscopic surgery, a flexible scope is used to secure the view. Furthermore, curved forceps, such as SILS™ (single incision laparoscopic surgery) forceps (Covidien, New Haven, CT, USA), are used to avoid interference among different forceps.

In the early stages of the introduction of SPLS we used the Roticulator graspers™ (Covidien). The release of dedicated SILS™ forceps (Covidien) has allowed SILS™ to be performed with superior manipulability. Furthermore, bendable automatic suturing devices, such as the SILS™ Stitch (Covidien), have also been made available. However, the use of disposable devices is disadvantageous in terms of the cost, and the SILS™ forceps (Covidien) are low in rigidity because they can be bent in the peritoneal cavity. As a solution, reusable, rigid, curved forceps, such as DAPRI forceps (Karl Storz–Endoskope, Tuttlingen, Germany) [13, 14] and YAMAGATA forceps (Adachi, Tokyo, Japan), have been introduced in the market. We have also developed and been using rigid forceps for gynecological use.

41.3.2.1 SPLS for the Uterine Adnexae

Salpingo-oophorectomy with the SLS technique is described here. Basically, ablation of ligaments with a sealing device facilitates the procedure. In this case, rigid forceps manufactured by Adachi industry were used (Fig. 41.4). Even for large cysts, the procedure can be applied after aspirating the contents of the cysts with a SAND balloon catheter (Hakko Co., Nagano, Japan). Because the incision in SPLS is of a certain size, it is easy to extract cysts from the body cavity.

41.3.2.2 Linear Salpingostomy with the SILS™ Stitch (Covidien)

Linear salpingostomy with the SILS™ Stitch (Covidien) refers to the surgery performed to resect pregnancy tumors and simultaneously to preserve the tubal patency in case of ectopic pregnancy [15]. Although extremely fine sutures are needed, the fascia and serosa are separately sutured using the SILS™ Stitch (Covidien) (Fig. 41.5).

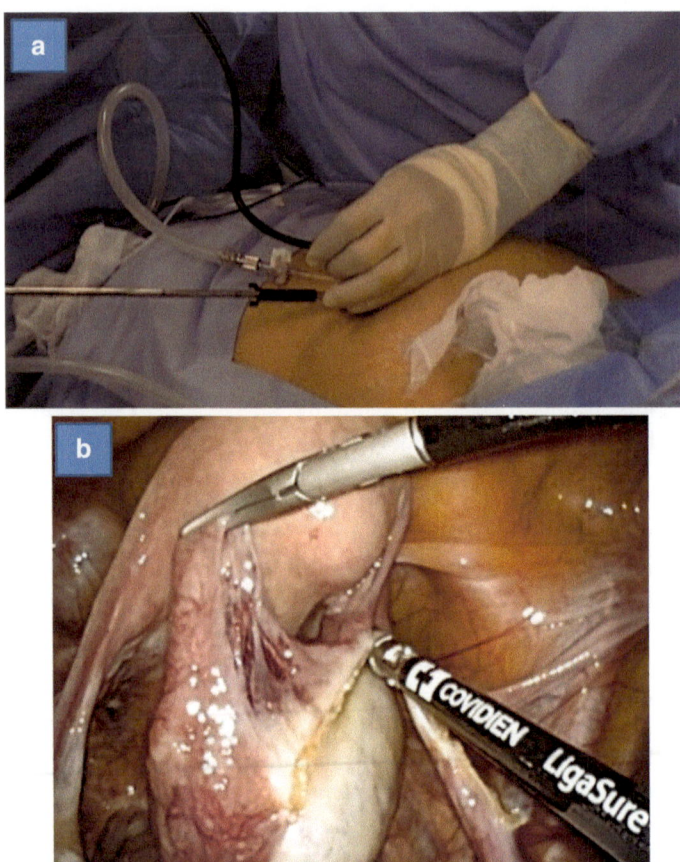

Fig. 41.4 (**a**) Direct insertion of reusable curved forceps ((Adachi) Industry Co. Ltd.) via SILS™ port (Covidien). (**b**) Salpingo-oophorectomy using vessel-sealing device and reusable curved forceps

41.3.2.3 Uterine Myomectomy (SPLS)

Uterine myomectomy also requires extremely fine sutures because the myometrium, which is somewhat hard, must be sutured with certainty. Thus, we also applied the 2-port laparoscopic technique to myomectomy in the early stages of the introduction of RPLS. At our institution, the indications for SPLS are as follows: myomas measuring 8 cm or less in size, the presence of 3 or fewer tumors, and the location of the largest myoma on the anterior wall of the uterus. Moreover, the use of barbed sutures, such as V-Loc 180 (Covidien), is helpful for suturing. Because the myometrium has a hard texture, sutures may be applied more easily if a surgeon controls the manipulator with one hand [16].

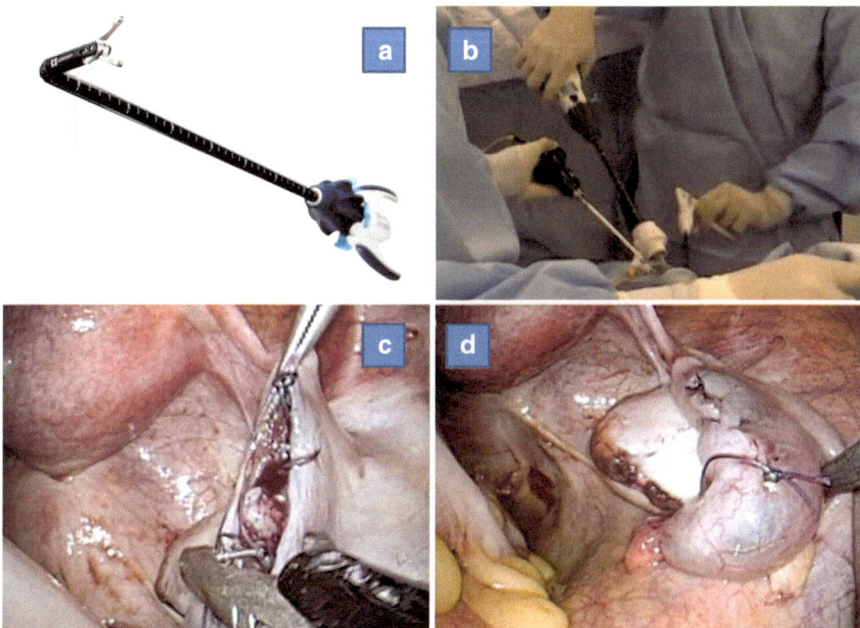

Fig. 41.5 (**a**, **b**) Use scenery of the SILS™ stitch (Covidien). (**c**, **d**) Linear salpingostomy using SILS™ stitch (Covidien)

41.3.2.4   Total Hysterectomy (SPLS)

Although total hysterectomy may require advanced techniques of gynecological surgery for benign diseases, it can be performed even by RPLS if the indications for the procedure are understood and the skill level is sufficient. Because the forceps inserted via the umbilical port can reach both the right and left sides of the uterus, manipulation may be rather easy, in some cases.

Total hysterectomy by SPLS is essentially the same as conventional laparoscopic surgery. From our experience, it may be better to treat the right side of the posterior wall first, which can be complex because manipulation in opening the vaginal canal may be extremely difficult. Closure of the vaginal wall may be facilitated by the use of V-Loc 180 (Covidien).

41.3.2.5   Promontory Fixation for Vaginal Prolapse
After Total Hysterectomy (SPLS)

Promontory fixation by the single-incision laparoscopic surgery (SLS) technique is described here. At present, it is considered a highly effective treatment for vaginal prolapse [17]. Although this procedure is commonly performed after supravaginal hysterectomy, this section describes vaginal prolapse after total hysterectomy. The

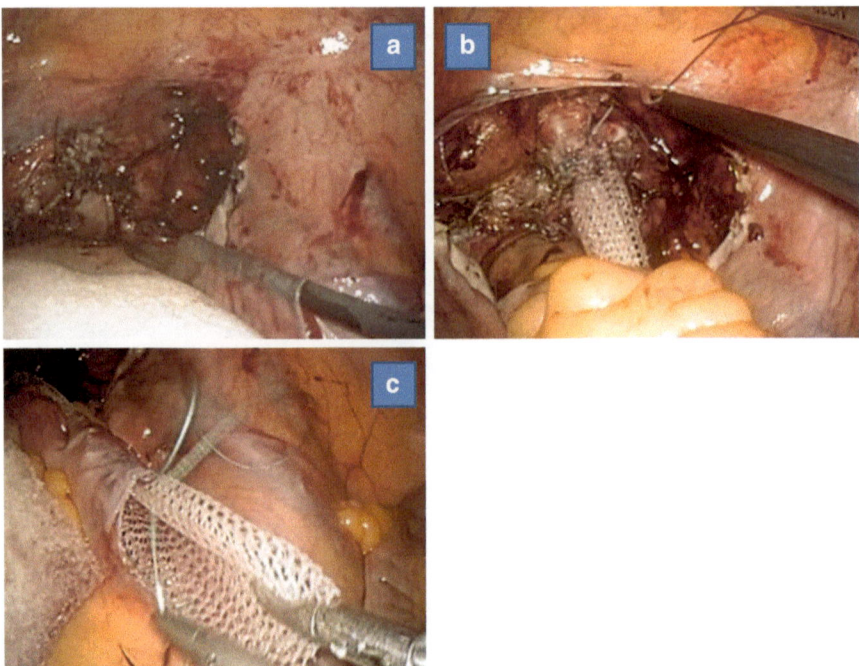

Fig. 41.6 (**a**) A subperitoneal tunnel is formed from the peritoneum. (**b**) The lower end of the mesh is sutured to the vaginal stump. (**c**) The upper end is sutured and fixed to the periosteum of the promontory

peritoneum over the promontory is first exposed. While the rectum is displaced to the left side, a subperitoneal tunnel is formed from the peritoneum, and a mesh is passed through the tunnel. The lower end of the mesh is sutured to the vaginal stump, and the upper end is sutured and fixed to the periosteum of the promontory (Fig. 41.6).

41.3.3 Change in Thinking: Another Interpretation of RPLS

What is the aim of RPLS? Is it to perform minimally invasive surgery so as to minimize the burden on the patients? Has the essence of this aim been lost amid concerns regarding the size and number of surgical wounds? If too much insistence on RPLS leads to prolongation of the operation time or a decrease in the quality of the surgery, true minimal invasiveness will not have been achieved.

The procedures described in the following sections are slightly different from those that have been described above. However, they share the same goal of achieving minimal invasiveness.

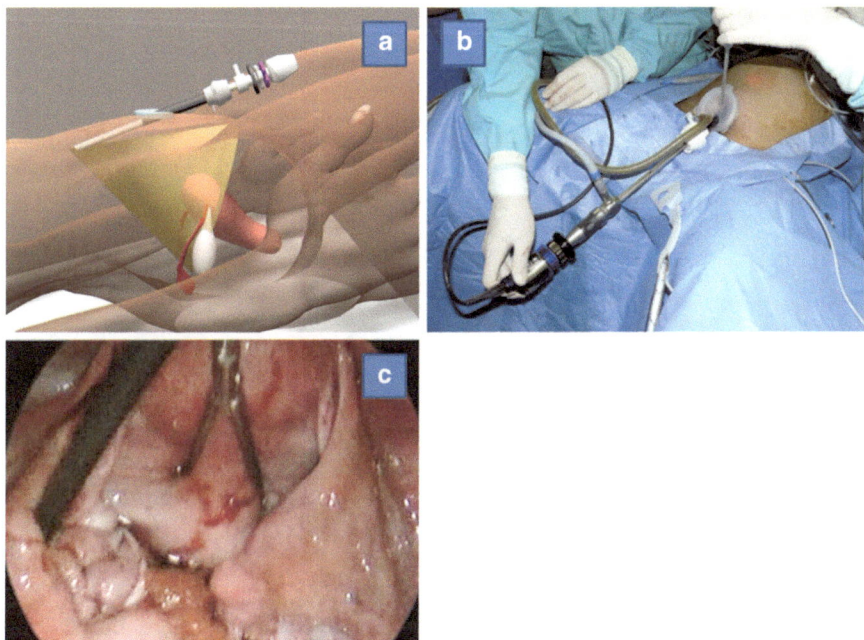

Fig. 41.7 (**a–c**): The field development only by the suprapubic wound using a special scope, EndoCAMeleon (Karl Storz–Endoskope)

41.3.3.1 Extra-Corporeal Ovarian Cystectomy (SPLS Through Only a Suprapubic Incision)

In the case of laparoscopic surgery for large ovarian cysts such as dermoid cysts that contain large solid materials, such as tooth, sebum, and hair, an incision of a certain size may sometimes be needed for retrieval of cysts. Salpingo-oophorectomy can be performed by SPLS, which has been described above. However, cystectomy requires the extra-corporeal abdominal technique, in which the ovary, once pulled out from the body cavity, is returned after the removal of a cyst. While an incision above the pubis that is close to the pelvis is often used for the extraction, an incision that can be covered by pubic hair may be more esthetically acceptable. Although the view was obtained with a scope inserted from the trocar at the umbilicus in the past, the use of Endo CAMeleon (Karl Storz–Endoskope) allows this procedure to be performed with only an incision above the pubis (Fig. 41.7) [18]. Can this procedure also be considered as SPLS or RPLS in a broad sense ?

41.3.3.2 Oophorectomy for Cryopreservation of Ovaries and Ovarian Transplantation by RPLS

Within the indications, RPLS can utilize an advantage of minimal invasiveness to the maximum. Because RPLS offers the benefit of minimal invasiveness, we have

Fig. 41.8 Back-
transplantation of ovarian
cortex: the surface of the
remaining ovary is resected
to form a basis for
transplantation of the ovarian
cortex, which is then sutured
and fixed

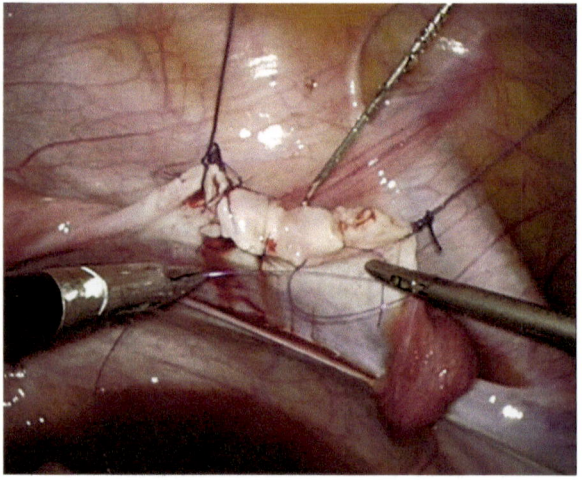

been performing oophorectomy for the cryopreservation of ovaries in patients who are scheduled for chemotherapy or radiotherapy for cancer and malignant tumors and will become infertile due to the loss of ovarian function as a result of adverse reactions to the therapies [19]. In this procedure, ovaries are extirpated by RPLS and cryopreserved for future pregnancies. Given the possibility of cases showing no loss of ovarian function because of few adverse reactions to chemotherapy, etc., one ovary is extirpated and cryopreserved by vitrification. The follicles in the remaining ovary are punctured, and the ova are cryopreserved at the same time. Because primordial ovarian follicles are located in the ovarian cortex, the latter is cut into 1 cm [2] and 1 mm thick pieces to be preserved. When they are transplanted, the surface of the remaining ovary is resected to form a basis for transplantation of the ovarian cortex, which is then sutured and fixed (Fig. 41.8). By postoperative day 173, the ovarian follicle had increased to 10 mm in diameter, and the patient's estradiol level had risen to 101 pg/mL, suggesting recovery of ovarian function [20].

41.4   Conclusion

RPLS has also been attempted for gynecological malignant tumors [21, 22], although this is not covered in this chapter. In addition, RPLS has also been performed using a robot [23]. However, SPLS currently represents surgery with low manipulability and many limitations. As mentioned before, situations must be avoided in which the quality of the surgery is sacrificed for the sake of completing SPLS. For safe introduction of this procedure, it is important to add incisions for insertion of trocars and to implement up-conversion without hesitation.

Because of the remarkable advances in the development of medical devices, it is quite probable that more user-friendly devices may be developed in the future, leading to expansion of the indications for this procedure. Further developments in the future are awaited.

Acknowledgments We would like to express our appreciation to Prof. Motoo Yamagata for giving us the opportunity to write this chapter.

References

1. Kikuchi I, Takeuchi H, Shimanuki H et al (2008) Questionnaire analysis of recovery of activities of daily living after laparoscopic surgery. J Minim Invasive Gynecol 15(1):16–19
2. Navarra G, Pozza E, Occhilnlrelli S et al (1997) One-wound laparoscopic cholecystectomy. Br J Surg 84:695
3. Piskun G, Rajpal S (1999) Transumbilical laparoscopic cholecystectomy utilizes no incisions outside the umbilicus. J Laparoendosc Adv Surg Tech A 9:361–364
4. Langebrekke A, Qvigstad E (2009) Total laparoscopic hysterectomy with single-port access without vaginal surgery. J Minim Invasive Gynecol 16(5):609–611
5. Myong Cheol Lim Æ, Tae-Joong Kim Æ, Kang S et al (2009) Embryonic natural orifice transumbilical endoscopic surgery (E-NOTES) for adnexal tumors. Surg Endosc 23(11):2445–2449, Epub 2009 Apr 3
6. Esposito C (1998) One-trocar appendectomy in pediatric surgery. Surg Endosc 12:177–178
7. Romanelli JR, Earle DB (2009) Single-port laparoscopic surgery: an overview. Surg Endosc 23:1419–1427
8. Pelosi MA, Pelosi MA 3rd (1991) Laparoscopic hysterectomy with bilateral salpingo-oophorectomy using a single umbilical puncture. N J Med 88(10):721–726
9. Mettler L (2011) From air insufflation to robotic endoscopic surgery: a rocky road. J Minim Invasive Gynecol 18(3):275–283
10. Kalloo AN, Singh VK, Jagannath SB, Niiyama H, Hill SL, Vaughn CA et al (2004) Flexible transgastric peritoneoscopy: a novel approach to diagnostic and therapeutic interventions inthe peritoneal cavity. Gastrointest Endosc 60:114–117
11. Kikuchi I, Kumakiri J et al (2009) A novel modification of traditional 2-port laparoscopic surgery using a 5-mm flexible scope. J Minim Invasive Gynecol 16(6):734–738
12. Kikuchi I, Kumakiri J, Matsuoka S, Takeda S (2012) Learning curve of minimally invasive two-port laparoscopic myomectomy. JSLS 16(1):112–118
13. Dapri G, Bron D, Himpens J, Casali L, Carnevali P, Koustas P, Cadière GB (2011) Single-access transumbilical laparoscopic splenectomy using curved reusable instruments. Surg Endosc 25(10):3419–3422
14. Dapri G (2012) Specially designed curved reusable instruments for single-access laparoscopy: 2.5-year experience in 265 patients. Minim Invasive Ther Allied Technol 21(1):31–39
15. Kumakiri J, Kikuchi I, Kitade M, Matsuoka S, Tokita S, Takeda S (2010) Linear salpingotomy with suturing by single incision laparoscopic surgery for tubal ectopic pregnancy. Acta Obstet Gynecol Scand 89(12):1604–1607
16. Kumakiri J, Kikuchi I, Sogawa Y, Jinushi M, Aoki Y, Kitade M, Takeda S (2013) Single-incision laparoscopic surgery using an articulating monopolar for juvenile cystic adenomyoma. Minim Invasive Ther Allied Technol 22:312, 2013 Apr 17
17. Bacle J, Papatsoris AG, Bigot P, Azzouzi AR, Brychaet PE, Piussan J, Mandron E (2011) Laparoscopic promontofixation for pelvic organ prolapse: a 10-year single center experience in a series of 501 patients. Int J Urol 18(12):821–826

18. Kumakiri J, Kikuchi I, Ozaki R, Jinushi M, Kono A, Takeda S (2013) Feasibility of laparo-scopically assisted extracorporeal cystectomy via single suprapubic incision using an adjustable-view laparoscope to treat large benign ovarian cysts: comparison with conventional procedure. Eur J Obstet Gynecol Reprod Biol 168(1):64–67
19. Kikuchi I, Kagawa N, Silber S, Kuwayama M, Takehara Y, Aono F, Kumakiri J, Kato O, Takeda S (2013) Oophorectomy for fertility preservation via reduced-port laparoscopic sur-gery. Surg Innov 20(3):219–224
20. Kikuchi I, Kawaga N, Silber S et al. Successful ovarian vitrification and back-transplantation to preserve fertility in a patient requiring chemotherapy for malignant lymphoma. J Blood & Lymph (In press)
21. Fagotti A, Boruta DM 2nd, Scambia G, Fanfani F, Paglia A, Escobar PF (2012) First 100 early endometrial cancer cases treated with laparoendoscopic single-site surgery: a multicentric retrospective study. Am J Obstet Gynecol 206(4):353, e1–6
22. Carvalho L, Flyckt RL, Escobar PF, Falcone T (2012) Single port laparoscopy. Fertil Steril 97(5):e17
23. Weinberg L, Rao S, Escobar PF (2011) Robotic surgery in gynecology: an updated systematic review. Obstet Gynecol Int 2011:852061, Epub 2011 Nov 28

Chapter 42
Breast Surgery

Koji Yamashita

Abstract Breast-conserving surgery with sentinel node (SN) biopsy is recognized as the standard treatment for early breast cancers. We have reported the cosmetic merits and reduced complication rate achieved with video-assisted breast surgery (VABS). We devised a trans-axillary retro-mammary (TARM) approach to VABS. This approach requires only a single skin incision in the axilla and can be used to treat any tumor, even in the medial or caudal part of the breast, without incising and thus scarring the breast skin or altering sensation.

We have performed VABS in 300 patients since December 2001. The TARM approach was used in 120 patients with early breast cancer (stage I or II). After endoscopic sentinel node biopsy, the axillary skin incision was extended to 2.5 cm. The pectoral fascia behind the tumor was then dissected. The proximal side of the tumor was excised vertically, and the skin overlying the tumor was dissected. The tumor was then excised on the opposite side and extracted. Breast reconstruction was done with oxidized cellulose.

This approach was successful in all cases. All surgical margins were negative. There was no significant difference in the complication rate between the TARM method and the conventional VABS method. The reconstruction procedure required no excessive detachment of the skin outside the surgical margin. The natural shape of the breast was maintained in all 120 patients. The aesthetic results were excellent, and sensory disturbance was minimal. All patients were satisfied with the operation.

VABS performed via the TARM approach in patients with breast cancer provides an excellent cosmetic outcome and is rated favorably by patients.

Keywords Axilla • Breast cancer • Endoscopic surgery • Single-port laparoscopic surgery

K. Yamashita (✉)
Department of Breast Surgery, Nippon Medical School,
1-5, Sendagi-1, Bunkyo-ku, Tokyo 113-8602, Japan
e-mail: yamasita@nms.ac.jp

T. Mori and G. Dapri (eds.), *Reduced Port Laparoscopic Surgery*,
DOI 10.1007/978-4-431-54601-6_42, © Springer Japan 2014

42.1   Introduction to the Technique

Breast-conserving surgery has gained popularity for early breast cancer. Oncoplastic surgery methods are applied in the pursuit of an aesthetic ideal. That is, a wide area of breast skin is detached, the mammary gland is mobilized, and autografting is done. However, these procedures are aimed simply at maintaining the natural shape of the breast and do not address the need for restoration of natural skin sensation. Many patients complain of postoperative pain and discomfort, sensory disturbances, skin problems, and ugly granulating wounds such as keloids [1, 2]. A laparoscopic technique, video-assisted breast surgery (VABS), has been applied to resolve these issues. We have reported the usefulness and the aesthetic benefit of VABS [3–4] and have since devised a single-port surgery for the breast. A small, 2.5-cm, skin incision is made in the axilla. The pectoral fascia behind the tumor is then dissected, and part of the mammary gland, including the tumor and safety margin, is excised and removed through the axillary incision. This technique can be applied to tumors in any part of the breast, even in the caudal or medial part. The technique is commonly called the trans-auxiliary retro-mammary (TARM) approach [5]. The subcutaneous dissection is restricted to the area of lumpectomy. Sensory disorders are thus minimized.

42.2   Indications and Contraindications

The indications for VABS performed via TARM approach are a single small tumor (> 3 cm) or multiple small tumors in a restricted area, tumor in any area of the breast without extension to the nipple, tumor without skin invasion or massive lymphovascular invasion, patient age <75 years, and patient choice.

 The contraindications for VABS performed via TARM approach are a serious visceral complication such as heart failure, severe liver damage, or renal dysfunction; patient age >75 years, ipsilateral implantation of a pacemaker(although the surgery is possible if the pacemaker is reimplanted contralaterally); and presence of a contraindication for radiotherapy (such as collagen disease).

42.3   Description of the Technique

42.3.1   Three-Dimensional-Computed Tomography (3D-CT) Mammary Lymphography (LG)

3D-CT LG [8] is performed before surgery for precise localization of the nearby sentinel node and then marking this node on the skin. A conventionally used contrast media is injected intracutaneously at the peripheral margin of the areola and

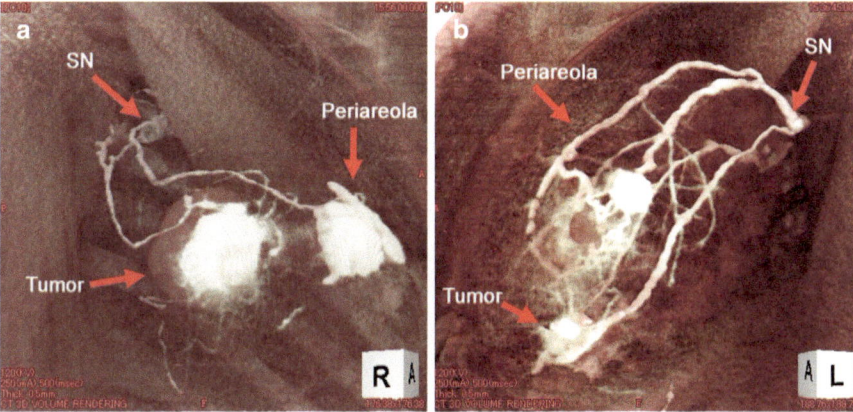

Fig. 42.1 Visualization of sentinel nodes (SNs) and lymph ducts (LDs) by means of three-dimensional computed tomographic lymphography (3D-CT LG). Iopamidol is injected into the periareolar skin and the skin above the tumor. The 3D-CT LG procedure reveals the precise lymphatic flow from the tumor to the SN. In the case depicted here, the lymphatic flow from the tumor is branched to the periareolar direction and directly to the axilla. Lymph drains from the tumor, encircles the nipple, and travels to the lymph nodes of the axilla. A second duct carries lymph directly from the tumor to the axilla

over the tumor. The injected contrast media enters the lymph ducts and drains into the sentinel node in the axilla [6]. A typical drainage pattern revealed by 3D-CT LG is shown in Figure 42.1. Dye travels from 2 injection sites to 3 different lymph ducts and then to a single lymph node, which is thus identified as the sentinel node.

3D-CT LG reveals the sentinel node within 1 min after contrast injection. By 3 min and 5 min after injection, the flow of dye beyond the sentinel node can be tracked to the second and third nodes toward the venous angle with the complex plexus [7, 8]. An example is shown in Figure 42.2, which reveals 5 bead-like grouped nodes beyond the sentinel node and the communicating lymphatic plexuses.

42.3.2   Endoscopic Sentinel Node Biopsy

Sentinel node biopsy is performed endoscopically by the dye-staining method. In the periareolar region and over the tumor, 2 mL of 1% indocyanine green is injected subcutaneously. After 20 min, a 1-cm incision is made along the skin cleavageline in the axilla, along the marks placed with the aid of 3D-CT LG. A Visiport optical trocar is inserted into the incision. The view is obtained through the Visiport with a

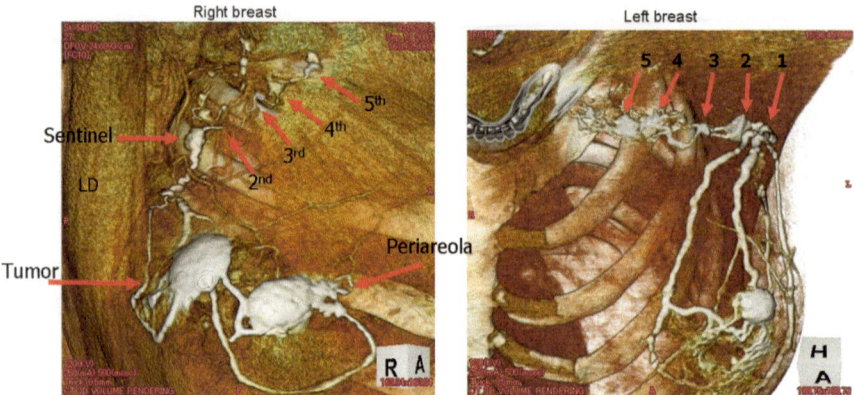

Fig. 42.2 Examination of a right and left breast by means of three-dimensional computed tomographic lymphography (3D-CT LG). Examination is performed chronologically 1, 3, and 5 min after iopamidol injection.Iopamidol flows into the sentinel node (SN) and then into successive nodes. Here, a string of five bead-like grouped lymph nodes is seen in the axilla after partial removal of the pectoral muscle. These successive nodes are thought to indicate the path of lymph metastasis. The *arrows* point to lymph nodes 1–5, which receive lymph from the SN

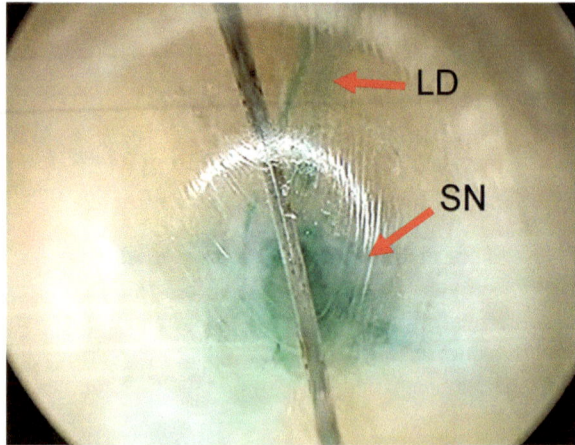

Fig. 42.3 Endoscopic view (through the Visiport) of the sentinel node (SN) and the draining lymph duct (LD). Both the SN and LD are stained green. The SN is found by tracking the flow of dye through the LD

10-mm-diameter, rigid, oblique-viewing endoscope, and the stained lymph nodes are found by tracking the dye in the lymph ducts (Figure 42.3). The nodes are sampled, and the samples are sent out for intraoperative frozen section pathology.

42.4 VABS by TARM Approach

42.4.1 Skin Incision

Conventional endoscopic surgery for the breast is performed via skin incisions in the axilla and in the periareolar region. However, with the TARM approach, the skin incision is made in the axilla, horizontally about 2.5 cm along the natural skin fold. A LapProtector for the breast is inserted. The surgical margins are marked by injection of blue dye at 8 points.

42.4.2 Dissection Behind the Mammary Gland

First, the adipose tissue is cut deeply to the shallow lateral chest fascia, and the cut is extended to the lateral edge of the pectoral muscle. The pectoral muscle fascia is bluntly dissected beyond the back of the tumor by UltraRetractor vein harvest under video assistance. The penetrating vessels are cut and coagulated with a Harmonic Scalpel (Ethicon, Cincinnati, OH, USA) and electrocoagulator.

The mammary gland is lifted to create a retromammary space. 2 0 Vicryl sutures are placed in the gland via the skin, and attached to a lifting device, anchoring the mammary gland. The anchor point is 1 cm away from the cut margin. This step creates a large working space behind the mammary gland and facilitates vertical cutting of the gland.

The cut is initiated at the point marked at the proximal margin. The proximal margin is recognized by the blue dye markings as well as a straight needle inserted through the skin. The gland is cut vertically toward the skin, as illustrated in (Figure 42.4). The distance between the end of the cut and the skin above is easily evaluated by touching the patient's skin.

42.4.3 Dissection of the Subcutaneous Tissue Overlying the Tumor

A skin flap over the tumor is made by the tunnel method. Many penetrating tunnels are created at 1-cm intervals in the subcutaneous tissue at a fixed depth with the use of an endodissector. Blood vessels collect in the septa between these tunnels, and the septa are cut with a Harmonic Scalpel (Ethicon). This minimizes blood loss.

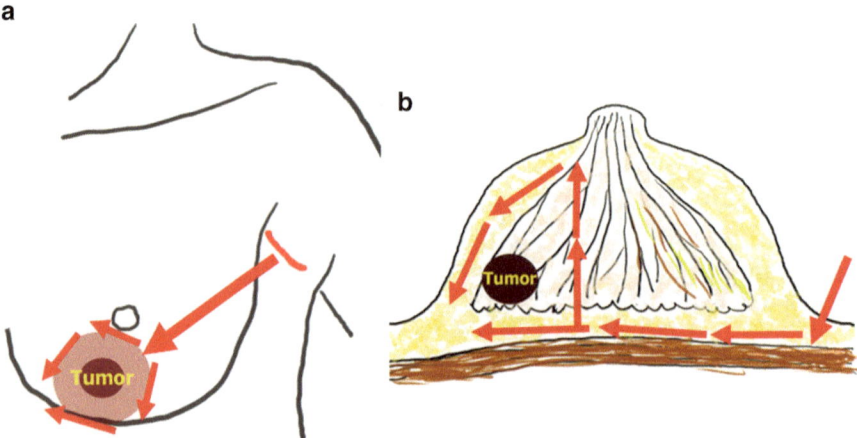

Fig. 42.4 Diagram of the trans-axillary retro-mammary (TARM) approach (**a**) Frontal view of the surgical procedure. Arrows show the axillary skin incision, dissection route, and partial resection of the mammary gland, for breast cancer in the left caudal medial quadrant. (**b**) Cross-sectional view of the retro-mammary route. Arrows show the approach from the axillary skin incision, dissection of the major pectoral muscle fascia, upward cutting to subcutaneous tissue at the proximal surgical margin, and dissection of subcutaneous tissue over the tumor

42.4.4 Partial Excision of the Gland Along With the Tumor and Safety Margin

To excise the tumor with an adequate safety margin, the 8 dye-marked points are very important because we cannot touch the tumor directly. The gland is cut with a Harmonic Scalpel (Ethicon) or bipolar scissors to minimize blood loss. For a clear view, mist and smoke are evacuated with the suction probe. The resected part of the gland is pulled out through the axillary port in an Endo Catch specimen pouch (Covidien, New Haven, CT, USA). When the specimen is larger than the port, the wound can be widened or the gland cut into pieces within the pouch so that the pouch can be easily pulled out. After careful hemostasis and warm saline lavage, breast reconstruction is performed.

42.4.5 Breast Reconstruction

For breast reconstruction, we usually mobilize the mammary gland and fill the lateral defect with a skin flap. However, when there is a shortage of subcutaneous fat tissue, absorbable synthetic cotton fiber, oxidized cellulose (Surgicel Absorbable Hemostat), can be used effectively to fill the defect. This absorbable hemostat can be unravelled like cotton.

An MR image obtained 6 months after a patient's breast surgery is shown in Figure. 42.5. The absorbable fiber fills the defect; thus the breast retains its original shape.

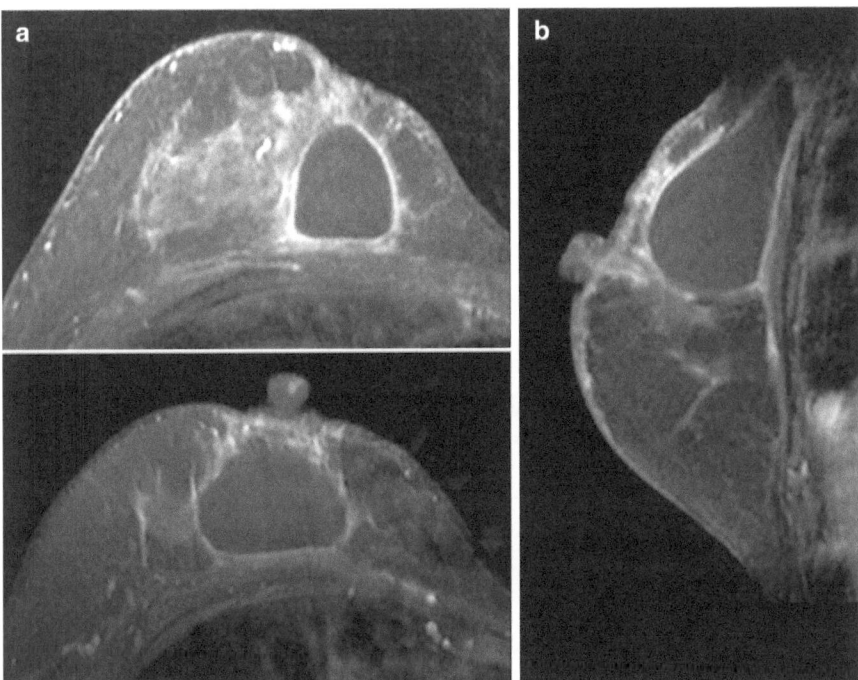

Fig. 42.5 MR images of the breast 6 months after the operation. Contrast-enhanced subtraction MR images of the breast in the axial (**a**) and sagittal (**b**) planes show capsule wall-like contrast enhancement surrounding a homogenous nonenhanced mass, which is thought to be the breast reconstruction material.

The material "melts" into the tissue to become a solid fibrous mass surrounded by a granulated capsule. A good aesthetic outcome can be achieved, regardless of the size of the defect.

42.4.6 Axillary Clearance

When the sentinel node biopsy shows cancer metastasis, axillary clearance can be performed from level I to III through the same port.

42.5 Tips and Tricks

The port incision is made only in the axilla. It is 2.5 cm long and follows the skin cleavageline. Thus, it is quite inconspicuous. The procedure is based on the lifting method and does not require infusion of CO_2. In comparing the TARM approach with

Table 42.1 Clinical characteristics of our "TARM" and "periareolar" patients

	TARM approach (n=120)		Periareolar approach (n=180)		
	Mean	Range	Mean	Range	p value*
Age (years)	50.2	26–82	52.5	28–78	0.893
Tumor size (cm)	2.2	0.1–6	1.9	0.3–5	0.693
SN metastasis (n)	27 (22.5 %)		46 (25.6 %)		0.243
Resected volume (%)	27.2	15–30	24.3	13–33	0.143
Operation time (min)	172	65–210	149	55–180	0.081
Blood loss (mL)	114	5–150	93	0–135	0.189

TARM trans-axillary retro-mammary, *SN* sentinel node
*obtained by Chi-square test

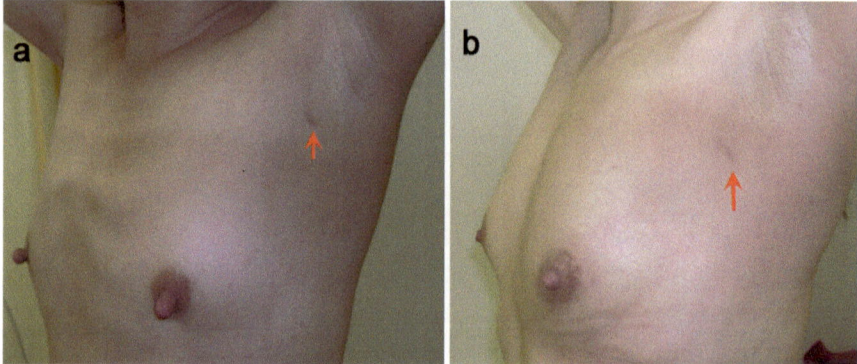

Fig. 42.6 Photographs obtained 1 year after the TARM procedure. Patients **a** and **b** were 42- and 39-year-old women. Each had noticed a mass in the left breast. The tumors were smooth, round masses, 1.3-cm and 1.5-cm in diameter, both in the caudal medial quadrant. Fine-needle aspiration biopsy revealed a malignant c-T1cN0M0, i.e., stage I, tumor in both cases. Pathology results: invasive ductal carcinoma, papillotubular carcinoma, and scirrhous carcinoma, g, n0, ER+, PgR +, HER2-

the periareolar approach, we found that the TARM approach extends the operation time (Table 42.1); however, the total time includes the wait time for the pathology results. The actual procedure time is only 1 hour.

The aesthetic results are evaluated by means of a Japanese Breast Cancer Society-approved scoring system, which is used to evaluate 5 items: asymmetry, breast shape, nipple shape, skin condition, and wound scar (ABNSW system). Each item is evaluated on a scale of 0 to 3. The scores are then totaled, with a possible total of 15. A total score of 12 to 15 is considered good to excellent. The cosmetic results are evaluated 6 months after the operation (Fig. 42.6). As shown in Table 42.2, the average total score for our "TARM patients" was 13.8 (vs. 13.0 for our "periareolar patients"), and more than 90% of our "TARM patients" realized a good-to-excellent outcome. Therefore, VABS performed by the TARM approach is thought to be very effective in terms of aesthetics.

Table 42.2 Aesthetic outcomes in our two patient groups

ABNSW score*	TARM approach (n=120)	Periareolar approach (n=180)	Combined total no. of patients
9	0	9	9
10	2	13	15
11	5	32	37
12	12	9	21
13	27	21	48
14	26	37	63
15	48	59	107

Note that outcomes are shown as total ABNSW (asymmetry, breast shape, nipple shape, skin condition, and wound scar) scores, and the table breaks down the group outcomes by the numbers of patients receiving specific scores.Note that no patient had a total score <9.
*Average score per patient group: 13.8 and 13 (TARM and Periareolar, respectively; p=0.007. Obtained by Chi-square test).

42.6 Recommendations from the Author

The TARM approach to VABS is very useful for early breast cancer patients. We recommend this approach for patients with a small mass and no extension into the nipple.

References

1. Penzer RD, Patterson MP, Lipsett JA (1992) Factors affecting cosmetic outcome in breast conserving cancer treatment-objective quantitative assessment. Breast Cancer Res Treat 20:85–92
2. Bajaj AK, Kon PS, Oberg KC, Miles DA (2004) Aesthetic outcomes in patients undergoing breast conservation therapy for the treatment of localized breast cancer. Plast Reconstr Surg 114:1442–1449
3. Yamashita K, Shimizu K (2006) Endoscopic video-assisted breast surgery: procedures and short-term results. J Nippon Med Sch 73:193–202
4. Tamaki Y, Sakita I, Miyoshi Y et al (2001) Transareolar endoscopy-assisted partial mastectomy: a preliminary report of six cases. Surg Laparosc Endosc Percutan Tech 11:356–362
5. Yamashita K, Shimizu K (2008) Transaxillary retromammary route approach of video-assisted breast surgery enables the inner-side breast cancer to be resected for breast conserving surgery. Am J Surg 196:578–581
6. Suga K, Ogasawara N, Okada M et al (2003) Interstitial CT lymphography-guided localization of breast sentinel lymph node: preliminary results. Surgery 133:170–179
7. Yamashita K, Shimizu K (2009) Evaluation of sentinel lymph node metastasis alone guided by three-dimensional computed tomographic lymphography in video-assisted breast surgery. Surg Endosc 23:633–640. doi:10.1007/s00464-008-9809-z
8. Yamashita K, Shimizu K (2009) 3D-CT lymphography for mapping metastatic breast sentinel node and axillary nodes. In: Leong S (ed) From local invasion to metastatic cancer: involvement of distant sites through the lymphovascular system. Humana, Springer, Totowa, pp 159–168, Chapter 14

Chapter 43
Pediatric Surgery

Manabu Okawada, Geoffrey J. Lane, and Atsuyuki Yamataka

Abstract Endoscopic surgery is the standard approach for most surgical procedures in both adults and children as a consequence of widely recognized benefits, in particular, improved postoperative recovery as a consequence of less pain, less risk for wound infection, and improved cosmesis. In order to further improve the perceived benefits of minimally invasive surgery (MIS), surgeons have tried smaller instruments, and decreasing the size and number of ports to the extent that endoscopic surgery is now being attempted using a single incision through which all instruments are placed. Single-incision laparoscopic surgery (SLS) is emerging as an alternative technique to conventional laparoscopy for the treatment of common surgical conditions. Despite widespread use, adoption of SLS in children has been slow, just as the general application of MIS in children has historically lagged behind that in adults. However, with more experience and improved instrumentation, MIS techniques are being applied in pediatric surgery to further decrease the invasiveness of surgery in children.

Keywords Children • Minimally invasive surgery (MIS) • Scarless • Single-incision laparoscopic surgery (SLS)

43.1 Introduction

The advent of laparoscopy significantly advanced minimally invasive surgery (MIS) as a field of surgery allowing surgeons to perform major procedures through several tiny incisions, rather than one large incision with decreased requirement for analgesia and enhanced wound cosmesis. Single-access site MIS [1, 2] was developed

M. Okawada • G.J. Lane • A. Yamataka (✉)
Department of Pediatric General and Urogenital Surgery, Juntendo University
School of Medicine, 2-1-1 Hongo, Bunkyo-ku, Tokyo 113-8421, Japan
e-mail: yama@juntendo.ac.jp

T. Mori and G. Dapri (eds.), *Reduced Port Laparoscopic Surgery*,
DOI 10.1007/978-4-431-54601-6_43, © Springer Japan 2014

because surgeons strove to improve MIS, with innovations ranging from decreasing the size of ports and instruments to a variety of techniques termed "scarless" surgery [3]. The rationale for reducing the number of access sites to the bare minimum is that surgical trauma will be decreased as much as possible with less likelihood for postoperative complications and shorter hospitalization. The most common application of this is SLS, which utilizes a single umbilical incision, with or without a specialized port. Recently, reports about the application of SLS to a number of procedures such as appendectomy, cholecystectomy, gastrectomy, adrenalectomy, colorectal procedures, bariatric procedures, and urologic procedures have appeared in the adult literature, and recent reports in children include appendectomy, cholecystectomy, splenectomy, intestinal procedures, gastrostomy, and urologic procedures [4].

43.2   SLS in Children

SLS was introduced in children much later than in adults. This delay may be attributed partly to the perception that the small scars left by pediatric laparoscopic instruments are acceptable. But there is a fairly universal belief that MIS is challenging in children because of space limitations, even with multiple trocars [5], so SLS would be expected to further limit instrument maneuverability because there is only one incision. In adults, multichannel ports are popular for SLS procedures, but their use is limited in small children due to their large size. Instead, many pediatric surgeons often prefer to place several 3/5-mm ports through a single umbilical wound with/without multichannel ports (Fig. 43.1), as well as transabdominal sutures. These sutures are used to encircle the round ligament for liver retraction and often include seromuscular bites through the wall of various hollow organs including the gallbladder, stomach, mesoappendix, uterus, or bladder. These "retraction" sutures are a common practice among pediatric surgeons and are particularly useful in small children with thin abdominal walls.

We believe that single-incision surgery has the potential to become a technique of choice in MIS provided devices, equipment, and instrumentation can allow procedures to be performed with the same ease of safety and effectiveness as multiple incision laparoscopic surgery.

43.3   Devices, Equipment and Instruments

As SLS has evolved, devices have been developed to assist surgeons in overcoming technical challenges. These range from access devices to flexible instruments and scopes. Multiple access devices currently exist that allow multiple instruments to be inserted at one site, with variable degrees of flexibility which may improve maneuverability and allow adjustment of angulation to overcome external parallel instrumentation [6].

Fig. 43.1 Multitrocar port inserted for SILA using a Lap Protector with EZ access system (Hakko)

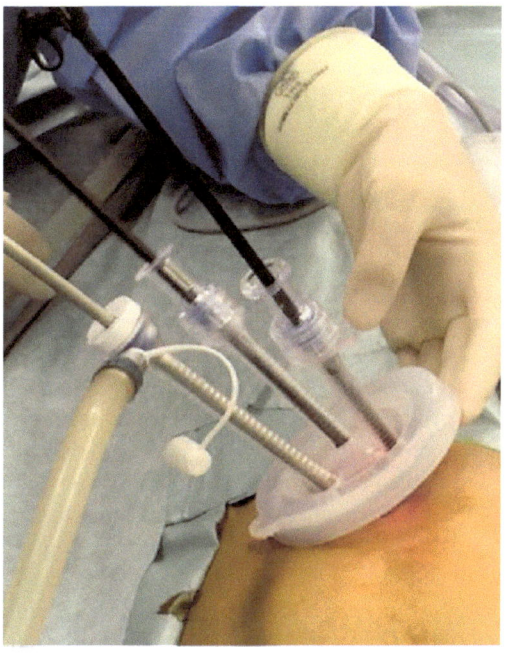

To date, surgeons have used various methods to improve the cosmetic results of laparoscopic surgery. Smaller instruments are available, such as the Stryker MiniLap instrument line (Kalamazoo, MI, USA), which is 2.3-mm and uses a retractable needle tip for percutaneous entry, leaving only a needle sized skin defect. Retraction has been accomplished with transabdominal sutures that decrease the number of port site incisions. At our institute, we prefer to use a Lap Protector with EZ access system (Hakko Co., Tokyo, Japan) and insert small head trocars because these trocars can be placed as required to prevent incision related trauma (Fig. 43.1). Furthermore, Covidien (New Haven, CT, USA) developed several 5-mm laparoscopic instruments that have flexible tips that can be angled relative to the shaft, but there is some loss of rigidity because of this added flexibility. The Autonomy Laparo-Angle (Cambridge Endo, Framingham, MA, USA) offers 360-degree flexibility, but has a larger handle. RealHand (Novare Surgical Systems, Cupertino, CA, USA) also has a wide range of motion tip and ergonomic handle. Olympus (Tokyo, Japan) has curved instruments which are not fully adjustable, but have the benefit of being more rigid [6]. Although standard laparoscopic instrumentation can still be used for single site surgery, especially for simple procedures, more specialized instruments may help overcome some of the technical challenges that are encountered when single site surgery is applied to more advanced procedures.

43.4 Applications of SLS

Today, SLS is being used widely in children for appendectomies and cholecystectomies to minimize surgical trauma and scarring and adopted for selected cases of pyloromyotomy, splenectomy, choledochal cystectomy [7], nephrectomy, inguinal hernia repair, high ligation of varicocele, Nissen fundoplication, and endorectal pull-through procedures.

Despite the potential benefits to patients, the single site approach has potential risks. The operative challenges imposed are unique to SLS and differ from those encountered in general surgery. The proximity of instruments restricts the range of movement of both a surgeon's hands and the instruments themselves; in particular, parallel alignment of instruments during SLS limits triangulation which is a founding principle of safe and effective laparoscopic surgery [6], and in line placement of the scope narrows the visual field, with the result that the view is both dependent on and limited by instrument mobility. These factors could affect the safety of a procedure, be implicated in longer operating times, and increase the risk for complications. With SLS a substantial fascia-splitting incision is required, which may be associated with more surgical infections, more pain, and an increased risk for postoperative hernias. These disadvantages would be counter to the progressive spread of MIS. Thus, the relative advantages of single-site procedures would appear to be few, compared with standard laparoscopy, and might prove only to be improved cosmesis. Reports in the literature focus primarily on feasibility and there are no reports comparing benefits currently available.

43.5 Conclusions

SLS is a developing technique in the field of MIS, aiming to be "less invasive" with expected benefits of further improvement in cosmesis, fewer requirements for analgesia, and shorter convalescence. SLS is generally considered safe and effective and may come to replace traditional multiport endoscopic surgery, as issues such as limited triangulation and tissue handling are resolved. In addition, the development of smaller, low-profile SLS ports will enhance the maneuverability of laparoscopic instruments and alleviate crowding of trocars apt to occur with reduced operative fields typical of surgery in children. The ultimate challenge of truly "scarless" surgery may be closer to realization due to the development of SLS and the creative diligence of pediatric surgeons.

References

1. Ponsky TA, Diluciano J, Chwals W, Parry R, Boulanger S (2009) Early experience with single-port laparoscopic surgery in children. J Laparoendosc Adv Surg Tech A 19(4):551–553
2. St Peter SD, Ostlie DJ (2011) The necessity for prospective evidence for single-site umbilical laparoscopic surgery. Semin Pediatr Surg 20(4):232–236

3. Garey CL, Laituri CA, Ostlie DJ, St Peter SD (2010) Single-incision laparoscopic surgery and the necessity for prospective evidence. J Laparoendosc Adv Surg Tech A 20(5):503–506
4. Garey CL, Laituri CA, Ostlie DJ, Snyder CL, Andrews WS, Holcomb GW 3rd et al (2011) Single-incision laparoscopic surgery in children: initial single-center experience. J Pediatr Surg 46(5):904–907
5. Blanco FC, Kane TD (2012) Single-port laparoscopic surgery in children: concept and controversies of the new technique. Minim Invasive Surg 2012:232347
6. Garey CL, Laituri CA, Ostlie DJ, St Peter SD (2010) A review of single site minimally invasive surgery in infants and children. Pediatr Surg Int 26(5):451–456
7. Diao M, Li L, Li Q, Ye M, Cheng W (2013) Single-incision versus conventional laparoscopic cyst excision and Roux-Y hepaticojejunostomy for children with choledochal cysts: a case–control study. World J Surg 37(7):1707–1713

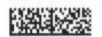